HAROLD G. SCHEIE, M.D.

William F. Norris and George E. de Schweinitz Professor of
Ophthalmology and Chairman of the Department, University of
Pennsylvania School of Medicine. Chief of Ophthalmology Service,
Philadelphia General Hospital. Ophthalmologist, Senior Surgeon and
Head, Division of Ophthalmology, Department of Surgery, The
Children's Hospital of Philadelphia. Chief of Ophthalmology Service
and Consultant, Philadelphia Veterans Administration Hospital,
Philadelphia, Pennsylvania.

DANIEL M. ALBERT, M.D.

Associate Professor of Ophthalmology and Chief, Ophthalmic Pathology
Laboratory, Yale University School of Medicine; Attending Physician
in Ophthalmology, Yale-New Haven Hospital; Consultant in
Ophthalmology, West Haven Veterans Administration Hospital.
Formerly Associate in Ophthalmology, University of Pennsylvania
School of Medicine, Philadelphia General Hospital, Philadelphia
Veterans Administration Hospital, and Children's Hospital of Philadelphia.

EIGHTH EDITION • 565 ILLUSTRATIONS • 38 COLOR PLATES

Adler's
Textbook
of
Ophthalmology

W. B. SAUNDERS COMPANY · Philadelphia · London · Toronto

W. B. Saunders Company: West Washington Square
Philadelphia, Pa.   19105

12 Dyott Street
London, WC1A   1DB

833 Oxford Street
Toronto, Ontario M8Z 5T9, Canada

Listed here is the latest translated edition of this book together with the language of the translation and the publisher.

Spanish (*8th Edition*) — NEISA, Mexico City,
                Mexico

Adler's Textbook of Ophthalmology   ISBN 0-7216-7950-1

Print No.:   9   8   7   6

Dedicated to

our wives and children

Collaborating Authors

From the Department of Ophthalmology of the
University of Pennsylvania Hospital and Medical School
and the Children's Hospital of Philadelphia

Chapter 2–Anatomy – *Myron Yanoff, M.D.*

Chapter 3–Embryology – *David M. Kozart, M.D.*

Chapter 4–Genetics and Ophthalmology – *David B. Schaffer, M.D.*

Chapter 5–Pediatric Ophthalmology – *David B. Schaffer, M.D.*

Chapter 7–Neuro-ophthalmology – *Alan M. Laties, M.D.*

Appendix IV–Physiology – *Arthur M. Goldstein, M.D.*

Appendix V–Pharmacology – *Charles W. Nichols, M.D.*

Medical Illustrator: *Jean E. Wolfe*   Photographer: *Herbert C. Ulrich*
Editorial Assistant: *Margaret J. Patton*

PREFACE TO THE EIGHTH EDITION

This book aims to provide the medical student and the practicing physician with a concise and profusely illustrated current text, organized in a convenient and useable manner, on the eye and its disorders. It is hoped that the beginning, or even practicing, ophthalmologist may find it of value. To have been invited to continue the tradition of excellence and usefulness of the Gifford-Adler textbook is a strongly felt responsibility.

In the years that have passed since the previous edition, new observations have been made regarding ocular changes in disease states and the normal function of the eye. Additional techniques of diagnosis and modes of therapy have been introduced. It was the belief of the authors that rewriting, rather than revising and updating, the last edition was desirable together with the inclusion of a vast number of new color and black-and-white illustrations.

The decision to produce a radically new volume was largely influenced by the revolution in curricula which has been sweeping through many of our medical schools. Among the basic changes introduced in the teaching of students are the following:

1. Curtailment of the blocks of time scheduled for formal instruction in clinical subjects, including ophthalmology, and increases in the time available for participating in elective courses and research activities.

2. Earlier introduction of clinical material.

3. Integration of the clinical and basic medical sciences.

Although such a curriculum has advantages for the medical student, it leads to lack of exposure to many specialties such as ophthalmology. These changes also make the familiar ophthalmology textbook, consisting of disease entities arranged in an anatomic sequence, a less effective teaching tool.

In this new edition, therefore, ophthalmology is approached from the standpoint of basic science and medical disciplines rather than structures and coats. To avoid repetition and to serve as a reference, an introduction to ophthalmologic terminology is presented in the first chapter, Ophthalmic Entities. Since a knowledge of the anatomy of the eye is fundamental to an understanding of ophthalmology, this subject is dealt with in the second chapter. Chapters on embryology of the eye and genetics are essential to, and therefore precede, the section on pediatric ophthalmology. A correlation is made with general pediatrics. In a similar manner, medical ophthalmology and neuro-ophthalmology are organized to complement the study of neurological and medical disorders. Glaucoma, ocular injuries, and eye surgery, topics unique to ophthalmology, are arranged in independent chapters and are directed toward the general physician and embryo ophthalmologist. The appendix offers supplemental sections on symptomatology, ocular physiology, and ocular pharmacology.

In addition to conforming to the modern curriculum, the authors believe this new arrangement should have a more general appeal than was possible by the rigid listing of diseases by organ system. The 565 new illustrations, 275 of which are in color, should make the book more valuable and enjoyable.

This reorganization of *Adler's Textbook of Ophthalmology* does not represent merely the packaging of "old wine in new bottles." The text has been almost entirely rewritten and reillustrated, with new topics added and others shortened or modified. The subjects stressed and the organization followed are adapted from the series of lectures given to the medical and graduate students at the University of Pennsylvania by the senior author. The major portion of the illustrations are from a lifetime collection of clinical slides. The basic science chapters represent a cooperative effort with other members of our Department of Ophthalmology who have particular knowledge of and interests in the subjects covered.

The authors express their appreciation and gratitude to numerous members of our staff and to our residents for their suggestions, criticism, and help in the preparation of this book. Particular mention should be made of former chief resident, Dr. Clifford J. Mullen, Jr., who expedited the revision of various chapters in the appendix and provided certain illustrations; Domenic A. Fuccillo, Jr., who helped with editing and proofreading; Dr. Ben S. Fine, of the Armed Forces Institute of Pathology and assistant professor of ophthalmology, George Washington University, Washington, D.C.; Dr. Gertrude Kohn, instructor in pediatrics, University of Pennsylvania Medical School; Dr. William J. Mellman, associate professor of pediatrics and medical genetics, University of Pennsylvania Medical School; and James Loftus, who supplied the photographs for the genetics chapter.

HAROLD G. SCHEIE

DANIEL M. ALBERT

CONTENTS

CONTENTS

xiv

Chapter One

OPHTHALMIC ENTITIES

SKULL AND ORBIT
Developmental Abnormalities

Abnormal development of the skull and face occurs in a number of conditions. The skull deformity may result from premature closure of a cranial suture, and the skull may assume several shapes depending upon the sutures involved. The *craniofacial dysostoses* are discussed in the chapter on pediatric ophthalmology (p. 105). Included in these disorders are:

1. *Oxycephaly* ("tower skull"), in which the frontal, parietal, and occipital bones ascend steeply, and the vertex is dome-shaped. Associated ocular complications are shallow orbits, wide-set eyes, optic atrophy, papilledema, and strabismus.

2. *Craniofacial dysostosis of Crouzon,* a dominantly inherited disorder with characteristic froglike facies and a variety of ocular and other disorders.

3. *Apert's syndrome,* a somewhat similar disease to the aforementioned that includes syndactylism.

4. *Hypertelorism,* a familial condition characterized by abnormally wide-spaced orbits and considerable broadening of the root of the nose.

The *mandibulofacial dysostoses* include a number of syndromes in which ocular findings are prominent.

Facial Hemiatrophy. This condition is a progressive disease commencing before puberty and occurring more often in females than in males. The skin, subcutaneous fat, muscles, cartilage, and bone of one half of the face atrophy. The principal ocular findings are enophthalmos, trichiasis, narrowing of the palpebral fissure, and atrophy of the lids and globe. Congenital, nonprogressive facial hemiatrophy has also been described. Facial hemiatrophy may be associated with von Recklinghausen's disease (p. 170). *Facial hemihypertrophy,* a much rarer condition, may be associated with ipsilateral enlargement of the globe and exophthalmos.

Meningocele. The membranes covering the brain, sometimes together with brain substance (encephalomeningocele), may herniate through defects in the walls of the orbit, usually along suture lines. This appears as a flocculent mass and is most commonly found at the upper inner angle of the orbit. Such herniations must be differentiated from *mucoceles,* which are noncongenital cystic formations arising from chronic inflammations of the frontal sinus. Mucoceles are filled with a thick, gelatinous material.

Exophthalmos

The eye lies in, and the anterior portion fills, the palpebral fissure and the anterior

1

portion of the orbit, and may be considered to behave much like a tampon. Exophthalmos denotes forward displacement (proptosis) of the eyeball from the orbit. This can occur with the appearance of any mass in the orbital cavity (e.g., tumor or varix), or with a reduction in orbital volume (e.g., hyperostosis of bone). Acute exophthalmos may occur when fracture of the medial orbital wall allows air from the sinus to enter the orbit, or when there is traumatic or spontaneous hemorrhage. Intermittent exophthalmos results when the eyeball is displaced by the individual changing posture or coughing, or by events leading to stasis of blood in the head. It usually follows trauma, but may come on gradually without any apparent cause. The primary cause is a varix in the orbit.

Pulsating exophthalmos generally is due to a communication of the carotid artery with the cavernous sinus, a condition resulting either from trauma or secondary to rupture of a carotid aneurysm within the cavernous sinus. Other causes of pulsating exophthalmos are orbital aneurysms, orbital angiomas, meningoceles, and the absence of a large part of the orbital roof.

Unilateral exophthalmos frequently is the result of a local lesion. Orbital inflammations such as *periostitis* and *orbital cellulitis* (p. 202), however, may produce bilateral involvement. Other causes of unilateral exophthalmos are: vascular abnormalities (hemorrhages, varicosities, and aneurysms); trauma; tumors, pseudotumors, and cysts (p. 272); and relaxation of retractors of the eyeball, which occurs with paralysis of the extraocular muscles.

General diseases which cause exophthalmos, e.g., endocrine disease (p. 250), xanthomatosis and blood dyscrasia are apt to produce bilateral exophthalmos. However, exceptions are frequent, especially with endocrine ophthalmopathy, which is often unilateral at the start. Thyrotoxic and thyrotropic types of endocrine ophthalmopathy and their associated physical signs are discussed elsewhere (p. 250). Conditions that can lead to prominence of the eyes simulating exophthalmos—marked lid retraction, shallow orbits, congenital macrophthalmos, and high myopia—are referred to as *pseudoexophthalmos*.

Enophthalmos

Enophthalmos is a backward displacement of the eyeball into the orbit. Its most common cause is trauma, but the condition may be congenital or arise from inflammation. When present at birth, it is commonly bilateral and associated with other congenital defects such as microphthalmos and ptosis. Any absorption of orbital fat will produce enophthalmos and hollow-eyed appearance. Enophthalmos is the chief facial expression of fatigue and probably has to do with dehydration of the orbital contents. Enophthalmos has been described with paralysis of the sympathetic nerve supply. Actual measurements, however, have shown that it is apparent only, and is simulated because of the ptosis produced by the paralysis of the sympathetically innervated smooth muscle in the lids. Traumatic enophthalmos is caused mostly by fracture of the orbital floor so that the globe and its contents herniate into the maxillary sinus.

THE EYELIDS

Alterations in Size, Form, and Position

The *epicanthus*, a concave skin fold at the inner angle of the lids, gives the eye a mongoloid appearance. It is the most frequent malformation of the eyelids in Caucasians. *Blepharophimosis* is a decrease in the overall size of the palpebral apertures, probably resulting from the formation of cicatricial tissue after trauma or disease. Occasionally a congenital form is seen that usually is familial and associated with ptosis and epicanthus (p. 114).

In *entropion* the lid margin turns in and results in the eyelashes rubbing on the conjunctiva and cornea. It usually is seen in elderly patients with chronic lid inflammation (spastic entropion) (p. 275), but also may be congenital (p. 113). Scars causing traction on the posterior layers of the lid result in cicatricial entropion. *Ectropion* is a disorder in which the lid margin turns out, exposing the palpebral conjunctiva. Four types generally are referred to: cicatricial, spastic, paralytic, and senile.

Alterations in Movements of the Lid

Fibrillation of the orbicularis muscle results in an involuntary twitching of one or both lids. When marked, it is called *myokymia* of the lids. It often results from nervous tension, eyestrain, and occasionally a local ocular irritation. Improper refraction may be a factor contributing to eye fatigue. Another cause is anticholinesterase compounds taken topically or systemically. Although the condition is annoying, it generally is of minor significance.

Blepharoclonus is an exaggerated form of reflex blinking. The closure phase may persist excessively or the blinking rate may increase. Blepharoclonus may be associated with ocular inflammation, long lashes, and other causes. It also may occur as a tic with other facial muscles involved, or as a symptom of hysteria. *Blepharospasm* is forcible closure of the lids and frequently accompanies inflammatory diseases of the anterior segment of the globe.

Lagophthalmos is an inadequate closure of the eyelids that leaves the cornea exposed. This abnormality may result from orbicularis muscle disease or facial nerve paralysis. Other causes are proptosis, lid retraction, and enlargement of the globe.

Bell's phenomenon, which consists of the eyes reflexly turning upward above the horizontal with closing of the lids, is an important protective mechanism particularly during sleep. It is present and protects the cornea in peripheral facial palsy, but the phenomenon is absent in nuclear lesions of the seventh cranial nerve.

Ptosis, or drooping of the upper eyelid, may be congenital (p. 114) or acquired. A combination of ptosis, miosis, anhidrosis, and usually dilatation of vessels, resulting from paralysis of the superior cervical sympathetic chain on the side involved, is known as *Horner's syndrome*.

Widening of the palpebral fissure occurs with exophthalmos, but also may result from spasm of the levator or smooth muscle fibers of the lid and orbit. The condition occurs following the administration of drugs such as cocaine, phenylephrine, and epinephrine. Irritative lesions of the sympathetic nerves in the neck also may produce a widening of the fissure. Most authors consider the widened fissures in thyrotoxicosis to be the result of spasm of the smooth muscle in the orbit. Widened fissures also are seen in essential hypertension, in suprasellar meningiomas, and in lesions near the posterior commissure. The upper lids frequently retract in infants with meningitis or hydrocephalus.

Diseases of the Skin of the Lids

Hemorrhages in the lids vary from small petechiae to massive ecchymoses (p. 257). Edema of the lids may result from trauma, from inflammatory diseases of the globe and other tissues in the orbit, and from various general conditions. Emphysema of the lids usually is due to a communication between the orbit and the nose or the sinuses.

The skin of the lids may be involved in a large variety of inflammatory and infectious diseases. These may be limited to the skin of the ocular region or may be part of a generalized dermatosis (p. 258). Among the infections that may involve the lids are a variety of bacterial, fungal, and viral disorders (p. 203). Allergic disorders (p. 183), collagen diseases, and other disorders affecting the tissue (p. 226), and a number of dermatoses, have important lid manifestations. *Blepharitis* (inflammation of the lid margin) has several forms (p. 203).

Xanthelasma palpebrarum are flat, yellow lesions of the lids, which are composed of masses of lipid laden histiocytes that may contain scattered Touton giant cells. These lesions occur in systemic lipoidoses, in patients with increased serum lipids, and in apparently normal individuals.

Diseases of the Cilia

The cilia are subject to a number of diseases. Absence of the lashes frequently is the result of chronic inflammatory disease of the lid margin. It occurs after some severe, generalized infection and after excessive x-ray therapy. A congenital lack of lashes is rare. *Alopecia areata* is a trophic disorder in which lashes, eyebrows, and patches of hair are lost without any sign of inflammation of the lid margin.

Distichiasis generally is a congenital anomaly in which lashes grow from an abnormal position along the posterior border of the lid margin, apparently from the openings of the meibomian glands (p. 115). *Trichiasis* is an acquired condition in which the lashes turn in after chronic inflammation of the lids. Both conditions may cause severe irritation and corneal ulceration with decreased vision. Treatments consist of plastic procedures, surgical removal of the lashes, and electrolysis.

Pigment Abnormalities

In albinos there is a congenital lack of pigment in the lids. Decreased pigmentation also occurs after severe, generalized infection. One form of this condition is *vitiligo*, in which there are oval, usually symmetrical, depigmented areas on both lids and their cilia. *Poliosis*, a whitening of the lashes, may be associated with uveitis and other findings (Vogt-Koyanagi syndrome).

Chloasma is a large, ill-defined, brown spot that occurs on the skin of the brow and on the lids during pregnancy. Dermatoses due to photosensitivity include xeroderma pigmentosum (p. 262), hydroa vacciniforme, and acute solar dermatitis (p. 262).

Diseases of the Glands of the Lids

Absence of sweating (anhidrosis) of the lids, excessive sweating (hyperhidrosis) of the lids, cysts of the sweat glands and sebaceous glands, and retention cysts are discussed in Medical Ophthalmology—Diseases of the Skin (p. 257).

An *external hordeolum* is a purulent infection of a sebaceous or sweat gland along the lid margin. It is localized and points on the skin surface. An *internal hordeolum* is a similar infection with the swelling appearing on the conjunctival side and intermarginal space of the lids. A *chalazion* is a chronic inflammation of a meibomian gland. Histopathologic examination of this lesion shows a granulomatous reaction to liberated fat. This lesion may develop spontaneously or may follow a hordeolum. These lesions are discussed in Medical Ophthalmology—Infections Limited Primarily to the Eye (p. 202).

Tumors and Related Lesions of the Lids

Tumors of the lids, including basal cell carcinoma, squamous cell carcinoma, senile keratoses, Bowen's disease, meibomian gland carcinoma, nevi, hemangiomas, and pseudocancerous lesions, are discussed in Medical Ophthalmology—Tumors (p. 263). Verrucae and molluscum contagiosum are described in Medical Ophthalmology—Infections Limited Primarily to the Eye (p. 202). Neurofibromas (p. 170) and xanthoma also are considered later.

THE LACRIMAL APPARATUS

Diseases of the Lacrimal Gland

Diseases of the lacrimal gland may be revealed by hyposecretion or hypersecretion of tears and by enlargement of the gland, with or without signs of inflammation. Measurement of tear secretion is carried out by insertion of standardized strips of filter paper into the lower cul-de-sac (Schirmer Test).

Decreased tear secretion sometimes develops with aging. A more serious insufficiency in lacrimal secretion occurs in a general systemic disease of unknown etiology called *Sjögren's syndrome*. This consists of atrophic changes in the lacrimal glands that lead to scanty lacrimal secretion, a feeling of dryness of the eyes, deficient salivary secretion with dryness of the mouth and tongue, rheumatoid polyarthritis, and various other complications. Sjögren's syndrome occurs almost exclusively in women past their menopause.

Conjunctival cicatrization from chemical burns, erythema multiforme, trachoma, and other diseases may result in occlusion of the orifices of the lacrimal gland and a diminished quantity of tears. Congenital alacrima occurs in the *Riley-Day syndrome* (familial autonomic dysfunction) (p. 175). Instillation of methyl cellulose or other types of artificial tears may relieve some of the dryness, burning, and discomfort resulting from decreased tear secretion. Surgical measures include obstructing the puncta and transplanting Stensen's duct into the conjunctival sac.

Excessive tear formation may result from reflex stimulation of the lacrimal gland, from irritation of the conjunctiva or cornea, and from excessive stimulation of the retina by light. In patients with facial nerve paralysis, the nerve may regenerate abnormally by diverting fibers from the salivary to the lacrimal gland. This results in tearing associated with salivation ("crocodile tears").

Acute inflammation of the lacrimal gland (*dacryoadenitis*) is seen as a complication of mumps, measles, infectious mononucleosis, and other systemic diseases. It may also develop secondary to an extension of inflammation from the lids or conjunctiva, or following a perforating injury to the lacrimal gland. In acute dacryoadenitis there is swelling, pain, and redness over the upper temporal aspect of the eye. The treatment is the same as that of any acute, localized infection.

Chronic dacryoadenitis, a painless, slowly developing swelling of one or both lacrimal glands, is usually due to chronic granulomatous diseases such as syphilis, tuberculosis, or sarcoid. Chronic enlargement of the salivary and lacrimal glands is frequently termed *Mikulicz's syndrome*. Besides the granulomatous diseases just referred to, the syndrome should arouse suspicion of reticulocytoses, leukemia, and lymphosarcoma. If there is associated uveitis, the condition is termed *Heerfordt's disease*. Tumors of the lacrimal gland are discussed elsewhere (p. 272).

Diseases of the Lacrimal Ducts

Epiphora is an overflow of tears due to excessive tear secretion and defective tear drainage. Causes of impaired tear drainage include poor apposition of the lacrimal puncta to the lacrimal lake (p. 366), scarring or stenosis of the puncta, paresis or paralysis of the orbicularis oculi muscle, and occlusion of the common canaliculus, or tear sac (p. 206).

Canaliculitis is an inflammation of the canaliculi occurring because of infection. It is often associated with obstruction by the fungus Streptothrix (p. 208). *Dacryocystitis* is an inflammation of the lacrimal sac. It is almost always unilateral and results from an obstruction of the nasolacrimal duct. Acute dacryocystitis results from a secondary bacterial infection of the lacrimal sac. This is made manifest by an acute swelling, with redness and tenderness below the lid margin on the side of the nose. The eyelids may swell because of edema.

Chronic dacryocystitis usually occurs in infants (p. 116) and in middle life. In many patients the cause of obstruction is not apparent, but in adults it may follow injury or nasal disease in the region of the lacrimal sac. The chief symptoms are epiphora and the appearance of pus through the puncta, with pressure on the lacrimal sac.

DISEASES OF THE ENTIRE GLOBE

Developmental Abnormalities

Anomalies of the eyeball result from disturbances in the development of the optic vesicles and include the following:

Anophthalmos is a term used clinically to denote cases in which the eye appears to be absent. The deformity is generally bilateral. Typically the orbits are small and the lids are concave and closed (p. 116). *Cyclopia* is a rare anomaly in which the elements of the two eyes are fused to form an apparently single eye in the middle of the forehead (p. 116). Affected fetuses are usually stillborn since this condition is associated with other abnormalities that are incompatible with life. A *congenital cystic eyeball* is another rare condition in which invagination of the anterior part of the primary optic vesicle (the presumptive retina) is arrested (p. 116). At birth, instead of the globe, a cystic structure is present.

Microphthalmos is a condition in which the eye is smaller than normal (p. 116). The term includes a great variety of abnormalities, most of which result from involution of the primary optic vesicle or failure of the fetal fissure to close. The underlying cause is most frequently a genetic defect or some type of infection of the embryo. Microphthalmos frequently is associated with other ocular anomalies. Enlargement·of the eye at birth or during the neonatal period may occur in congenital glaucoma (p. 354), in Sturge-Weber syndrome (p. 172), in von Recklinghausen's neurofibromatosis (p. 170) and in myopia (p. 446).

Pigment Disturbances

Albinism is a genetically determined metabolic defect in which melanin is either scarce or absent. The metabolic defect consists of a failure to convert tyrosine to DOPA (3,4-dihydroxyphenylalanine), a precursor of melanin. Albinism occurs in a variety of forms and may affect the eyes alone or the skin, hair, and eyes. The iris appears pink and translucent. Pigment is absent from the choroid and retina, revealing clearly the choroidal vascular network. The macula may be difficult to identify on ophthalmoscopic examination. Poor vision, nystagmus, photophobia, and high errors of refraction are prominent features.

Excessive melanin pigmentation occurs among dark races whose eye tissues are frequently heavily pigmented. *Melanosis oculi* is a condition in which there is congenital hyperpigmentation of the uveal tract of one eye, usually occurring with increased pigmentation of the sclera, episclera, and disc region. When the eyelid or adjacent skin is involved, the condition is known as *oculodermal melanocytosis*, or the *nevus of Ota*. Oculodermal melanocytosis may be present at birth, or can occur at puberty or later.

Inflammation and Infection

Panophthalmitis designates those inflammations involving all three coats of the eye and Tenon's capsule. In *endophthalmitis* the inflammation is in the ocular cavities and their immediately adjacent structures. The inflammatory changes are similar in both entities, and the clinical distinction is one of degree. Signs and symptoms are pain, a hazy cornea, and exudate in the anterior chamber. In panophthalmitis the lids and conjunctiva are congested and edematous, and exophthalmos is present. Panophthalmitis and endophthalmitis are caused by pyogenic bacteria and, less frequently, by fungi. These infections may follow penetrating wounds, intraocular surgery, and corneal ulcers. Infection may spread directly from the adjacent tissues or through the bloodstream from a focus elsewhere in the body. Necrosis of intraocular tumors and retained intraocular foreign bodies may also cause endophthalmitis. When the cause is infection, treatment is with systemic antibiotics. Evisceration may be necessary in panophthalmitis. Atrophy of the eyeball is the sequela of panophthalmitis and endophthalmitis. *Phthisis bulbi* denotes atrophy with hypotony.

THE CONJUNCTIVA

Abnormalities of the Conjunctiva

Congestion. Irritation of the conjunctiva causes congestion ·of the superficial conjunctival vessels. Inflammation within the eye itself usually is associated with congestion of the deeper vessels. Superficial congestion is characterized by the following: pink or light red color of the enlarged vessels; tortuosity of the vessels; congestion that is greater near the periphery of the bulbar conjunctiva and becomes less marked as the limbus is approached; vessels that when emptied of their contents by pressure through the lids can be seen to refill with blood from the periphery; and enlarged vessels that are movable with the conjunctiva. Deep congestion, known as ciliary injection or ciliary flush, is described elsewhere (pp. 11, 17).

Hyperemia of the Conjunctiva. Chronic dilatation of the conjunctival vessels occurs commonly, especially among people who do a considerable amount of close work. These patients complain of their eyes being red most of the time and of exacerbated redness after long periods of close work, especially at night or after they have been exposed to wind and dust. They are aware of a foreign body sensation. There is no significant discharge, either in the conjunctival cul-de-sac or dried on the lid margins in the form of scales. Examination shows a generalized hyperemia of the conjunctiva that can be distinguished from conjunctivitis only by the absence of secretion. The symptoms may be mild, or severe and persistent.

When no cause for congestion can be found, it must be assumed that there is a local hypersensitivity to all noxious agents, with dilation of the conjunctival vessels occurring to an abnormal degree, probably as an axon reflex. The patients should be protected from wind and dust, and errors of refraction should be corrected with spectacles.

Subconjunctival Hemorrhages. These usually appear spontaneously as bright red areas, resulting from rupture of a conjunctival blood vessel (Plate 1*A*). They may come on without any apparent cause, but frequently a history of coughing, or of exertion such as lifting a heavy weight or straining at a bowel movement, is elicited. The patient generally is alarmed by the appearance of the hemorrhage, so he should be reassured that, although frightening, it is harmless. The blood usually takes from one to two weeks to become absorbed and may go through all the characteristic color changes caused by breakdown of blood pigments. Occasionally a large hemorrhage lifts up the conjunctiva and may have to be incised to let out the blood that has not clotted.

Most conjunctival hemorrhages are significant only in the disfigurement they cause, but some are associated with more serious disorders, such as hemorrhagic blood dyscrasia, acute febrile infections, local vascular anomalies, and local acute inflammation.

Edema or Chemosis of the Conjunctiva. Edema of the lids is usually associated with this condition. A filtration chemosis occurs with the presence of a fistula into the anterior chamber, as is made in glaucoma surgery or results from injury. Certain general conditions, such as nephritis, cardiac disease, the anemias, Graves' disease, and angioneurotic edema, that cause an increased capillary permeability also cause edema of the conjunctiva and lids. Chemosis may arise with inflammation of surrounding ocular structures, or on blockage of the venous lymphatic drainage.

Conjunctivitis

Conjunctivitis is an inflammation of the conjunctiva, generally consisting of conjunctival hyperemia associated with a discharge. Edema, cellular infiltration, and other changes also may occur. The broad underlying causes of conjunctivitis are bacterial, viral, rickettsial, spirochetal, fungal, parasitic, allergic, and traumatic. The clinical appearance, diagnosis, and treatment of conjunctivitis caused by specific agents are discussed in Medical Ophthalmology (p. 183).

In addition to classification by their etiology, various types of conjunctivitis are distinguished clinically according to course and associated findings. These are summarized in Table 1-1. Conjunctivitis may be acute or chronic. Chronic conjunctivitis also may represent changes resulting from repeated attacks of acute inflammation or senile degenerative changes, in which symptoms referable to the conjunctiva are present almost constantly.

Most cases of conjunctivitis are associated with a discharge. Accordingly, *catarrhal conjunctivitis* is spoken of when there is excessive mucous secretion. *Purulent conjunctivitis* is an inflammation of the conjunctiva in which pus has formed. In certain types of viral conjunctivitis no discharge is associated with the conjunctival hyperemia; this is sometimes referred to as a serous inflammation. With acute inflammation of the conjunctiva, an exudate

TABLE 1-1   CLINICAL CLASSIFICATION OF CONJUNCTIVITIS

Acute and subacute catarrhal conjunctivitis (hyperemia of the conjunctiva with
   an excessive mucous secretion, "pink eye")
   Diplococcus pneumoniae
   Hemophilus conjunctivitidis
   Hemophilus aegyptius (Koch-Weeks bacillus)
   Staphylococcus aureus
   Streptococcus viridans
   Streptococci
Chronic catarrhal conjunctivitis
   Staphylococcus aureus
   Moraxella lacunata (Morax-Axenfeld bacillus)
   Neisseria catarrhalis
   Proteus vulgaris
   Escherichia coli
   Mimeae
   Deficiency of lacrimal secretion
   Excessive meibomian secretion
   Toxic or allergic factors
Purulent conjunctivitis
   Neisseria gonorrhoeae (gonococcus)
   Neisseria meningitidis (meningococcus)
   Staphylococcus aureus, Streptococcus hemolyticus,
      Diplococcus pneumoniae, Hemophilus aegyptius,
      Escherichia coli, Corynebacterium diphtheriae,
      Borrelia vincentis, fusiform bacilli, and many other organisms
Pseudomembranous and membranous conjunctivitis
   Corynebacterium diphtheriae
   Streptococcus hemolyticus
   Neisseria gonorrhoeae
   Epidemic keratoconjunctivitis (adenovirus 8)
   Trachoma
   Herpetic keratoconjunctivitis
   Can occur with many other acute bacterial and viral infections, as well as a
      result of allergic or toxic factors
Papillary conjunctivitis
   Subacute stages of many types of infective conjunctivitis
   Vernal catarrh
   Contact allergies
Follicular conjunctivitis
   Epidemic keratoconjunctivitis (adenovirus 8)
   Pharyngoconjunctival fever (adenovirus 3 and 7)
   Inclusion conjunctivitis virus
   Trachoma
   Primary herpetic keratoconjunctivitis
   Influenza A virus
   Newcastle disease
   Molluscum contagiosum irritation
   Cat-scratch fever
   Toxic (including prolonged use of eserine and pilocarpine)
   Etiology undetermined: conjunctival folliculosis
   Angular conjunctivitis (hyperemia most marked near the angle of the lids)
   Staphylococcus aureus
   Moraxella lacunata (Morax-Axenfeld bacillus)
   Vitamin B deficiency (particularly pyridoxine)
   Neisseria meningitidis
   Diplococcus pneumoniae
   Hemophilus conjunctivitidis

TABLE 1-1   CLINICAL CLASSIFICATION OF CONJUNCTIVITIS *(Continued)*

Parinaud's oculoglandular syndrome
    Leptotrichosis conjunctivae *(Leptothrix)*
    Cat-scratch fever
    Mycobacterium tuberculosis
    Pasturella tularensis
    Lymphogranuloma venereum
    Hemophilus ducreyi
    Treponema pallidum (chancre)
    Glanders
    Vaccinia
    Sporotrichosis
Newborn conjunctivitis
    Staphylococcus aureus
    Inclusion conjunctivitis virus
    Diplococcus pneumoniae
    Hemophilus influenzae
    Neisseria gonorrhoeae

rich in fibrin is formed on the surface of the conjunctiva and *pseudomembranous conjunctivitis* results. The pseudomembrane characteristically can be easily peeled off, leaving the epithelium intact. If the exudate is firmly fixed to the epithelial cells, attempted removal results in a raw, bleeding surface; this is the situation in *membranous conjunctivitis.*

A characteristic feature of the subacute stage of many types of conjunctivitis is the formation of small elevations (papillae) on the conjunctival surface that contain newly formed capillaries infiltrated with lymphoid cells. Inflammations in which these elevations are numerous are termed *papillary conjunctivitis.* Follicles are dense, localized infiltrations of lymphoid tissue that occur as a response to irritation. If an excessive formation of follicles accompanies conjunctivitis, it may be termed a *follicular conjunctivitis.* These typically are of viral origin. *Parinaud's oculoglandular syndrome* consists of a conjunctivitis associated with marked preauricular gland enlargement.

OTHER INFLAMMATIONS AND DEGENERATIONS OF THE CONJUNCTIVA

Pemphigus.   Pemphigus can involve the conjunctiva. Bullae form, which upon rupturing leave ulcerated areas. Cicatrization and atrophy of the conjunctiva ensue with resultant severe ocular complications.

This disease is serious, both from the point of view of vision and of life itself. *Ocular pemphigoid* is a chronic condition in which newly formed connective tissue invades the submucous tissue. There is subsequent contraction and shrinkage of the conjunctiva. Other mucous membranes usually are affected, but the disease is not fatal.

Erythema Multiforme Bullosum.   Erythema multiforme is characterized by varied erythematous, urticarial, bullous, and purpuric lesions that appear suddenly and are self-limited. Stevens-Johnson disease is a term often applied to an extremely serious form of the disease that often occurs in childhood and that may be fatal (p. 230).

Symblepharon is an adhesion between the palpebral and bulbar conjunctiva that fixes the eyelids against the globe. The major causes are chemical burns, infection, and inflammation, including trachoma, Stevens-Johnson disease, and pemphigus. *Ankyloblepharon* is an adhesion of the eyelids to each other.

New Growths on the Conjunctiva

Pinguecula.   At either side of the limbus, but especially the nasal side, a raised yellow-gray area frequently is seen, particularly in patients in middle life or later. This is a benign lesion.

Pterygium.   This is a growth on the cornea, usually extending from the nasal limbus. Histologically it resembles a pinguecula and frequently is preceded by one. Repeated irritation of the conjunctiva and of the cornea by ultraviolet light, dust, and wind is the only known important cause. Humidity may play a part. The condition is common in the southwestern United States. Men working out-of-doors are most commonly affected. A well developed pterygium resembles a wing extending from the limbus toward the center of the cornea.

Pseudopterygium. This is a conjunctival overgrowth of the cornea caused by a burn or other injury. A probe can be passed beneath the head of a pseudopterygium, whereas the tight attachment of a true pterygium does not permit a probe to be passed.

Lymphangiectasis. In this condition, small, clear, localized, cystlike dilatations of lymph vessels, which are occasionally irritating, appear in the conjunctiva.

Conjunctival lithiasis. This is seen as small, yellow or white, calcareous deposits in the tarsal conjunctiva or the inferior fornix. When they irritate the cornea, they can be easily excised.

Tumors. A discussion of tumors of the conjunctiva is given elsewhere in this book (p. 269).

Pigmentation of the Conjunctiva

Patients with alcaptonuria *(ochronosis)* and Addison's disease develop pigmentation of the conjunctiva (p. 218). The prolonged topical use of silver salts in the eye results in a dark gray discoloration of the conjunctiva most marked in the lower cul-de-sac *(argyrosis)*. Mercury salts also can cause discoloration. Patients receiving atabrine for the treatment of malaria may develop a reversible discoloration of the conjunctiva. Prolonged use of antiglaucoma medication containing epinephrine compounds may result in localized black deposits of melanin pigment in the palpebral conjunctiva (Plate 1*B*).

Congenital Anomalies

Megalocornea. This term denotes bilateral, nonprogressive, congenitally enlarged corneas (p. 118). The diameter may reach 16 mm. Myopia, dislocation of the lens, and posterior subcapsular cataracts are frequently associated findings. Normal intraocular pressure helps to distinguish this condition from congenital glaucoma.

Microcornea. In this condition, which often is associated with microphthalmos, the cornea is abnormally small (10 mm. or less). Patients often are highly hyperopic and predisposed to glaucoma.

Dermoids. These congenital tumors involve tissue of mesodermal and ectodermal origin and are seen as yellow raised lesions situated usually at the limbus (p. 272).

Posterior Embryotoxon. This congenital, hyaline-appearing, ringlike opacity occurs within the limbus at the terminus of Descemet's membrane (Schwalbe's line), which is displaced centrally. The cornea therefore is clear peripheral to the opacity. The root of the iris is usually adherent to the opacity, and abnormal development of the angle structures and trabecular area with an elevated intraocular pressure (Axenfeld's syndrome) is common (p. 120).

Birth Injuries

Corneal birth injuries usually result from compression of the globe, most commonly by the blade of an obstetrical forceps. The abrupt folding in of the cornea results in tears in Descemet's membrane and striae. Immediately after birth the cornea is steamy, as in interstitial keratitis, but during ensuing weeks it appears partially clear to gross examination. With focal illumination and magnification, however, fine striae may be seen, usually running diagonally across the cornea at the site of the tear in Descemet's membrane. These striae persist throughout life and frequently impair vision.

Vascularization of the Cornea

The normal cornea has no blood vessels. In inflammatory conditions of the cornea the perivascular loops dilate at the limbus, causing a characteristic pericorneal injection that is called a *ciliary flush*. During many inflammatory conditions the cornea is invaded by newly formed blood vessels. After the inflammation subsides, the blood vessels empty or contain little blood and are difficult to detect. They remain in the cornea, however, and are called "ghost" vessels. Their presence always signifies a previous pathologic condition.

Corneal vascularization may be superficial or deep. If the vessels are situated at or near the level of Bowman's membrane, they have been derived from the conjunctival circulation and cross the limbus in direct continuity with the conjunctival vessels. If they are found below the area of Bowman's membrane in the substantia propria, they come from the deep ciliary vessels and disappear at the limbus. Superficial vessels are bright red, usually irregular, and branch frequently to form an anastomotic network; deep vessels are dark purple and tend to run in straight lines.

Superficial vascularization usually accompanies severe inflammations of the epithelium and Bowman's membrane. It is particularly prominent in acne rosacea keratitis, trachoma, phlyctenular keratoconjunctivitis, and herpetic keratoconjunctivitis. Deep vascularization occurs in the forms of keratitis that involve the substantia propria, the most common form being interstitial keratitis.

When infiltration of granular tissue accompanies superficial vascularization, the condition is termed a *pannus*. It frequently is found in trachoma where it occurs at the upper limbus beneath the upper lid. Pannus often is observed also in severe phlyctenular disease (p. 187) and in degenerated eyes that have been afflicted with any serious intraocular inflammation.

Edema of the Cornea

If the epithelium, and especially the endothelium, of the cornea is damaged, corneal edema results. Nearly all inflammatory conditions of the cornea are accompanied by some corneal edema. Corneal edema also occurs if the intraocular pressure increases, i.e., in glaucoma. If fluid collects under the epithelium, blebs form that may cause photophobia and irritation. When the blebs break, foreign body sensation and pain may be excruciating. Edema of the epithelium or stroma causes blurring of vision.

Inflammation of the Cornea: Keratitis

Keratitis (inflammation of the cornea) may be superficial or deep. Superficial keratitis affects primarily the corneal epithelium and Bowman's membrane. Most types of superficial keratitis take the form of punctate epithelial opacities or erosions. The extent and depth of de-epithelialized areas can be gauged on the slit lamp biomicroscope after instillation of fluorescein dye. These lesions may have a variety of shapes and sizes. In many disorders several different types are present simultaneously or appear in succession. On gross examination a decrease of the usual corneal luster often is observed, with dilatation of the limbal vessels.

Acute, diffuse, epithelial keratitis commonly occurs in association with bacterial conjunctivitis, particularly those forms caused by Staphylococcus, pneumococcus, and *Hemophilus aegyptius* (Koch-Weeks bacillus). Many viral diseases of the eye give rise to punctate lesions. *Superficial punctate keratitis (SPK)* is a somewhat confusing term that was used originally in the nineteenth century to describe spots on the cornea that could be seen with the naked eye or a loupe, the spots occurring secondary to acute conjunctivitis. Presently, the term superficial punctate keratitis is used to denote a specific condition characterized by coarse, punctate, epithelial lesions occurring bilaterally and in the absence of conjunctivitis. The etiology probably is viral and the course usually is a chronic, remittent one. In vaccinia, and occasionally in other viral diseases, a large area or the entire corneal epithelium may be involved. Keratitis is a major feature of herpes simplex virus infection of the eye. An epithelial lesion having a dendritic pattern is seen characteristically.

Decreased tear secretion results in epithelial erosions (keratitis sicca) and mucus-like strands and threads of nonviable epithelium, which are attached firmly to the cornea and stain brilliantly with the instillation of Bengal rose dye (filamentary keratitis). Such filaments also are seen in viral keratitis, following trauma, in edematous states, as after wearing a contact lens, and in chronic uveitis, particularly that caused by sarcoid. When the cornea is not protected adequately by the lids, the corneal epithelium dries, and punctate, or in severe cases blotchy, lesions develop (exposure keratitis). A similar picture may occur as a result of corneal anesthesia (neurotrophic keratitis). A superficial keratitis may develop secondary to ocular medications, as a result of x-ray and ultraviolet exposure, and as a complication of a number of diseases of the skin.

Xerophthalmia refers to the ocular changes caused by vitamin A deficiency. In the late stages of xerophthalmia, exfoliation of the epithelium, corneal clouding, ulceration, and liquefaction are seen (p. 273).

Bitot's spots are gray-white, oval to triangular lesions occurring predominantly on the temporal side of the limbus. They have a cheeselike or foamy appearance and are not wetted by tears; if removed by scraping, they quickly re-form. Bitot's spots usually are associated with a deficiency of vitamin A, but they also have been observed in pellagra and in other nutritional deficiencies.

Keratitis nummularis is a rare form of subepithelial keratitis of unknown etiology. The principal findings are 10 to 20 small, disc-shaped opacities located in the central cornea just beneath Bowman's membrane. Vascularization of the affected areas may occur. Generally the lesions disappear over a period of years. Treatment is symptomatic.

Dellen are shallow, saucer-like depressions at the periphery of the cornea, usually on the temporal side. They probably are due to an insufficiency of the limbal circulation. These lesions may appear spontaneously in the aged, may follow ocular inflammation with swelling of the perilimbal tissues, may

develop after ocular muscle surgery or cataract operation, may occur in lagophthalmos, or may be seen after prolonged cocaine administration. Dellen usually are asymptomatic and transient, regressing spontaneously within about 48 hours after their onset.

Central corneal ulcers and marginal corneal ulcers of bacterial, viral, and fungal etiology, as well as ring ulcers and Mooren's ulcer (chronic serpiginous ulcer), are discussed in Medical Ophthalmology, Infections of the Eye (p. 189).

Deep keratitis, or interstitial keratitis, is an inflammation of the cornea stroma. It is typically seen as a late manifestation of congenital syphilis (p. 136), but sometimes it is a result of acquired syphilis. In these latter patients the disease is usually limited to one eye and frequently is milder than the congenital form. Interstitial keratitis can occur also as a complication of tuberculosis, leprosy, and sarcoid, as well as following mumps, influenza, herpes zoster, and smallpox vaccination.

Cogan's syndrome consists of vertigo, tinnitus and deafness, pain in the eyes, and impaired vision due to interstitial keratitis. Usually both eyes are involved. A patchy infiltration of the deep corneal stroma, a slight but deep vascularization, and a small amount of inflammation of the anterior segment are seen. Vestibuloauditory and ocular symptoms generally begin within a few weeks of each other. This rare syndrome affects young adults. Presumably a generalized hypersensitivity reaction, it may be related to polyarteritis nodosa.

Trauma to the Cornea

Corneal foreign bodies, abrasions, and lacerations are commonly seen. Their treatment and diagnosis are considered elsewhere in this book (p. 367). When a corneal wound penetrates deeper than the epithelium, the healing is by scar formations. Nebulae are slight scars that can be seen only with oblique illumination. They seldom interfere with the patient's vision. Maculae are denser scars that can be seen without special optical aids. If located in the pupillary space, maculae may interfere with the patient's vision. Leukoma is a dense, white, opaque scar. When the iris adheres to such a scar, the condition is called adherent leukoma.

Pigmentation of the Cornea

Foreign substances such as silver *(argyrosis)*, iron *(siderosis)*, and copper *(chalcosis)* cause pigmentation of the cornea. The cornea may develop black areas as a result of frequent instillation of epinephrine drops. The *Hudson-Stahli line,* a fine, somewhat sinuous, horizontal, brown line seen with a slit lamp biomicroscope in the inferior third of the cornea of older persons, may represent deposits of hemosiderin in the cornea at the site of tears in Bowman's membrane. Brown pigment, possibly iron, also deposits in the epithelium at the base of the cone in keratoconus *(Fleischer's ring).* The *Kayser-Fleischer ring* is seen in the cornea of patients with Wilson's hepaticolenticular degeneration (p. 222). This completely or partially pigmented ring is red or bright green, about 2 mm. wide, and encircles the cornea near the limbus. It appears to be composed of a copper compound deposited in the periphery of Descemet's membrane. In some patients it can be seen only with slit lamp biomicroscope examination. In Negroes, melanin pigment may be seen in the superficial layers of the limbus and peripheral cornea.

Krukenberg's spindle is a vertical, spindle-shaped deposition of uveal pigment on the endothelial surface of the cornea. Sometimes it can be seen grossly, but it may require a loupe or slit lamp biomicroscope examination. Although it has been described in a number of ocular diseases, it is especially important as a sign of pigmentary glaucoma (p. 360).

Blood staining of the cornea is a result of anterior chamber hemorrhage associated with increased intraocular pressure. Under such circumstances the corneal epithelium usually is damaged, and blood pigment may pass into the cornea. Clinically, the color of the cornea may vary from a dark brown — almost black, to yellow.

Keratic precipitates (K.P.) are deposits of inflammatory cells on the posterior surface of the cornea. They are seen with the slit lamp biomicroscope or loupe in patients with inflammation of the anterior segment of the eye.

Degenerative Processes of the Cornea

Corneal degeneration denotes chemical and histologic changes that occur in the cornea during aging, following local inflammatory disturbances, and in systemic disorders. Corneal degenerations are distinct from corneal dystrophies (see following section).

Arcus senilis is found bilaterally in most persons past 50 years of age. It appears as a gray, opaque ring about 1 to 1.5 mm. wide following the contour of the limbus but separated from it by a clear zone. The outer edge of the ring is a sharp line, but the inner edge shades off gradually.

Arcus juvenilis, or *anterior embryotoxon,* is identical in appearance to arcus senilis, but either is present at birth or develops before or during middle age. Arcus juvenilis may occur as an isolated phenomenon or in association with other congenital anomalies. It has been described as the result of premature corneal degeneration, irritation to the cornea, other corneal diseases such as interstitial keratitis, and familial hypercholesterolemia.

A *staphyloma* is an ectasia or bulging of weakened cornea or sclera lined with uveal tissue. It occurs after corneal disease or injuries that are accompanied by prolapse or incarceration of iris. The weak areas that result may bulge and appear blue. Secondary glaucoma may be a causative factor. Descemet's membrane resists trauma and pathologic processes more than does the rest of the cornea. When an ulcer destroys the stroma, Descemet's membrane may remain and protrude forward under the effect of intraocular pressure, forming a *descemetocele.*

Bullous keratopathy is characterized by epithelial bullae or blebs and occurs in the late stages of chronic corneal edema. Consequently, this condition is seen in severely diseased eyes, especially those with long-standing glaucoma. It is common also after perforating wounds or complicated surgery, and in the late stages of Fuchs' dystrophy (p. 281). The condition is persistent, with the bullae enlarging, bursting, and reappearing, and is associated with *tumors of the cornea* (p. 269), are discussed elsewhere in this book.

severe pain and irritation. Modes of treatment include chemical cauterization of the cornea, placement of the conjunctival flap over the cornea, and penetrating cautery. In blind, painful eyes, retrobulbar alcohol injection or enucleation may be resorted to.

In *band-shaped keratopathy* there is a gradual development of a gray-white opaque band starting at the limbus and extending across the cornea at a level slightly below the middle of the pupil. Histopathologically there is a deposition of calcium salts in the superficial cornea and replacement of Bowman's membrane by fibrous tissue. This disorder usually occurs secondary to severe ocular disease, especially chronic iridocyclitis in young persons. Band-shaped keratopathy also may develop in hypercalcemia from hyperparathyroidism or vitamin D poisoning. Reportedly, this lesion occasionally has occurred without apparent cause in otherwise healthy eyes. The most effective treatment is the application of a chelating agent, disodium ethylene diamine tetraacetate (EDTA), after the epithelium has been removed. Calcium deposition in the cornea sometimes is seen in patterns other than a band.

Corneal Dystrophies

Corneal dystrophy is a term applied to developmental, frequently hereditary, conditions affecting the cornea. Dystrophies usually are bilateral. They are not associated with inflammation, vascularization, and common changes of aging. The distinction between corneal degeneration and corneal dystrophy often is not clear.

These disorders include Meesmann's corneal dystrophy; Cogan's microscopic cystic epithelial dystrophy; granular, macular, and lattice dystrophies; Salzmann's nodular dystrophy; keratoconus; cornea guttata; and the combined dystrophy of Fuchs (p. 281).

Other Corneal Diseases

Drug induced changes in the cornea, including chloroquine keratopathy and

THE ANTERIOR CHAMBER

The anterior chamber is bounded anteriorly by the cornea and (corneoscleral) trabecula and posteriorly by the iris and pupillary space (p. 70). It is filled with aqueous humor that under normal conditions is clear and optically empty. It contains a very low concentration of protein (0.01 per cent), but when the blood vessels of the inflamed iris and ciliary body leak protein, the aqueous humor then contains amounts approximating that of blood (7 per cent), causing the aqueous humor to cloud. This *Tyndall phenomenon* (i.e., the visibility of floating particles in gases or liquids when illuminated by a ray of sunlight) is called an *aqueous flare* (p. 420) and can be seen with the beam of the slit lamp biomicroscope. With adequate magnification, white blood cells and minute protein aggregates that form floaters also can be seen. In severe and more prolonged inflammation, groups of cells may form a yellow mass known as *hypopyon* on the inferior portion of the anterior chamber. Aggregations of cells and debris may adhere to the back surface of the cornea, appearing as small yellow or white dots (*keratic precipitates*).

Blood in the anterior chamber is called a *hyphema* and usually is the result of trauma to the eye (p. 375). Under certain conditions the vitreous humor may prolapse into the anterior chamber or there may be an ingrowth of conjunctival epithelium cells into the anterior chamber.

THE SCLERA

Inflammation: Scleritis and Episcleritis

Inflammation of the sclera proper (scleritis) is distinct from inflammation of the episclera, the thin layer of vascular elastic tissue between the sclera and the conjunctiva (episcleritis).

Scleritis. Types of scleritis may be classified according to etiology:

1. Infections and systemic diseases such

as syphilis, sarcoidosis, gout, and other granulomatous disorders.

2. Toxic chemical and physical irritants.
3. Allergic and hypersensitivity reactions.

Collagen and its ground and cement substances are prone to hypersensitivity reactions. The so-called collagen diseases involve tissues such as the sclera, the dermis, and the walls of the blood vessels. In rheumatoid arthritis lesions frequently appear in the sclera.

Scleritis is also classified according to clinical and pathological features:

Anterior scleritis is seen most frequently in young people, particularly females. Characteristic nodular swellings are dark red and more extensive than the milder diffuse areas characteristic of episcleritis. They may eventually fuse. When the cornea is involved, a secondary parenchymal sclerosing keratitis occurs, transforming the cornea into a structure closely resembling the sclera. In annular scleritis the entire corneoscleral limbus is affected. Brawny scleritis is a progressive and severe scleritis characterized by remissions and exacerbations. It usually results in the loss of the affected eye.

In posterior scleritis the cornea and anterior part of the globe are usually normal in appearance. Depending upon the severity of the scleritis, there may be associated edema of the lids, protrusion and immobility of the globe, and inflammation of the choroid and retina. *Scleromalacia perforans* is discussed in Medical Ophthalmology (p. 228).

The *treatment of scleritis* depends upon the etiology. Most important is a thorough physical examination to reveal the underlying systemic condition. Possible foci of infection must be considered. Syphilis and tuberculosis should be ruled out. Blood uric acid should be determined. Salicylates may relieve symptoms during the acute stages. Treatment may include heat, instillation of antibiotic or sulfonamide drops, and, if signs of uveitis are present, the use of atropine and local corticosteroids. In the forms allied with the collagenous diseases, ACTH or corticosteroids given systemically are sometimes effective. Conjunctival and Tenon's capsule flaps have been helpful in some cases.

Episcleritis. This condition is a common, localized inflammation involving the episclera, usually of one eye, between the insertion of the rectus muscle and the corneoscleral limbus. In *circumscribed episcleritis* nodules form with purple oval elevations of a few millimeters in diameter. The inflammation involves the sclera internally and Tenon's capsule and the conjunctiva externally. The symptoms are pain and photophobia. The process tends to recur and involve adjacent areas. Treatment is the instillation of local corticosteroid drops.

A more diffuse inflammation is termed *episcleritis periodica fugax* and is characterized by a transient congestion and edema of a quadrant of the episclera. The disease tends to recur regularly. It usually does not affect the vision or leave serious sequelae. The etiology of episcleritis is obscure.

Pigmentation

The normal sclera is porcelain white with occasional pigment spots. Pigmentation of the sclera may vary, however, with the general pigmentation of the individual. In the colored races, collections of brown pigment at the points of exit of the anterior ciliary arteries may be mistaken for malignant melanomas.

Jaundice. The yellow discoloration occurring in jaundice characteristically affects the sclera, the skin, and the mucous membranes.

Blue Sclera. This apparent scleral pigmentation results from thinning and alteration in the character of the sclera. This allows the pigment of the choroid to be prominently seen, thereby giving the sclera a blue appearance. Blue sclera occurs in disorders of connective tissue and is a prominent feature of *osteogenesis imperfecta* (p. 222). It also has been described in other disorders, including Marfan's syndrome (p. 222) and pseudohypoparathyroidism (p. 255).

Ectasia and Staphyloma

Ectasia. The sclera is constantly subjected to intraocular pressure and, under certain conditions, may become stretched and thinned (ectatic). Such changes are frequently seen in congenital glaucoma and may also occur later in life following prolonged elevation of intraocular pressure. Ectasia may also follow scleritis and injuries.

Staphyloma. When, as usually happens, uveal tissue is pressed into a scleral ectasia, the condition is termed staphyloma. Staphylomas are seen as thin, dark blue, bulging areas. When the entire globe enlarges as in congenital glaucoma or in myopia, the condition is sometimes called total staphyloma. A partial staphyloma involves a localized segment of the globe, usually as the result of injuries or inflammation of the sclera. Partial staphylomas are described according to their anatomical position. The anterior staphylomas may occur between the ciliary body and the cornea (intercalary) or over the ciliary body (ciliary). Equatorial staphylomas are those at the anatomic equator and are sometimes associated with retinal detachment. Posterior staphylomas are located between the equator and the optic nerve, most commonly at the lamina cribrosa, and often follow prolonged and severe glaucoma, with optic atrophy or with high degrees of myopia. Donor grafts of scleral tissue and fascia lata have been used to treat ectasia and staphyloma, but the prognosis is poor.

IRIS, CILIARY BODY, AND PUPIL

Congenital and Developmental Defects

Aniridia. Absence of the iris (aniridia) is never total. The degree of hypoplasia varies, but a thin strip of iris tissue almost always persists in the angle. Aniridia generally is bilateral and transmitted as a dominant trait. Other defects occurring with this condition are glaucoma, cataract, microphakia, underdevelopment of the macula, and retinal aplasia (p. 120).

Coloboma of the Iris. This is a congenital cleft of the iris in the inferior nasal sector that occurs when the optic cup fails to close in the region of the fetal fissure. The defect may vary from a mere notch in the pupillary part of the iris to a severe sector defect in the uveal tissue that extends from the iris to the optic nerve. Surgical resection of a piece of iris in the course of an intraocular surgical procedure is a common cause of iris coloboma (Fig. 1-1).

Heterochromia. This denotes a difference in color between the two irides (Plates 1C and 1D), e.g., brown on one side and blue on the other. Heterochromia is sometimes found in normal eyes. It may also occur in abnormal conditions (p. 122).

Essential iris atrophy is a patchy degeneration and disappearance of the iris stroma and is of unknown etiology (p. 282).

Freckles and Nevi in the Iris

Freckles are clusters of pigmented melanocytes, a few cells thick, occurring along the anterior surface of the iris. Although probably present from birth, they usually are not observed clinically until after puberty, when all melanocytic cells of the body may become active. Studies indicate that about 50 per cent of people have freckles in one or both irides.

Nevi are more extensive lesions than freckles. They vary in size and shape, are slightly elevated, extend into the iris stroma, and may involve a segment of the iris. A nevus of the iris is often referred to as a "benign melanoma," but it may be difficult to distinguish from a malignant melanoma of the iris and, indeed, may give rise to such a neoplasm (p. 263).

Trauma to the Iris and Ciliary Body

In *iridodialysis* the iris is torn from its root at the ciliary body. As a result the iris moves away from its insertion, flattening the corresponding pupil margin. A dark

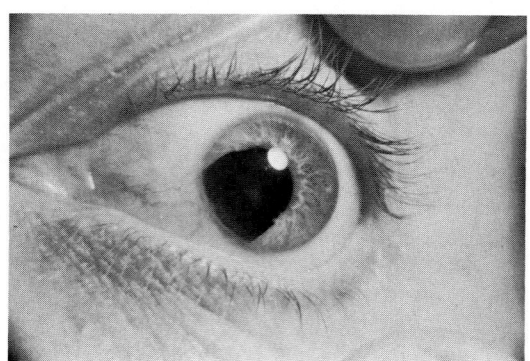

Figure 1-1 Surgical coloboma resulting from resection of iris melanoma.

space bounded by a straight line on the side toward the pupil margin may be seen at the site of the tear. The condition usually occurs following a blunt injury to the globe.

Iridodonesis is a tremulousness of the iris seen with movements of the eye. It indicates subluxation or dislocation of the lens (p. 376).

A contusion angle deformity is a tear into the face of the ciliary body resulting from blunt trauma. When this deformity is present, gonioscopic examination shows a wide and deep peripheral anterior chamber with the iris displaced, giving the characteristic appearance of a cleft or recess. Some patients with this lesion develop late chronic glaucoma (p. 360).

Prolapse of the iris denotes protrusion of the iris into a wound in the cornea or sclera. It occurs following injury or surgery.

Sympathetic ophthalmia is a bilateral inflammation of the entire uveal tract almost invariably caused by a perforating wound that involves uveal tissue. This condition is considered in detail elsewhere in this book (p. 373).

Inflammation of the Iris, Ciliary Body, and Choroid

The iris, ciliary body, and choroid together form the uveal tract. The intimate anatomic, physiologic, and pathologic relationships of the parts of this coat of the eye require that inflammation of all three be considered together. Other abnormalities of the choroid are discussed in a later section (p. 129).

Classification of Uveal Tract Inflammation. Certain diseases have a predilection for the anterior part of the uveal tract, whereas others chiefly affect the choroid. Inflammation of the iris and ciliary body is called *iridocyclitis;* inflammation of the iris alone is called *iritis;* inflammation of the uveal tract may be referred to as a *panuveitis.*

Inflammation of the uveal tract can be classified broadly as *granulomatous* and *nongranulomatous.* Granulomatous inflammation is characterized by a proliferation of large mononuclear cells, particularly the epithelioid giant-cell type. These inflammations also may be exogenous and endogenous. A broad etiologic classification is presented in Table 1-2.

SIGNS AND SYMPTOMS OF IRIDOCYCLITIS (Plate 1*E*). *Ciliary flush* refers to a deep,

diffuse, dull red injection around the limbus, resulting from dilatation of the vessels supplying the iris and ciliary body. Aqueous flare and floaters, as well as keratic precipitates (K.P.), have been defined previously (p. 14). *Posterior synechiae* are adhesions of the iris to the anterior capsule of the lens with irregularly shaped pupils (Plate 1*F*). If they form around the entire pupillary margin (occlusion of the pupil), they can prevent the normal passage of aqueous humor from the posterior into the anterior chamber. This causes the midportion of the iris to bulge forward toward the inner surface of the cornea, a condition called *iris bombé.* Elevated intraocular pressure results. Adhesions of the iris anteriorly to the cornea or angle structures (*anterior synechiae*) also can impede the outflow of aqueous and cause glaucoma. *Koeppe's nodules* are small, white nodules in the stroma or at the pupillary margin found in certain types of uveitis, particularly that associated with tuberculosis.

Findings Associated with Chorioretinitis. A variety of fundoscopic findings may occur with different types of choroiditis. In the acute phase one may see a solitary white patch of exudate situated deep to the retinal vessels, diffuse inflammation of a large area of the fundus, multiple scattered foci of choroidal infiltration, edema of the retina, retinal hemorrhages, edema of the optic nerve, and vitreous opacification. After the acute phase the choroidal lesion may undergo fibrosis and atrophy. The resulting choroidal scar may be seen as a flat, white area, sometimes traversed by larger

TABLE 1-2 ETIOLOGIC CLASSIFICATION OF UVEITIS

Uveitis due to infection
Uveitis due to allergy
Uveitis due to trauma (including sympathetic ophthalmia)
Uveitis due to irritants and toxic agents
Uveitis associated with noninfective systemic diseases
 Collagen diseases, sarcoidosis, and related diseases
 Diseases of the central nervous system
 Diseases of the skin
 Diabetes
Uveitis of unknown etiology

choroidal vessels, and associated with pigment clumps. The pigment epithelial cells are disintegrated, phagocytized, and carried into the retina.

In *peripheral uveitis* or *pars planitis* exudate is seen over the most anterior portion of the retina. This portion can be seen only with scleral indentation. This type of uveitis frequently is accompanied by macular edema and posterior polar cataract.

In *Jensen's choroiditis juxtapapillaris* there are circumscribed inflammatory changes of the choroid adjacent to the disc. This may be confused with optic neuritis (p. 304). An important feature is the sector-shaped defect in the field of vision that spreads fanlike from the blind spot.

Specific Types of Uveitis. *Behçet's syndrome* is a rare disorder of unknown cause, consisting of a severe uveitis and retinal vasculitis, optic atrophy, and aphthous-like lesions of the mucous membrane of the mouth and genitalia. Numerous other signs have been described, most possibly due to a diffuse vasculitis. The most serious complication is central nervous system involvement which may be fatal. The ocular involvement tends to be chronic and recurrent, and results in severe loss of vision. *Vogt-Koyanagi-Harada disease* is a clinical complex consisting of a prodromal meningismal episode followed by bilateral uveitis, vitiligo, alopecia, poliosis, and hearing defects. The etiology has not been determined.

Reiter's syndrome, a disorder of unknown etiology, consists of recurrent conjunctivitis, sterile urethritis, polyarthritis; and skin and mucous membrane lesions. Uveitis may occur. Additional ocular complications are scleritis and interstitial keratitis.

Fuchs' heterochromic cyclitis usually is a unilateral condition in which a mild anterior uveitis occurs in association with depigmentation of the pigment layer of the iris. The disease occurs insidiously, usually between 20 and 35 years of age. Clinical signs are heterochromia; fine, nonpigmented precipitates on the corneal endothelium; flare and cells in the anterior chamber; and dustlike opacities in the vitreous. Cataract and mild open angle glaucoma develop frequently in the involved eyes. External evidence of inflammation and ocular discomfort usually are absent. The etiology of Fuchs' heterochromic uveitis is unknown. Steroid therapy has little influence on the uveitis. In this condition cataract extraction usually can be performed without difficulty.

Cysts and Tumors of the Iris

Two types of cysts occur, intraepithelial and pupillary. These are discussed in Medical Ophthalmology, Degenerative Diseases and Ocular Changes in the Aging (p. 274). Tumors of the iris, including malignant melanoma, nevoxanthoendothelioma, hemangioma, leiomyoma, medulloepithelioma, and metastatic carcinoma, are described elsewhere in this book (p. 263).

Other Conditions Involving the Iris and Ciliary Body

New blood vessels formed on the anterior surface of the iris are known as *rubeosis iridis*. This condition is particularly associated with diabetes mellitus (p. 255) and retinal vein occlusion (p. 246). These new vessels lead to a severe glaucoma that rarely responds to medical or surgical treatment.

The Pupil

Dilatation of the pupil is called *mydriasis* and contraction of the pupil, *miosis*. *Anisocoria* denotes a difference in the size of the two pupils and is seen in about 25 per cent of normal individuals. *Corectopia* denotes a congenital displacement of the pupil resulting in its eccentricity. In *polycoria* the iris has more than one opening (i.e., there are multiple pupils). *Hippus* refers to a very marked "play" or variation in pupil size under normal conditions when the individual is awake.

The *Argyll Robertson pupil* consists of a miotic pupil that shows complete or partial absence of constriction to light, either direct or consensual, but contraction of the pupil to near stimulus (p. 327).

Adie's, or *tonic pupil*, is characterized by a sluggish, prolonged contraction to light; when constricted, the pupil takes an abnormally long time to dilate in darkness or on looking into the distance. These syndromes are discussed in detail elsewhere in this book (p. 328).

Ophthalmoplegia interna denotes the paralysis of all of the fibers of the third nerve supplying the internal muscles of the eye, i.e., the pupil, as well as the ciliary muscle. As previously noted, Horner's syndrome consists of a constricted pupil together with ptosis of the lid, apparent enophthalmos, and frequently a dilatation of the vessels, with loss from sweating on the homolateral side. These disorders, as well as paralysis and other pupillary disturbances, are considered elsewhere in this book (p. 329).

Pupillary block denotes a resistance to the passage of aqueous humor at the site of contact between the pupillary border of the iris and the anterior lens capsule. Seclusion of the pupil is an annular posterior adhesion or synechia resulting from iritis and shutting off the anterior from the posterior chamber. Severe glaucoma results. Occlusion of the pupil is an obstruction of the pupil by a pupillary membrane. The membrane results from organized connective tissue and usually is connected to the pupillary margin of the iris.

THE CHOROID

Congenital Anomalies of the Choroid

Coloboma of the Choroid. In this condition the pigment epithelium and choroid usually are absent from an area below the disc extending peripherally to the ora serrata. Through an ophthalmoscope the involved area appears as a large, sharply demarcated, oval lesion that is white in color as a result of its exposed sclera and surrounded by choroidal pigment. Some retinal vessels may cross the coloboma. The visual field will show a defect corresponding to the affected area. When colobomas occur at the macula, central vision is poor or absent. They are primarily of interest to the physician for differential diagnosis from conditions such as toxoplasmosis.

Vascular and Atrophic Disorders of the Choroid

Choroidal Hemorrhage. Localized choroidal hemorrhages usually occur as dark circular areas and are seen in a number of conditions (p. 246). Massive hemorrhage from the choroid is a rare complication of intraocular surgery. Sclerosis of the choroidal vessels due to aging results in a fundus picture in which the choroidal vessels are seen to be sheathed. This may vary from the presence of two parallel white borders outlining the blood column to the disappearance of the blood column completely (p. 283).

Primary choroidal sclerosis, an uncommon, degenerative condition possibly related to the tapetoretinal degenerations, is discussed in Medical Ophthalmology, Degenerative Diseases and Ocular Changes of Aging (p. 274).

Other Abnormalities of the Choroid

Detachment of the Choroid. This is usually a complication of intraocular surgery. Ophthalmoscopic examination or oblique illumination through a widely dilated pupil shows a smooth, round, dark gray–brown elevation. It is highly translucent with normally appearing retinal vessels passing over it. Choroidal detachment is most frequent in the lower temporal segment. It is associated with hypotony and usually resolves spontaneously without any residual abnormality.

Contusion Injury or Rupture of the Choroid. The characteristic picture of a choroidal rupture is a white, crescent-shaped lesion concentric with the disc and usually situated 3 or 4 mm. from it. These lesions may be single or multiple and are most commonly seen on the temporal side. The white color is due to exposed sclera.

Tumors of the Choroid

Nevi (benign melanomas), malignant melanomas, hemangiomas, and metastatic tumors of the choroid are discussed in the section on tumors (p. 263).

Vitreous Degeneration and Opacities

THE VITREOUS

CONGENITAL ANOMALIES

Persistence of the Primary Vitreous. This abnormality consists of a complete or partial persistence of the embryonic hyaloid vascular system (p. 127). A remnant of the lenticular portion of the hyaloid artery may be attached to the posterior lens, and may also persist as a small opacity slightly inferior to and nasal to the posterior pole of the lens *(Mittendorf dot)*. A hyaloid artery may remain in the vitreous as a threadlike structure and may even contain blood. The posterior portion of the hyaloid artery either may persist as a vascular loop extending into the vitreous, or may be occluded and surrounded by glial tissue on the disc *(Bergmeister's papilla)*. These changes generally cause no serious ocular problems.

Persistent Hyperplastic Primary Vitreous (PHPV). This abnormality develops from remnants of the fibrovascular tunic of the lens and part of the hyaloid vascular system. The anomaly is also referred to as persistent tunica vasculosa lentis and persistent fetal fibrovascular sheath of the lens (p. 127).

Inflammation and Infection of the Vitreous

The vitreous may be the site of both exogenous and endogenous infection. The causative agents may be bacteria, fungi, or parasites (p. 218). Pathologic reactions of the vitreous to infection are liquefaction, opacification, and shrinkage.

In severe and chronic inflammation, fibrin and inflammatory exudates may accumulate in the posterior chamber and anterior vitreous. This may subsequently organize into a connective tissue membrane *(cyclitic membrane)* in the anterior region of the vitreous cavity, most frequently across the vitreous face behind the lens. Contraction of the cyclitic membrane may result in detachment of the retina.

Vitreous Detachment. Detachment of the vitreous from the retina commonly occurs after middle life and may cause flashes of light and other annoying symptoms. More serious complications, such as retinal tears, may predispose to retinal detachment (p. 390).

Liquefaction and shrinkage are additional aging changes of the vitreous (p. 281), but these also may occur with injury, inflammation, or high myopia. *Asteroid hyalitis* is a condition in which spherical and stellate calcium-containing opacities are present in the vitreous. When illuminated by an examining light they appear to sparkle. Asteroid hyalitis is unilateral and does not give rise to symptoms (p. 281). In *synchysis scintillans* crystals composed of cholesterol develop as a degenerative change in the vitreous following inflammation and other ocular diseases (p. 281). The crystals are noted to settle to a dependent position when there is no movement of the globe. There is no effective treatment.

Vitreous Hemorrhage. Vitreous hemorrhage usually originates from the retinal blood vessels and may occur with diabetic retinopathy, with hypertensive retinopathy, with perivasculitis, with trauma, in subarachnoid hemorrhages, or as an initial sign of retinal hole formation. A sudden loss of vision in the affected eye usually is the chief symptom. The blood may appear in sheets or evenly distributed throughout the vitreous. On ophthalmoscopic examination fundus detail is obscured, and if the hemorrhage is severe even the red reflex may be absent. Absorption may be rapid or the hemorrhage may persist for many months. The final outcome is variable. In many instances vitreous hemorrhage recurs and eventually there is fibroblastic organization. Medication will not facilitate absorption of the vitreous hemorrhage.

OTHER VITREOUS OPACITIES

Inflammatory cells, epithelial cells from the ciliary body, pigment particles, tumor cells, mycotic "snowball" opacities, cysticercus, and echinococcus may all occur in the vitreous body.

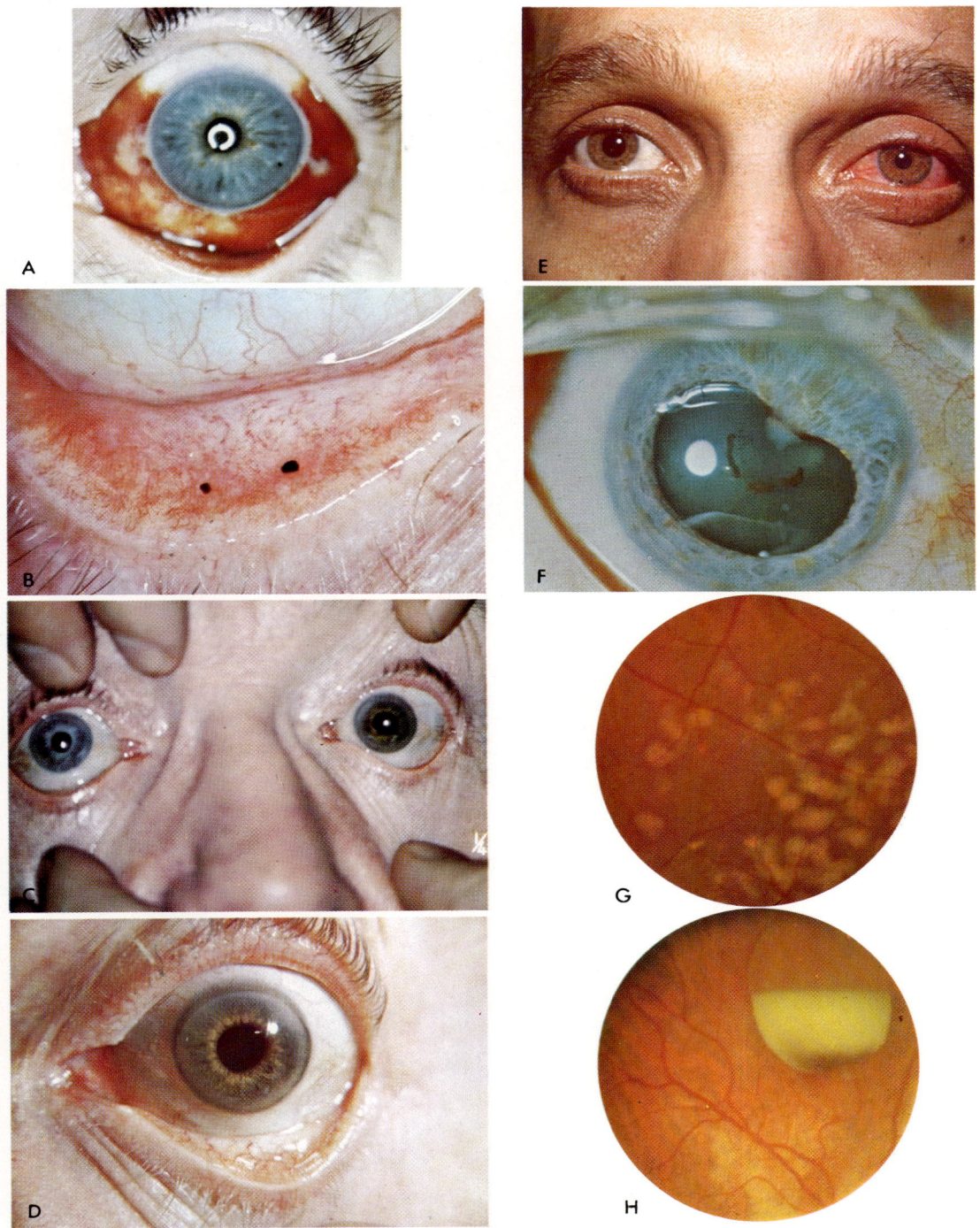

Plate 1 *(A)* Subconjunctival hemorrhage. *(B)* Conjunctival pigmentation resulting from long-term instillation of epinephrine drops. *(C)* Heterochromia irides. *(D)* Close-up of left eye of same patient as shown in 1*C*. *(E)* Acute iritis. *(F)* Posterior synechia resulting from iritis. *(G)* Giant drusen of the retina. *(H)* Retinal cyst.

THE LENS

Congenital Anomalies (Excluding Cataract)

Anomalies in the Formation of the Lens. Congenital absence of the lens (*primary aphakia*) has only rarely been reported. More commonly the lens is absent because of degeneration or absorption (*secondary aphakia* or *pseudoaphakia*). A small notch in the inferior nasal equator of the lens, a *coloboma*, occurs in association with a failure of the zonular fibers to develop in that sector. Incomplete separation of the lens vesicle from the surface ectoderm may result in a deep corneal opacity and an anterior polar cataract (*Peters' anomaly*).

Anomalies in the Size and Shape of the Lens

Abnormal development may result in a lens that is smaller than normal (*microphakia*) and also spherical (*spherophakia*). When the pupil is fully dilated, the edges of such a lens and its zonular fibers can be seen. In microphakia the lens may occlude the pupil and cause glaucoma. The spherical shape results in increased refractive power and myopia. This abnormality may be an isolated finding or may occur as part of an hereditary syndrome (Marchesani's syndrome) (p. 123). *Lenticonus* is a congenital abnormality in which there is a conical protrusion from the central portion of the anterior and posterior surface of the lens. On ophthalmoscopic examination this is seen as an "ora globule" or dark disc. Lenticonus appears to be a familial, usually bilateral, abnormality occurring predominantly in males.

Cataract

A cataract usually is defined as an opacification of the lens or its capsule. In this sense almost every adult has cataracts, for some fine lens opacities are frequently visible during slit lamp biomicroscope examination. Cataracts are not considered to be of serious clinical significance unless they interfere with vision.

Not all cataracts progress. Many opacities, particularly congenital ones, remain stationary. Most cataracts are bilateral, but the severity and rate of progression in each eye may vary.

Causes of Opacification of Lens Fibers. Cataracts develop through alteration of the physical and chemical states of the lens proteins. Denaturation of protein and imbibition of water may each play a role. It is known that in cataractous lenses sodium and calcium content are higher than normal; potassium, ascorbic acid, and protein content are lower than normal; and glutathione is absent.

A vast amount of experimental work has been done with animals on the production of cataracts, but the cause of senile cataracts in human beings is still unknown.

Symptoms of Cataracts. The only symptom of a cataract is impaired vision. A patient usually complains of things seeming misty. Cataracts, like glaucoma, may cause the patient to see halos around lights. He may notice some changes in color values, particularly a loss of blue and yellow; in some instances monocular diplopia may be present. Difficulty with night driving due to scattering of light from headlights is another common complaint. Early in development, opacities in the central portion of the lens will cut down acuity. A patient with this type of cataract will complain of poor vision in bright illumination (when the pupil is contracted), but he will report better vision in dim light. If the opacities are in the periphery of the lens, visual impairment occurs late in the course of the disease. This patient will often state that his vision is better in bright light than in dim light with the pupil dilated.

Age of Development. Congenital lens opacities are extremely common and may be mild or severe, and may or may not impair vision. They are usually bilateral. The commonest cause is heredity, but there are many others.

On slit lamp biomicroscope examination, congenital cataracts usually are seen as multiple, fine, irregularly shaped densities in the center level at the periphery of the lens. They may, however, involve all or only a tiny part of the lens. When total, they give the appearance of a white pupil. Causes and types are discussed in the chapter on pediatric ophthalmology (p. 126).

Cataracts may occur at any time after birth, but are a common ocular problem in elderly patients. Senile cataracts are discussed in Medical Ophthalmology (p. 282). Cataracts developing during infancy, childhood, and adolescence are relatively uncommon and may represent an inherited abnormality or may be a manifestation of a systemic disorder.

Secondary or After Cataract. In certain forms of cataract extraction, either planned or unplanned, the anterior capsule is opened and the cataractous lens is expressed. The lens capsule and epithelium remain inside the eye. The epithelial cells may proliferate and form grapelike clusters called *Elschnig bodies* and *Soemmering's spot.* If the capsular remains are dense and interfere with vision, or if the capsular epithelium proliferates, a secondary, or after cataract, forms. A second operation is necessary to cut through the membrane in order to allow a clear image to fall on the retina.

Complicated Cataract. This term describes lens opacification resulting from some intraocular disease process. Among the causes of complicated cataracts are diseases of the uveal tract, pigmentary retinal degeneration, absolute glaucoma, retinal detachment, and old injuries. The opacities usually occur at the posterior pole. After an attack of acute glaucoma, anterior subepithelial deposits (diffuse, small, and white) may develop (glaucomaflecken). Nuclear cataracts are common in patients with high myopia. Cataracts are an associated finding in certain systemic diseases, particularly those involving the skin.

Traumatic Cataracts. A cataract may result from blunt injury to the eye. Rosette-shaped opacities, located in the anterior or posterior subcapsular region, are characteristic of this type of cataract, although lamellar cataracts and diffuse punctate opacities may also occur. In addition, contusion of the eye may give rise to a ring of pigment granules deposited on the surface of the anterior lens capsule. This pigment possibly derives from the iris pigment epithelium *(Vossius' ring)*. Penetrating injuries of the eye with a rent in the lens capsule usually result in total opacification of the lens. Occasionally, however, only a small localized area may opacify at the site of a capsular injury.

Intraocular foreign bodies may cause cataracts in the absence of direct injury to the lens as they slowly oxidize within the eye. The products of oxidation slowly impregnate the ocular tissues including the lens. Iridocyclitis and loss of the eye may result. Should copper impregnate the lens, there appears in the subcapsular area a green-gray, almost metallic, disciform opacity, which often has serrated edges and radiating opacities *(sunflower cataract; chalcosis lentis)*. An iron foreign body will cause a characteristic rust brown or yellow opacity of the lens *(siderosis lentis)* together with the more widespread *siderosis bulbi* (p. 369).

Phacolytic glaucoma may occur with traumatic cataract and senile cataract. Perforation of the lens capsule may in addition result in the development of phacoanaphylaxis. Radiation (neutron, gamma, X, infrared, and microwave) and high voltage electricity may also cause cataracts.

Toxic Cataracts. Certain drugs are cataractogenic, such as ergot, dinitrophenol, naphthalene, phenothiazines, and triparanol (MER/29). Patients on long-term corticosteroid therapy are prone to develop posterior subcapsular cataracts.

Displacement of the Lens (Ectopia Lentis)

Subluxation of the lens denotes partial separation from the zonules. A luxated lens is completely separated from its zonular and vitreous attachments. Displacement of the lens may occur spontaneously at birth or traumatically. Marfan's syndrome (p. 222) accounts for 70 per cent of congenital ectopic lenses and homocystinuria (p. 218) for about 5 per cent of spontaneously displaced lenses. Spherophakia is an additional cause. Dislocation may occur from contusion of the globe. Most frequently a luxated lens is displaced into the vitreous. Iridodonesis, a tremulousness of the iris with movements of the eye, is an important sign of dislocation. Management is difficult. Cataract, iridocyclitis, and glaucoma may ensue, and lens extraction may become necessary.

Exfoliation and Pseudoexfoliation of the Lens Capsule

True exfoliation, which occurs in welders and glassblowers, is caused by infrared heat. A thickening and lamination of the anterior lamellae of the anterior lens capsule are seen clinically as a curling of the capsule, the free ends of which float in the anterior chamber. This is associated with a characteristic posterior cortical (glassblowers') cataract. In pseudoexfoliation particles of flaky, translucent material of unknown origin are found on the lens capsule, most markedly between the pupillary area and the equator, as well as on the zonules, ciliary body, and trabecular meshwork. This abnormality often is associated with excessive pigmentation of the anterior chamber angle. It has been frequently noted in patients with glaucoma.

THE RETINA

Congenital and Developmental Abnormalities

Myelinated (Medullated) Nerve Fibers. Myelination of the optic nerve fibers begins centrally at the lateral geniculate body during embryonic life and extends peripherally. By about the seventh month of fetal life it reaches the lamina cribrosa where the deposit of myelin usually stops, but occasionally it may extend beyond to the nerve fibers in the retina. Myelinated nerve fibers are seen in the fundus as white, glistening patches with characteristic feathered margins that cover and partly obscure the retinal vessels. Generally these patches extend to the retina from one or two quadrants of the optic disc. Sometimes they surround the entire disc, and

occasionally they may occur as isolated patches in the peripheral retina. Myelinated nerve fibers produce no symptoms and require no treatment. They can be confused with pathologic conditions such as chorioretinitis, exudate at the disc margin, optic neuritis, and edema of the optic nerve.

Grouped Pigmentation of the Retina. This is a nonprogressive, nonheritable condition in which clusters of pigmented spots either are present in a sector of the fundus or, as occurs less often, are scattered throughout it. These are sharply outlined lesions ranging from gray to black. They tend to be paired and "bean shaped." They have also been compared to "bear tracks." They result from proliferation of the cells of the pigment epithelium.

Congenital Retinal Fold (Falciform Fold). In this rare anomaly a gray or white ridge of elevated retina extends from the disc toward the periphery of the fundus, displacing the macula. Usually a persistent hyaloid artery or some of its branches are also present. In some instances congenital retinal folds may be an aborted form of retrolental fibroplasia (see below). The eye usually is myopic (p. 136).

Retrolental Fibroplasia (Retinopathy of Prematurity). This is an oxygen-induced retinopathy in premature infants who weigh less than four pounds. The disease is primarily the response of an immature retinal vascular system to a high concentration of oxygen. The eyes appear normal at birth, but swelling and necrosis of the capillary endothelium, with subsequent occlusion of the vessels, occur. The earliest clinical changes are dilatation and tortuosity of the retinal vessels at about one month. The retinal veins may enlarge to three or four times their normal diameter, and the arterioles may bend sharply. Displacement of the retinal vessels may occur with temporal migration of the macula. Generalized retinal edema and neovascularization commence in the peripheral retina. New vessels and connective tissue may proliferate into the vitreous and detach the retina.

Ultimately the retina is converted into a fibrous mass which can be seen as a dense membrane behind the lens. At this stage of the disease a white pupil will be present. The growth of the eye usually is arrested, and microphthalmos may result. The anterior chambers are extremely shallow and secondary glaucoma may be present. The course of the disease may become arrested early, but 20 per cent of afflicted eyes go on to the last stage, resulting in blindness. It is bilateral and usually symmetrical. Retrolental fibroplasia has, to a great extent, been eliminated by careful regulation of oxygen therapy (p. 148).

Pseudoglioma, a general term that is sometimes applied to conditions other than retinoblastoma, also gives rise to a white pupil (p. 152).

Ocular Findings Related to Hematologic Abnormalities

Diseases of the blood may be associated with alteration in the color of the fundus, changes in the appearance of the retinal and choroidal vessels, the presence of hemorrhages and exudates, and retinal edema. With certain changes in the viscosity and composition of the blood, sludging and segmentation ("boxcarring") of the blood column in the retinal vessels may be seen. This sign indicates a slow circulation of the red blood cells.

The characteristic changes associated with specific diseases of the blood are discussed elsewhere in this book (p. 233) and include anemias, sickle cell and related retinopathies, hemorrhagic disorders, polycythemia, leukemias, multiple myeloma, and macroglobulinemia and cryoglobulinemia.

Lipemia retinalis is an unusual condition in which the blood vessels of the retina appear cream-colored or yellow-white because of an elevated blood lipid level. This complication may accompany diabetes mellitus, essential hyperlipemia, secondary hyperlipemia from such causes as lipoid nephrosis, pancreatitis, and von Gierke's disease.

Changes in the Retinal Vessels

Arterioles. Narrowing of the retinal arterioles and constrictions and variations in caliber occur in hypertension. In diseases in which the retina has degenerated, such as end-stage glaucoma, optic atrophy, and pigmentary degeneration of the retina, the vessels narrow as a result of regenerative intimal thickening. Changes in the wall in arteriolar sclerosis result in broadening of the light reflex, changes in the color of the vessels, and tortuosity of the arterioles, particularly in the macular region. Profound tortuosity of the retinal arterioles is associated with coarctation of the aorta. *Sheathing*, a white cuff surrounding the blood column, may occur in arteriolar sclerosis, especially after obstruction of the vessel. It is seen also in inflammatory conditions, resulting from perivascular collections of white blood cells. Ocular changes due to hypertension (p. 240), arteriolar sclerosis (p. 240), and diabetes (p. 255) are discussed in detail elsewhere in the book.

Occlusion of the Retinal Arteries. This may be caused by emboli, spasm, or thrombosis. Occlusion of the retinal arteries may result from a number of underlying causes, the most common of which is atherosclerosis. The causes and clinical features are discussed in Medical Ophthalmology, Cardiovascular Diseases (p. 250).

Retinal Veins

Dilatation of Retinal Veins. Pathologic changes in retinal arterioles usually result in constriction, but in the veins the result is dilatation. Such enlargements are sometimes associated with aneurysms or varicosities. They may also occur in diabetic retinopathy (p. 256) and blood dyscrasias (e.g., anemia, polycythemia, and leukemia), or when there is stasis of the venous circulation (such as in cardiac insufficiency), or with increased intraocular pressure.

Tortuosity of Retinal Veins. An abnormal degree of tortuosity of the retinal veins is sometimes seen as a congenital anomaly, as in hereditary hemorrhagic telangiectasis. In papilledema it is noted in the vessels on or near the disc.

Sheathing of the veins occurs as a result of inflammation (phlebitis). Prominent causes are syphilis (both congenital and acquired), endophthalmitis, Behçet's disease (p. 18), and Eales' disease (p. 190). Sheathing may also result from degenerative or sclerotic changes of the wall of the vein, such as those seen following venous occlusion, and from diabetic retinopathy. In leukemia sheathing is due to infiltration of the vein wall by leukemic cells. In patients with retinitis pigmentosa (p. 130), pigment sheathing results from pigment infiltration of the vessel walls.

Occlusion of Retinal Veins. This disorder is caused by a number of conditions and results in reduction of vision and widespread retinal hemorrhage (p. 246).

Changes in the Arteriovenous Crossings

The retinal arterioles and venules share a common sheath at arteriovenous crossings. Many abnormal changes in the crossings have been described in arteriolar sclerosis. These include tapering of the vein, banking of the vein (Gunn's sign), and deflection of the vein (Salus' sign).

Retinal Hemorrhages

Most retinal hemorrhages arise from capillaries. The etiology may be trauma, obstruction, inflammation, acute febrile diseases, vascular retinopathies, senile atherosclerosis, hematopoietic diseases, and many other conditions. Some hemorrhages may originate in arterioles. These may be associated with atheromatous degeneration, septicemia, venous obstruction, and phlebitis. Often no explanation is found.

Location and Appearance of Retinal Hemorrhages. The physical appearance of retinal hemorrhages depends upon their location. Preretinal hemorrhages (subhyaloid hemorrhages) lie in front of the retina between the internal limiting membrane and the hyaloid membrane. Characteristically these hemorrhages are keel-shaped, with a straight upper border and a hemispherical lower margin. There are several types within the retina itself. Flame-shaped hemorrhages occur in the nerve fiber layer and follow the striated pattern of the nerve fiber bundles. Small hemorrhages in the deep layers of the retina appear as isolated, round spots. On histologic examination, these are commonly found in the outer molecular layer. Round or flame-shaped hemorrhages having a pale center are seen, particularly in subacute bacterial endocarditis, septic retinitis, anemia, and blood dyscrasias. The white centers may signify white blood cells or amorphous deposits.

Microaneurysms are small, round, red spots closely resembling deep hemorrhages. Most are too small to be seen with the ophthalmoscope. Frequently, however, groups of these tiny punctate dots, arranged in the form of grape clusters, are found at the ends of the small vascular twigs. In patients with diabetes these are characteristically located at the venous end of the capillary in the macular area (p. 256). Occasionally they accompany hypertension, phlebitis, and venous stasis, but in these and similar conditions the microaneurysms usually are situated in the periphery of the fundus.

Subretinal hemorrhages lie between the pigment epithelium and Bruch's membrane, and appear as dark, slate-colored areas.

Neovascularization. In certain pathological conditions, particularly when the normal blood supply has been compromised, many "newly formed" vessels appear. These occur most commonly within the retina or on its anterior surface; they may also occur beneath the retina, as chorioretinal anastomotic vessels, and on the optic disc. When present on the surface of the retina they may form a dense, web-like network *(rete mirabile)*. This network probably represents dilatation and proliferation of preexisting vessels. Neovascularization often extends into the vitreous and is followed by the formation of a fibrous tissue membrane *(retinitis proliferans)*, as occurs in the end stages of diabetic retinopathy. In another type the connective tissue membrane extending into the vitreous either is not vascularized or becomes vascularized later (e.g., Eales' disease or periphlebitis retinae). Retinitis proliferans is frequently the sequela of massive retinal hemorrhage. The prognosis is poor. Other diseases in which the retinal vessels proliferate abnormally are angiomatosis retinae (von Hippel-Lindau disease) (p. 179), retrolental fibroplasia (p. 148), aortic arch syndrome, Coats' disease (p. 154), and disorders giving rise to vitreous hemorrhage.

Inflammation of the Retinal Vessels (Vasculitis Retinae)

Eales' disease is a syndrome of recurrent hemorrhages into the retina and vitreous, affecting mainly males in the second and third decades of life. These patients usually show no evidence of systemic disease. Ophthalmoscopic findings are sheathing of the retinal veins with scattered hemorrhages and sometimes exudate, new vessel formation, and capillary aneurysms. The patient complains of recurrent attacks of decreased vision caused by vitreous hemorrhage. These hemorrhages may resorb at first, but eventually retinitis proliferans, chronic uveitis, and secondary glaucoma may result in permanent loss of vision. In about 50 per cent of patients, both eyes are affected. Surface diathermy or photocoagulation of affected vessels retards regression, but in general treatment is ineffective.

Similar changes to those described for Eales' disease have been noted in sickle cell disease (p. 234), tuberculosis (p. 190), and foci of infection.

Deposits and Exudates

In the early years of the ophthalmoscope, lesions that were lighter in color than the normal fundus were thought to be products of inflammation and were called "exudates." This term has persisted and is presently used to describe lesions varying from barely visible dots to abnormalities occupying a large portion of the fundus. *Cotton-wool exudates* are soft-edged, white or gray opacities that are round or oval and usually less than one disc diameter in size. Histologically they are composed of globular structures called *cytoid bodies*, which resemble cell nuclei in size and shape, and stain with eosin. These lesions are probably microinfarcts in the nerve fiber layer of the retina. Cotton-wool exudates are most often seen in hypertensive retinopathy, but they may also occur in lupus erythematosus, dermatomyositis, anemia, diabetes, bacterial endocarditis, occlusion of the central retinal vein, and papilledema.

In a number of pathologic conditions, transudate or exudate may leak from retinal vessels. This forms discrete, white to yellow, isolated or clustered, lesions. The final deposit may be hyaline, amyloidal, colloidal, fatty, lipoidal, or even calcareous, depending on the nature of the exudate, as well as on the secondary changes that it undergoes. In diabetic retinopathy, exudates rich in lipids and mucopolysaccharides seep out to the external plexiform layer. This forms characteristic yellow, waxy, hyaline lesions. Necrosis of retinal tissue with accumulation of masses of fat-laden cells and other secondary changes may produce white or gray patches of exudate. Areas of cellular infiltration in leukemia, neoplasms, syphilis, tuberculosis, and sarcoidosis may give an ophthalmic picture of opacities in the retina. Glial proliferation occurring after injury, inflammation, and degenerative processes may appear clinically as a white or gray veil that can resemble exudates.

Some exudates have a characteristic shape. In *circinate retinitis* they are seen as a wreath, usually around the fovea. Exudates may radiate from the macular area in all directions forming a "macular star," such as is seen in severe hypertensive retinopathy, intracranial disease, and thrombosis of the vein.

Drusen (colloid or hyaline bodies) usually are small, round, yellow spots but may be quite large (Plate 1G). They usually occur in the macular area of elderly patients. They are a benign, degenerative change. Histologically they are seen as homogeneous or hyaline outgrowths of Bruch's membrane. *Gunn's dots* are fine, round, metallic-appearing spots in the disc and macula. They probably represent a reflex from the surface of the retina and should not be confused with punctate exudates.

Edema of the Retina

In generalized retinal edema, which is observed in severe hypertensive retinopathy, one sees an increased luster of the retinal reflexes and an accentuation of the nerve fiber pattern. The retina usually looks thicker and more opaque than normal. When the edema is marked, retinal folds concentric with the disc, and also folds radiating from the macula, develop. Except for the macula, which appears as a cherry red spot, the retina may be white.

Commotio retinae (Berlin's edema) is a condition in which a milky white area of edema appears in the retina within 24 hours following traumatic injury to the globe, usually by a blunt object (p. 377). The posterior retina is most often involved, with the macula standing out as a red spot. The ophthalmoscopic picture is somewhat similar to that of retinal artery occlusion. The central vision is considerably reduced. Edema usually clears within a few days, and vision returns to normal. In other types of posttraumatic or postconcussive edema of the macula, a cyst or hole may form, causing loss of central vision.

Inflammatory and Infectious Diseases of the Retina

Inflammations of the retina may occur as a primary disease, as part of a systemic disorder, and as an extension of disease in neighboring tissues. Retinal changes may be local or widespread. Inflammation may result in dilatation of retinal vessels, accumulation of leukocytes in the perivascular spaces (sheathing), hemorrhage, edema, degeneration of retinal elements, and migration and proliferation of glial tissue and new blood vessels. Inflammations affecting the retina or choroid usually involve both structures simultaneously.

Retinitis Associated with Infection. Septic retinitis occurs when circulating organisms reach the retina through the bloodstream. In the most virulent infections inflammation can progress to an endophthalmitis or panophthalmitis, resulting in a blind, shrunken eye. Infective material may settle at a single point leading to a local massive lesion. Most often in embolic retinitis, however, the changes consist of cotton-wool exudates, retinal hemorrhages, some with white centers *(Roth's spots)*, vascular sheath-

ing, and retinal edema. Often this picture is seen in patients with subacute bacterial endocarditis. Antibiotics have lowered the incidence of this type of retinitis. Virus infections, such as cytomegalic inclusion disease and nematode infections, may affect the retina primarily. In toxoplasmosis there is also primary retinal involvement with subsequent choroidal changes (p. 200). The retina may be a primary site of granulomatous inflammation in syphilis (p. 193), tuberculosis (p. 190), and sarcoidosis (p. 232). The retina is affected in *collagen diseases,* particularly disseminated lupus erythematosus (p. 226) and periarteritis nodosa (p. 228).

Coats' disease is an ambiguous term that probably includes a number of conditions characterized by massive exudation between the retina and the choroid. Generally Coats' disease applies to a chronic, progressive, exudative retinopathy occurring in male children and young adults. It is usually unilateral, the principal symptom being a sudden onset of blurred vision. Ophthalmoscopic examination reveals yellow-white exudate beneath the retina. Eventually this may appear as large, elevated masses. In addition, retinal vessels are tortuous and dilated; microaneurysms, neovascularization, and subretinal hemorrhages are frequent. Its progressive course usually leads to retinal detachment, iritis, glaucoma, and cataract. Photocoagulation and surface diathermy, although used to treat Coats' disease, appear to be of limited effect.

Familial Lipoid Degeneration

Amaurotic Familial Idiocy. This group of diseases has in common a lipoid degeneration of cells in the central nervous system and retina with the formation of large numbers of vacuolated "foam" cells. The group is divided according to age of onset (p. 134).

Tay-Sachs disease is largely confined to Jewish infants. The fundus picture is characteristic: the central retina is opaque white from lipid-filled ganglion cells. The fovea is seen as a cherry red spot due to the absence of ganglion cells, and hence, absence of opacification. The optic nerve usually is pale. As the disease progresses, a flaccid paralysis of all the limbs develops. There is no effective treatment, and death almost always occurs before the third year.

A late infantile form of amaurotic familial idiocy that affects non-Jewish children between the second and fourth years of life has also been described. The ophthalmoscopic picture is not as marked as in Tay-Sachs disease. Frequently the cherry red spot is not seen in the macular area, but pigmentary changes occur instead. The prognosis is equally poor, and these children generally die in one to two years after the onset of symptoms.

Juvenile amaurotic familial idiocy makes its appearance in children between 5 and 10 years of age. The first clinical symptoms are those of mental retardation and visual disturbance. Ophthalmoscopic examination reveals abnormal pigmentation of the macula, consisting of fine peppering of the retina with pigment ("salt and pepper" pigmentation). Loss of the foveal reflex, pallor of the optic disc, and narrowing of vessels may also be seen, but a cherry red spot does not develop. Death usually occurs in adolescence.

It appears that amaurotic familial idiocy is a heredofamilial degeneration and not a systemic lipoidosis. A fundus picture identical with that seen in Tay-Sachs disease may occur in *Niemann-Pick disease*, a generalized, systemic, lipoid histiocytosis (p. 135).

Retinitis Pigmentosa and Allied Diseases (Tapetoretinal Degeneration)

This category includes a group of degenerative diseases of the retina and choroid. The rod and cone layer of the retina is principally affected, usually with a marked disturbance of the pigment epithelium (tapetum). Night blindness (nyctalopia) is a principal symptom, and electroretinographic examination shows early abnormality. These diseases are, for the most part, inherited. They include:

1. Retinitis pigmentosa (pigmentary degeneration of the retina (p. 130).
2. Fundus albipunctatus (p. 132).
3. Fundus flavimaculatus (p. 132).
4. Oguchi's disease (p. 130).
5. Choroideremia (p. 129).

6. Gyrate atrophy of the choroid and retina (p. 129).

Retinitis Pigmentosa. This group of primary degenerations of the rod and cone layer is the most common of the tapetoretinal degenerations. The classic ophthalmoscopic findings are spider-shaped clumps of pigment, appearing first in the midperiphery, and distributed particularly around and over vessels; severe attenuation of the retinal vessels; and pallor of the optic disc. The associated findings and course of the disease are more completely discussed in Pediatric Ophthalmology.

A number of variants of retinitis pigmentosa have been described. In the macular type, or *inverse retinitis pigmentosa*, the disturbance is limited to, or most marked at, the macula. In *retinitis pigmentosa sine pigmento* little or no pigment occurs in the peripheral fundus in spite of the occurrence of other features. Atypical forms are common when the disease is associated with other systemic defects.

Secondary Retinitis Pigmentosa, or Pseudoretinitis Pigmentosa. In secondary syphilis (p. 193), in rubella retinitis, and following measles and vaccination, pigmentary degeneration occurs and may closely resemble that seen in retinitis pigmentosa. Electroretinography is useful in the differential diagnosis.

Macular Degeneration

Heredomacular degeneration refers to a group of diseases that shows a strong familial incidence but usually appears to be recessive in inheritance (p. 132). The principal symptom is loss of central vision, sometimes termed daylight blindness (hemeralopia) to distinguish it from the night blindness of retinitis pigmentosa. Macular lesions vary from bilateral cysts having a "fried egg" appearance (*vitelliform macular degeneration*) to massive drusen bodies or pigmentary mottling about the macula. The lesion may change with age and vary within the same family. The time of onset may be used to describe the types of disease:

congenital, or occurring during the first few years in life (Best's disease); infantile, between 6 and 8 years of age; juvenile, about the time of puberty; and adult, presenile and senile. Macular changes occurring in late infantile or juvenile amaurotic family idiocy and the macular type of retinitis pigmentosa are considered by some authors to be types of heredomacular degeneration.

Senile macular degeneration is an acquired degenerative process that frequently causes loss of vision in the elderly. It frequently begins as a subtle disturbance of pigmentation in the macular area with loss of the normal foveal reflex. Later, gross clumps of pigment and drusen may be seen.

Cystic degeneration of the macula, characterized by the formation of a sharply outlined, round, red, cystic defect in the macula, may also occur as an aging change, or as the result of edema or inflammation, myopic degeneration or vascular disease.

Disciform macular degeneration (Kuhnt-Junius disease) begins as a dark, round, raised extravasation in or near the macular area, and usually in persons over 40 years of age. The final result appears ophthalmoscopically as a model dome-shaped elevation.

Circinate retinopathy is characterized by yellow exudates in a circular or horseshoe pattern around the macula. This disorder may occur in middle age or later without any apparent cause, or may develop secondary to diabetic retinopathy, chronic, recurrent central serous retinopathy, and other disorders.

No effective treatment for these disorders is presently available and the end result usually is a dense, central scotoma. These types of adult and senile macular degenerations are discussed in greater detail in Medical Ophthalmology (p. 284).

Degeneration of the macula may accompany changes in Bruch's membrane (see angioid streaks, colloid bodies, and Doyne's honeycomb choroiditis. The latter, a bilateral, familial disease, develops in its early stages discrete yellow or white deposits around the macula. Later the spots

coalesce and hemorrhages appear. Other causes of macular degeneration are inflammation of the choroid or retina, venous and arterial occlusion, trauma, exposure to excessive radiant energy (e.g., eclipse burns), and myopia.

Other Degenerative Retinal Conditions

Angioid streaks denote red to black irregular bands running outward from the region of the disc. They occur bilaterally. These streaks may resemble retinal vessels in their appearance and course. The lesions probably represent ruptures in Bruch's membrane. Associated ocular lesions, not the streaks themselves, cause visual loss in about one third to one half of affected patients. These abnormalities are pigmentary disturbances of the macula, hemorrhages and exudates, atrophy of the choroid, and proliferation of pigment and connective tissue. Angioid streaks occasionally are found in several members of the same family. Streaks may be associated with pseudoxanthoma elasticum, Paget's disease of the bone (osteitis deformans), less commonly with occlusive arterial disease in the extremities, and sickle cell disease.

Central serous retinopathy (central angiospastic retinopathy; central serous chorioretinitis) is a well recognized clinical syndrome that is more common in men than in women. It usually occurs between the ages of 30 and 50 years. The ophthalmoscopic finding is a distinct, round or oval, slightly raised area of the retina in the macular region. The elevation is dark red and surrounded by a ring-shaped light reflex. The foveal reflex is decreased or absent, and frequently a number of small white dots are present in the involved area. Symptoms include blurred vision, which is usually associated with a distortion of viewed objects (metamorphopsia), and a central scotoma. With fluorescein fundus examination, dye leaks from the choriocapillaris and pools beneath the pigment epithelium. The disease is often self-limited; the lesion usually resolves and vision returns to normal within three to six weeks. Recurrences, however, are common, and pigment changes in the macular region or chronic edema may result. In some cases the final picture is circinate retinopathy or disciform degeneration of the macula. Emotional factors sometimes play a role. Among treatments advocated have been vasodilators such as nicotinic acid, sedatives, vitamins, antihistamines, and corticosteroids. Avoiding stress, exposure to cold, and tobacco also have been suggested, but the effectiveness of these measures is questionable.

Serous detachment of the retina in the macular region, with a clinical picture similar to that just described, can occur as a secondary process. It may be associated with trauma, uveitis, optic neuritis, papilledema, ocular hypotony, systemic hypertension, vitreous traction, a macular hole, and an optic pit.

Retinoschisis and retinal cysts (Plate 1*H*) result from the sensory retina splitting into two layers. This is discussed in Medical Ophthalmology (p. 286), as are also lattice degeneration and peripheral cystoid degeneration.

Retinal Detachment

In retinal detachment (retinal separation) the neural layer of the retina detaches from the pigment epithelium layer which is left attached to Bruch's membrane of the choroid. Normally the neural retina is attached firmly to the underlying layer only at the ora serrata and the rim of the optic nerve. The retina is kept in position by capillary attraction and by the intra-ocular pressure, which is distributed uniformly through the vitreous body. A potential space that once formed the primary optic vesicle is present between the neural retina and the pigment epithelium layer. Accumulation of fluid exudate or other material within this potential space results in a retinal detachment.

Types of Retinal Detachments. In most detachments the retina is separated by serous fluid that contains considerably more protein than the vitreous and is derived from the blood. These are termed *serous detachments*, and usually occur secondary to some local ocular abnormality that predisposes to hole formation in the retina. Few can be termed "idiopathic" or "primary." The pathogenesis and signs and symptoms of serous detachments are dis-

cussed in Medical Ophthalmology (p. 287).

Conditions in which retinal detachments may be a prominent feature, and in which there are no holes or breaks in the retina, are:
1. Inflammation of the choroid and retina
   a. Vogt-Koyanagi syndrome (uveitis, alopecia, poliosis, vitiligo, and deafness)
   b. Harada's disease (bilateral diffuse exudative choroiditis occurring with headache, vomiting, and an increase of lymphocytes in the cerebral spinal fluid)
   c. Vasculitis of the retina, including Eales' disease
2. Disturbances in retinal and choroidal circulation
   a. Retinal vein occlusion
   b. Papilledema (peripapillary detachment of retina may occur)
   c. Serous detachment of choroid
   d. Primary or metastatic neoplasm of the choroid (retinal detachment of the ordinary serous type may occur, in addition to elevation from the tumor)
3. Detachment associated with the retinopathy of systemic diseases
   a. Severe hypertension (particularly with the hypertensive toxemia of pregnancy)
   b. Chronic glomerulonephritis
   c. Periarteritis nodosa
   d. Angiomatosis retinae (von Hippel-Lindau disease)

When retinal detachment occurs in the absence of holes or breaks, spontaneous reattachment usually occurs following improvement of the underlying conditions, and surgery is contraindicated. *Treatment* of retinal detachments is discussed in the chapter on ocular surgery (p. 390). If a detachment secondary to a retinal break is untreated, the entire retina usually becomes involved over a period of weeks or months, resulting in a blind eye.

Other Disorders of the Retina

Tumors of the retina (see neoplasms of the pigment epithelium, retinoblastoma, astrocytoma, glioneuroma, metastasis, and pseudoglioma) are discussed in the section on ocular tumors (p. 263). The phakomatoses (tuberous sclerosis, neurofibromatosis, Sturge-Weber disease, and retinal angiomatosis) are covered in the chapter on pediatric ophthalmology (p. 105). Color blindness is included in the appendix section on the physiology of the eye.

THE OPTIC NERVE

Congenital Malformations and Anatomic Variations

Aplasia and Hypoplasia. Complete failure of the optic nerve to develop (aplasia) is extremely rare (p. 128, Pediatric Ophthalmology), although a partial deficiency in growth (hypoplasia) may occur as a hereditary defect, or as a sporadic developmental abnormality. This may range from a slight reduction in size to an almost total absence of the nerve, and correspondingly, vision may be reduced or completely absent.

Colobomas. Defects in the optic nerve can result from incomplete closure of the fetal cleft. Located in the lower portion of the disc, they may be associated with defects in the retina and choroid. Vision usually is impaired.

Pits of the Optic Disc. "Pits" are discrete, isolated holes, usually located on the temporal edge of the disc. Mostly congenital and stationary, they probably represent atypical coloboma. When the pits interrupt the macular fibers passing through this area, acute arcuate scotoma results. They also reportedly occur in association with central serous retinopathy. Generally, however, they are of no clinical significance.

Drusen of the Optic Disc. Drusen (hyaline bodies) of the nerve head can be considered a variant from the normal, and are seen with the ophthalmoscope as translucent, waxy irregularities on the surface of the disc. They may be single or multiple and often are bilateral (p. 299).

Congenital and Myopic Crescents (Conus). The ophthalmoscopic appearance of the optic nerve border is determined by the relative distance from the disc margin to the terminal points of the pigment epithelium, Bruch's membrane, and the choroid. Most often the choroid and retina terminate adjacent to the optic disc margin. Occasionally these tissues are absent along the temporal side, and a white crescent of sclera is seen adjacent to the disc. A similar crescent may be seen in myopia, possibly due to chorioretinal atrophy or traction of the retina on the nasal side. Occasionally the optic nerve enters obliquely through the sclera, whereas the retina and choroid terminate at varying distances below the optic disc, giving rise to an inferior conus. This latter condition often is associated with hyperopic astigmatism. In some patients the pigment epithelium increases in thickness at its terminal point, resulting in a pigment ring surrounding the disc.

Optic Atrophy

Symptoms of atrophy of the optic nerve fibers are pallor of the nerve heads, as seen ophthalmoscopically, loss of visual acuity, and changes of the visual fields. Pallor of the disc results from two factors: a loss of the smaller blood vessels of the disc, and a deposit of fibrous or glial tissue. Some ophthalmologists use a decrease in the number of arterioles crossing the disc margin (Kestenbaum's sign) as a criterion for optic neuritis. Usually about ten such arterioles are seen; the presence of only six or seven indicates optic atrophy.

Primary optic atrophy refers to an ophthalmoscopic picture of a pale, white nerve head with well-defined borders. The physiologic cup and the lamina cribrosa are visible, and the arteries either show little change or are constricted. This indicates that little edema or inflammation preceded atrophy. Primary atrophy is typical in tabes or taboparesis. *Secondary optic atrophy* denotes a pale disc with blurred edges, and the physiologic cup frequently is filled in with gray tissue. This type of atrophy results from previous inflammation or edema of the nerve head. Although the terms primary and secondary optic atrophy are used frequently, they have no etiologic significance.

Lesions of the retina that cause degeneration of the ganglion cells and nerve fiber layers may produce an *ascending* or *consecutive optic atrophy*. When limited to the papillomacular bundle, these lesions result in a pallor confined to a wedge-shaped area of the disc on the temporal side (*papillomacular atrophy*). *Descending optic atrophy* results from lesions or injuries located in the intraorbital, intracanalicular, and intracranial portions of the nerve. Causes of the optic atrophy are discussed in Neuro-ophthalmology (p. 310).

Papilledema (Choked Disc)

Papilledema, a noninflammatory swelling of the nerve head, is seen clinically as an abnormal elevation of the disc and an obliteration of its margins. This abnormality is most often caused by increased intracranial pressure. In its early stages papilledema is seen ophthalmoscopically as a blurring of the disc margin. The upper and lower borders of the disc on the nasal side change earliest; the temporal margin is less involved. Although edema usually covers the physiologic cup, in some instances the cup may be retained. The disc surface becomes elevated above the rest of the fundus. By moving the ophthalmoscope from side to side, one may elicit parallax between the top of the disc and the retina beneath. The amount of papilledema may be measured with the ophthalmoscope.

Edema extends into the retina adjacent to the disc, and concentric folds are frequently seen. Retinal edema may occur in the macular region. White exudates, which in late stages form a star-shaped figure, may be seen. Vascular changes are prominent in papilledema, particularly when the onset is acute. Venous pulsations, which under normal conditions are frequently seen in the vessels emerging from the disc, can be elicited only by pressure on the globe. The veins are overfull; the capillaries are engorged and appear as red streaks in the edematous retina. When the disc is elevated, the vessels are seen to bend sharply at its borders. Numerous flame-shaped and globular hemorrhages may be seen on and about the disc. They may even extend into the overlying vitreous. The papilledema of advanced hypertension sometimes may be indistinguishable from that of other causes. The more extensive distribution of hemorrhages in hypertension and the appearance of the peripheral arterioles, however, may help in the differentiation.

Papilledema is usually bilateral. A notable exception is papilledema in patients with meningiomas of the sphenoid ridge (*Foster Kennedy syndrome*) (p. 320), in which there is primary optic atrophy on the side of the tumor and papilledema in the other eye.

Since papilledema results from passive edema and not from inflammation, usually only minor visual disturbance occurs in the early stages. Massive or prolonged edema may damage the nerve fibers at the disc, with serious visual loss or complete blindness. The causes, pathogenesis, differential diagnosis, and management of papilledema are discussed in Neuro-ophthalmology (pp. 300 to 304).

Optic Neuritis

Optic neuritis is a general term applied to inflammatory and demyelinative diseases of the optic nerve. That type of optic neuritis in which changes can be seen ophthalmoscopically on the nerve head or optic disc is called *papillitis*. When the surrounding retina is inflamed, the condition is sometimes called *neuroretinitis*. When the nerve is affected behind its entrance into the globe, and when the ophthalmoscopic picture of the disc is entirely normal, it is called *retrobulbar neuritis*.

Although numerous and diverse diseases can cause optic neuritis, multiple sclerosis is probably the most frequent cause. Opticomyelitis, or Devic's disease, is a well defined entity in which there is a bilateral optic neuritis and symptoms of transverse myelitis. Diffuse sclerosis, including Schilder's disease and the leukodystrophies, may affect the optic nerve. Optic neuritis may result from vasculitis, inflammatory processes, metabolic diseases, and intoxication.

Clinical Features of Optic Neuritis. Characteristically, there is a sudden onset of poor vision. Other prominent symptoms are pain when the eye moves, and tenderness when pressure is applied to the globe.

A central scotoma usually forms as a result of the involvement of the papillomacular bundle; in some instances total blindness ensues.

If the part of the optic nerve lying within the globe becomes inflamed (papillitis), the ophthalmoscopic picture closely resembles that of papilledema. The disc is hyperemic, the margins are blurred, and all the vessels are dilated. Unlike papilledema, however, disc elevation rarely exceeds two diopters. The physiologic cup is obliterated, and fine, diffuse opacities frequently appear in the overlying vitreous. There may be edema of the retina (neuroretinitis), particularly in the macular region. Exudates and hemorrhages may be scattered around the retina, and a "star figure" may be present in the macula. If the papillitis is mild and of short duration, recovery may be complete. It is common, however, for a secondary optic atrophy to occur. Causes, differential diagnosis, and treatment of optic neuritis are considered in Neuro-ophthalmology (p. 300).

Toxic Amblyopias

The toxic amblyopias are a group of diseases in which ingested toxic agents damage the retinal or optic nerve, producing a visual defect. Such poisons as methyl alcohol produce a picture of optic neuritis; other substances, such as quinine and organic arsenicals, cause damage to the ganglion cells of the retina with secondary optic atrophy. The toxic amblyopias are usually divided into two groups: those causing central scotomas, and those with peripheral visual field loss.

Tobacco or tobacco and alcohol are the most common causes of toxic amblyopia. The patient usually gives a history of excessive smoking and drinking. He complains that his vision has gradually become misty and that he is unable to read or to do close work. Nearly all cases are bilateral, although one eye usually is affected more severely. A diagnosis can be made from a characteristic change in the visual fields, which consists of an egg-shaped scotoma involving an area from fixation over to and including the blind spot (cecocentral scotoma). The scotoma is present to both white and colored test objects, but is disproportionately greater for red and green. The fundus is usually normal at first. If the patient discontinues tobacco and alcohol, his vision improves, but only after considerable time. Late in the disease, especially in patients who persist in using tobacco and alcohol, one sees atrophy of the portion of the optic nerve corresponding to the central fibers (papillomacular atrophy). Considerable evidence suggests that associated vitamin B_{12} deficiency, other dietary deficiencies, and hepatic disease may all play roles in this disease.

In the majority of persons who survive ingestion of methyl alcohol, or wood alcohol, the result is optic atrophy and permanent blindness. The ocular manifestations of lead poisoning are varied. Some patients develop sudden loss of sight in both eyes without changes in the fundus. In others, however, a papillitis develops, followed by atrophy. Tumors of the optic nerve (melanocytoma, glioma, meningioma, and metastatic carcinoma) are discussed in Neuro-ophthalmology (p. 317).

GLAUCOMA

In glaucoma the intraocular pressure is elevated. The disease is characterized by pathologic changes in the optic disc and typical defects in the field of vision. Glaucoma is discussed further in Chapter 8. Certain ophthalmic entities included in that chapter are briefly defined below.

Primary Glaucoma

This is a type of glaucoma unrelated to other ocular disease. It may occur at any time of life and can be conveniently divided into glaucoma in the adult and congenital glaucoma.

On the basis of gonioscopic and tonographic studies of aqueous outflow, two clinical types of primary glaucoma may occur in the adult: *chronic simple* (open wide angle) *glaucoma,* and *narrow angle (angle closure, iris block, acute congestive) glaucoma.*

Chronic Simple Glaucoma. This type of primary adult glaucoma is characterized by an open filtration angle and a chronic, insidious course. It occurs more frequently than acute glaucoma and its incidence increases significantly after 40 years of age.

Narrow Angle Glaucoma. In this disorder there is a very narrow or closed angle resulting in episodes of elevated intraocular pressure associated with acute congestion, pain, and blurred vision.

Congenital Glaucoma. This term denotes glaucoma occurring in individuals under 30 years of age and is separable into infantile and juvenile types.

OTHER OPHTHALMIC ENTITIES PERTAINING TO GLAUCOMA

Secondary Glaucoma. This category includes glaucoma resulting from associated ocular disease such as uveitis, intraocular tumors, trauma, hemorrhage, and others.

Absolute Glaucoma. This term is used to describe an eye, usually causing pain, that is blind as a result of glaucoma of any type or cause.

ABNORMALITIES OF OCULAR MOTILITY

Ocular disorders of this type are discussed in the chapters Neuro-ophthalmology and Pediatric Ophthalmology (p. 156). Some of the more common entities are defined below.

Nystagmus

This is a disorder of eye movements usually characterized by a regular, rapid, involuntary oscillation or rotation of the eye. Nystagmus has been classified in several ways. The etiologic causes are considered in Neuro-ophthalmology (p. 324).

Classification Based on Severity. Three degrees of nystagmus are recognized, as described in the following sections.

FIRST DEGREE. Nystagmus is manifest only when the patient looks in the direction of the quick component (i.e., nystagmus to the right when looking to the right).

SECOND DEGREE. Nystagmus is present when the patient looks straight ahead in addition to looking in the direction of the quick component.

THIRD DEGREE. The nystagmus continues to be manifest even when the patient looks to the side opposite the quick component (e.g., nystagmus to the right in all horizontal positions of gaze). First degree nystagmus may be physiologic or pathologic. Second and third degree nystagmus always are pathologic.

Classification by Characteristics of Eye Movements

PENDULAR NYSTAGMUS. This type of nystagmus almost always is horizontal and is characterized by rotations that are approximately equal in rate for the two directions.

JERK NYSTAGMUS. The oscillations in this type are faster in one direction than the other, resulting in a characteristic jerky rhythm. The direction of the nystagmus is described according to the direction of the fast component. The causes of pendular and jerk nystagmus are discussed in Neuro-ophthalmology (p. 325).

Orthophoria and Heterophoria

It is customary to measure the position that the two eyes assume when the fusional impulses are either totally or partially removed. This measurement is said to determine the patient's muscle balance, or *phoria.* If, under these conditions, the visual axes remain in such a position that the image of the object of regard still falls on the two foveas, *orthophoria* is said to be present. On the other hand, if the two images do not fall on the two foveas, a *heterophoria* is apparent, and the character and degree of deviation is then determined and measured.

Depending upon which way the visual axes turn after the visual stimuli have been eliminated, i.e., whether they turn in or out, or one above the other, the following types of heterophoria are recognized:

1. Esophoria, when the visual axes turn in after the fusional stimuli have been eliminated.

2. Exophoria, when the visual axes turn from each other.

3. Right and left hyperphoria. If the right eye turns higher than the left, the condition is spoken of as right hyperphoria; if the left eye turns up above the right, the condition is spoken of as left hyperphoria.

Etiology, symptoms, and treatment of the phorias are discussed in Pediatric Ophthalmology (p. 161).

Strabismus (Squint; Heterotropia)

If the visual axes are not straight in the primary position, or if the eyes do not follow one another normally in any of the conjunctive or disjunctive movements, the condition is spoken of as strabismus. This is a manifest deviation of an eye, in contrast to the phorias, in which the deviation of the eyes is latent and is seen only after the fusional impulses have been partially or fully removed. There are two kinds of strabismus, comitant and noncomitant.

Comitant Strabismus. In this type the amount of strabismus (angle of squint) is always the same, no matter what the direction of gaze (i.e., right or left, up or down, or oblique).

Noncomitant Squint. In this type the amount of strabismus (angle of squint) is not the same in the various positions of gaze.

Esotropia, Exotropia, and Hypertropia. Strabismus may be convergent (esotropia) or divergent (*exotropia*). If one eye is manifestly higher than the other, the condition is a hypertropia; and, as with the phorias, the condition is usually named from the higher eye (i.e., right or left hypertropia).

Paralysis of Ocular Movements

Supranuclear Paralysis. Any lesion from the frontal oculogyric cortex down to the pontine gaze center will produce a paralysis of associated movements to the right or left (see chapter on neuro-ophthalmology).

Internuclear Paralysis. This syndrome, also discussed in the chapter on neuro-ophthalmology, results from a lesion in the medial longitudinal bundle, somewhere between the third and sixth nuclei.

Other Paralyses. Paralyses of the third nerve (the ophthalmoplegias), fourth nerve, and sixth nerve are also considered in the chapter on neuro-ophthalmology.

OPTICAL DEFECTS OF THE EYE

The eye functions as an optical system. A knowledge of the disorders of the eye requires some familiarity with the theory and practice of the correction of optical defects of the eye. Appendix III presents simplified and essentially nonmathematical descriptions of these defects and of ocular refraction. Certain of these entities are introduced here.

Accommodation. Accommodation is the process by which the dioptric power or refractive power of the eye is increased for seeing at close distances by changing the curvature of the crystalline lens. The gradual loss of accommodation with age is known as *presbyopia.*

Emmetropia and Ametropia. If the eye is optically normal, rays of light coming from a distance of 6 meters or more from the eye should be focused on the retina. Such an eye is called an *emmetropic* eye. If an optical defect is present which does not permit parallel rays of light to fall exactly on the retina, the eye is termed *ametropic,* i.e., having a refractive error.

HYPEROPIA (HYPERMETROPIA; FARSIGHTEDNESS). This is a refractive error in which rays of light from distant objects (parallel rays of light) come to a focus in back of the retina when the eye is at rest. The fault could be that the eyeball is relatively too short from front to back, or that there is a decreased curvature of the refracting surfaces or a change in the refractive index.

MYOPIA. Myopia (nearsightedness) is that form of refractive error in which parallel rays of light come to a focus in front of the retina when the eye is at rest. The myopic eye usually is relatively too large. In rare instances there is an increase in the curvature of the refracting surfaces or a change in the refractive index resulting in myopia.

ASTIGMATISM. In this condition refraction in different meridians of the eye is not the same, thereby preventing light rays from coming to a single focus (point focus) on the retina. This abnormality is nearly always the result of the curvature of the cornea; curvature astigmatism of the lens occurs only rarely.

BIBLIOGRAPHY

Skull and Orbit

Boyd, R. W.: Radiologic findings in exophthalmos. Canad. J. Ophth. *1*:44, 1966.

Cleasby, G. W.: The orbit. Arch. Ophth. *78*:676, 1967.

Cleasby, G. W.: The orbit. Arch. Ophth. *76*:450, 1966.

Cleasby, G. W.: The orbit. Arch. Ophth. *74*:412, 1965.

Johnson, W. A., and Christensen, R. D.: Pseudotumor of the orbit. Am. J. Ophth. *61*:334, 1966.

Zimmerman, L. E., and Font, R. L.: Congenital malformations of the eye: some recent advances in knowledge of the pathogenesis and histopathologic characteristics. J.A.M.A. *196*:684, 1966.

Eyelids

Burns, R. P.: Eyelids, lacrimal apparatus, and conjunctiva. Arch. Ophth. *79*:211, 1968.

Burns, R. P.: Eyelids, lacrimal apparatus, and conjunctiva. Arch. Ophth. *74*:850, 1965.

Fox, S. A.: The palpebral fissure. Am. J. Ophth. *62*:73, 1966.

Lacrimal Apparatus

Barraquer, J. I.: Localized discontinuity of precorneal lacrimal film: cause of Fuchs' dellen, progression of pterygium, and certain necrosis adjacent to keratoprosthesis and keratoplastics. Ophthalmologica *150*:111, 1965.

Burns, R. P.: Eyelids, lacrimal apparatus, and conjunctiva. Arch. Ophth. *79*:211, 1968.

Burns, R. P.: Eyelids, lacrimal apparatus, and conjunctiva. Arch. Ophth. *74*:850, 1965.

Campbell, H. S., Smith, J. L., Richman, D. W., and Anderson, W. B., Jr.: A simple test for lacrimal obstruction. Am. J. Ophth. *53*:611, 1962.

Cassady, J. W.: Abnormalities and treatment of conditions of the lacrimal sac and duct. Tr. Am. Acad. Ophth. *62*:687, 1958.

Flynn, F., and Schulmeister, A.: Keratoconjunctivitis sicca and new techniques in its management. Med. J. Aust. *1*:33, 1967.

Jones, L. T.: An anatomical approach to problems of the eyelids and lacrimal apparatus. Arch. Ophth. *66*:111, 1961.

Lemoine, A. N., Jr.: The lacrimal system. Surv. Ophth. *7*:325, 1962.

Vers, E. R.: The Lacrimal System, Clinical Applications. New York, Grune & Stratton, 1955.

Conjunctiva

Allen, H. F. (ed.): Infectious Diseases of the Conjunctiva and Cornea. Symposium of New Orleans Academy of Ophthalmology. St. Louis, The C. V. Mosby Co., 1963.

Burns, R. P.: Eyelids, lacrimal apparatus and conjunctiva. Arch. Ophth. *79*:211, 1968.

Burns, R. P.: Eyelids, lacrimal apparatus, and conjunctiva. Arch. Ophth. *74*:850, 1965.

Cornea

DeVoe, A. G.: The management of endothelial dystrophy of the cornea. Am. J. Ophth. *61*:1084, 1966.

Donn, A.: Cornea and sclera. Arch. Ophth. *73*:278, 1965.

Forgacs, J., and Franceschetti, A.: Histologic aspects of corneal changes due to hereditary, metabolic and cutaneous affections. Am. J. Ophth. *47*:191, 1959.

Gass, J. D. M.: The iron lines of the superficial cornea. Arch. Ophth. *71*:348, 1964.

Jones, S. T., and Zimmerman, L. E.: Histopathologic differentiation of granular, macular, and lattice dystrophies of the cornea. Am. J. Ophth. *51*:394, 1961.

Smelser, G. K., and Gzanics, V.: Morphology and functional development of the cornea. In Transparency of the Cornea: A Symposium. Duke-Elder, S., and Perkins, E. S. (eds.). Oxford, Blackwell Science Publishers, Ltd., 1960.

Thomas, C. I.: The Cornea. Springfield, Illinois, Charles C Thomas, 1955.

Trotter, R. R.: Cornea and sclera. Arch. Ophth. *79*:338, 1968.

Tschetter, R.: Arcus senilis. Arch. Ophth. *76*:325, 1966.

Sclera

Lyne, A. J., and Pitheathley, D. A.: Episcleritis and scleritis. Arch. Ophth. *80*:171, 1968.

Trotter, R. R.: Cornea and sclera. Arch. Ophth. *79*:338, 1968.

Watson, P. G.: Management of scleral disease. Tr. Ophth. Soc. U. Kingdom *86*:151, 1966.

Choroid, Iris, Ciliary Body, Pupil

Ferry, A. P.: Lesions mistaken for malignant melanoma of the iris. Arch. Ophth. *74*:9, 1965.

Goren, S. B.: Expulsive subchoroidal hemorrhage. Am. J. Ophth. *62*:536, 1966.

Hogan, M. J., Kimura, S. J., and O'Connor, G. R.: Ocular toxoplasmosis. Arch. Ophth. *72*:592, 1964.

Kaufman, H. E.: The uvea. Arch. Ophth. *73*:420, 1965.

Kaufman, H. E.: The uvea. Arch. Ophth. *75*:407, 1966.

Kurz, G. H.: Uveitis: its varied manifestations and causes. Med. Clin. N. Am. *48*:1529, 1964.

Maumenee, A. E., and Silverstein, A.: Immunopathology of Uveitis. Baltimore, Williams & Wilkins Co., 1964.

Norton, E.: Fluorescein in fundus photography. An aid for the differential diagnosis of posterior ocular lesions. Tr. Am. Acad. Ophth. *68*:755, 1964.

Smith, J. L.: Seronegative ocular and neuro-syphilis. Am. J. Ophth. *59*:753, 1965.

Sugar, H. S.: Heterochromic irides. Am. J. Ophth. *60*:1, 1965.

Lens and Vitreous

Davis, M. D.: Vitreous contraction in proliferative diabetic retinopathy. Arch. Ophth. *74*:741, 1965.

Haik, G. M.: Cataract extraction by cryosurgery. Arch. Ophth. *76*:426, 1966.

Haney, W. P.: Posterior lenticonus. Am. J. Ophth. *61*: 1134, 1966.

Linder, B.: The vitreous body and retinal detachment. Acta Ophth. *84*:77, 1966.

Raskind, R. H.: Persistent hyperplastic primary vitreous. Necessity of early recognition and treatment. Am. J. Ophth. *62*:1072, 1966.

Roche, J.: Pseudoexfoliation of the lens capsule. Brit. J. Ophth. *52*:265, 1968.

Straatsma, B. R.: The lens and vitreous. Arch. Ophth. *73*:559, 1965.

Tolentino, F. I., Pei-Tei, L., and Schepers, C. L.: Biomicroscopic study of vitreous cavity in diabetic retinopathy. Arch. Ophth. *75*:238, 1966.

Winter, F. C.: The lens and vitreous. Arch. Ophth. *78*: 229, 1967.

Retina and Optic Nerve

Adams, S. T.: Retina and optic nerve. Arch. Ophth. *73*:724, 1965.

Duke-Elder, S., and Dorbee, J. H.: A System of Ophthalmology. Vol. X: Diseases of the Retina. St. Louis, The C. V. Mosby Co., 1967.

Klien, B. A.: Comments on the cotton-wool lesions of the retina. Am. J. Ophth. *59*:17, 1965.

Lee, P. F., McNeel, J. W., Schepens, C. C., and Field, R. A.: A new classification of diabetic retinopathy. Am. J. Ophth. *62*:207, 1966.

Manschot, W., and de Bruijn, W. O.: Coats' disease: definition and pathogenesis. Brit. J. Ophth. *51*: 145, 1967.

Maumenee, A. E.: Further advances in the study of the macula. Arch. Ophth. *78*:151, 1967.

Rucker, C. W.: Papilledema. Arch. Ophth. *71*:454, 1964.

Sabates, F. N.: Juvenile retinoschisis. Am. J. Ophth. *62*:683, 1966.

Schepens, C. L., and Marden, D.: Natural history of retinal detachment. Am. J. Ophth. *61*:213, 1966.

Zimmerman, L. E.: Embolism of central retinal artery. Arch. Ophth. *73*:822, 1965.

Chapter Two

ANATOMY OF THE HUMAN EYE

THE ORBIT

The pear-shaped orbital cavity has its apex directed posteriorly, medially, and slightly upward (Fig. 2-1), and is enclosed anteriorly by the eyeball and lids. The orbital contents include the eye and lacrimal gland, along with fat, blood vessels, nerves, smooth and striated muscles, and elastic, collagenous, and cartilagenous tissue. The walls of the orbit are lined by periosteum and consist of a roof, a floor, and a medial and a lateral wall.

Roof. The roof is formed by the orbital process of the frontal bone and, to a lesser extent posteriorly, by the sphenoid (Fig. 2-1). The orbital roof is so thin that the ridges and depressions formed by the sulci and gyri of the frontal lobe of the brain can be demonstrated by holding the bone up to light. In older people portions of this thin, fragile roof may be absorbed at times and show deliquescence. Long instruments entering the orbit may easily pierce the roof and enter the cranial cavity.

Floor. The floor of the orbit (the roof of

Figure 2-1 The orbit from in front.

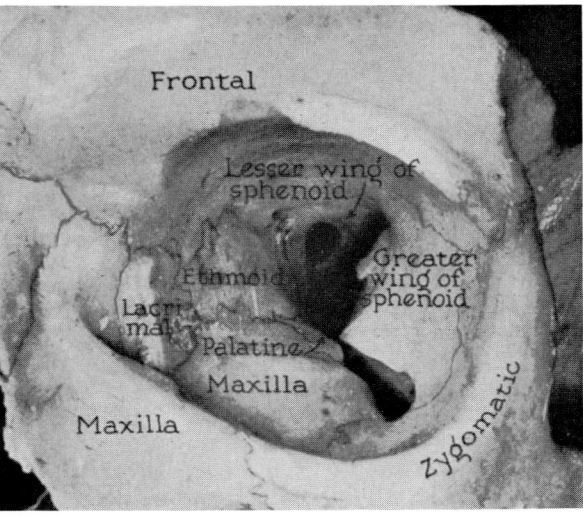

the antrum) is formed by the orbital plate of the superior maxilla, the orbital surface of the zygomatic bone, and the orbital process of the palatine bone (Fig. 2-2). The infraorbital fissure, located in the floor, separates the greater wing of the sphenoid from the maxilla (Fig. 2-1). The infraorbital groove runs from the anterior aspect of this fissure and conducts the infraorbital nerve and artery, and occasionally the vein, through the infraorbital canal to the infraorbital foramen, where they emerge onto the anterior aspect of the face to supply the skin. After trauma to the orbit, anesthesia of the skin of the cheek in

the distribution of the infraorbital nerve suggests a fracture of the floor of the orbit. The floor of the orbit consists of very thin bone, sometimes only 0.5 to 1 mm. thick, which fractures easily. Tumors in the antrum readily enter the orbit by traversing or invading the floor.

Walls. The medial wall runs parallel to the longitudinal fissure of the brain and to the medial wall of its fellow orbit. This wall is formed by the frontal process of the superior maxilla, the lacrimal bone, the very thin lamina papyracea of the ethmoid, and a small portion of the body of the sphenoid (Fig. 2-3). The lacrimal fossa, lying anteriorly and containing the lacrimal sac, is formed by the lacrimal bone and the frontal process of the maxilla.

The lateral wall of one orbit forms a 90-

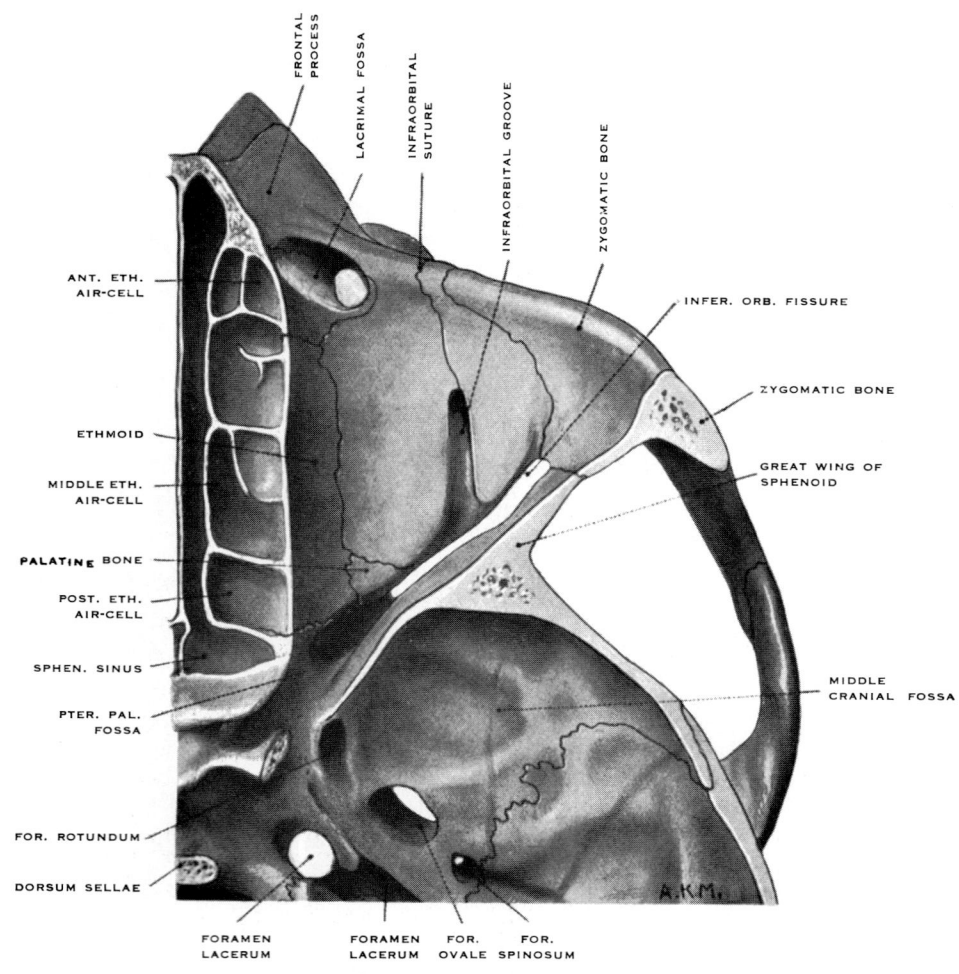

Figure 2-2   The floor of the orbit. (Wolff: *Anatomy of the Eye and Orbit.* H. K. Lewis & Co., Ltd., London.)

degree angle with the lateral wall of the opposite orbit. The anterior third of the wall is formed by the zygomatic bone; this separates the orbit from the temporal fossa. The posterior two thirds is formed by the greater wing of the sphenoid bone, which separates the orbit from the temporal lobe of the brain in the middle cranial fossa. The lateral orbital wall, the thickest wall, is especially strong anteriorly at the orbital rim. The superior orbital fissure, actually a gap between the lesser and greater wings of the sphenoid, is found posteriorly between the lateral wall and the roof. The third, fourth, and sixth nerves, the first division of the fifth nerve, the sympathetic nerves, and the superior ophthalmic veins pass through this fissure (Fig. 2-4). A lesion near the fissure is likely to catch all of these structures as they enter the orbit and to produce total ophthalmoplegia, as well as anesthesia of the cornea (the cavernous sinus syndrome). Where the roof and the lateral wall join anteriorly, a fossa houses the orbital portion of the lacrimal gland. The trochlea, or pulley, through which the tendon of the superior oblique muscle runs, is found anteriorly, where the roof and the medial wall join.

Optic Canal.   The optic canal, at the apex of the orbit, is formed by the two roots of the lesser wing of the sphenoid. From 8 to 9 mm. long, it connects the middle cranial

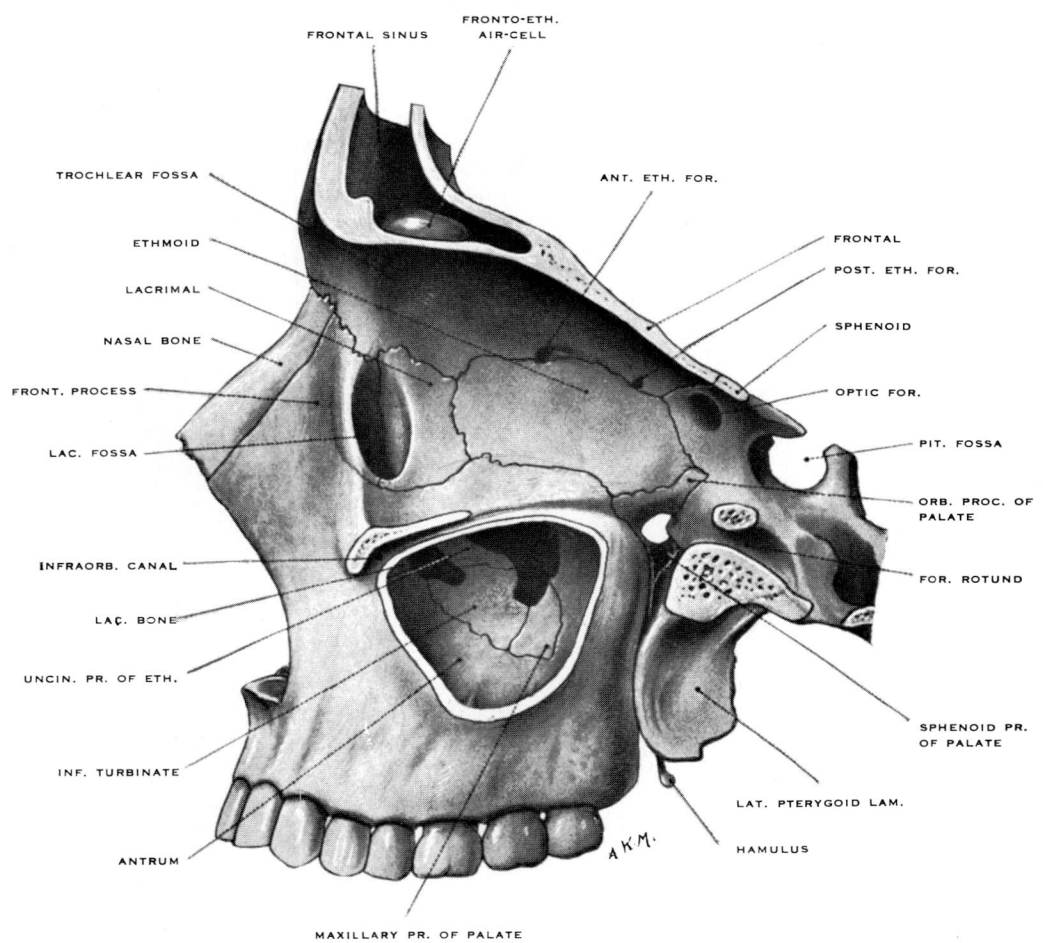

Figure 2-3   The medial wall of the orbit. (Wolff: *Anatomy of the Eye and Orbit.* H. K. Lewis & Co., Ltd., London.)

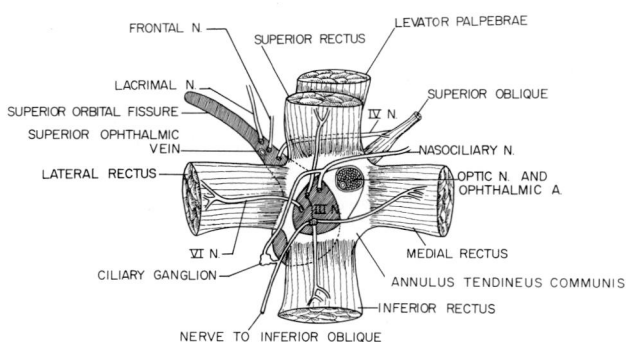

FRONTAL N.
SUPERIOR RECTUS
LEVATOR PALPEBRAE
LACRIMAL N.
SUPERIOR OBLIQUE
SUPERIOR ORBITAL FISSURE
IV N.
SUPERIOR OPHTHALMIC VEIN
NASOCILIARY N.
LATERAL RECTUS
OPTIC N. AND OPHTHALMIC A.
VI N.
MEDIAL RECTUS
CILIARY GANGLION
ANNULUS TENDINEUS COMMUNIS
INFERIOR RECTUS
NERVE TO INFERIOR OBLIQUE

Figure 2-4 Diagram of apex of orbit showing structures passing through the optic foramen and superior orbital fissure.

fossa with the orbit. Medially, the canal is adjacent to, and sometimes surrounded by, the sphenoidal sinus and, occasionally, by a posterior ethmoidal air cell. The canal transmits the optic nerve and the ophthalmic artery.

Lymphatics and Veins. Although no lymphatics have been demonstrated in the orbit, the occurrence of lymphangiomas and perivascular and perineural infiltration by certain neoplasms suggest their presence. There are no lymph nodes. The superior and inferior ophthalmic veins drain the area. These anastomose with the anterior facial vein and empty into the cavernous sinus and pterygoid plexus. Because orbital veins have no valves and anastomose fully with one another, orbital venous congestion is rare.

Periosteum and Orbital Septum. Periosteum (periorbita) lines the orbit. It firmly adheres to the bones along sutures, at various fissures or foramina, and at the trochlear fossa where it unites with the cartilagenous trochlea of the superior oblique muscles. Elsewhere it is loosely attached to the orbital bones. The periosteum is continuous with the dura mater through the orbital (optic) foramen. A thin membrane of fibrous and elastic connective tissue, the orbital (lid) septum, arises from the periosteum of the orbital rim and extends beneath the orbicularis oculi to attach to the tarsal plates. The orbital septum is an essential supporting structure of the eyelids.

THE LACRIMAL APPARATUS

Secretory System

The secretory portion of the lacrimal apparatus consists largely of the lacrimal gland, which secretes tears that flow across the eye and drain into the nose. The larger orbital portion, or lacrimal gland proper, lies in the lacrimal fossa in the upper, outer wall of the anterior portion of the orbit. A smaller palpebral portion is located in the upper lid. Tiny tubules (excretory ducts) from the orbital gland pierce the palpebral gland and are joined by tubules from it. These tubules, about eight in number, plus independent ones from the palpebral portion, empty into the conjunctival sac just in front of the fornix. In some normal people having prominent eyes, particularly among Negroes, the palpebral portion herniates in front of the tarsus and can be seen through the conjunctiva when the upper lid is everted. In most people, however, it can be seen only when the tissues of the upper fornix are pushed downward with an applicator after the lid has been everted. The lacrimal branch of the ophthalmic artery and the infraorbital branch of the internal maxillary artery supply blood to the gland. The lacrimal vein flows into the ophthalmic vein. Lymphatics drain into the preauricular lymph nodes. Both sympathetic and parasympathetic fibers innervate the lacrimal gland. If the parasympathetic fibers are severed, tear secretion is immediate_y impaired. The sympathetics have little to do with tear formation. Besides the main lacrimal gland, numerous, structurally identical, accessory lacrimal glands (p. 47) can be found in the subepithelial tissue of the conjunctiva.

Excretory System

Tears, which are formed constantly in small amounts, flow downward and medially over the surface of the cornea and conjunctiva to the lacrimal lake near the inner canthus. Here they enter the superior and inferior canaliculi through the lacrimal puncta, then flow on to the lacrimal sac, the lacrimal duct, and into the nose (Fig. 2-5). The lacrimal sac occupies the lacrimal fossa in the medial aspect of the orbital rim. It is surrounded by periosteum and the medial canthal ligament. The lacrimal duct carries tears and runs through the medial wall of the maxillary sinus to empty beneath the inferior turbinate. Its inferior opening is loosely covered by a flap of nasal mucosa called the valve of Hasner.

THE EYELIDS

The upper lid extends from the free lid margin upward to the brow; the lower lid extends from the free lid margin down-

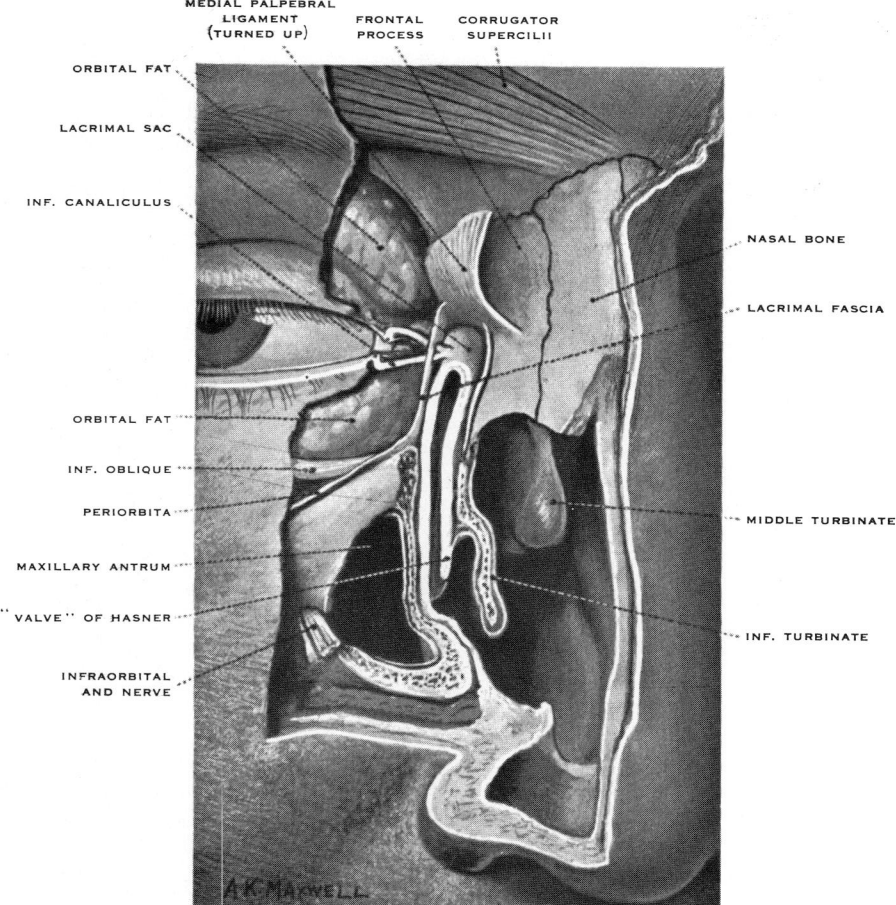

Figure 2-5 Dissection to show relations of the lacrimal sac and the nasolacrimal duct from in front (Wolff's preparation). (Last: *Wolff's Anatomy of the Eye and Orbit*, 5th ed. H. K. Lewis & Co., Ltd., London.)

ward to a semicircular furrow. Each eyelid, from anterior to posterior, has four basic layers: skin, muscle, tarsus, and conjunctiva (Fig. 2-6). The free margin of the lid is rectangular. The anterior border of the lid margin gives rise to the lashes. The openings of the meibomian glands can be seen just in front of the posterior border. The area between the anterior and posterior borders is called the intermarginal space.

The Skin Layer. The skin of the lids, the thinnest in the body, is covered with fine, downy hairs. Since the subcutaneous tissue is areolar, the skin is freely movable and can be picked up readily with the fingers. For the same reason the eyelids may swell dramatically when blood or other effusions

occur; these fluids, however, are confined to the lids themselves, because they are limited by the tight attachment of the skin to the underlying periosteum at the orbital margins. The skin continues over the lid margin to fuse with the conjunctiva near the posterior border. The so-called gray line runs across the entire intermarginal space of the lid and can be seen at the junction of the posterior and middle thirds of the lid margin, just anterior to the tarsal plate. Its color probably is due to the relative avascularity of the area. The lid can be split along this line for surgical purposes. Numerous tubular and rather deeply placed sweat glands are embedded in the sub-epithelial tissue of the skin of the eyelid.

The Muscle Layer. The orbicularis muscle, a sheet of subcutaneous, elliptical, striated muscle fibers that encircle the palpebral fissure, acts as a sphincter and is

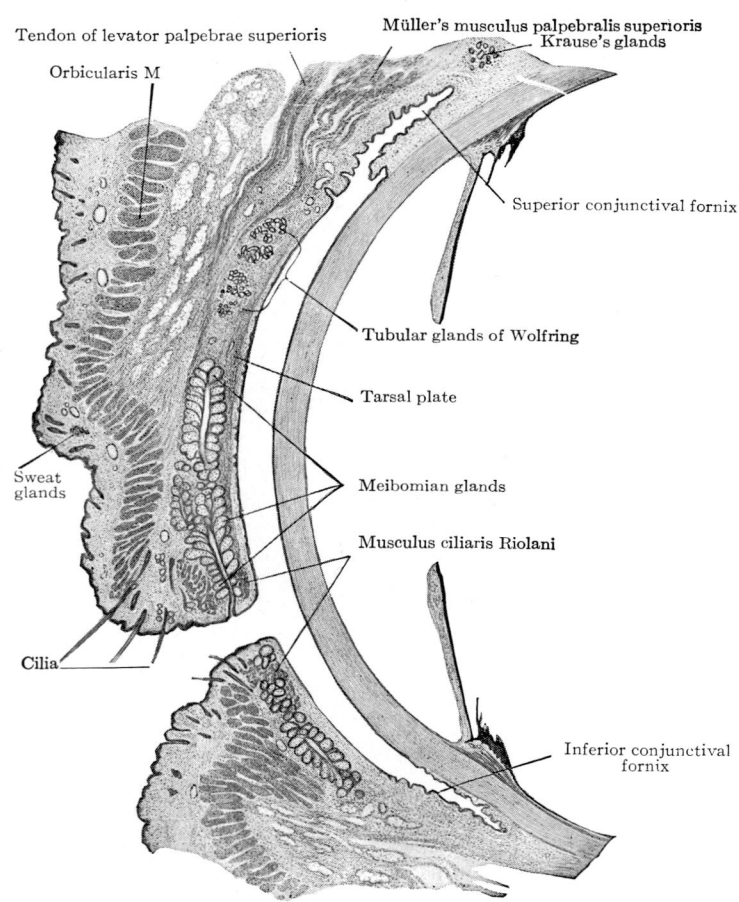

Tendon of levator palpebrae superioris
Müller's musculus palpebralis superioris
Krause's glands
Orbicularis M
Superior conjunctival fornix
Tubular glands of Wolfring
Tarsal plate
Sweat glands
Meibomian glands
Musculus ciliaris Riolani
Cilia
Inferior conjunctival fornix

Figure 2-6 Cross section of the upper lid and the structures contained therein.

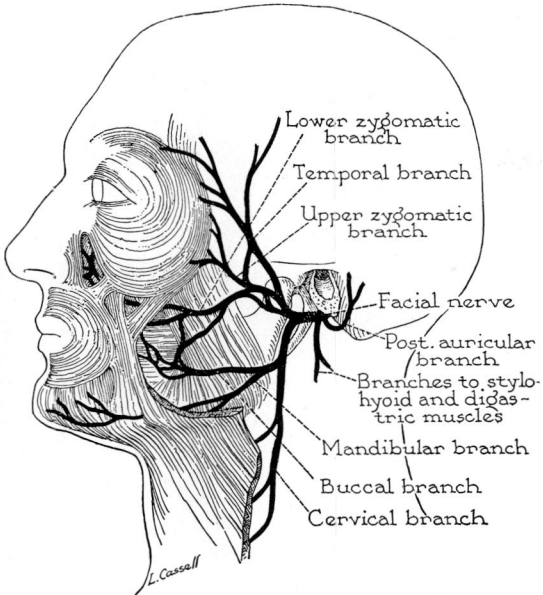

Figure 2-7 Innervation of the orbicularis muscle by the seventh nerve. (Millard, King, and Showers: *Human Anatomy and Physiology*, 4th ed. W. B. Saunders Co., Philadelphia.)

supplied by the seventh nerve (Fig. 2-7). When contracted, it closes the lids. Orbicularis fibers spread out like a sheet extending onto the temple, cheek, and forehead. The levator palpebrae superioris arises from the apex of the orbit at the annulus of Zinn and inserts into the upper border of the tarsal plate (Fig. 2-8). It also sends fibers that traverse the orbicularis muscle to insert into the subcutaneous tissue of the skin in front of the tarsus. This muscle supports and elevates the upper lid. If the levator muscle is paralyzed or severed, the result is a droopy upper lid that cannot be elevated (ptosis). Müller's muscle, a non-

striated accessory levator muscle, lies just beneath the conjunctiva. It runs from the inner aspect of the levator palpebrae to insert into the upper portion of the tarsal plate. It is innervated sympathetically.

The Tarsal or Fibrous Layer. The tarsal plate gives form and firm consistency to the half of the lid adjacent to the palpebral fissure. It is a dense matrix of connective tissue and some elastic tissue. The upper tarsus is considerably larger than the lower. About 30 meibomian glands in the upper eyelid, and somewhat fewer in the lower, run into the tarsal plate perpendicularly from the free border of the lid (Fig. 2-6). Their opening ducts can be seen on the intermarginal space immediately anterior to the posterior lid border. The tarsal layer continues into the orbital portion of the lids as the orbital septum.

Lid Appendages. The cilia, with their follicles and modified sebaceous and sweat glands, are found on the anterior (ciliary) border of the lid margin (Fig. 2-9). They usually are arranged in two rows curving outward from the surface of the eyeball. The sebaceous glands of the cilia (the glands of Zeis) are holocrine, i.e., they have no lumen. Their secretion, formed by decomposition of the cells, empties into hair follicles. The glands of Moll are modified apocrine sweat glands whose secretions empty into the lash follicles. Originally these glands were thought to secrete by releasing parts of their cytoplasm into their lumen (hence the name apocrine), but recent histochemical studies do not support this concept. The cells probably

Figure 2-8 Diagram of the levator palpebrae superioris. A, aponeurosis; M, superior palpebral involuntary muscle of Müller; T, tarsal plate; P, pretarsal space; S, septum orbitale. (Whitnall: *Anatomy of the Human Orbit.* Oxford Medical Press, Henry Frowde & Hodder & Stoughton, London.)

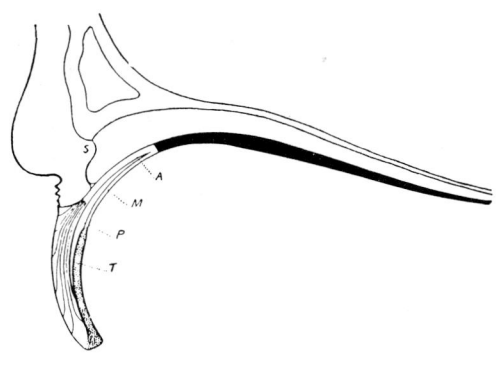

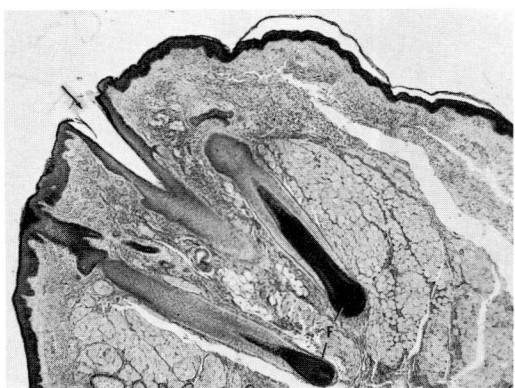

Figure 2-9 Cilium arises from follicle, F, and exits through the skin at the anterior (ciliary) border of the anterior lid margin (arrow) (hematoxylin and eosin, ×36).

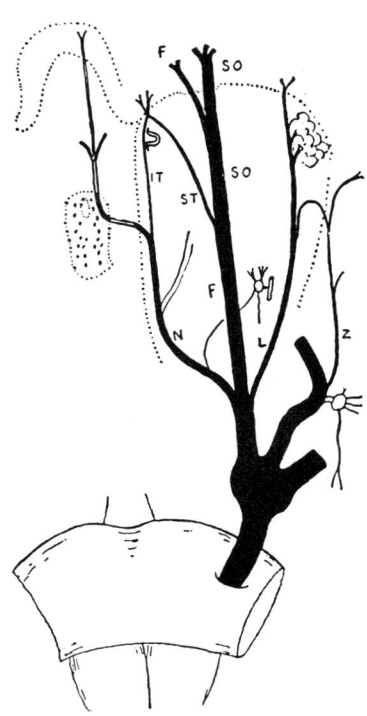

Figure 2-10 Diagram of the distribution of the ophthalmic division of the fifth nerve. F, frontal nerve gives off the supratrochlear branch, ST; SO, supraorbital nerve; N, nasociliary nerve gives off the sensory root to the ciliary ganglion and two long ciliary nerves to the eyeball, and just before leaving the orbit it gives off the infratrochlear nerve, IT. Anastomosis is shown between L, the lacrimal nerve, and a branch of the zygomatic nerve, Z. (Whitnall: *Anatomy of the Human Orbit.* Oxford Medical Press, Henry Frowde & Hodder & Stoughton, London.)

release secretory material from their cytoplasm into the lumen.

Palpebral Fissure. When the eye is open normally, an elliptical space, the palpebral fissure, separates the lids. The temporal and nasal angles of this space are spoken of as the external and internal canthus, respectively. The caruncle, an island of modified skin, appears as a slightly elevated area just within the internal canthus. It helps to form the lacrimal lake, where the tears collect before they pass into the upper and lower canaliculi. At the lateral border of the caruncle is a semilunar fold of conjunctiva, the plica semilunaris, a structure that is a vestigial remnant of the third eyelid, or nictitating membrane, of many lower vertebrates. Above and below the semilunar fold on the lid margin are relatively avascular, moundlike elevations topped with small openings, the puncta. These puncta, one in the upper lid and one in the lower, mark the openings of the lacrimal canaliculi. The canaliculi are fine, epithelial tubes extending along the medial aspect of the portion of the lid margin where no lashes are present; this is the canalicular portion of the lid margin.

Blood Vessels and Lymphatics of the Lids. The main blood supply of the lids comes from superior and inferior palpebral arches (tarsal arcades) that are formed by a rich plexus of anastomotic vessels derived largely from the posterior conjunctival arteries (Fig. 2-15). The palpebral arches receive blood from the internal carotid artery through the ophthalmic and lacrimal arteries, and from the external carotid artery through twigs from the superficial temporal, transverse facial, and infraorbital arteries. These arches send fairly large vessels to the edge of the lid, to the anterior surface of the tarsus, and back through the midportion of the tarsal plate to the conjunctiva as perforating branches. When the lids are injured, this rich blood supply causes them to bleed profusely; the rich blood supply also greatly facilitates healing and helps to prevent infection. The lid veins, larger and more numerous than the arteries that they follow, form a dense

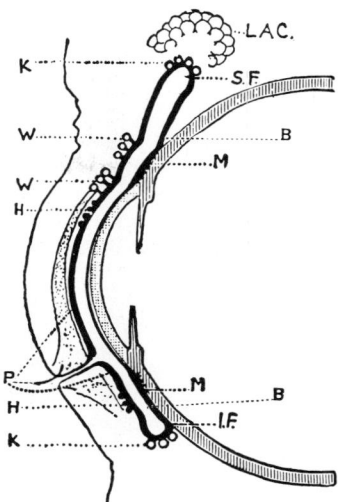

Figure 2-11 Scheme of a sagittal section through the eyelids and eyeball to show the conjunctival sac and the position of its glands. SF and IF, the conjunctiva of the superior and inferior fornices, respectively; B, the bulbar conjunctiva; P, the palpebral conjunctiva; LAC, the lacrimal gland proper; K, the accessory lacrimal glands of Krause; W, the accessory lacrimal glands of Wolfring; H, the crypts of Henle; M, the "glands" of Manz. (After Dubreuil, 1908.) (Whitnall: *Anatomy of the Human Orbit.* Oxford Medical Press, Henry Frowde & Hodder & Stoughton, London.)

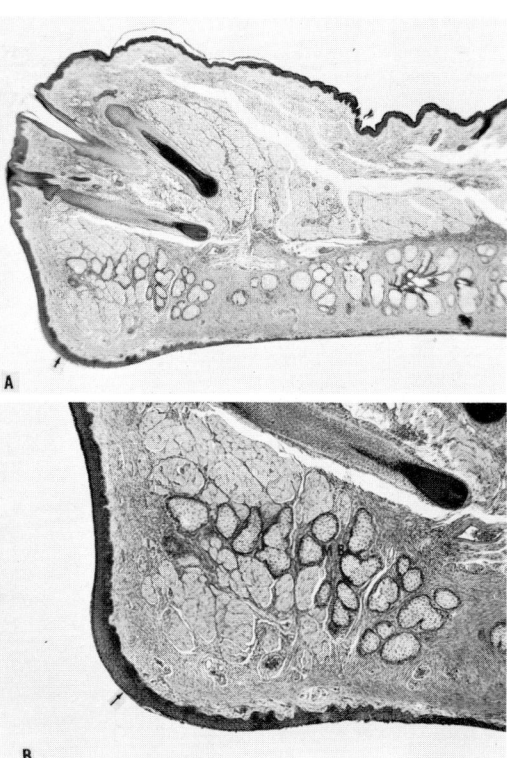

Figure 2-13 *(A)* Conjunctival epithelium is continuous with the keratinized squamous skin epithelium (arrow) near the posterior border of the lid's intermarginal space (hematoxylin and eosin, ×22). *(B)* Higher power of Part *A* showing the junction of conjunctival epithelium with skin epithelium (arrow). MB, meibomian glands in fibrous tarsus (hematoxylin and eosin, ×44).

plexus in the lids. They drain into the veins of the forehead, but some pass through the orbicularis muscle to reach the ophthalmic vein and thence the cavernous sinus. Spasm of the orbicularis muscle, therefore, may compress the branches that traverse it and result in venous engorgement. Also, infection may reach the cavernous sinus via this route.

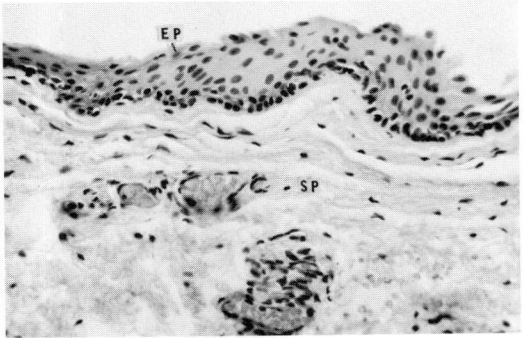

Figure 2-12 Multilayered, nonkeratinized, columnar epithelium, EP, covers the vascularized substantia propria, SP, of the conjunctiva (hematoxylin and eosin, ×315).

Nerve Supply of the Lids. The first, or ophthalmic, division of the fifth nerve transmits sensation to the upper lid, largely through the supraorbital nerve that emerges from the skull through the supraorbital foramen (Fig. 2-10). Both the first and second division of the fifth nerve transmit sensation to the lower lid. The seventh cranial nerve supplies motor fibers to the orbicularis muscle (Fig. 2-7). The upper division of the third nerve supplies motor fibers to the levator palpebrae. Sympathetic fibers supply Müller's muscles.

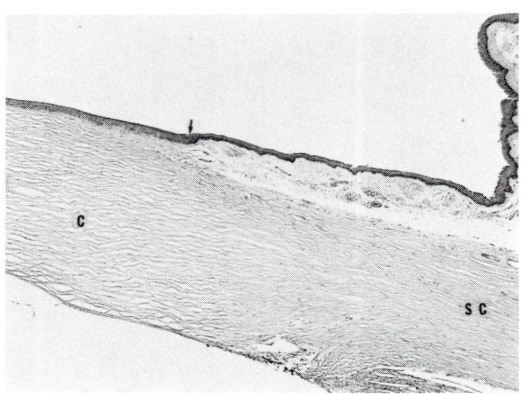

Figure 2-14 Conjunctival epithelium becomes continuous with the nonkeratinized squamous corneal epithelium (arrow) at the limbus. C, cornea; SC, sclera (hematoxylin and eosin, ×40).

THE CONJUNCTIVA

The conjunctiva, a mucous membrane, lines the eyelid (palpebral portion) and covers the eyeball (bulbar portion) except for the cornea (Fig. 2-11).

Palpebral Conjunctiva.   The palpebral portion of the conjunctiva forms the inner layer or lining of the eyelids and reflects over the eyeball at the upper and lower cul-de-sacs. Since it contains little subepithelial connective tissue over the tarsal plate, it is firmly attached to, and not movable over, this structure. Except over the tarsal plate, the subconjunctival tissue is areolar and the conjunctiva is freely movable, a situation helping to ensure mobility of the eyeball.

Bulbar Conjunctiva.   The bulbar conjunctiva is so extremely thin and transparent that subconjunctival and even episcleral vessels shine through. It also is easily grasped and freely movable except at the corneoscleral limbus, where it becomes continuous with the corneal epithelium.

Structure of the Conjunctiva.   As with all mucous membranes, the conjunctiva is composed of nonkeratinizing epithelium overlying a substantia propria (Fig. 2-12). The multilayered columnar epithelium of the palpebral conjunctiva has as its innermost layer a single row of cylindrical basal cells. Each cell contains a central or internally placed nucleus in a slightly basophilic cytoplasm and rests on a delicate basement membrane that is argyrophilic and positive to the periodic acid–Schiff (PAS) reaction. The columnar epithelial cells contain

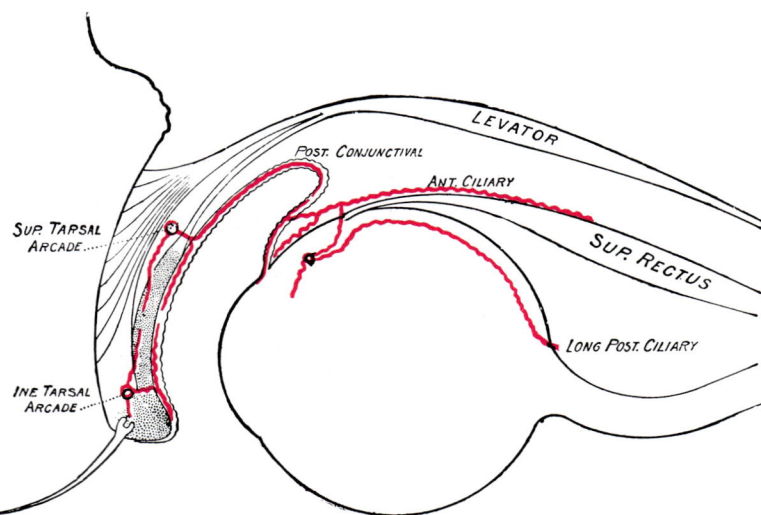

Figure 2-15   Diagram to show the deep arteries of the upper eyelid and conjunctiva and their anastomoses with those of the forepart of the eyeball. (Whitnall: *Anatomy of the Human Orbit*, 2nd ed. Oxford Medical Press, Henry Frowde & Hodder & Stoughton, London.)

numerous goblet (mucous) cells near the cul-de-sac, but few are seen near the cornea or lid margin.

The epithelium of the palpebral conjunctiva becomes keratinized as it becomes continuous with the squamous epithelium of the skin on the intermarginal space of the lid near the posterior border (Fig. 2-13). The underlying substantia propria near the cul-de-sac is loose collagen and elastic tissue containing blood vessels, lymphatics, and nerves. Lymphoid collections are frequent. At the limbus the multilayered, columnar epithelium becomes squamous and covers the cornea (Fig. 2-14). Papillas form from the interdigitation of the substantia propria with the overlying epithelium.

Glands. The glands of the conjunctiva consist of a few, simple invaginations (crypts) in the bulbar and retrotarsal portions that secrete a mucinous fluid (Figs. 2-6 and 2-11). The accessory lacrimal glands of Krause are found in the upper (about 40) and lower (about six) fornices. Three or more glands of Wolfring lie at the superior margin of the upper tarsus. These accessory glands secrete a fluid resembling tears that flows through tiny ducts onto the conjunctiva.

Vasculature. Beneath the conjunctiva of both eyelids the blood vessels form a system of arcades that sends branches to the conjunctival folds in the cul-de-sac and to the bulbar conjunctiva (Fig. 2-15). On the globe this system is seen beneath the thin conjunctiva as a series of rather tortuous, light pink vessels. Near the limbus the conjunctival vessels anastomose with deeper branches of the long, ciliary vessels.

THE EXTRAOCULAR MUSCLES

Six extraocular muscles rotate the eyeball: the superior and inferior recti, the medial and lateral recti, and the superior and inferior obliques. The recti arise from a fibrous ring, the anulus tendineus communis, which surrounds the optic foramen and bridges part of the superior orbital fissure (Figs. 2-16 and 2-17). The four recti muscles are inserted into the sclera over the anterior portion of the globe by broad, flat tendons (Fig. 2-18). The superior oblique arises from the periosteum of the

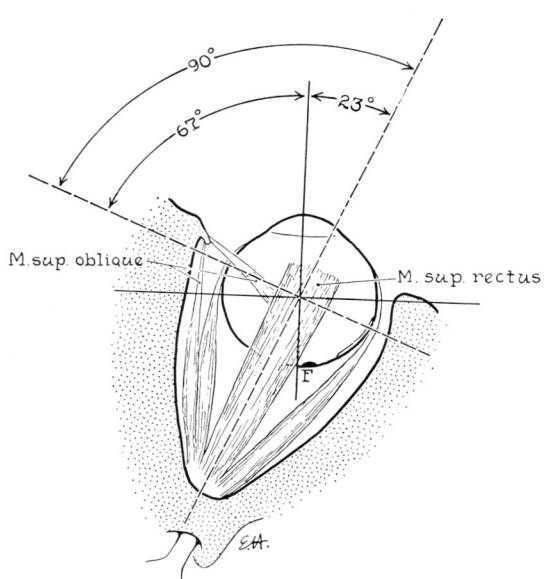

Figure 2-16 Diagram of the muscles seen from above, showing the origin and insertion of the right superior rectus.

body of the sphenoid bone, medially and a little anteriorly to the optic foramen and to the origin of the medial rectus. It passes along the nasal, or medial, wall of the orbit to the trochlea, a cartilaginous ring just behind the upper, inner angle of the orbit (Fig. 2-18). Here the muscle becomes tendinous and runs through the trochlea to pass under the superior rectus and to attach to the sclera above and slightly lateral to the posterior pole of the eye. The inferior oblique muscle, the only muscle to arise from the anterior part of the orbit, originates from a shallow depression just inside the lower, orbital margin, where it adjoins the lacrimal fossa laterally. It passes back below the inferior rectus muscle to insert below and somewhat lateral to the posterior pole of the eye.

Fascial sheaths which are connected intimately with Tenon's capsule of the globe, surround all the muscles and form prolongations, known as check ligaments, that attach to the periosteum of the adjacent orbital wall (Fig. 2-19). The check ligaments insure normal limits to eye movements.

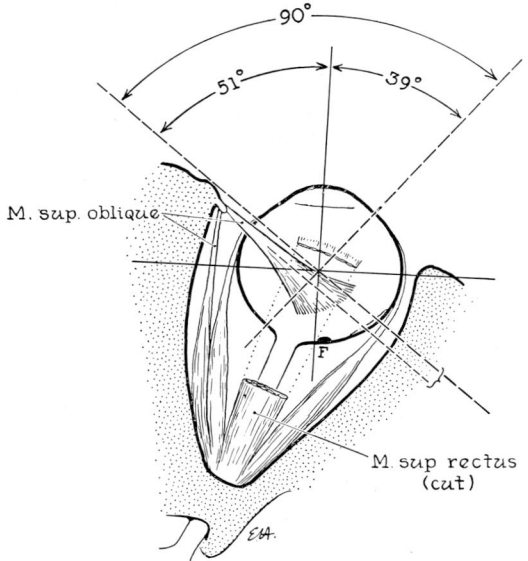

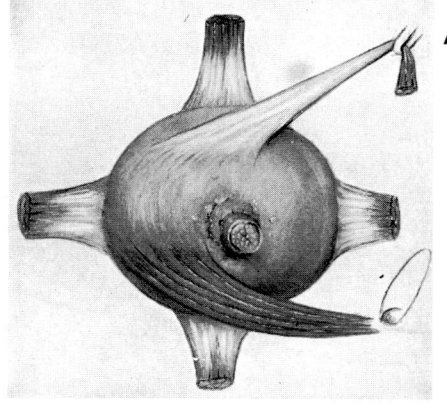

Figure 2-17 Diagram showing the origin and insertion of the muscles from above with the superior rectus cut away. The physiologic origin of the superior oblique is at the trochlea.

M. sup. oblique

M. sup. rectus (cut)

Figure 2-18 Insertions of the extraocular muscles, showing the trochlea, A, of the superior oblique.

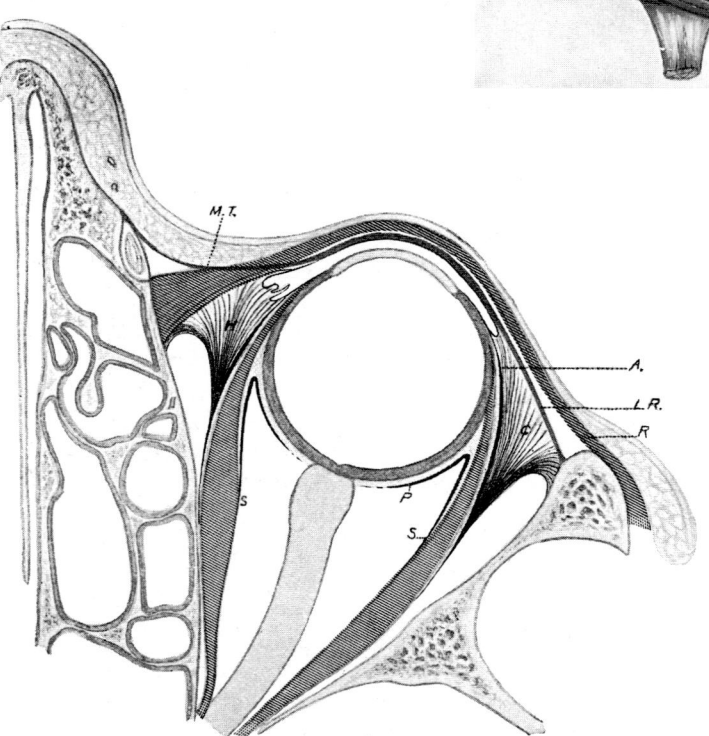

Figure 2-19 Schematic view of a horizontal section through the right orbit to illustrate the fascia of the orbit. The fascia bulbi, or Tenon's capsule, is shown by A, its anterior part, and P, its posterior part. The fascial sheaths of the muscles are marked by S, and their offshoots form the lateral, C, and the medial, H, "check ligaments." The drawing also illustrates certain points in the anatomy of the eyelids: MT, the medial palpebral ligament with its two limbs passing in front of and behind the fossa for the lacrimal sac; LR, the lateral palpebral ligament; and R, the lateral palpebral raphe. (Whitnall: *Anatomy of the Human Orbit.* Oxford Medical Press, Henry Frowde & Hodder & Stoughton, London.)

Branches of the third nerve supply all the extraocular muscles except the lateral rectus, which is innervated by the sixth nerve, and the superior oblique, which is supplied by the fourth nerve.

THE EYEBALL

The eye, considered simply, consists of a retinal-lined, fibrovascular sphere containing the aqueous humor, the lens, and the vitreous body (Fig. 2-20). Covering the anterior one sixth of the surface of the eye is the normally transparent cornea. The remainder of the fibrous coat, the sclera, is white and opaque. The cornea, which has a smaller radius of curvature (about 8 mm.) than the sclera (12 mm.), is demarcated externally at its posterior limit by a circumferential groove called the external scleral sulcus. The center of the cornea is regarded as the anterior pole of the eye; the

posterior pole is opposite at the back of the eye. An imaginary line connecting the two is called the geometric, or optic, axis of the eye, and the distance between them is the anteroposterior diameter. The visual axis is an imaginary line connecting the fovea centralis (macula) of the retina with the nodal point of the eye, and continuing anteriorly through the cornea. Since the fovea centralis is temporal and slightly inferior to the posterior pole, the visual axis and the optic axis do not coincide (Fig. 2-20).

The average anterior to posterior dimensions of the adult eyeball lie between 24 and 25 mm., and the average vertical and horizontal dimensions are between 23 and 24 mm. The horizontal distance is slightly greater than the vertical. At birth the eyeball averages about 14 mm. anteropos-

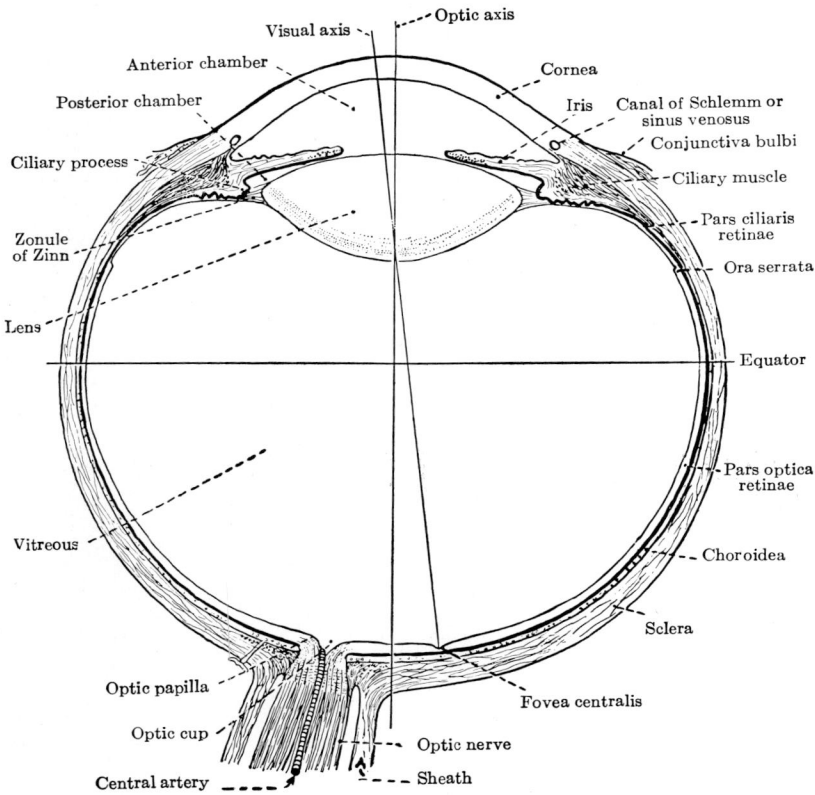

Figure 2-20 Schematic section along the horizontal meridian of the right eyeball (×4). (Whitnall modified from *Toldt's Atlas.*)

teriorly, and the vertical and horizontal meridians are slightly larger. The eye, especially the anterior segment, grows most rapidly in the first year of life, with subsequent growth mainly involving the posterior segment.

Directional Terms. Many directional terms are used to describe the eye. A meridional line is the direction of an arc that passes through the anterior and posterior poles (Fig. 2-21). The equatorial plane is the locus of points equidistant from the two poles. A transverse section through the eye parallels or follows the equatorial plane and divides the eye into anterior and posterior parts. A radially placed structure within the eye also parallels the equatorial plane and is perpendicular to the meridional plane. A sagittal section is synonymous with a vertical meridional section. A frontal or coronal section is synonymous with a transverse or equatorial section and is at right angles to a sagittal section.

Topographic Anatomy of the Opened Eye. Two unequal compartments can be seen within an eye bisected along the meridional plane: a smaller, or aqueous, compartment that lies mostly in front of the lens, and a larger, or vitreous, compartment that lies behind the lens (Fig. 2-22). The iris diaphragm further subdivides the aqueous compartment into two chambers, an anterior and a posterior. Each chamber con-

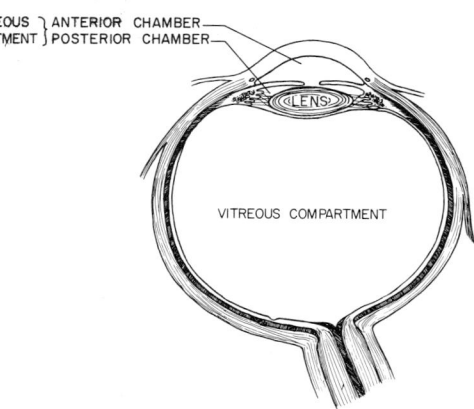

Figure 2-22 Diagram of opened eye showing aqueous and vitreous compartments.

tains the watery, structureless aqueous that is formed by the ciliary epithelium and flows from the posterior to the anterior chamber through the pupil. It leaves the eye through a drainage mechanism at the periphery of the anterior chamber in the region of the iridocorneoscleral angle (anterior chamber angle). The large, vitreous compartment is filled by an exquisitely delicate, markedly hydrated connective tissue.

The coverings of the eye have two layers in addition to the cornea and sclera: (1) the uveal tract, consisting of heavily pigmented, vascular tissue (choroid) with its anterior modifications into ciliary body and iris, and (2) the retina, or sensory layer. The retina, by gross appearance, ends abruptly at the heavily pigmented pars plana of the ciliary body. The posterior border of the pars plana (ora serrata) is a scalloped zone of

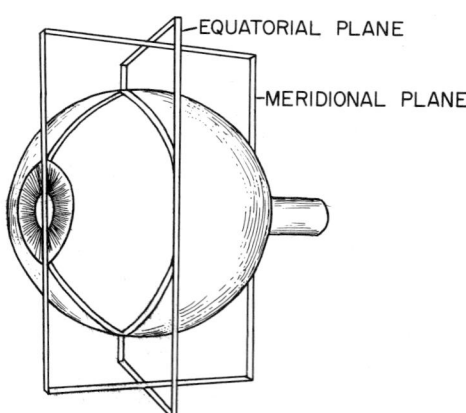

Figure 2-21 Diagram of equatorial and meridional planes of the eye.

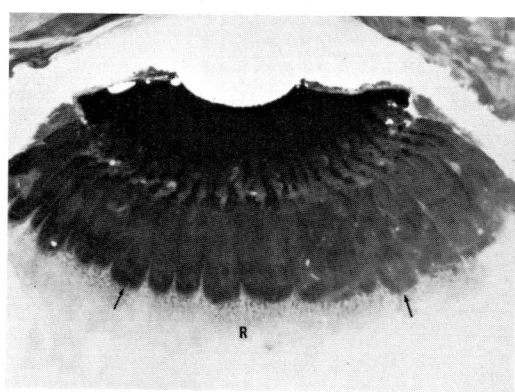

Figure 2-23 Scalloped zone of ora serrata (arrows) marks the junction of the multilayered sensory retina, R, with the single-layered, nonpigmented epithelium of the ciliary body.

transition which marks the histologic termination of the multilayered, sensory retina and its continuation as a single layer of non-pigmented epithelium covering the ciliary body (Fig. 2-23). The periphery of the retina is scalloped, or serrated, in outline, with long, forward projections that extend further anteriorly and are more prominent on the nasal side where the pars plana is shortest. On the temporal side the serrations are poorly developed and difficult to see. The temporal side of the pars plana usually is more heavily pigmented than the nasal side.

Ocular Blood Supply. Several groups of blood vessels, some accompanied by nerves to be described later, supply the eyeball and its contents (Fig. 2-24). They traverse the sclera anteriorly, just posterior to the equator, near the optic nerve. Conveying the vessels and nerves into and out of the globe are scleral emissaria, or canals. These frequently contain uveal melanocytes, especially in deeply pigmented persons. These melanocytes often are visible anteriorly through the conjunctiva as dark pigment spots.

CENTRAL RETINAL ARTERY AND VEIN. These vessels penetrate the optic nerve 8 to 15 mm. posterior to the globe. Along its course within the optic nerve, the central

retinal artery gives off numerous branches to the nerve fibers. It then enters the eye through the scleral foramen near the center of the optic nerve, where it branches outward within the retina.

VORTEX VEINS. Although veins accompany many of the arteries entering the eye anteriorly and posteriorly, veins alone exit the midportion of the globe. The latter, called vortex veins, are usually four in number, and can be seen emerging from the sclera 5 to 8 mm. behind the equator on either side of the vertical meridian superiorly and inferiorly. They quickly join to form the superior and inferior ophthalmic veins.

SHORT POSTERIOR CILIARY ARTERIES. Branches of the ophthalmic artery, numbering about 15 vessels, accompanied by nerves, form a circle around the optic nerve as they pass almost perpendicularly through the sclera to supply the choroid. They are most abundant on the temporal side of the nerve near the posterior pole.

LONG POSTERIOR CILIARY ARTERIES. These two vessels enter the eye on each side of the optic nerve slightly more

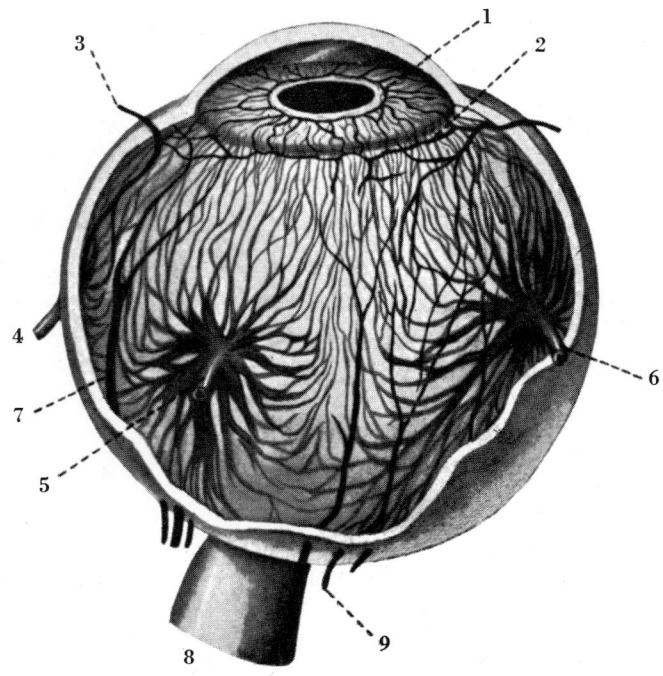

Figure 2-24 Blood vessels of the globe. 1, minor arterial circle; 2, major arterial circle; 3, anterior ciliary artery; 4 to 6, vortex veins; 7, long posterior ciliary artery; 8, optic nerve; 9, short posterior ciliary arteries.

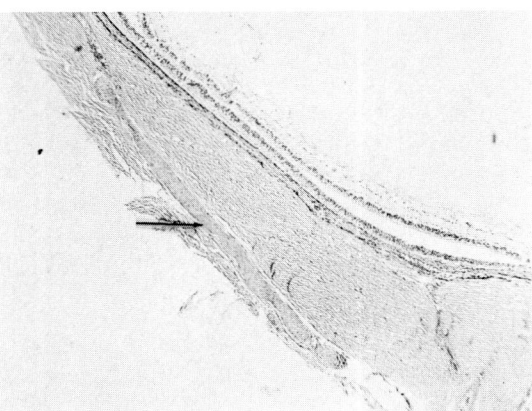

Figure 2-25 Long posterior ciliary artery and nerve (arrow) running an oblique course through the sclera to reach the suprachoroidal space (hematoxylin and eosin, ×22).

anterior than do the short posterior ciliary vessels. They run an oblique course through the sclera to reach the suprachoroidal space just posterior to the equator (Fig. 2-25). They then continue forward to the ciliary body where they anastomose with the anterior ciliary arteries to form the major arterial circle of the iris, which supplies the ciliary body and iris (Fig. 2-15). The nerves and vessels that pass through the canals in the sclera are surrounded by a loose, connective-tissue stroma.

ANTERIOR CILIARY ARTERIES. These are anterior branches of the vessels supplying the rectus muscles. From the tendinous insertions of the muscles, the muscular arteries send branches forward that run a short distance on the surface of the sclera and enter the eyeball at approximately 4 mm. behind the limbus. These vessels, and their site of entrance into the eye, often are visible through the conjunctiva. They may be surrounded by pigment.

THE CORNEA

The transparent cornea forms the window of the eye. Mainly a fibrous tissue, the cornea contains relatively few cells. It is continuous with the sclera at the limbus, the opaque scleral fibers overlapping the cornea fibers slightly at the anterior corneoscleral junction. Corneal transparency is due largely to the special arrangement of cells and collagenous fibrils in an acid mucopolysaccharide environment, and also to an absence of a nutrient vascular bed. The diameter in the adult eye averages 12 mm.; it is about a millimeter greater horizontally than vertically when viewed from the front. The cornea is more circular when seen from behind (in the open eye).

Structure. The cornea is composed of six distinct layers: (1) tear film, (2) epithelium, (3) Bowman's membrane, (4) stroma, (5) Descemet's membrane, and (6) endothelium (Fig. 2-26). The tear film, which covers the eye, is made up of three layers: a posterior layer rich in glycoproteins derived from the goblet cells of the conjunctival epithelium; a middle, watery layer secreted by the lacrimal gland and the accessory lacrimal glands; and an anterior, oily layer secreted by the meibomian glands and the glands of Moll and Zeis. This tear film maintains the proper optical qualities of the cornea. The non-keratinized squamous epithelium of the cornea consists of approximately five layers of stratified cells that are more regularly arranged than squamous epithelium else-

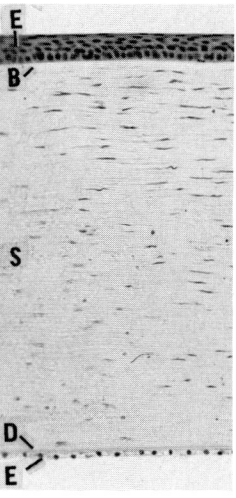

Figure 2-26 Section of normal cornea. E, epithelium; B, Bowman's membrane; S, stroma; D, Descemet's membrane; E, endothelium. The tear film cannot be demonstrated in histologic sections (hematoxylin and eosin, ×115).

where in the body. The most posterior, or basal layer, rests upon a thin, delicate basement membrane, and consists of cuboidal cells with centrally placed nuclei in a slightly basophilic cytoplasm (Fig. 2-27). The cells of this layer may be slightly pigmented in the peripheral area of the cornea, particularly in darkly pigmented races. The layers tend to flatten as they migrate anteriorly until the surface cells are markedly flattened in their anteroposterior diameter, although they may be quite broad across the surface. The epithelial layer is continuous with the epithelial layer of the bulbar conjunctiva that changes appearance at the limbus (Fig. 2-14).

The epithelium and its basement membrane rest on Bowman's membrane, which is a modified layer of the anterior corneal stroma (Fig. 2-28). A homogeneous layer without cells, Bowman's membrane has no capacity to regenerate.

The remainder of the stroma is made up of collagenous lamellae that are slightly oblique to one another beneath Bowman's layer, but with an increasingly parallel

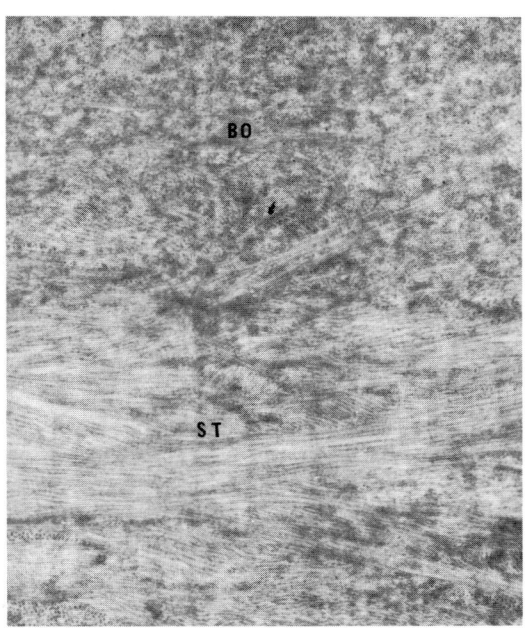

Figure 2-28 Electron micrograph showing the transition between the "homogeneous" Bowman's membrane, BO, and the first regularly arranged bundles of collagen (anterior) that make up the corneal stroma, ST (×16,500). (Courtesy of Ben S. Fine, M.D.)

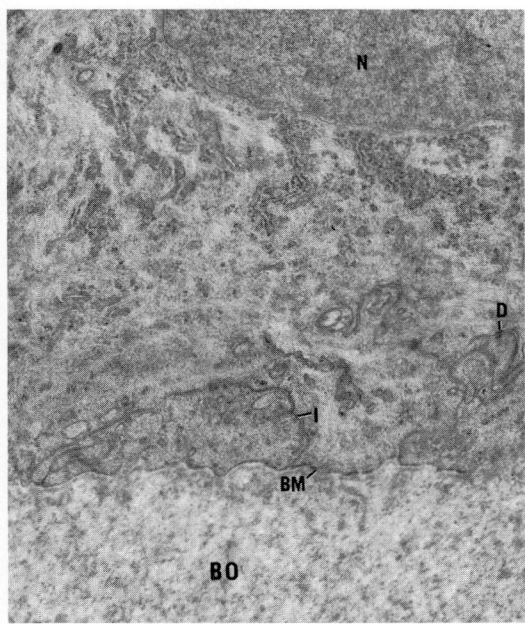

Figure 2-27 Electron micrograph showing a corneal basal epithelial cell with its basement membrane, BM, separating the cell from Bowman's membrane, BO. N, portion of cell nucleus; I, intercellular spaces; D, desmosomal attachment plaque (×16,000). (Courtesy of Ben S. Fine, M.D.)

arrangement as they approach Descemet's membrane. The corneal cells ("keratocytes" or "corneal corpuscles") are relatively few and lie between the stromal lamellae. They are marked by their prominent, elongated nuclei and generally are considered to be fibrocytes.

Descemet's membrane is totally different from Bowman's membrane in that it is a cuticular product developed from the endothelial cells and can be regenerated. Like other basement membranes, Descemet's has a strong affinity for PAS stain. It is somewhat elastic and is more resistant than the remainder of the cornea to trauma and disease.

The corneal endothelium is actually a mesothelium. It consists of a single layer of flattened cuboidal cells that ends as a cuboidal layer at Schwalbe's line.

Blood Vessels and Nerves. There are no blood vessels in the cornea except at the limbus where fine capillary loops from the anterior ciliary vessels pass into the cornea to form the limbal arcade. The size of this arcade varies in normal individuals, and it is difficult to distinguish some early pathologic processes from slight, normal variations. Any other blood vessels found in the cornea, with or without blood in their lumen, are pathologic.

The corneal nerves are branches of the ciliary nerves. They enter the cornea at the limbus and, under magnification, can be followed for some distance into the cornea. As they radiate toward the center, fine branches penetrate Bowman's membrane and terminate between the epithelial cells. Although the cornea is extremely sensitive, the corneal nerves do not supply it with all forms of sensation. Pain and cold receptors are abundant, but not heat or touch receptors.

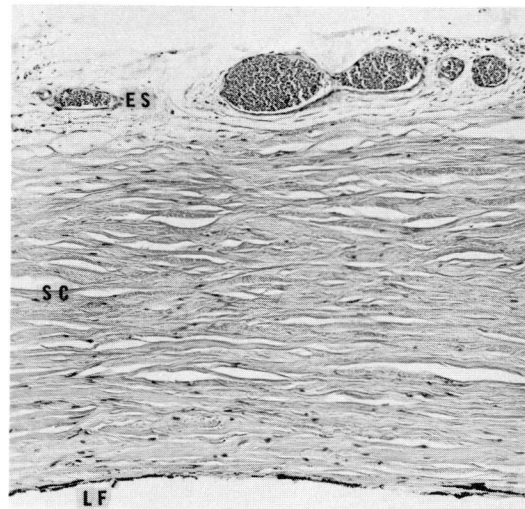

Figure 2-29 Section of normal sclera. ES, episclera; SC, sclera; LF, lamina fusca (melanocytic layer) (hematoxylin and eosin, ×100).

THE SCLERA

The sclera is opaque and white, rather than clear like the cornea, due to the haphazard large collagen fibrils and to its relatively hydrated state (turgescence). Turgescence can be demonstrated by a large degree of clearing with considerable transparency after a dehydrating substance is used.

Structure. The sclera is composed of three layers: (1) the outer, or episclera; (2) the sclera proper; and (3) the inner lamina fusca (melanocytic layer) (Fig. 2-29). The episclera, a filmy, highly vascular, connective tissue, loosely attaches Tenon's capsule (the fascia bulbi) to the sclera. The episclera is thickest and best developed anterior to the attachments of the recti muscles. It is differentiated from the sclera by its looser texture, and from Tenon's capsule by its rich vascularity.

The sclera proper is a relatively avascular, thick, fibrous tunic of collagen that contains considerable elastic tissue. This strong outer coat supports and protects the inner structures of the eye. The sclera is basically extracellular tissue having a rich, and apparently endless, random interdigitation

of collagen fibers. The space, or interstitium, between the collagen fibers is occupied by a ground substance that contains acid mucopolysaccharides. Occasional scleral cells (fibrocytes) are seen between the collagen bundles. These cells probably secrete not only the collagen but also the ground substance. Uveal melanocytes often are seen within the scleral stroma, particularly in deeply pigmented people.

If the sclera is dissected from the choroid, its inner surface is seen as a light brown color; hence the name lamina fusca. This lamina marks the transition zone from the inner layers of the sclera to the outer layers of the uvea or suprauvea. The brown color is due to numerous uveal melanocytes adhering to, and within, the internal scleral collagen bundles.

The thickness of the sclera varies considerably in individual eyes and in different regions of the same eye. It is approximately 1 mm. thick posteriorly, and gradually thins to about 0.3 mm. just posterior to the insertions of the recti muscles. Just anterior to the area of the insertion of the recti muscles, it swells to 0.6 mm. and remains so to the limbus. The anterior sclera adjacent to the limbus contains part of the drainage mechanism for aqueous humor. The optic nerve leaves the eye at the posterior aspect of the globe, nasal to the posterior pole, through the scleral canal or foramen.

This canal is about 1.5 mm. in diameter anteriorly and 3 to 4 mm. posteriorly and, therefore, appears as a short segment of a cone with the narrow end facing anteriorly.

THE UVEAL TRACT

The uveal tract, made up of the iris, ciliary body, and choroid, runs from the pupillary border to the optic nerve. Its most important function is to supply nourishment to the globe.

The Iris

The iris is a layer of delicate tissue that arises from the ciliary body and divides the aqueous compartment into an anterior and a posterior chamber (Fig. 2-30). Many dehiscences or holes (iris crypts) are found in the loose iris stroma (Fig. 2-31). Frequently the stroma is more compact at the anterior surface than elsewhere in the iris and forms an anterior border layer, which, in heavily pigmented persons, has an easily visible, abrupt termination at the iris root. Normally the anterior surface has no lining of any sort (Fig. 2-32), allowing the stroma to communicate freely with the aqueous in

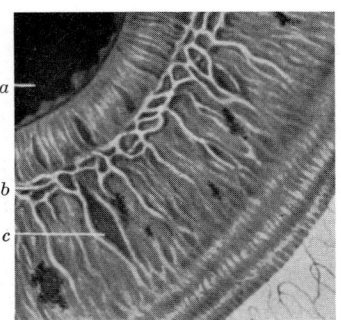

Figure 2-31 Surface of normal iris. A, pigment seam; B, collarette; C, iris crypt.

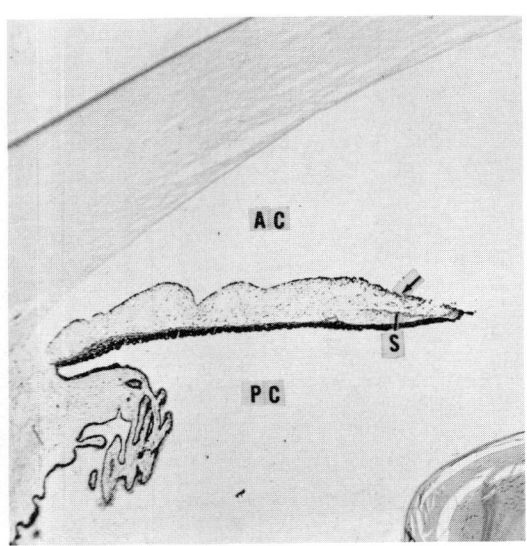

Figure 2-30 The iris (arrow) divides the aqueous compartment into an anterior chamber, AC, and a posterior chamber, PC. S, sphincter pupillae (hematoxylin and eosin, ×22).

the anterior chamber. The posterior surface of the iris is lined by two layers of epithelium: a partially pigmented anterior layer, and a completely pigmented posterior layer (Fig. 2-33). Both layers run forward to the pupillary margin of the iris, where the pigment layer may be seen from the front as a ring forming the pigment seam, or ruff, of the pupil. Nodular thickenings of this seam can be seen in normal eyes.

The iris forms a diaphragm whose aperture, the pupil, changes size, thereby controlling the amount of light admitted to the eye. The size of the pupil varies widely among persons and at different ages. In infancy the pupils are small; they reach their largest size during childhood and early adulthood, and shrink again in old age. In general, eyes with light irides have wider pupils than those with dark. The pupil is never at rest, and, because of constant changes of tonus of the sphincter and dilator muscles, the pupil shows what is called the "normal play of the pupil." Marked play of the pupil is spoken of as hippus. Factors offsetting pupillary size are: illumination, changes of gaze, vascular filling, and psychic factors. In evaluating such pupillary reactions as light reflex, care must be taken to eliminate extraneous factors. During sleep the pupil contracts because the cortical impulses that inhibit the sphincter or stimulate the dilator are diminished. Dilatation of the pupil is called mydriasis; contraction is called miosis. Both pupils usually are the same size, but in 20

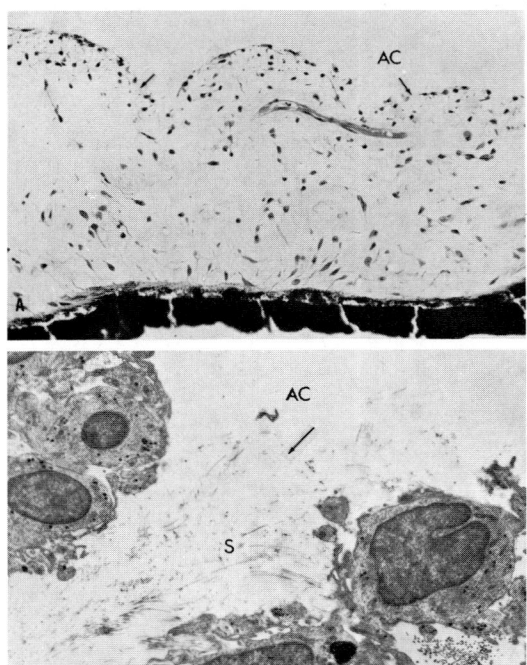

Figure 2-32 *(A)* No lining is present on anterior surface of iris (arrows) (hematoxylin and eosin, ×200). AC, anterior chamber. *(B)* Electron micrograph of the anterior surface of iris to show one of the many apertures (arrow) that may be present in the anterior border layer. Stroma (S) communicates freely with anterior chamber (AC). The surface cells are discontinuous and resemble the cells of deeper iris stroma (×5400). (Courtesy of Ben S. Fine, M.D.)

pupillary border (Fig. 2-30). Of neuroectodermal origin, as are the erector pili of the skin, this muscle is innervated by parasympathetic nerve fibers that originate in the Edinger-Westphal nucleus, a small-celled nucleus at the anterior aspect of the third nerve nucleus. The fibers accompany the third nerve into the orbit and are carried by the branch that goes to the inferior oblique muscle. They shortly branch off like a small twig to arrive at the ciliary ganglion, where a synapse occurs. Fibers from the ciliary ganglion enter the eye by way of the short ciliary nerves. There is some evidence that the sphincter muscle is also supplied with inhibitory fibers by way of the sympathetic nerves.

The dilator muscle is composed of smooth muscle fibers derived from the anterior part of the partially pigmented, or anterior, layer of iris epithelium (Fig. 2-33). Also of neuroectodermal origin, it runs radially in the peripheral portions of the iris, and when it contracts the pupil dilates. It is supplied by sympathetic nerves that probably arise in the cortex, descend into the hypothalamus, and enter the central gray matter around the aqueduct of Sylvius. The fibers reach Budge's ciliospinal center and then leave the spinal cord with the eighth cervical and first thoracic segments to enter the cervical sympathetic chain. They then ascend in this chain to the superior cervical ganglion, where a new synapse is located. Fibers from this ganglion ascend with the internal carotid plexus to

to 25 per cent of normal individuals the size differs slightly. If the change is marked, the condition is called anisocoria. In corectopia there is congenital displacement of the pupil so that it is eccentric. In polycoria there are multiple pupils, because the iris has more than one opening.

The size of the pupil depends to a great extent upon the balance of tone between two opposing muscles that obey the rule of reciprocal innervation: the sphincter pupillae, supplied by the third nerve, or the parasympathetic nervous system; and the dilator pupillae, supplied by the sympathetic nervous system (Figs. 2-34 and 2-35). The sphincter muscle, a 1 mm. band of smooth muscle that encircles the pupil, is embedded in the iris stroma close to the

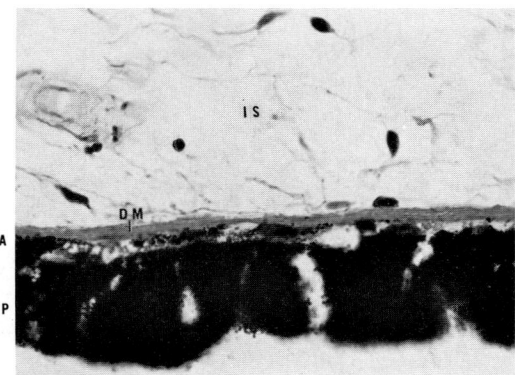

Figure 2-33 Pigment epithelium of the iris consists of: A, a partially pigmented anterior layer containing dilator muscle, DM, in the anterior portion, and P, a completely pigmented posterior layer. IS, iris stroma (hematoxylin and eosin, ×750).

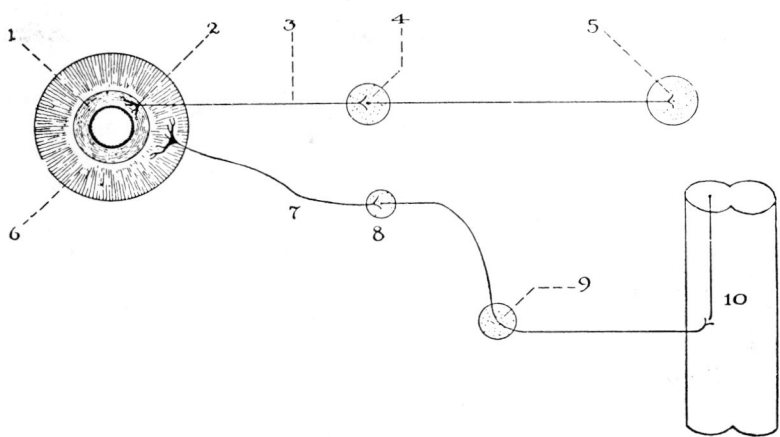

Figure 2-34 The nerve supply to the iris. 1, sphincter muscle; 2, myoneural junction of third nerve; 3, third nerve fiber; 4, ciliary ganglion; 5, cells in third nerve nucleus governing the sphincter; 6, dilator muscle; 7, sympathetic nerve supply; 8, superior cervical ganglion; 9, thoracic sympathetic ganglion; 10, spinal cord. (Adler: *Clinical Physiology of the Eye*. The Macmillan Co., New York.)

Figure 2-35 The sympathetic nerve supply to the eye. a, subthalamic center; b, cortical center in the frontal lobe; c, sensory nucleus of the 5th cranial nerve; d, unstriped muscle in the orbit; e, fiber to the dilator pupillae; f, superior and inferior palpebral unstriped muscle; g, plexus around carotid artery; h, superior cervical sympathetic nerve; i, superior cervical ganglion; k, middle cervical ganglion; l, inferior cervical ganglion; m, Budge's ciliospinal center; gg, gasserian ganglion. (Adler: *Clinical Physiology of the Eye*. The Macmillan Co., New York.)

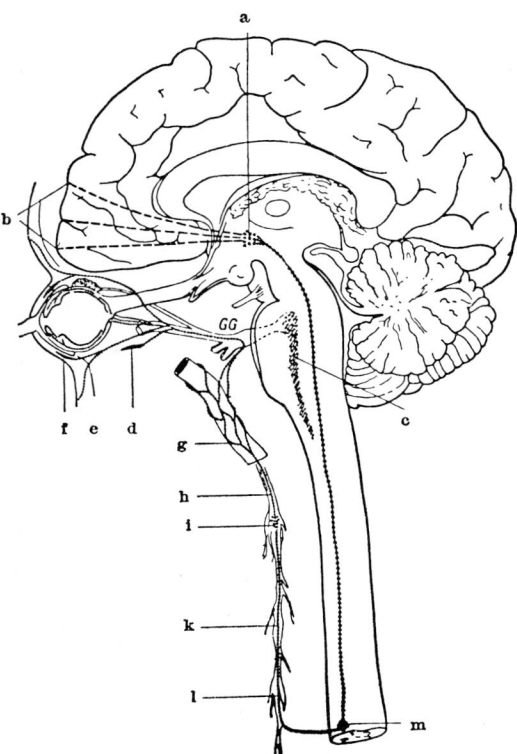

enter the skull. Intracranially they join the first division of the fifth nerve and form part of the nasociliary nerve with which they travel to the orbit; there they are given off as the two long posterior ciliary nerves, which enter the eye on each side of the optic nerve.

The Ciliary Body

The ciliary epithelium produces aqueous humor, and the ciliary muscle enables accommodation, or the changing of the focus of the eye, to take place. The ciliary body is triangular in shape, 6 to 6.5 mm. long, with its apex at the ora serrata and its base facing anteriorly, the latter forming the anterior face of the ciliary body (Fig. 2-36) from which the iris originates. Posteriorly at the ora serrata, the ciliary body becomes continuous with the choroid. Uveal melanocytes are present in the stroma and within the muscles of the ciliary body.

The two parts of the ciliary body are the corona ciliaris (pars plicata), which occupies the anterior 2 mm. and contains the ciliary processes, and the orbicularis ciliaris (pars plana), which forms the posterior 4 to 4.5 mm., or flat part, of the ciliary body. The ciliary body is covered on its inner as-

pect by two layers of epithelium; the inner, nonpigmented layer is continuous with the sensory retina, and the outer, pigmented layer is continuous with the retinal pigment epithelium. At the anterior aspect of the ciliary body, the same two layers continue forward to form the epithelial layers of the iris. In the region of the first ciliary process, however, the inner layer of nonpigmented ciliary epithelium abruptly becomes, and remains, pigmented over the iris.

The ciliary body (Fig. 2-36) is made up of at least six layers: (1) the suprachoroidal potential space, (2) the ciliary muscle, (3) the layer of vessels, (4) the external basement membrane, (5) the epithelium, and (6) the internal basement membrane ("membrane limitans interna"). The muscles consist of two distinct groups and a third, vaguely defined group. The innermost layer is the round, or radial, muscle. This lies just posterior to the iris root. The outermost layer is the meridional, or longitudinal, muscle that runs from its fixed point at the scleral spur to the nonfixed choroid. Between these two prominent muscle bands are the oblique muscles of the ciliary body. When the round muscle contracts, it acts as a sphincter and shortens the diameter from the ciliary processes on one side of the eye to the other, thereby relaxing the zonular fibers. Likewise, when the meridional muscle contracts (since the scleral spur is the fixed point), it shortens the ciliary body and also relaxes the zonular fibers; the oblique muscles have a similar action. All three muscle bundles, therefore, by relaxing the zonular fibers, release the tension on the elastic lens capsule and allow the lens to become more spherical. This increases the optic power of the eye (more "plus") and permits focusing on near objects (accommodation). By pulling on the trabecula beyond the scleral spur, the ciliary muscle may also play a significant role in the normal drainage of aqueous humor from the eye.

The Choroid

The choroid, whose gross structure resembles a honeycomb of blood channels, includes the remainder of the uveal tract extending from the ora serrata to the optic

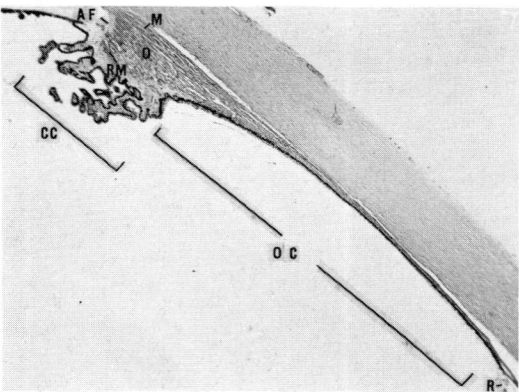

Figure 2-36 Section of normal ciliary body. AF, anterior face; CC, corona ciliaris (pars plicata); OC, orbicularis ciliaris (pars plana); M, meridional muscle; O, oblique muscle; RM, round muscle; R, retina (hematoxylin and eosin, ×26).

nerve. It nourishes the outer layers of the retina and conducts nerves and arteries to the anterior portions of the eye. Excess light may be absorbed by the pigment of the choroid. In times of inflammation the entire uveal tract, including the choroid, may act as a lymph node to combat infection via the proliferation of lymphocytes and plasma cells, and the elaboration of antibodies.

The choroid varies from 0.22 mm. in the region of the posterior pole to 0.1 to 0.15 mm. toward the periphery. At least five layers can be recognized: (1) the suprachoroid, which loosely attaches the choroid to the sclera; (2) a layer of large vessels (Haller's layer), which is fed by the fifteen or more short ciliary arteries; (3) a layer of vessels of medium caliber (Sattler's layer); (4) the choriocapillaris; and (5) Bruch's membrane (Fig. 2-37). The choroid is most loosely attached to the sclera anteriorly, where choroidal detachments are most apt to occur. Although muscular arteries are present in the two outermost vessel layers of Haller and Sattler, veins predominate and empty into the four vortex veins. There is free anastomosis between the anterior and posterior ciliary arteries. The caliber of the capillaries of the choriocapillaris is probably the largest of any in the body. In the posterior aspect of the eye, especially at the posterior pole, the capillaries are somewhat smaller, more compact, and more numerous than they are in the peripheral portion of the eye.

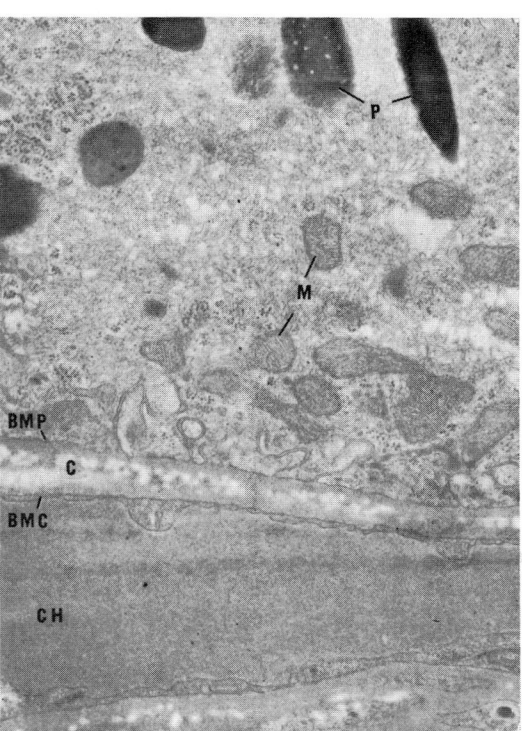

Figure 2-38 Electron micrograph showing region of Bruch's membrane (rabbit). Basement membranes of the retinal pigment epithelial cells, BMP, and of the endothelial cells of the choriocapillaris, BMC, are separated by collagenous material, C. CH, choriocapillaris; M, mitochondria in retinal pigment epithelial cell; P, pigment granules (×24,000). (Courtesy of Ben S. Fine, M.D.)

Bruch's membrane is a thin membrane of three parts. Outermost is the basement membrane of the endothelium of the choriocapillaris. The innermost, or cuticular, portion is the basement membrane of the pigment epithelium of the retina (Fig. 2-38). Between the two is mesenchymal tissue, mainly composed of loose collagen and elastin.

Uveal melanocytes, fibroblasts, and mast cells are scattered throughout the choroid, as well as the entire uveal tract. The degree of choroidal pigmentation varies considerably. Negroes, Asiatics, and other heavily pigmented people tend to have deeply pigmented choroids. Lightly pigmented people with blond hair and blue

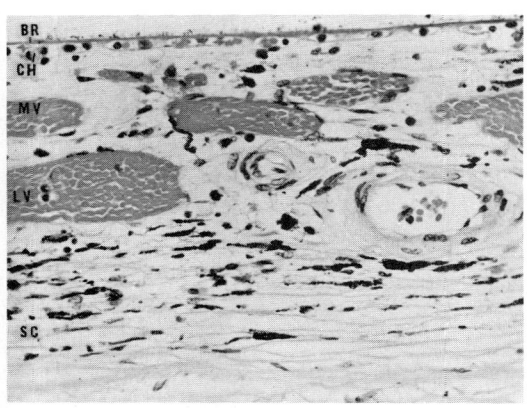

Figure 2-37 Section of normal choroid. SC, suprachoroid; LV, large vessels (Haller's layer); MV, medium vessels (Sattler's layer); CH, choriocapillaris; BR, Bruch's membrane (hematoxylin and eosin, ×360).

eyes tend to have lightly pigmented choroids. The nerve supply is derived from the short posterior ciliary and also from some of the long anterior ciliary nerves. Cells resembling those of ganglia of the central nervous system also are found scattered through the choroid.

THE RETINA

The retina, or innermost layer of the eye, is a thin, delicate, transparent sheet of tissue derived from neuroectoderm. A sensory structure, it contains cells that respond to visual stimuli by a photochemical reaction. The retina measures about 0.4 mm. at the border of the optic nerve and tends to become thinner toward the periphery until it reaches approximately 0.14 mm. at the ora serrata. This increasing thinness is rather continuous in all quadrants of the retina except temporally over the macula, where, except for the thin avascular fovea, it stays 0.4 mm. until it reaches the peripheral portions of the macula; it then thins to correspond to the other retinal quadrants.

Layers of the Retina. The retina has at least ten recognizable layers: (1) pigment epithelium; (2) visual cells, i.e., rods and cones; (3) external limiting membrane; (4) outer nuclear layer; (5) outer plexiform layer, which includes the Henle nerve fiber layer, the middle limiting membrane, and the plexiform portion; (6) inner nuclear layer; (7) inner plexiform layer; (8) layer of ganglion cells; (9) nerve fiber layer; and (10) internal limiting membrane (Fig. 2-39).

The pigment epithelium, derived from neuroectoderm, is continuous with the pigment epithelium of the ciliary body at the ora serrata. It is a single layer of hexagonal cells having a remarkably regular, mosaic pattern when viewed in flat preparations (Fig. 2-40). They adhere to one another by a series of strong attachments called terminal bars, and they secrete the cuticular portion of Bruch's membrane (basement membrane). The large elliptical pigment granules are densest in the macular area

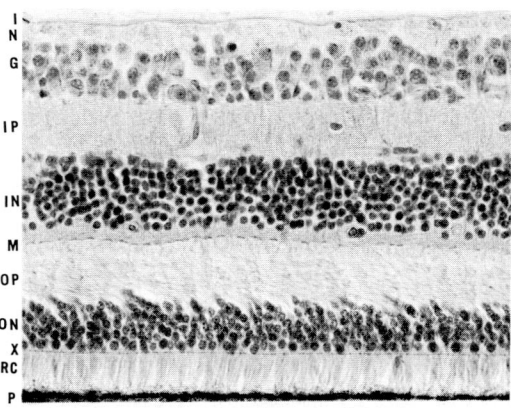

Figure 2-39 Section of normal retina. P, pigmentary epithelium; RC, rods and cones; X, external limiting membrane; ON, outer nuclear layer; OP, outer plexiform layer containing M, middle limiting membrane; IN, inner nuclear layer; IP, inner plexiform layer; G, ganglion cell layer; N, nerve fiber layer; I, internal limiting membrane (hematoxylin and eosin, ×300).

and in the periphery. Pleomorphic cells, including binucleate forms, may be present in the periphery.

Light must traverse most of the retinal layers in order to reach and to stimulate the second layer, the layer of rods and cones. Cones function best in bright light and mediate not only vision but also color. In the central areas of the retina, cones are more numerous than rods. In the fovea itself, the area of most acute vision, only special cones are present. In contrast, rods are most numerous in the periphery of the retina, except at the extreme periphery where they are replaced by poorly formed cones. Since rods are extremely light sensi-

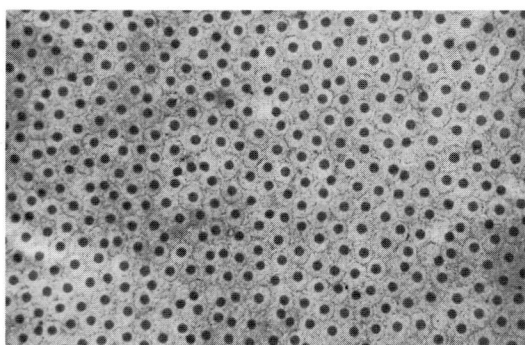

Figure 2-40 Flat preparation of retinal pigment epithelium (adult monkey) (×250). (Ts'o, M.O.M., and Friedman, E.: *Arch. Ophth. 78*:642, 1967.)

tive, they function best in reduced illumination.

The external limiting membrane is not a true membrane but a series of dashes formed by the terminal bar attachments of the cell bodies of rods, cones, and Müller's cells (Fig. 2-41*A*). The parts of the rods and cones that extend beyond this external limiting membrane are generally subdivided into two segments, the outer and the inner (Fig. 2-41*B*). The outer nuclear layer is actually the nuclei of these rods and cones. The outer plexiform layer, composed of the axons of the rods and cones, contains synapses in its inner third only; this inner zone is the only truly plexiform portion of the layer. For the axons of the rods and cones to reach their respective bipolar cells from the area of the fovea, they must take a tangential or oblique course. This unique axonal orientation often is referred to as the nerve fiber layer of Henle, and helps to explain the peculiar arrangement of exudates (a star figure) that radiate out from the fovea in certain pathologic conditions such as malignant hypertension. The

middle limiting membrane is not a continuous membrane but a series of dots and dashes formed by synaptic and desmosomal attachments in the plexiform region of the inner third of the outer plexiform layer (Fig. 2-42).

The nuclei of the bipolar cells, Müller's cells, horizontal cells, and amacrine cells form the inner nuclear layer. The inner plexiform layer is composed of the axons of the bipolar cells and the dendrites of the ganglion cells. The ganglion cells form a continuous, single layer of cells throughout most of the retina. In the area of the macula they form a four- to six-cell layer. The layers diminish abruptly at the fovea where ganglion cells and all layers of the retina, except for the layer of rods and cones, the external limiting membrane, and the outer nuclear layer, have been displaced.

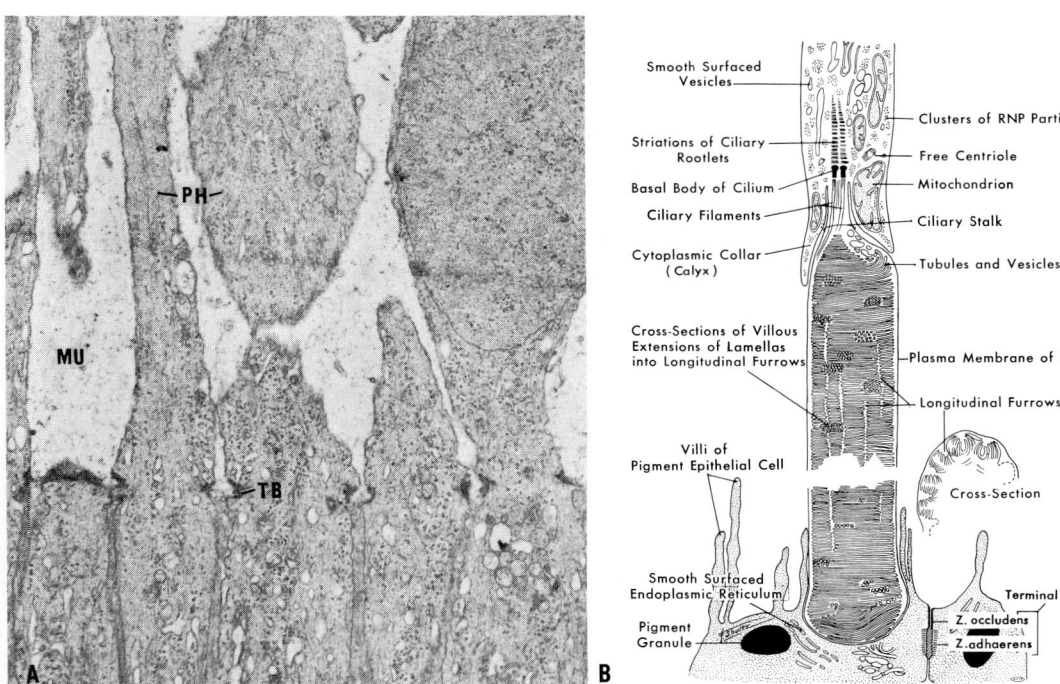

Figure 2-41 *(A)* Electron micrograph showing external limiting membrane made up of terminal bars, TB. Internally, the Müller cell cytoplasm, MU, is easily distinguished from the photoreceptor cells, PH, in the outer nuclear layer (×7,000). (Courtesy of Ben S. Fine, M.D.) *(B)* Diagram showing parts of the photoreceptors that extend beyond (are external to) the external limiting membrane. (Fine, in McPherson: *New and Controversial Aspects of Retinal Detachment.* Hoeber Medical Division, Harper and Row, New York.)

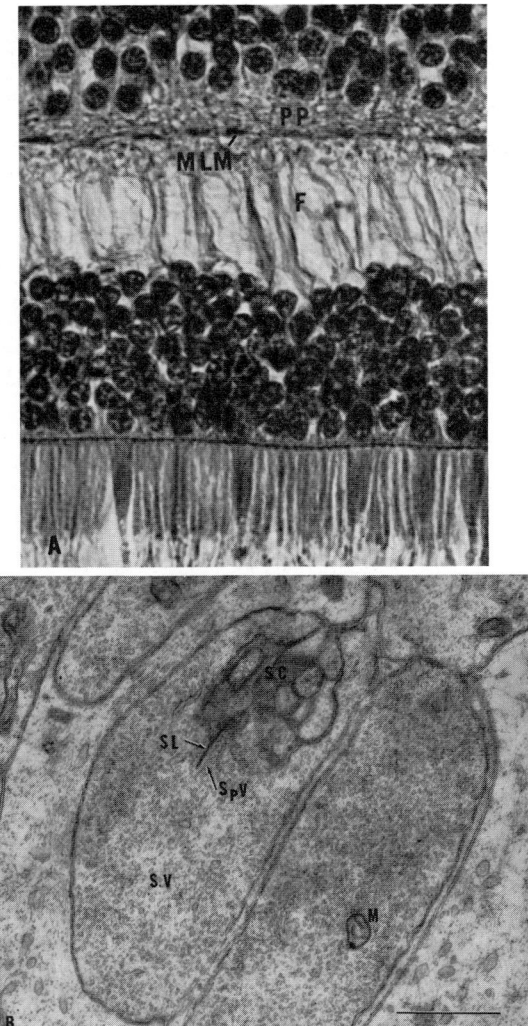

Figure 2-42 *(A)* Middle limiting membrane, MLM, seen as a series of dashes, limits the outer boundary of the plexiform portion, PP, of the outer plexiform layer. The remainder of this layer is predominantly seen as fibers, F, (hematoxylin and eosin, ×520). (Courtesy of Ben S. Fine, M.D.) *(B)* Electron micrograph showing rod spherule synaptic terminal expansion from the nasal retina. The complex synaptic invagination by the connector cell is seen at the inner pole, SC. The synaptic expansion is filled with small vesicles, called synaptic vesicles, SV. The dense plate, or lamella, SL, is seen in cross section. A specially segregated grouping or layer of synaptic vesicles, SpV, forms a "halo" around this synaptic lamella (×22,860). (Fine, B. S.: *J. Neuropath. & Exper. Neurol. 22*:255, 1963.)

The ganglion cells send their fibers toward the optic disc to form the nerve fiber layer of the retina. Ultimately these fibers make up the optic nerve. The internal limiting membrane of the retina is a basement membrane, presumably secreted by the retinal Müller's cells. These cells, which are modified astrocytes, are oriented perpendicular to the surface of the retina. Their cytoplasm is more fibrous in their inner aspects, and much more loosely arranged in their outer aspects. They store glycogen and may give structural support to the retina.

Visual Pathway. The neurons in the visual pathway may be compared with those of common sensation (Fig. 2-43). For example, three neurons form the pathway of such common sensations as the sense of pain and of temperature. Special end organs in the skin conduct the sensations to the first neuron of this pathway, which is located in the spinal ganglion. The first neuron connects the sensory end organ to a cell in the gray matter of the posterior gray column of the spinal cord. Dorsal root fibers transmit the impulses, sometimes mediated through one or more intercalated neurons, to the neurons of the second order found in the posterior gray column. Their axons cross almost immedi-

ately over the medial plane and ascend in the lateral spinothalamic tract to end in the posterolateral ventral nucleus of the thalamus. The third and last neuron begins with a cell in this thalamic nucleus; its fiber runs from this point by way of the thalamic radiation and the posterior limb of the internal capsule to its appropriate cell station in the cerebral cortex of the posterior central gyrus.

In the retinocalcarine pathway, three other neurons are associated in a similar combination. The sensory end organs, or receptors, consist of the rods and cones that transform light stimulation into nerve impulses. The first neuron, located in the outer nuclear layer, corresponds to the neuron of the spinal ganglion. The bipolar and ganglion cells can be considered the second order neurons; the bipolar cells would correspond to the intercalated neurons in the relay from the first order neurons in the spinal ganglion to the second order neurons in the gray matter of the spinal column; the retinal ganglion cells would correspond to the second main neu-

THE OPTIC NERVE

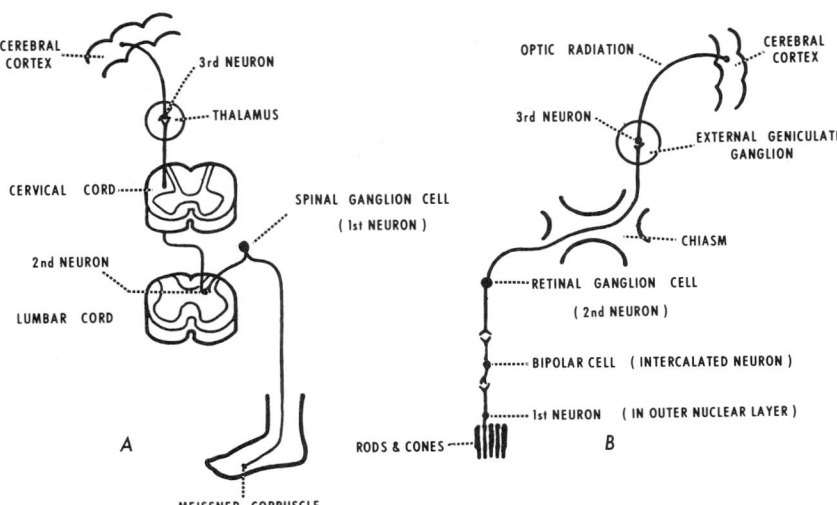

Figure 2-43 (*A*) Neurons in the pathway of common sensation. (*B*) Neurons in the visual pathway. (Modified from Adler, F. H.: *Ann. Surg. 101*:2, 1935.)

ron, whose fibers form the optic nerve and the optic tract. As these fibers ascend to the lateral geniculate body, about 60 to 85 per cent of them cross to the opposite side at the optic chiasm. These fibers form a retino-geniculate tract that is analogous to the spinothalamic tract of the common sensory pathway. The third order neurons are in the lateral geniculate body. Their fibers run by way of the optic radiation to the occipital cortex, ending in area 17 around the calcarine fissure. These geniculate neurons and their tract correspond to the thalamic neurons and the thalamic radiations of the common sensory pathway.

Vessels. The vessels of the retina are derived from the central retinal artery and vein. After entering the retina near the optic disc, the artery quickly loses its internal elastic lamina and its continuous muscular layer, and becomes an arteriole. The retinal arterioles tend to have right angle branching in the posterior portion of the eye, and dichotomous, or Y-shaped branching, toward the periphery. Between the arterioles and the venules is a rich capillary network (Fig. 2-44). The capillaries are freely anastomotic and most numerous posteriorly, particularly at the posterior pole. In the region of the fovea, however,

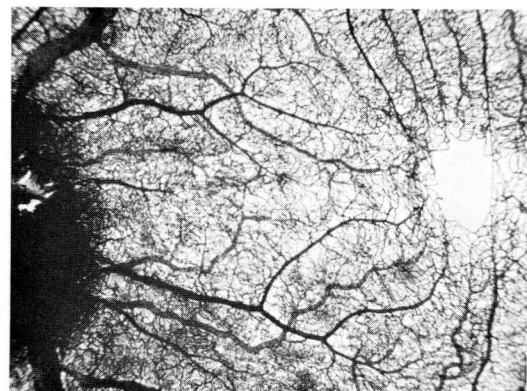

Figure 2-45 Trypsin-digested preparation of retina. The foveal area on the right is devoid of capillaries; the optic disc on the left appears black (periodic acid–Schiff, ×22).

there are no capillaries (Fig. 2-45). The foveal area is supplied entirely by the underlying choriocapillaris of the choroid and the surrounding capillaries of the macular region of the retina. If the retina surrounding the fovea becomes semi-opaque, such as in occlusion of the central retinal artery or in some of the lipid storage diseases (e.g., Tay-Sachs), the choroid underlying the thin avascular fovea then appears as a bright red spot, the so-called cherry red spot of the macula.

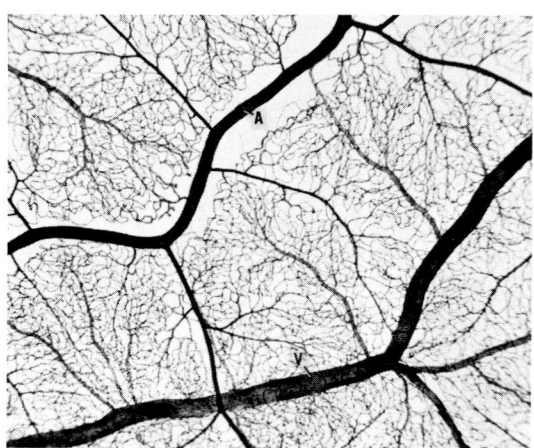

Figure 2-44 Trypsin-digested preparation of retina. Retinal arterioles, A, are distinguished from the retinal venules, V, by their darker color, smaller caliber, and characteristic capillary-free zone. A rich, anastomotic capillary network connects the arterioles to the venules (periodic acid-Schiff, ×26).

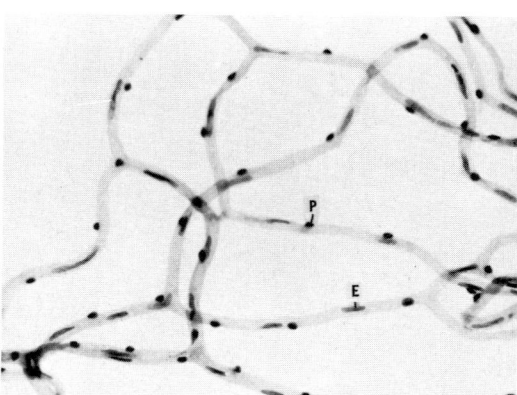

Figure 2-46 Trypsin-digested preparation of retina. There is an approximate 1:1 ratio of the smaller, darker, rounded pericytes, P, to the lighter, oval endothelial cells, E., of the capillaries (periodic acid–Schiff, ×325). (Yanoff, M.: *New England J. Med. 274:* 1348, 1966.)

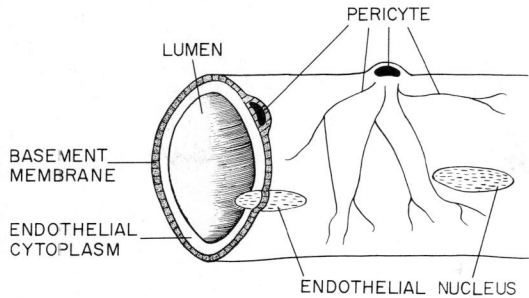

Figure 2-47 Diagram of a retinal capillary tube showing basement membrane material covering endothelial cells externally and surrounding pericytes completely.

The retinal capillaries contain two types of cells (Fig. 2-46). Innermost are endothelial cells, whose cytoplasm makes up the lining, or wall, of the capillaries. On the surface (outside) of the capillaries are the pericytes. When stained with silver, the cytoplasm of these cells appears to surround the capillary completely or partially. Basement membrane surrounds the endothelial cells externally and the pericytes completely. The capillaries, therefore, are tubes completely surrounded by basement membrane material (Fig. 2-47). The arterioles and venules course through the nerve fiber and ganglion cell layers parallel to the surface of the retina. The capillaries arise from the arterioles perpendicular to the surface of the retina and dip down into the retina as far as the middle limiting membrane of the outer plexiform layer. Around the arterioles is a wide, capillary-free zone. A similar, but much smaller, zone surrounds the venules.

THE OPTIC NERVE

Structure. The optic nerve is not a true nerve like a peripheral nerve, but is actually a nerve fiber tract whose fibers are derived from the ganglion cells of the retina. Although composed of the usual axons and myelin sheaths, these fibers entirely lack the neurolemmal sheaths characteristic of peripheral nerves. Instead of being separated from one another by neurolemmal sheaths, the optic nerve fibers are separated by scattered neuroglia cells. In this respect the fibers resemble the white substance of the brain and spinal cord, which also is formed by myelinated fibers devoid of any neurolemmal sheaths. Since the optic nerve is the second neuronal pathway (tract) along the path of conduction, it is subject to the same diseases that affect such tracts in the central nervous system and reacts similarly to disease processes.

Sheaths of the Optic Nerve. The optic nerve also differs from peripheral nerves in that it is surrounded by continuations of the meningeal sheaths that encase the brain: the dura, the pia, and the arachnoid. At the

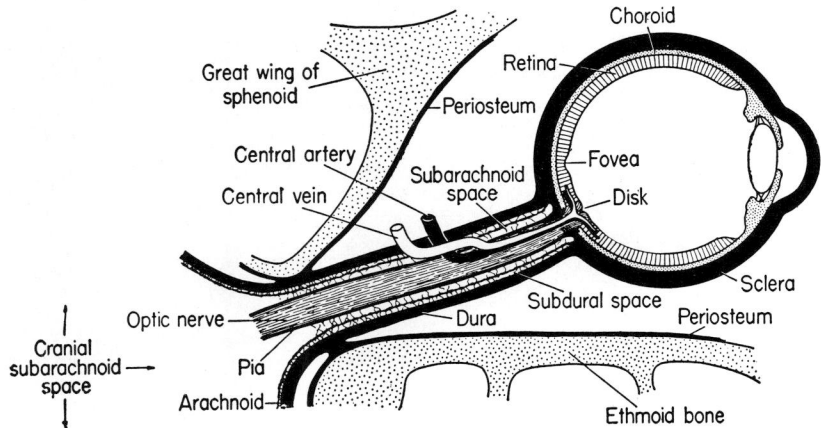

Figure 2-48 Diagram showing the continuity between the sheaths of the optic nerve and the sheaths of the brain, and the continuity between the cranial subarachnoid space and that around the optic nerve. Note how the central vessels cross the space and may be compressed if the intracranial pressure is raised, thus producing papilledema. (Adler: *Physiology of the Eye.* The C. V. Mosby Co., St. Louis, Mo.)

optic canal the dural sheath splits into two layers. One layer becomes continuous with the periosteum of the orbit, and the other adheres closely to, and follows, the optic nerve itself, finally becoming indistinguishable from the outer layers of the sclera (Fig. 2-48). The subarachnoid and the subdural spaces of the optic nerve communicate with those of the brain. The central retinal artery and vein cross these spaces to enter the nerve anywhere from 8 to 15 mm. behind the globe. Before entering the nerve, the vein frequently runs for some distance between the arachnoid and pia mater in the subarachnoid space whereas the artery generally takes a shorter course (Fig. 2-48).

FUNCTIONAL LOSS. Optic nerve fibers, like all other nerves, degenerate if the connections with their cell bodies are severed; their lack of neurolemmal sheaths, however, renders them incapable of meaningful regeneration. In addition, function may be interrupted without actual division or degeneration of the nerve. Great functional loss, even total loss of sight, may result from tumors in the orbit or inside the skull pressing on the nerve. When this pressure is removed, recovery of vision may be rapid, probably due to return of an adequate circulation.

Vascular Supply. The central retinal artery and vein penetrate the optic nerve posterior to the disc. In its course through the optic nerve, the artery gives off numerous branches that supply the nerve fibers. The vascular supply to the optic nerve is extraordinarily rich, especially at the intraocular end of the optic nerve where the retinal system anastomoses with branches of the ciliary or choroidal system to form the circle of Zinn-Haller. This network, located near the disc, helps to account for the characteristic pink color of the normal disc, as seen with an ophthalmoscope.

THE OCULAR CONTENTS

The space within the eye is occupied by the vitreous, the lens, and the aqueous humor.

The vitreous compartment contains the vitreous body and makes up the greatest volume of the eye. The body is a clear, jelly-like substance which not only offers support to the structures within the eye, but helps maintain the transparency of the media. The "face" of the vitreous (anterior hyaloid) and the lens separate the vitreous from the aqueous compartments.

Structure. A biphasic structure, the vitreous body is composed of a delicate, collagenous skeleton associated with a hydrophilic acid mucopolysaccharide, hyaluronic acid (Fig. 2-49). A precise balance between the acid mucopolysaccharide and the collagen preserves the structure of the vitreous. Any breakdown between these two components results in vitreous disease. Delicate collagen filaments attach the vitreous to the internal limiting membrane of the retina. The attachment is strongest near the optic disc and ora serrata. It is also strong in the macular area. The collagen filaments thicken anteriorly in the vitreous and are oriented anteroposteriorly, and they continue anteriorly to form the filamentous collagen framework of the zonular

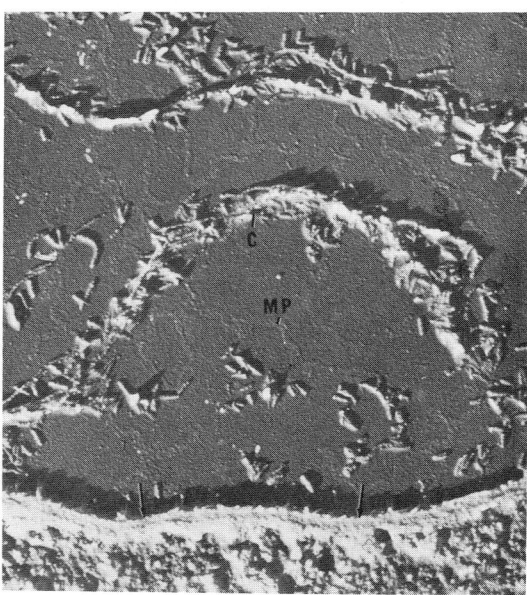

Figure 2-49 Electron micrograph showing the drying pattern of vitreous acid mucopolysaccharides, MP, between the aggregates of delicate collagenous filaments, C, of the vitreous framework. Below lies the inner surface of the retina (arrows) (×24,000). (Courtesy of Ben S. Fine, M.D.)

fibers of the lens. The nonpigmented, ciliary epithelium of the pars plana secretes most, if not all, of the acid mucopolysaccharide of the vitreous in the adult eye; the retina, possibly Müller's cells, may also play a role.

The anterior surface of the vitreous body is condensed to form a hyaloid membrane that helps to prevent the escape of vitreous during cataract extraction. No posterior limiting membrane of the vitreous is present unless the vitreous separates from the retina, as, for example, in posterior detachment of the vitreous. The posterior surface then tends to condense and gives the clinical impression of a posterior limiting membrane (posterior hyaloid membrane). This is not a true cellular, or cuticular, membrane, however, but is a condensation of the vitreous border layer, similar to the anterior hyaloid.

The Lens

The lens is a transparent, biconvex body enclosed in a capsule, lying directly behind the iris (Fig. 2-50). It has an anterior surface whose center is called the anterior pole, and a posterior surface with a central posterior pole. The radius of curvature of the anterior surface averages 10 mm., but it is subject to marked changes during accommodation. The radius of curvature of the posterior surface averages 6 mm. The place at which the anterior joins the posterior surface is called the equator. The equator

is not smoothly curved, but shows numerous irregularities resulting from the pull of the zonular fibers. When the ciliary muscle contracts, the pull of these zonules is relaxed and the lens becomes more spherical with an increase in power (accommodation).

Structure. Under the light microscope the lens capsule appears as a clear, structureless membrane of varying thickness. The capsule is thickest anteriorly to the equator and is thinnest posteriorly (Fig. 2-51). With special stains, or in the electron microscope, the lens capsule often appears to have a lamellar arrangement. The capsule stains brilliantly with the PAS reaction, and seems to be composed of a glycoprotein-collagen complex, analogous to the composition of basement membranes found elsewhere in the body.

Immediately beneath the entire capsule and extending to the equator is a single layer of cells, the epithelium of the lens (Fig. 2-51). The equatorial cells give rise to new lens fibers that are formed throughout life. Persisting nuclei of the youngest lens "fibers" form the lens bow going into the interior of the lens. After birth all of the lens fibers arise from the epithelial cells

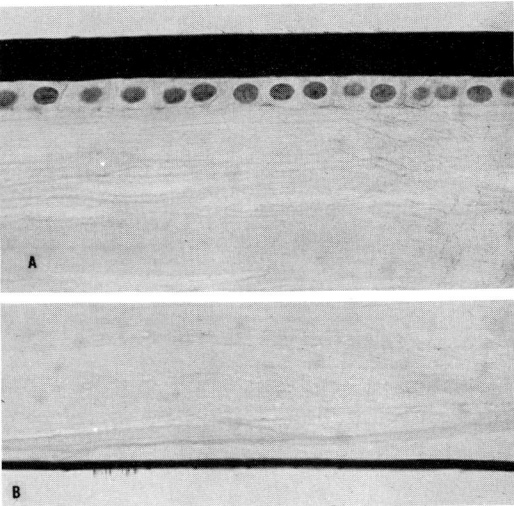

Figure 2-51 (*A*) Thick anterior capsule of a lens with underlying epithelium. (*B*) Thin posterior capsule of the same lens. (Both, periodic acid–Schiff, ×730.)

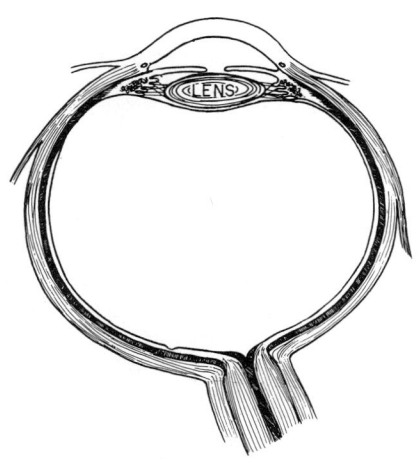

Figure 2-50 Diagram showing position of biconvex lens.

in the region of the equator. The cytoplasm of the cells makes up the lens substance. As cells are formed, they move slowly toward the inside of the lens and become more compact. A urochrome deposit gives them a yellow to brown color, which may become marked in adult life giving the typical senile nuclear cataract its yellow-brown color. The outer fibers of the cortex are much softer than the more compact inner fibers of the nucleus.

Attachments. The lens is suspended from the ciliary body around its entire circumference by the zonules of Zinn. These delicate but strong fibers hold the lens in place, allowing it to swing like a hammock between the ciliary processes. When the eye is at rest, the zonules are taut and exert a pull on the lens capsule that flattens its surface. During accommodation the zonules are relaxed by the contraction of the ciliary muscles. This laxity of the zonules allows the inherently elastic lens capsule to bulge, making the lens more convex. The lens also is supported by the hyaloideocapsular ligament that unites it to the vitreous body. This union probably is due to the posterior zonules (such an attachment would be indistinguishable from that of the vitreous). When the zonular fibers rupture, gravity causes the lens to sink and the lens is said to be subluxated. The lens is said to be dislocated when it is found outside the posterior chamber, in either the anterior chamber or the vitreous compartment.

Aqueous

Secretion and Flow of Aqueous. Aqueous appears to be actively secreted by the ciliary epithelium of the ciliary body. The aqueous is secreted into the posterior chamber from which it exits into the anterior chamber through the pupil. Convection currents are set up in the aqueous by the differential temperature gradient from the warm posterior aqueous to the anterior aqueous cooled by the corneal surface. Thus, aqueous flows not only from the posterior to the anterior, but also in a circular fashion,

tending to rise posteriorly and fall anteriorly. The aqueous subsequently leaves the interior of the eye, mainly through drainage channels located in the drainage area of the anterior chamber.

The Drainage Area of the Anterior Chamber. The angle of the anterior chamber formed by the union of the uveal tract with the corneoscleral coat is the most important region for aqueous drainage. The iridocorneoscleral angle describes an arc whose concavity points back toward the ciliary body, thereby forming the angular sinus. Anatomically this arc begins at the end of Descemet's membrane (Schwalbe's line or ring) and terminates at the iris root where the anterior border layer of the iris ends abruptly (Fig. 2-52).

This drainage angle is occupied mainly by perforated, collagenous, trabecular sheets that comprise the trabecular meshwork. An imaginary line from the scleral spur to the end of Descemet's membrane (Schwalbe's line) divides this meshwork into two main parts (Fig. 2-53): the inner, or uveal, layer; and the outer, or corneoscleral, layer. The region of the corneoscleral meshwork that abuts on the canal of Schlemm is modified into a specialized zone of variable thickness that is known as juxtacanalicular connective tissue (Fig. 2-54). The beginning of this zone marks the theoretical terminus of the anterior chamber, which is continuous to this point via the nonsuperimposed spaces of descending diameter across the trabecular sheets (Fig. 2-55). The trabecular sheets of uveal meshwork pass the scleral spur and are continuous posteriorly with the ciliary muscle and the tissues at the root of the iris.

A single beam from the trabecular sheet is composed of a twisted bundle of collagen as a core, surrounded by an endothelial covering separated from the core by basement membrane of variable thickness and appearance (Fig. 2-56).

The canal of Schlemm is a large, branching, circumferential vessel lying deep within the internal scleral sulcus. It is composed of a single lining of endothelial cells resembling those that line a capillary or a lymphatic (Fig. 2-57). Neither apertures ("pores") nor attenuations ("fenestrae") are found within these endothelial cells. The canal is drained directly and obliquely through the corneosclera by large collector channels whose endothelial lining is con-

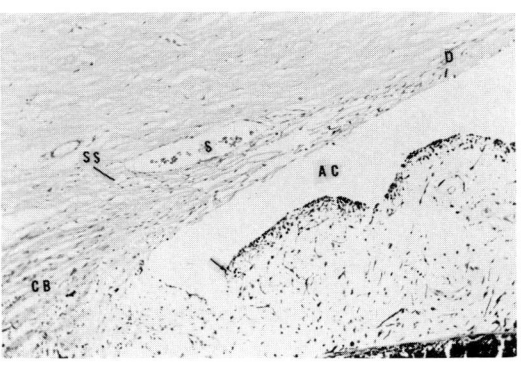

Figure 2-52 Iridocorneoscleral angle begins at the end of Descemet's membrane, D, and terminates at the iris root (arrow). S, Schlemm's canal; CB, ciliary body; SS, scleral spur; AC, anterior chamber (hematoxylin and eosin, ×100).

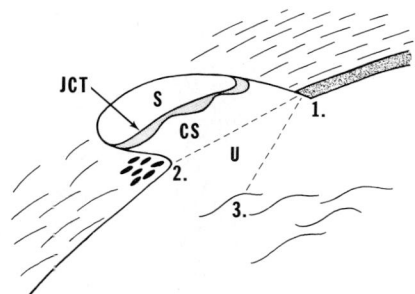

Figure 2-53 Schematic drawing of anatomic relationships within the drainage angle. Canal of Schlemm, S, is separated from the bulk of trabecular meshwork by a thin zone of juxtacanalicular connective tissue, JCT. Remainder of trabecular meshwork is divisible into: an anterior corneoscleral portion, CS, and a posterior uveal portion, U, by an imaginary line drawn from 2, the scleral roll, or spur, to 1, the end of Descemet's membrane. The inner boundary of uveal meshwork is demarcated by a line drawn from 1, the end of Descemet's membrane, to 3, the iris root. (Fine, B. S.: *Tr. Am. Acad. Ophth. & Otol.* 70:785, 1966.)

Figure 2-54 Electron micrograph of a portion of endothelial cell lining, EN, from the inner wall of the canal of Schlemm, CS, and a thin portion of the juxtacanalicular region, JCT. Cells, C, and extracellular materials, varying in morphologic appearance from fibrillar to homogeneous, are found in this region. IT, intertrabecular spaces; RBC, portion of red blood cell (×11,700). (Fine, B. S.: *Tr. Am. Acad. Ophth. & Otol.* 70:784, 1966.)

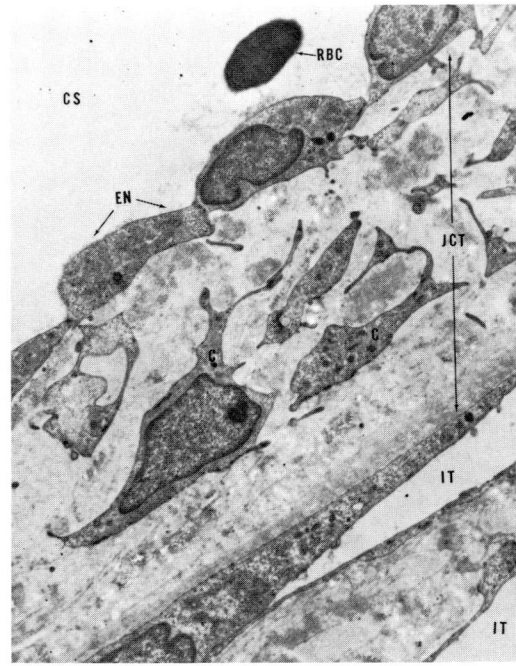

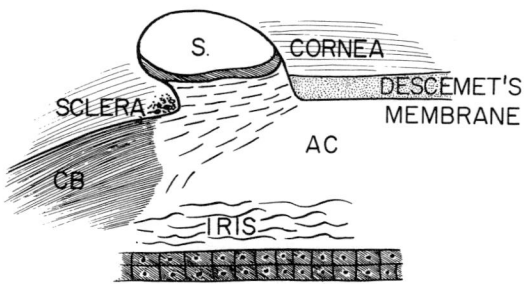

Figure 2-55 Diagram showing that the anterior chamber, AC, is continuous via the nonsuperimposed spaces of the trabecular sheets up to the juxtacanalicular connective tissue that abuts on the outer wall of the canal of Schlemm, S. CB, ciliary body.

Figure 2-56 Electron micrograph of a portion of uveal trabecular meshwork. Collagenous cores, C, of the beams are separated from their endothelial cell coverings by a basement membrane, BM. The free surfaces of the endothelial cells that are not lined by basement membrane limit the intertrabecular spaces, IT, that comprise the interconnected diverticuli of the anterior chamber (×12,000). (Fine, B. S.: *Tr. Am. Acad. Ophth. & Otol. 70*:779, 1966.)

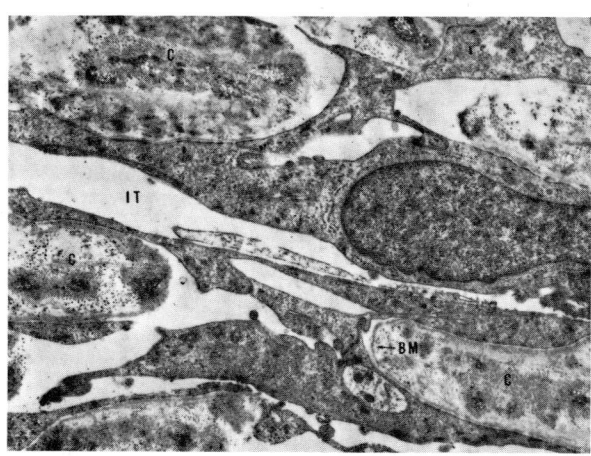

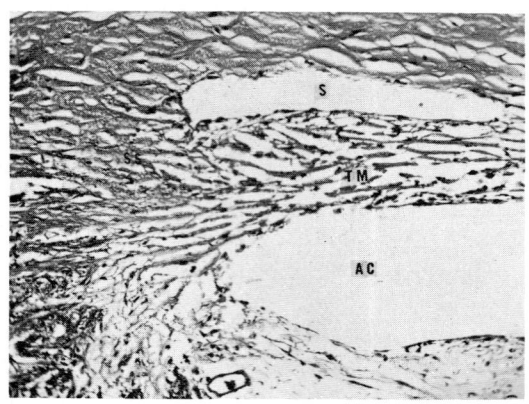

Figure 2-57 Canal of Schlemm, S, seen deep within the scleral sulcus. SS, scleral spur; TM, trabecular meshwork; AC, anterior chamber (hematoxylin and eosin, ×200).

tinuous with that of the canal. These large, aqueous-filled channels drain into the vessels of the corneoscleral plexus. Those that reach the surface of the sclera before making such connection can be directly observed in vivo as "aqueous veins."

BIBLIOGRAPHY

Adler, F. H.: Physiology of the Eye. 4th ed. St. Louis, The C. V. Mosby Co., 1965.

Adler, F. H.: Physiology of the Eye. 3rd ed. St. Louis, The C. V. Mosby Co., 1959.

Adler, F. H.: Physiological aspects of diseases of the optic nerve. Ann. Surg. 101:2, 1935.

Fine, B. S.: Retinal structure: light and electron microscopic observations. In McPherson, A. (ed.): New and Controversial Aspects of Retinal Detachment. New York, Hoeber Medical Division, Harper & Row, 1968.

Fine, B. S.: Structure of the trabecular meshwork and the canal of Schlemn. Tr. Am. Acad. Ophth. 70: 777, 1966.

Fine, B. S.: Synaptic lamellas in the human retina: an electron microscopic study. J. Neuropath. & Exper. Neurol. 22:255, 1963.

Garron, L. K., and Feeney, M. L.: Electron microscopic studies of the human eye. II. Study of the trabeculae by light and electron microscopy. Arch. Ophth. 62:966, 1959.

Millard, N. D., King, B. G., and Showers, M. J.: Human Anatomy and Physiology. 4th ed. Philadelphia, W. B. Saunders Co., 1956.

Salzmann, M.: The Anatomy and Histology of the Human Eyeball in the Normal State. Chicago, The University of Chicago Press, 1912.

Tousimis, A. J., and Fine, B. S.: Ultrastructure of the iris: an electron microscopic study. Part II. Am. J. Ophth. 48:397, 1959.

Ts'o, M. O., and Friedman, E.: The retinal pigment epithelium. I. Comparative histology. Arch. Ophth. 78:641, 1967.

Whitnall, S. E.: The Anatomy of the Human Orbit and Accessory Organs of Vision. London, The Oxford University Press, 1921.

Wolff, E.: Anatomy of the Eye and Orbit. 5th ed., revised by R. J. Last. London, H. K. Lewis & Co., Ltd., 1961.

Yanoff, M.: Pigment spots of the sclera. Arch. Ophth. 81:151, 1969.

Yanoff, M.: Diabetic retinopathy. New England J. Med. 274:1348, 1966.

Chapter Three

EMBRYOLOGY OF THE HUMAN EYE

The embryo develops from the nearly flat embryonic plate, an area of cellular proliferation at the zone of contact of the amnion and yolk sac. Of the three germinal layers in the plate, only the ectoderm and mesoderm are involved in the development of the eye. The longitudinal neural groove arises at the center of the embryonic plate, and as cellular proliferation proceeds, the groove forms a valley bounded on each side by ridges of thickened neural ectoderm called the neural folds (Fig. 3-1). The folds become more elevated, and their apices

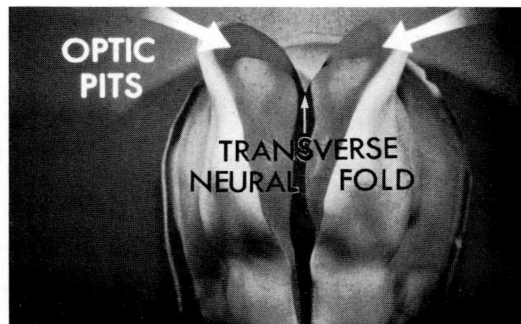

Figure 3-2 Model—24 days. Anterior edges of neural folds have begun to fuse, forming the transverse, or anterior, neural fold. Behind this fold, a small depression, or lateral outpouching, in each neural fold forms an optic pit, forerunner of the optic vesicle. (Courtesy of American Academy of Ophthalmology & Otolaryngology.)

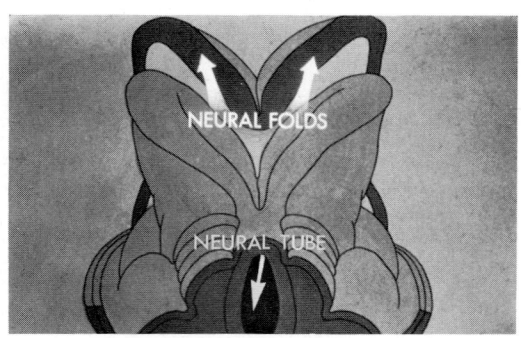

Figure 3-1 Drawing. Third week of gestation. Proliferating neural ectoderm forms prominent folds on each side of the primitive neural groove. Posteriorly, neural folds fuse at the midline, converting the neural groove into a neural tube. Anteriorly, neural folds remain unfused at this stage. (Courtesy of American Academy of Ophthalmology & Otolaryngology.)

grow toward the midline until they fuse to form the neural tube. Fusion begins near the center of the neural groove at the junction of the future spinal cord and brain, and extends both forward and backward. Toward the cephalic end of the embryonic plate, in the area of the future forebrain, the neural folds temporarily remain unfused and diverge from each other. At the extreme cephalic end of the neural groove, the ends of the neural folds fuse to form the transverse or anterior neural fold. With continued growth of the neural folds, the anterior neural fold heightens and a small

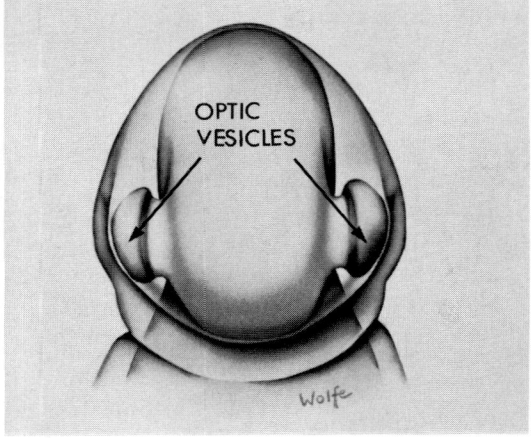

Figure 3-3 Drawing—25 days. Optic vesicles. (Courtesy of Medicolor Illustration and Editorial Service.)

recess forms behind it. Within the recess on each side a depression or outpouching of each neural fold forms the optic pits (Fig. 3-2) from which the primary optic vesicles are formed (Fig. 3-3).

THE OPTIC CUP

At about the 4.5 mm. stage the primary optic vesicle begins to invaginate to form the optic cup. If the optic vesicle fails to invaginate, a congenital cystic eye results in

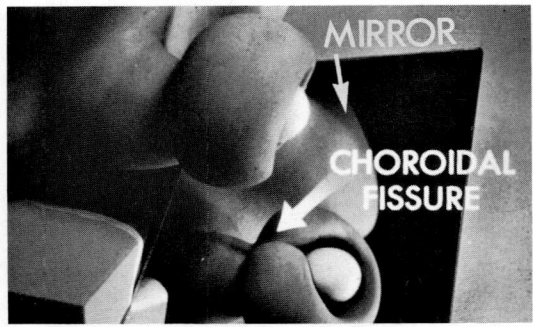

Figure 3-4 Model—33 days. The side and undersurface (ventral) of the optic vesicle invaginate to form the optic cup. The lens vesicle is seen in the mouth of the optic cup. The groove formed by invagination from below is termed the choroidal (fetal) fissure. The apposed margins of the choroidal fissure have begun to fuse near the middle of the fissure. (Mirror provides view of undersurface of optic cup.) (Courtesy of American Academy of Ophthalmology and Otolaryngology.)

which cystic material with traces of neural tissue is found in the orbit. Invagination takes place from the side and from below simultaneously, and the groove formed by this process is termed the fetal (choroidal) fissure (Fig. 3-4). It extends from the rim of the optic cup along the lower aspect of the optic stalk almost to the wall of the forebrain. Mesodermal tissue proliferates along the fetal fissure and ultimately forms the hyaloid system of vessels within the optic cup.

The optic cup is lined with a double layer of neural ectoderm (Fig. 3-5). The inner layer differentiates to form the sensory layer of the retina, the nonpigmented epithelium of the ciliary body, and the posterior epithelial layer of the iris; the outer layer gives rise to the pigment epithelium of the retina and ciliary body as well as to the anterior epithelial layer of the iris, including the sphincter and dilator muscles. Throughout life, a potential space repre-

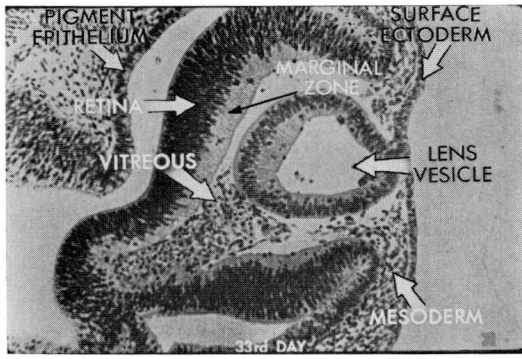

Figure 3-5 Photomicrograph—12 mm. stage. A double layer of neural ectoderm lines the optic cup. A potential space exists between the inner and outer neural ectodermal layers throughout life. This space is artifactitiously enlarged in the figure. The lens vesicle has pinched off from surface ectoderm, and posterior lens epithelial cells have begun to form primary lens fibers. Formation of primary vitreous is practically complete. Cells destined to form sensory retina have migrated outward to form an outer layer of proliferating cells, leaving an inner, nucleus-free marginal zone. Mesoderm has migrated around the rim of the optic cup and ultimately will form corneal and iris stroma, structures of the drainage system of the anterior chamber, and vascular layers of the uveal tract. (Courtesy of American Academy of Ophthalmology and Otolaryngology.)

TABLE 3-1 COMPARISON OF GESTATIONAL AGE AND EMBRYONIC LENGTH*

Age (wks.)	Length (mm.)
4	7.8
5	12.2
6	17.6
7	24.0
8	31.3
9	39.6
10	49.0
11	59.2
12	70.5
18	130.0
24	190.0
30	250.0
36	310.0
39	340.0

*Adapted from Mann, I.: The Development of the Human Eye. New York, Grune & Stratton, Inc., 1964.

senting the primary optic vesicle exists between the retinal pigment epithelium and the sensory portion of the retina. Under pathologic conditions these two layers may become separated, producing what is known clinically as a retinal detachment.

By the 7 mm. stage the fetal fissure has completely formed along the length of the optic cup, and by the 10 mm. stage its apposed margins begin to fuse (Fig. 3-4). Fusion begins first at the central portion of the cleft and then extends both anteriorly and posteriorly. By the 18 mm. stage the fetal fissure is completely closed except for two small areas, one anterior and another posterior along the under surface of the future optic nerve. The posterior defect allows the passage of the hyaloid artery into the eye (Fig. 3-17). If the fetal fissure fails to close, a typical coloboma or defect occurs in those structures (iris, choroid, and optic nerve) that are directly or indirectly related to the area of the fetal fissure. These defects are seen characteristically in the inferior nasal aspect of the globe.

THE LENS

The first sign of lens formation is seen at the 4 mm. stage. The lens plate (placode) appears as a thickening of the surface ectoderm overlying the neural ectoderm of the primary optic vesicle with which it has come in contact (Fig. 3-6). A slight depression known as the fovea lentis or lens pit appears in the lower part of the lens plate and eventually forms the lens vesicle. At the 9 mm. stage the lens vesicle closes and is pinched off from the surface ectoderm (Figs. 3-5, 3-7).

The wall of the lens vesicle consists of a single layer of short cuboidal cells. These cells give rise to a basement membrane which, by the 13 mm. stage, completely envelops the lens vesicle and forms the hyaline capsule of the lens.

After the lens vesicle closes, the cells covering its posterior half begin to elongate to form the primary lens fibers (Figs. 3-5, 3-8). These fibers encroach upon the lumen of the lens vesicle, and by the 16 mm. stage their ends have grown to meet the apices of the anterior lens epithelial cells, thus obliterating the lens cavity. With the formation of the primary lens fibers, the epithelium of the posterior one half of the lens vesicle disappears; only the anterior one half retains an epithelial layer. The lens grows by the subsequent formation of lens fibers from cells located at the equator of the lens (Figs. 3-9, 3-23).

The new fibers, formed in layers outside the primary lens fibers, are known as secondary lens fibers. The secondary fibers elongate and interlace anteriorly and posteriorly to produce suture lines. The suture lines provide a smooth lens surface that permits uniform refraction of light. The earliest visible sutures are the anterior up-

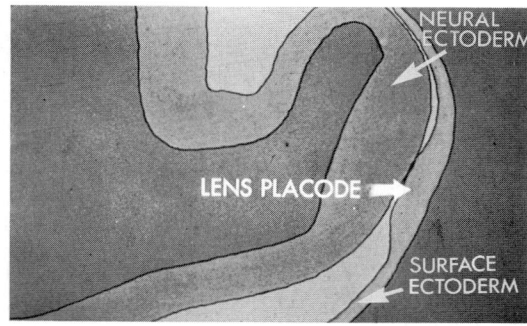

Figure 3-6 Drawing—26th day. Lens plate (placode) arises at the point of contact between neural and surface ectoderm. (Courtesy of American Academy of Ophthalmology and Otolaryngology.)

Figure 3-7 Model—30th day. Invagination of surface ectoderm produces the lens vesicle, a hollow sphere that protrudes into the mouth of the optic cup. Separation of the lens vesicle from surface ectoderm is complete by the 9 mm. stage (Figs. 3-5 and 3-8). (Courtesy of American Academy of Ophthalmology and Otolaryngology.)

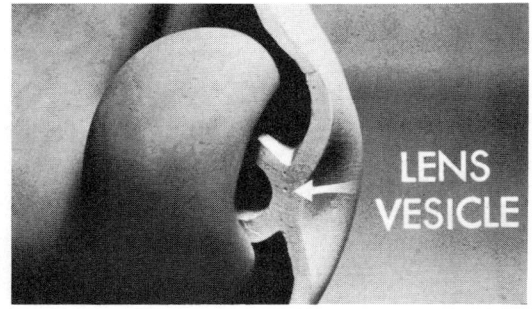

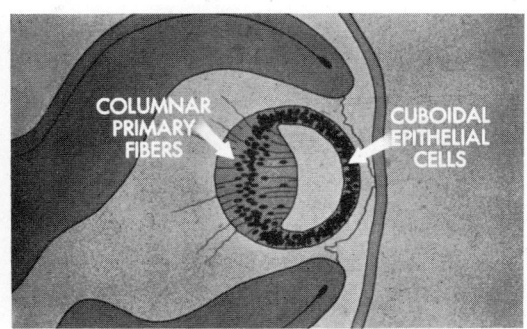

Figure 3-8 Drawing—36th day. The lens vesicle has separated from surface ectoderm. Posterior epithelial cells have begun to elongate to form primary lens fibers, which shortly will fill the cavity of the lens vesicle. Formation of the capsule excludes the lens from contributing further to vitreous formation. Mesoderm has grown between the lens vesicle and surface ectoderm. (Courtesy of American Academy of Ophthalmology and Otolaryngology.)

Figure 3-9 Drawing—38th day. Completion of primary lens fibers has resulted in the obliteration of the lens vesicle cavity and the disappearance of epithelial cells posterior to the lens equator. Formation of secondary lens fibers from cells at the lens equator causes further lens growth. (Courtesy of American Academy of Ophthalmology and Otolaryngology.)

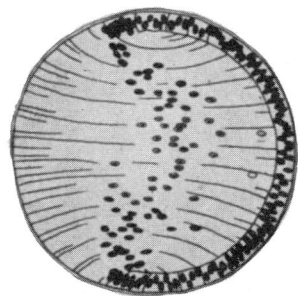

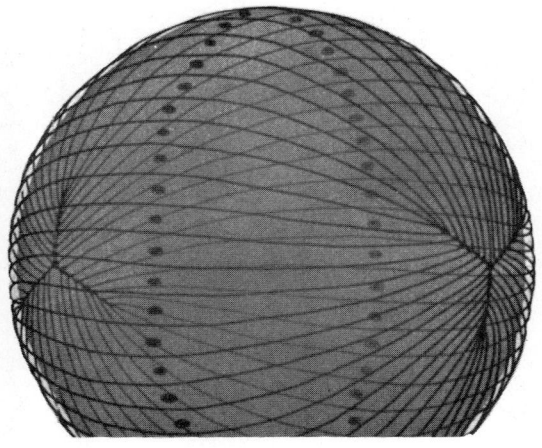

Figure 3-10 Drawing—seventh week. Secondary lens fibers arise from cells at the lens equator and interlace to form the anterior upright and posterior inverted Y sutures. (Courtesy of American Academy of Ophthalmology and Otolaryngology.)

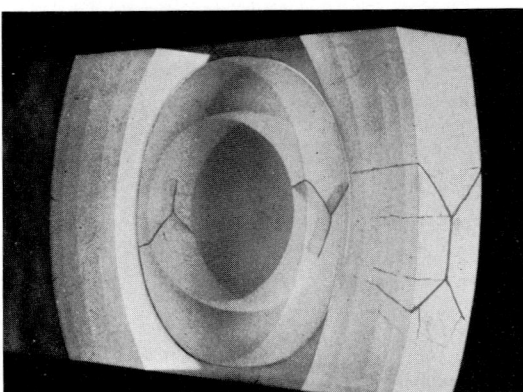

Figure 3-11 Drawing of the appearance of an adult lens in a slit lamp biomicroscope. Varying optical densities of lens fibers cause zones of discontinuity within the lens. Between the anterior and posterior Y sutures lies the embryonic nucleus (central dark space). The fetal nucleus encompasses the area of Y sutures. (Y sutures are three-dimensional.) Peripheral to the fetal nucleus lie several lamellae, which are designated infantile, adolescent, and adult nuclei. Lens cortex is located beneath the lens epithelium. (Lens epithelium and capsule not shown in figure.) (Courtesy of American Academy of Ophthalmology and Otolaryngology.)

opment of the retina occurs between the 4 mm. and the 7 month stages. At about the 4.5 mm. stage, the period during which the primary optic vesicle invaginates to form the optic cup, the cells destined to become the inner wall of the cup multiply, causing the inner wall to thicken. As the fetal fissure begins to close (10 mm.), the pigment epithelium acquires pigment granules, and the inner wall shows differentiation into the primitive layers of the sensory retina. At this stage nearly all of the nuclei of the future sensory retina have migrated toward the pigment epithelium to form an outer layer of proliferating cells, leaving an inner, nucleus-free marginal layer (Fig. 3-5). The outer, proliferating layer differentiates into an inner and an outer neuroblastic layer separated by the transient layer of Chievitz, which later disappears as the formation of the sensory retina is completed (Fig. 3-12). The inner layer differentiates early; its innermost cells migrate inward to produce the layer of ganglion cells from which processes (axons) arise to form the nerve fiber layer of the retina and the optic nerve. The space between the ganglion cells and the inner neuroblastic layer becomes the inner molecular (plexiform) layer, and the outer-

right and posterior inverted Y's. As secondary lens fibers continue to form, the Y sutures become more complicated and branched (Fig. 3-10).

The lens continues to grow throughout life by proliferation of secondary lens fibers. As the fibers are laid down, varying optical densities of the fibers produce zones of discontinuity which can be observed clinically with a slit lamp (Fig. 3-11). These areas have been designated as the central dark space (embryonic nucleus); the fetal nucleus; the infantile, adolescent, and adult nuclei superficial to the Y sutures; and the cortex. The lens gradually increases in size throughout life as new fibers develop.

THE RETINA

The retina develops from the two walls of the optic cup. The pigment epithelium arises from the outer wall and the sensory retina from the inner wall (Fig. 3-5). Devel-

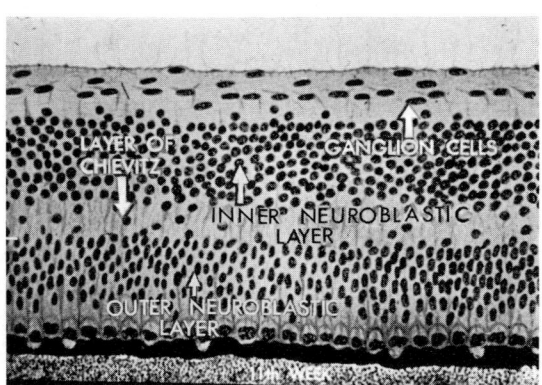

Figure 3-12 Drawing—11th week. The most central cells of inner neuroblastic layer have migrated inward to form the layer of ganglion cells. The inner molecular layer forms between ganglion cells and inner neuroblastic layer. The remaining cells of inner neuroblastic layer differentiate into amacrine cells and nuclei of fibers of Müller. These cells ultimately merge with bipolar and horizontal cells derived from outer neuroblastic layer to form a definitive inner nuclear layer and thereby obliterate the transient layer of Chievitz. The beginning of the outer nuclear layer (nuclei of rods and cones) and of pigment epithelium is depicted in the figure. (Courtesy of American Academy of Ophthalmology and Otolaryngology.)

most or remaining inner neuroblastic cells differentiate into amacrine cells and nuclei of the fibers of Müller.

The cells of the outer neuroblastic layer differentiate from within outward to form bipolar cells, horizontal cells, and the nuclei of the rods and cones. The horizontal cells and the nuclei of the rods and cones gradually separate, and the intervening zone becomes the outer molecular layer. The bipolar cells and the horizontal cells of the outer neuroblastic layer merge with amacrine cells and nuclei of Müller's fibers from the inner neuroblastic layer. This obliterates the transient layer of Chievitz and forms the definitive inner nuclear layer. The nuclei of the rods and cones constitute the outer nuclear layer, which is separated from the inner nuclear layer by the outer molecular layer. The outermost layer of the

sensory retina, the layer of rods and cones, arises from the outermost cells of the outer neuroblastic layer. This layer unites by extremely weak zones of attachment with the pigment epithelium (Table 3-2).

The retina is bounded internally by the internal limiting membrane, a true basement membrane formed by the Müllerian cells. An external limiting membrane lies between the outer nuclear layer and the layer of rods and cones.

By the seventh month of gestation all layers of the retina, except in the macular region, are complete and ready to function. Retarded during gestation, the macular

TABLE 3-2 DEVELOPMENT OF THE SENSORY RETINA*

4th to 5th Week	6th Week to 3rd Month	3rd to 7th Month	Adult
Surface of marginal layer			Internal limiting membrane
	Superficial portion of marginal layer	Nerve fiber layer	Nerve fiber layer
		Ganglion cells	Ganglion cells
			Inner molecular layer
Marginal layer free from nuclei	Inner neuroblastic layer	Amacrine cells	
		Müllerian fiber nuclei	
Primitive neuro-epithelium	Transient layer of Chievitz (deep part of marginal layer)	Bipolar cells	Inner nuclear layer
			Outer molecular layer
	Outer neuroblastic layer	Horizontal cells	
		Nuclei of rods and cones	Outer nuclear layer
			External limiting "membrane"
Cilia	Cilia	Primitive rods and cones	Rods and cones

*Adapted from Mann, I.: The Development of the Human Eye. New York, Grune & Stratton, Inc., 1964.

area is not complete until about four months postpartum.

THE CILIARY BODY

The neural ectodermal components of the ciliary body (ciliary epithelium) arise from a proliferation of cells of the two layers of the optic cup at its anterior margin or rim. At about the 48 mm. stage, the cells of these two layers advance forward to form a series of 70 to 75 radial folds around the circumference of the cup (Fig. 3-13). These folds, the future ciliary processes, consist of two layers of epithelium that are firmly united by a series of attachment bodies. The outer layer is pigmented; the inner layer, nonpigmented. Each fold develops a central mesodermal vascular core that supplies blood to the ciliary processes. As development of the eye continues, the folds slowly increase in size and depth and gradually move anteriorly. Immediately behind them a smooth region of the ciliary body (pars plana) is formed.

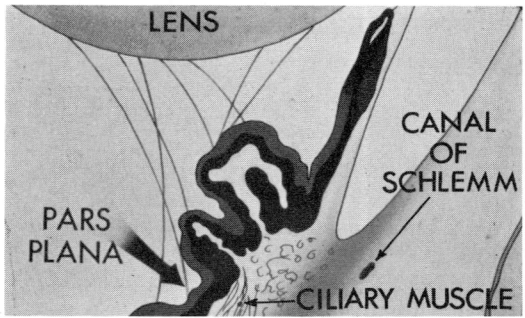

Figure 3-13 Drawing—fifth month. Proliferation of neural ectodermal layers at the rim of the optic cup results in formation of radially oriented folds, ciliary processes, and epithelial layers of iris. Pars plana develops in the smooth area between the roots of ciliary processes and the anterior extent of sensory retina. Mesoderm extends into epithelial folds to form the vascular core of ciliary processes and proliferates over the epithelial layers of the iris to form iris stroma. Mesodermal condensations in the area of the ciliary body mark the beginning of ciliary muscle. (Courtesy of American Academy of Ophthalmology and Otolaryngology.)

THE IRIS

The proliferating neuroectodermal cells at the rim of the optic cup extend beyond the area of the future ciliary body and form the two epithelial layers of the iris (Fig. 3-13). The inner cell layer forms the posterior epithelial layer of the iris and the outer cell layer forms the anterior epithelial layer of the iris. Both layers of the iris epithelium become pigmented by the seventh month. The sphincter muscle of the iris develops from the anterior layer of epithelium and eventually separates from it. At birth the sphincter is a separate mass of vascularized smooth muscle. The dilator muscle develops later than the sphincter as fine fibrils within the anterior part of the cells forming the anterior layer of the iris epithelium. Unlike the sphincter, it retains its embryonic form as part of the epithelium throughout life and is not vascularized (Fig. 3-14). The iris stroma is of mesodermal origin.

THE OPTIC NERVE

The axis cylinders (axons) of the retinal ganglion cells form the optic nerve. From the ganglion cell layer, the axons course in the nerve fiber layer of the retina and enter the optic stalk to travel to the forebrain (Fig. 3-15). The optic stalk cells derived from neural ectoderm contribute to neuroglial supporting tissue of the optic nerve. As the invaginated margins (fetal fissure) of the optic stalk fuse, the future central retinal artery, together with its perivascular mesodermal cells, is included with the substance of the optic nerve and supplies the nerve with blood. A mesodermal sheath of tissue surrounding the optic nerve becomes continuous with the meningeal layers of the central nervous system. Medullation of the optic nerve begins at about the seventh month. It begins centrally and extends peripherally up to the lamina cribrosa of the sclera (Fig. 3-16). In some lower animals (e.g., the rabbit) and occasionally in man, medullated nerve fibers may continue into the nerve fiber layer, producing a characteristic white patch on the retina, usually near the optic nerve.

Figure 3-14 Drawing—sixth month. The anterior epithelial cell layer of the iris gives rise to iris musculature. Sphincter muscle develops first and ultimately forms a smooth muscle mass distinct from the epithelium. Dilator muscle consists of smooth muscle fibers within cells of the anterior epithelial layer of the iris. (Courtesy of American Academy of Ophthalmology and Otolaryngology.)

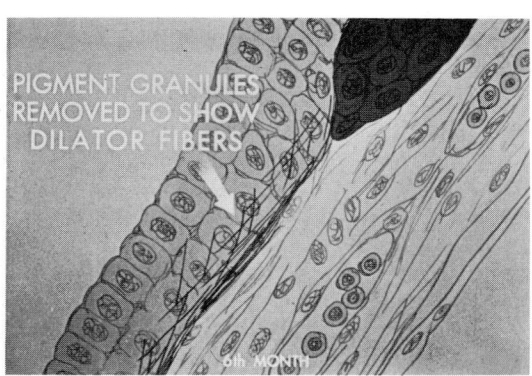

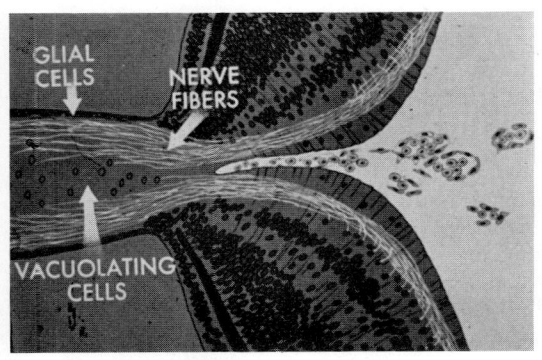

Figure 3-15 Drawing—40th day. Axons from ganglion cells form the nerve fiber layer and enter the optic stalk to comprise the optic nerve. Cells derived from the outer neural ectodermal layer of the optic vesicle form the glial (supporting) elements of the optic nerve. Cells from neuroblastic layers have begun to migrate and are obliterating the transient layer of Chievitz. Sections of the hyaloid vasculature are shown. (Courtesy of American Academy of Ophthalmology and Otolaryngology.)

Figure 3-16 Drawing—ninth month. Medullation of the optic nerve begins centrally at about the seventh month and reaches the lamina cribrosa by term. (Courtesy of American Academy of Ophthalmology and Otolaryngology.)

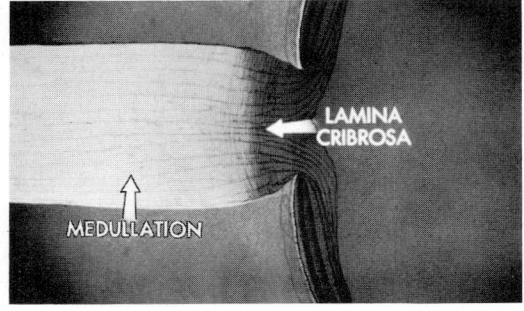

INTRAOCULAR CIRCULATION

The blood supply of the eye develops early from paraxial mesoderm that becomes vascularized by minute branches from the ophthalmic artery, a branch of primitive carotid artery. The ophthalmic artery grows along the ventral surface of the optic cup and gives off the hyaloid artery, a vessel that runs into the optic cup through the fetal fissure. Other branches migrate over the surface of the optic cup to its rim where they anastomose to form the annular vessel. The hyaloid artery, now enclosed within the eye by the closure of the fetal fissure, also sends anastomotic channels to the annular vessel. Simultaneously the future choriocapillaris begins to appear as a vascularized net over the outside of the optic cup (Fig. 3-17). This net communicates anteriorly with the annular vessel and empties posteriorly into the supra- and infraorbital plexuses, which, in turn, drain into the cavernous sinus. At the 18 mm. stage the future long posterior ciliary arteries arise from the ophthalmic artery, and in a short time, their terminal branches form a second anastomotic ring at the rim of the optic cup,

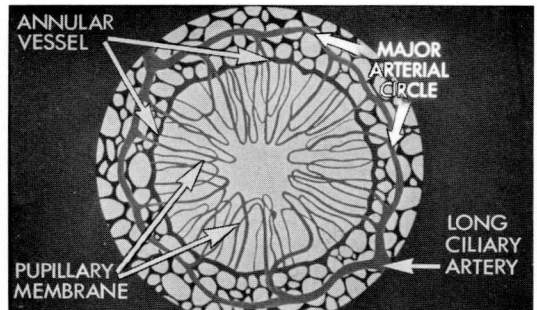

Figure 3-18 Drawing—45th day. The long posterior ciliary arteries anastomose to form the major arterial circle from which secondary channels arise to form the peripheral vascular arcades of the pupillary membrane. When the central portion of the pupillary membrane atrophies, the remaining peripheral vascular arcades form an incomplete vascular ring, the minor arterial circle. The annular vessel is incorporated into the future choriocapillaris and eventually disappears. (Courtesy of American Academy of Ophthalmology and Otolaryngology.)

the future major arterial circle of the iris (Figs. 3-18, 3-19). The annular vessel atrophies as it is incorporated into the choroidal net.

The main trunk of the hyaloid artery, after passing through the fetal fissure, runs forward to the posterior pole of the lens where it spreads over the posterior lenticular surface as a capillary net. These capillaries join others from the anterior surface of the lens given off by the annular vessel. This anastomosing vascular network, called the tunica vasculosa lentis, envelops the lens (Figs. 3-17, 3-19). The hyaloid trunk also gives rise to a large number of branches, the vasa hyaloidea propria, which at the height of their development almost

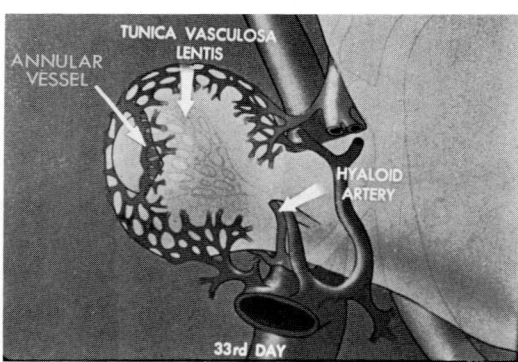

Figure 3-17 Drawing—33rd day. The hyaloid artery arises from the ophthalmic artery and enters the eye through a defect in the fetal fissure. Inside the eye, it contributes to the formation of the tunica vasculosa lentis and vasa hyaloidea propria (Fig. 19). A vascular network proliferates on the surface of the optic cup and forms the annular vessel. (Part of this network has been removed from the drawing to show the tunica vasculosa lentis.) Channels from the tunica vasculosa lentis also contribute to the annular vessel. (Courtesy of American Academy of Ophthalmology and Otolaryngology.)

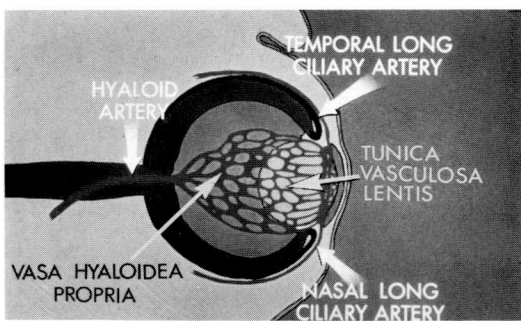

Figure 3-19 Drawing—46th day. The hyaloid artery gives rise to vasa hyaloidea propria from which posterior tunica vasculosa lentis is derived. These vascular channels ultimately resorb. (Courtesy of American Academy of Ophthalmology and Otolaryngology.)

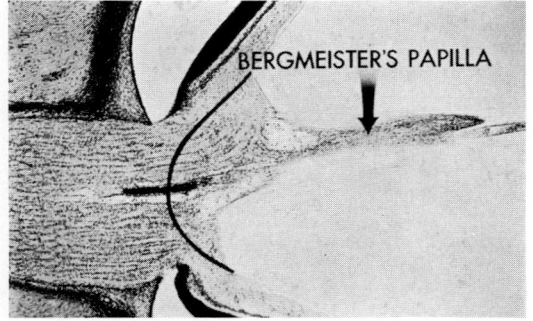

Figure 3-20 Photomicrograph—14th week. The posterior portion of the hyaloid artery and its enveloping glial tissue form Bergmeister's papilla, which atrophies simultaneously with the resorption of hyaloid vessels. The degree of atrophy of Bergmeister's papilla determines the depth of the physiologic cup of the adult disc. Curved line depicts the physiologic cup. (Courtesy of American Academy of Ophthalmology and Otolaryngology.)

fill the vitreous cavity (Figs. 3-17, 3-19). They also anastomose with the posterior part of the tunica vasculosa lentis. The hyaloid gives rise to the central retinal artery and its branches. These persist throughout life to nourish the inner one third of the retina.

After becoming this highly developed, the hyaloid vascular system begins to atrophy. (Atrophy is almost complete by the 8½ month stage.) The vasa hyaloidea propria and posterior tunica vasculosa lentis first disappear, followed later by the main trunk of the hyaloid, which first becomes occluded in its central part. Frequently the portion attached to the posterior pole of the lens remains as a remnant that is visible in adult life either as a Mittendorf dot on the posterior lens capsule or as an actual strand within Cloquet's canal. Posteriorly, the absorption of the hyaloid and its surrounding glial tissue (Bergmeister's papilla) produces the physiologic cup (Fig. 3-20). If posterior atrophy is incomplete, a vascularized glial membrane may persist, protruding from the disc into the vitreous cavity. Occasionally the anterior hyaloid system fails to atrophy and this leads to a developmental anomaly termed persistent hyperplastic primary vitreous.

THE VITREOUS

The vitreous develops in three stages. In the first stage the cavity of the optic cup, i.e., the vitreous space, is filled with a mass of ectodermal and mesodermal fibrils from which the primary vitreous forms (Fig. 3-5). The ectodermal components originate from the cells of the retina and lens vesicle; the mesodermal elements, including the hyaloid vessels, enter into the vitreous space through the fetal fissure. The primary vitreous is vascularized by the proliferating hyaloid system.

In the second stage, which occurs after the embryo reaches 13 mm., the lens capsule excludes the lens from participating further in vitreous formation. Vitreous now is formed by the inner layer of the optic cup at a time when the hyaloid vascular channels in the primary vitreous stop growing and begin to atrophy. Eventually the primary vitreous is surrounded by secondary vitreous and becomes limited to a cone-shaped region running through the vitreous space, its bases surrounding the posterior lens surface and its apex ending at the disc. Because the optical density of the primary and secondary vitreous differs, a line of demarcation (the wall of Cloquet's canal) can be seen at their interface. The hyaloid artery courses within Cloquet's canal to supply the vascular network surrounding the lens.

In the third stage the tertiary vitreous or the zonular fibers develop. This begins around the 65 mm. stage and is completed by the 110 mm. stage. The zonular fibers are derived both from the primary vitreous and from the basement membrane of the nonpigmented epithelium of the ciliary body. They eventually attach to the lens capsule, filling the gap between the rim of the optic cup and the lens (Fig. 3-13).

THE UVEAL TRACT

The uveal tract (choroid, ciliary body, and iris) is partly mesodermal and partly neural ectodermal in origin. The ectodermal components (epithelium of the ciliary body and iris) have been described previously. The choroid, derived from the paraxial mesoderm, appears early in gestation as a vascular net surrounding the primary optic vesicle. When pigment appears in the outer layer of the optic cup, Bruch's membrane begins to form and separates the future choriocapillaris from the retinal pigment epithelium. About the third month a second layer of relatively large venous channels (tributaries of the venae vorticosae) appears superficial to the choriocapillaris. At about the fourth month a third layer of vessels, derived from the short ciliary arteries, forms between the original two vascular networks. These vascular channels break up to supply the choriocapillaris. By the seventh month pigment-bearing cells (melanosomes) are evident in the outer layers of the choroid. Gradually the melanosomes migrate into the inner layers.

The ciliary muscle arises from paraxial mesoderm in contact with the outer surface of the optic cup in the region of the ciliary folds. By the third month muscle fibers begin to appear (Fig. 3-13). As they develop, they differentiate into longitudinal, meridional, and circular divisions. The muscle originates at the site of the future scleral spur. At its insertion posteriorly it is continuous with the connective tissue of the sclera and uvea.

The mesodermal tissue surrounding the margin of the optic cup, and the tunica vasculosa lentis form the iris stroma (Fig. 3-21). Initially this tissue forms the pupillary membrane, which stretches across the opening of the optic cup. As the epithelial margin of the optic cup grows forward, the pupillary membrane separates from the tunica vasculosa lentis. With further growth of the lips of the cup (epithelial layers of the iris), the peripheral portion of the pupillary membrane thickens and becomes vascularized by loops that also extend into its central (pupillary) zone (Fig. 3-18). The mesodermal iris is completely vascularized by about the seventh month. At this stage four tiers of vascular arcades can be recognized in the peripheral pupillary membrane (iris stroma). The central (pupillary) zone then begins to atrophy and eventually completely absorbs. Absorption extends peripherally beyond the pupillary aperture formed by

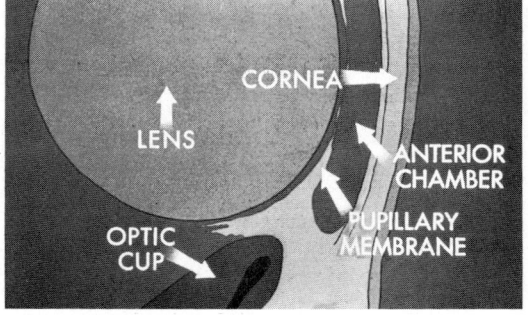

Figure 3-21 Drawing—seventh week. The tunica vasculosa lentis and mesoderm surrounding the optic cup form the pupillary membrane which stretches across the optic cup opening. As the neural epithelial portion of the iris advances forward from the optic cup margin, the tunica vasculosa lentis separates from the pupillary membrane. The iris epithelium then lies posterior to the portion of pupillary membrane that forms future iris stroma. (Courtesy of American Academy of Ophthalmology and Otolaryngology.)

the iris epithelium. As a result, a cleft called the iris collarette, or Fuchs' cleft, is formed in the iris stroma.

This cleft marks the location of an incomplete ring of arteriovenous anastomoses, sometimes called the minor arterial circle. The arterial channels which contribute to the minor arterial circle arise from the major arterial circle. Frequently in the adult, fine strands of tissue can be seen running from the collarette in one area of the iris to the collarette in another area, or from the collarette to the lens capsule. These strands represent the residual pupillary membrane which has failed to atrophy completely.

Pigment does not develop in the iris stroma until after birth. The amount of stromal pigmentation varies; if pigmentation is minimal, the iris is blue.

THE CORNEA AND ANTERIOR CHAMBER

The cornea is derived from both surface ectoderm and mesoderm. The surface ectoderm forms the corneal epithelium, and the mesoderm forms the rest of the cornea. After the lens vesicle forms, paraxial mesoderm from around the margin of the optic cup migrates between the lens vesicle and surface ectoderm. Part of this mesodermal sheet forms the pupillary membrane

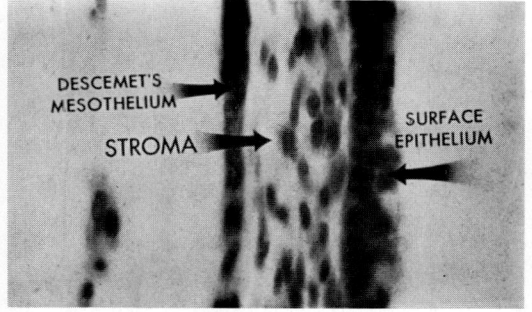

Figure 3-22 Photomicrograph—seventh week. Corneal epithelium is derived from surface ectoderm; the remainder of the cornea develops from mesoderm. Waves of mesoderm migrate between Descemet's mesothelium and surface ectoderm to form corneal stroma. (Courtesy of American Academy of Ophthalmology and Otolaryngology.)

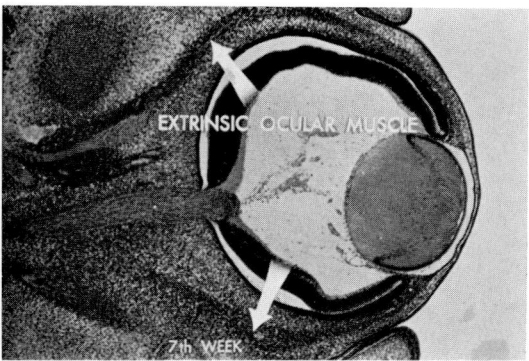

Figure 3-23 Photomicrograph—seventh week. Extraocular muscles initially appear as a single mass of paraxial mesoderm surrounding the optic vesicle. By the seventh week, mesoderm begins to separate into distinct muscle groups. (Courtesy of American Academy of Ophthalmology and Otolaryngology.)

and part forms a layer of mesothelium (future Descemet's mesothelium) parallel to the overlying surface ectoderm (Fig. 3-22). Successive waves of mesoderm migrate forward between the surface ectoderm and Descemet's mesothelium to form the substantia propria (stroma). Descemet's membrane, a true basement membrane, arises from Descemet's mesothelium. Bowman's membrane is a condensation of the anterior part of the substantia propria.

When the anterior chamber first becomes apparent, it is shallow and its angle is entirely filled with mesodermal tissue continuous with the pupillary membrane (Fig. 3-21). The ultimate configuration of the angle is attributed either to atrophy and resorption or cleavage of this tissue. The canal of Schlemm initially exists as a series of channels derived from the venous plexus at the margin of the optic cup (Fig. 3-13). By the third month, because of alteration in intraocular pressure dynamics, these channels begin to anastomose to form the definitive Schlemm's canal. Internal to the canal of Schlemm a small amount of mesodermal tissue persists as the trabecular meshwork of the angle.

THE SCLERA AND EXTRAOCULAR MUSCLES

The sclera arises as a condensation of paraxial mesoderm surrounding the optic cup. It first forms anteriorly near the future insertion of the rectus muscles and later spreads anteriorly and posteriorly. The posterior part develops later than the anterior. The sclera is fully differentiated at the fifth month.

The extraocular muscles also develop from paraxial mesodermal condensations surrounding the optic vesicle. Initially the extraocular muscles appear as a single, undifferentiated mass of mesoderm. By the 20 mm. stage the four recti and two obliques become recognizable as the mesodermal mass begins to separate into distinct muscle groups (Fig. 3-23). The separation occurs initially at the muscle insertions and then spreads proximally toward the origins. The levator palpebrae superioris arises last; it is derived from a separation within the mass of tissue that forms the superior rectus muscle.

THE ORBIT

The orbit forms early in the second month when the optic vesicle is being encircled by the lateral nasal process, which grows downward as the maxillary process extends upward. These two mesodermal masses join at the site of the future naso-lacrimal duct. The roof of the orbit forms from the capsule of the forebrain where the frontal bone develops. The floor and lateral orbital wall condense in the visceral mesoderm of the maxillary process. The medial wall originates from the lateral nasal process. Bones from the base of the skull complete the orbit posteriorly. At the two-month stage the optic axes make an angle of 160 degrees with each other, and at the 40 mm. stage this angle is reduced to 72 degrees, only about 10 degrees greater than in the adult.

THE EYELIDS AND ADNEXA

The rudiments of the eyelids appear as folds of surface ectoderm above and below the site of the eye at the 16 mm. stage. The skin of the lids arises from the outer layer of these folds, and the conjunctiva from the inner layer. Mesoderm grows in between the two layers of ectoderm and forms connective tissue elements, including the tarsal plates and the muscles of the lids. During the third month, the upper and lower lids fuse and remain adherent until the sixth month, when separation of the lid margins is complete. Cilia, meibomian glands, and lacrimal glands arise from the surface ectoderm.

POSTNATAL DEVELOPMENT

Although the eye is not completely developed at birth, it is a functioning sensory organ. Adult proportions are achieved early in life. The cornea, relatively large at birth, reaches adult size within the first two years of life. Pigment is absent from the iris stroma at term but appears at a variable time postpartum. The macula is poorly developed at birth and does not fully develop until four to six months of age.

DERIVATION OF OCULAR STRUCTURES*

Surface ectoderm gives rise to the following:

Lens.

Epithelium of the cornea.

Epithelium of the conjunctiva and hence to the lacrimal gland.

Epithelium of the lids and its derivatives, the cilia, the meibomian glands, and the glands of Moll and Zeis.

Epithelial lining of the lacrimal apparatus.

Neural ectoderm gives rise to the following:

Retina with its pigment epithelium.

Epithelium covering ciliary processes.

Pigment epithelium covering the posterior surface of the iris.

Sphincter and dilatator pupillae muscles.

Optic nerve (neuroglial and nervous elements only).

Adhesions between surface and neural ectoderm give rise to the following:

Vitreous.

Suspensory ligament of the lens.

Associated paraxial mesoderm gives rise to the following:

Blood vessels, i.e., the choroid, the arteria centralis retinae, ciliary vessels and other vessels of the orbit that persist, as well as the hyaloid artery, the vasa hyaloidea propria, and the vessels of the vascular capsule of the lens that disappear before birth.

Sclera.

Sheath of the optic nerve.

Ciliary muscle.

Substantia propria of the cornea and the endothelium of its posterior surface.

Stroma of the iris.

Extrinsic muscles of the eye.

Fat, ligaments, and other connective tissue structures in the orbit.

Upper and inner walls of the orbit.

Connective tissue of the upper lid.

Visceral mesoderm (maxillary process) below the eye gives rise to the following:

Lower and outer walls of the orbit. The structures lying behind and below the eye, i.e., the alisphenoid, malar, and orbital plate of superior maxilla.

Connective tissue of the lower lid.

*Adapted from Mann, I.: The Development of the Human Eye. 3rd ed. New York, Grune & Stratton, Inc. 1964.

During First Month

1. Formation of the optic pit and optic vesicle; invagination of the optic vesicle with formation of the optic cup and fetal fissure.

2. Presence of the lens pit in the lens plate and formation of the lens vesicle, which begins to detach from the surface ectoderm.

3. Pigmentation of the outer wall of the optic cup; formation of the primitive choroid.

4. Development of the inner nucleus free marginal zone and the outer proliferating cell layer of the retina.

5. Formation of the primitive vascular mesoderm (hyaloid artery) and posterior and lateral tunica vasculosa lentis.

During Second Month

1. Closure of the fetal fissure, except for the most anterior and posterior ends.

2. Separation of the lens vesicle from the surface ectoderm and obliteration of the lens vesicle cavity by primary lens fibers. Formation of the lens capsule (13 mm.); presence of secondary lens fibers (26 mm.); beginning formation of the Y sutures (35 mm.).

3. Completion of primary vitreous (13 mm.) and beginning of formation of secondary vitreous.

4. Formation of the inner and outer neuroblastic layers. Presence of nerve fibers coursing into the optic stalk; conversion of optic stalk into optic nerve and formation of chiasm; appearance of Bruch's membrane and internal limiting membrane.

5. Progression of the tunica vasculosa lentis and vasa hyaloidea propria to the height of their development; appearance of the long ciliary vessels.

6. Progression of the nasolacrimal system and lacrimal gland.

7. Presence of the anterior chamber and pupillary membrane; differentiation of Descemet's mesothelium.

8. Formation of the bony orbits.

9. Differentiation of the extraocular muscles.

During Third Month

1. Early development of retinal layers from the inner and outer neuroblastic layers.

2. Formation of neural ectodermal components of iris and ciliary body.

3. Atrophy of vasa hyaloidea propria; vascularization of the optic nerve and branching of central retinal artery on the disc; formation of the outer layer of the choroid.

4. Appearance of Descemet's and Bowman's membranes.

5. Appearance of canal of Schlemm.

6. Formation of the tertiary vitreous.

7. Presence of sclerotic condensations around the globe and appearance of the ciliary muscle.

8. Fusion of the eyelids.

During Fourth Month

1. Differentiation of sphincter pupillae muscle.

2. Atrophy of the tunica vasculosa lentis.

3. Formation of the middle layer of the choroid.

4. Early vascularization of the retina.

During Fifth Month

1. Differentiation of corneal curvature as distinct from curvature of the rest of the globe.

2. Completion of the choroid.

3. Formation of the meridional portion of the ciliary muscle.

4. Full differentiation of the sclera.

During Sixth Month

1. Formation of the circular portion of ciliary muscle.

2. Reopening of eyelids.

3. Differentiation of dilator pupillae muscle.

During Seventh Month

1. Formation of distinct pars plana.

2. Completion of vascularization of the mesodermal iris and beginning atrophy of the pupillary membrane in its central portion.

3. Medullation of the proximal end of the optic nerve.

4. Configuration of the filtration angle resembles that of the adult.

During Eighth Month

1. Completion of the sensory retina ex-

cept for the macular region, which begins to show differentiation.

2. Disappearance of hyaloid vascular system, except for remnants on the posterior lens surface.

During Ninth Month

1. Disappearance of pupillary membrane.

2. Medullation of the optic nerve up to the lamina cribrosa.

BIBLIOGRAPHY

Barber, A. N.: Embryology of the Human Eye. St. Louis, The C. V. Mosby Co., 1955.

Bock, L., and Seefelder, R.: Atlas zur Entwicklungsgeschichte des menschlichen Auges. Leipzig, 1914.

Duke-Elder, S., and Cook, C.: Normal and abnormal development. *In* System of Ophthalmology. Vol. IV, Part 1, Embryology. St. Louis, The C. V. Mosby Co., 1961.

Mann, I.: The Development of the Human Eye. 3rd ed. New York, Grune & Stratton, 1964.

Chapter Four

GENETICS AND OPHTHALMOLOGY

BASIC PRINCIPLES OF HEREDITY

In the past decade, much has been learned about human and animal genetics, but the *gene* is still useful as the basic unit of heredity. Each gene is a functional segment of a deoxyribonucleic acid (DNA) molecule, and together with other genes on a protein framework comprise the *chromosome*. Within each human cell there are about 100,000 different genes, and within any given population there is a multitude of alternative sets of genes. A gene's position on the chromosome is known as its locus, and for each of these functional loci a number of alternative units exist. The set of genes capable of occupying a given locus in a particular chromosome are known as *alleles*. The complement of a cell's genes is known as its *genotype*, whereas the ultimate expression of these genes in a physical, biochemical or physiological trait is considered a *phenotype*.

Within the nucleus of each cell, genes are united linearly into darkly staining chromosomes. They are invisible until cellular division begins when they align themselves to the mitotic spindle. The normal chromosomal complement of each human cell consists of 22 pairs of *autosomal* (nonsexual) chromosomes and one pair of *sex* chromosomes. Each cell, therefore, contains 46

chromosomes, which is the human *diploid* number.

Each chromosome is a particular size and has a characteristic constriction, the *centromere*. This can be centrally located (metacentric), slightly off center (submetacentric) or close to one end (acrocentric). Because of this consistency in size and position of

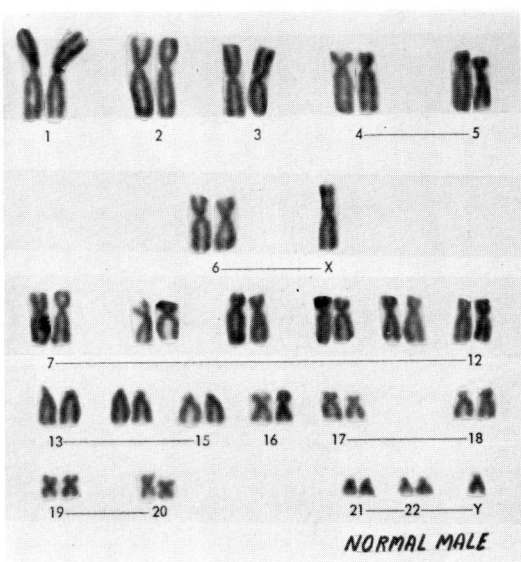

Figure 4-1 Chromosomal karyotype of a normal human male arranged according to the Denver classification. (Courtesy of Genetics Laboratory, Children's Hospital of Philadelphia.)

the centromere, cytogeneticists, in 1960, numbered and classified the chromosomes into standard groups. This arrangement is known as the Denver classification (Fig. 4-1).

MITOSIS AND MEIOSIS

Normal growth and development are accomplished by cellular division. Somatic cells multiply by mitosis (Fig. 4-2), a process in which the entire diploid number of chromosomes is duplicated and passed on to each daughter cell. This insures that each somatic cell contains the entire complement of chromosomes. Mature germinal cells, male spermatocytes and female oocytes, multiply by *meiosis* (Fig. 4-3), a process in which chromosomal material is duplicated only once, in two successive divisions. Thus, each mature gamete contains only one half (*haploid* number) of the total chromosomal complement that was present in the immature precursor gamete. When the male sperm and female egg unite at fertilization, they restore the normal diploid number. In this way, each individual receives half his genetic traits from his mother and the other half from his father.

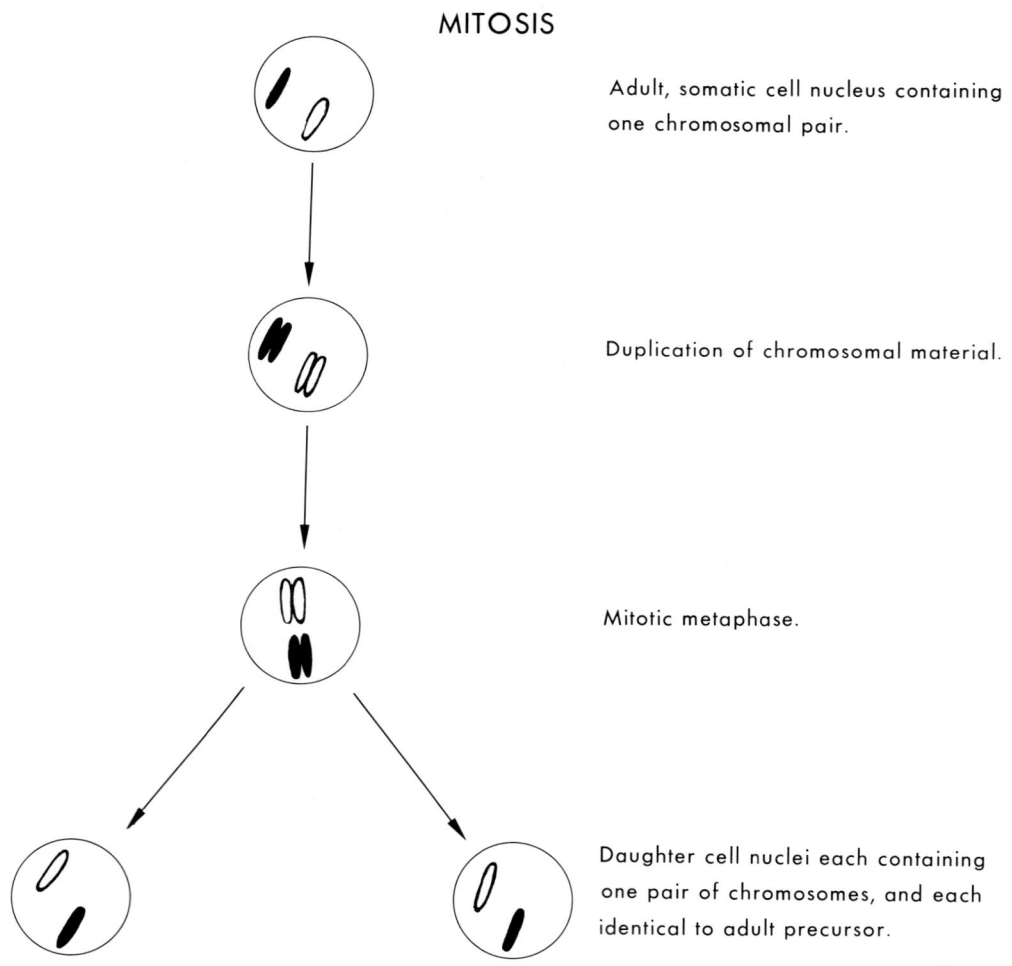

MITOSIS

Adult, somatic cell nucleus containing one chromosomal pair.

Duplication of chromosomal material.

Mitotic metaphase.

Daughter cell nuclei each containing one pair of chromosomes, and each identical to adult precursor.

Figure 4-2 Process of mitosis. Note that in the metaphase each duplicated chromosome lines up at the mitotic spindle by itself.

MEIOSIS

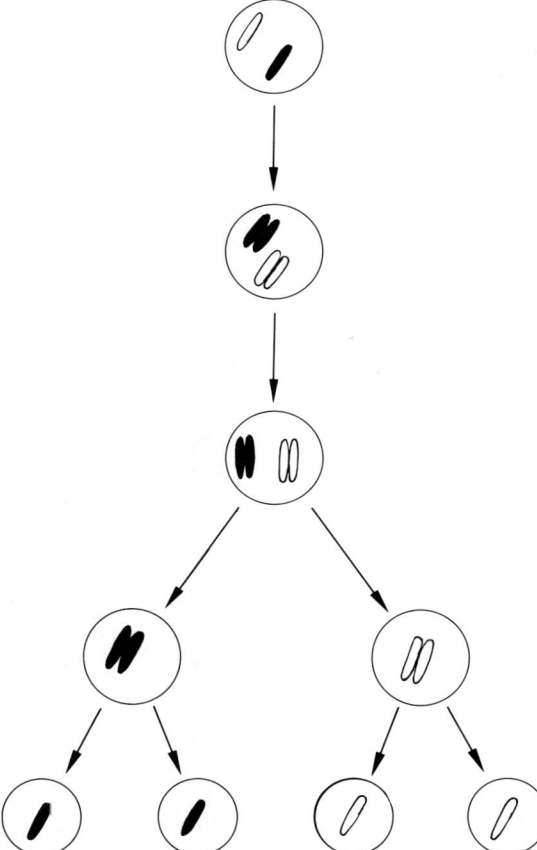

Immature male or female gamete nucleus containing one chromosomal pair.

Chromosomal duplication occurs as in mitosis.

Metaphase of first meiotic division. Each duplicated chromosome lines up at the spindle opposite its duplicated homologous chromosome.

First meiotic division: each pair of homologous chromosomes is separated.

Second meiotic division: each duplicated chromosome now divides, and mature gamete has one-half of its precursor's chromosomal complement.

Figure 4-3 Process of meiosis. Note that in the metaphase of the first meiotic division, each *pair* of duplicated homologous chromosomes lines up opposite the other.

GENETIC INHERITANCE PATTERNS

Although the actual transmission of the genetic material is governed by mitosis and meiosis, the genetically controlled traits may be expressed or depressed. To comprehend this, one should have a basic understanding of the concepts of dominance, recessiveness, autosomal versus sex-linked inheritance, penetrance, and expressivity. Modern geneticists have clarified and refined these concepts, but they still resemble the basic principles expounded by the brilliant Austrian monk, Johann Mendel, in 1865.

Each chromosome of a pair is identical to the other in that it contains genes controlling the same trait at the same locus. In any individual a simple trait can be controlled by a single pair of genes (alleles). There can be only two alleles for a simple trait in an individual, but a multitude of alleles for a chromosomal locus may exist in the entire population of the species. If two identical alleles are present, the individual is said to be *homozygous* for that gene or trait; if the genes are different, then the individual is *heterozygous*.

Autosomal Dominant Inheritance

When a gene expresses itself in an individual in either a single (*heterozygous*) or double (*homozygous*) dose, then it is said to be a dominant gene or trait. If the gene is located on one of the 22 pairs of autosomes, it is considered an autosomal dominant gene. For a simple hereditary trait governed by one pair of autosomal genes, there are three possible genotypes in an individual (Table 4-1). Since three genotypes could exist in each mate, there are six possible recombination patterns for any given pair of autosomal genes. These six patterns, along with the expected progeny, are shown in Table 4-2.

In medical genetics all of the possibilities do not need to be considered. Most of the genetically governed abnormalities and diseases in man are rare. This means that they generally exist, expressed or not

TABLE 4-1 GENOTYPES AND PHENOTYPES OF A SIMPLE DOMINANT HEREDITARY TRAIT*

Genes	Genotypes	Phenotypes
A	AA	Trait fully expressed
a	Aa	Trait fully or moderately expressed
	aa	Trait not expressed

*By convention, dominant genes are designated by capital letters and recessive genes by lower case letters.

expressed, in an individual in a heterozygous state. The most common recombination, then, for a rare, completely dominant autosomal gene is Aa × aa (Table 4-2). The criteria for making a diagnosis of a condition controlled by a rare dominant autosomal gene can be summarized by the following statements:

1. There is no "skipping" of generations (the trait appears in every generation).

2. Since this is an autosomal gene, the trait will be evenly distributed between males and females in each generation as well as in the entire geneologic tree.

3. An affected person will have an affected parent.

4. On the average, one half of the offspring of an affected parent will be affected.

TABLE 4-2 POSSIBLE RECOMBINATION PATTERNS OF A SIMPLE HEREDITARY TRAIT CONTROLLED BY A SINGLE PAIR OF GENES*

Genotypes of Parents	Genotypes of Offspring	
AA × AA	AA	100%
AA × Aa	AA	50%
	Aa	50%
AA × aa	Aa	100%
Aa × Aa	AA	25%
	Aa	50%
	aa	25%
Aa × aa	Aa	50%
	aa	50%
aa × aa	aa	100%

*See note Table 4-1.

The foregoing summary applies strictly to a completely dominant gene which, as mentioned before, is expressed every time it is present, even in a single dose. This is extremely rare, and more commonly the clear-cut patterns of inheritance as laid down by Mendel are modified, altered, or obscured by such factors as reduced penetrance, variable expressivity, intermediate inheritance, interaction of two or more gene pairs, and the influence of environment.

When a dominant gene is present in an individual but its trait is not expressed, the gene has reduced *penetrance* and is an *irregular* autosomal dominant. The individual's genotype would contain the abnormal dominant gene, but he would be phenotypically normal. Penetrance can be expressed as a percentage. For example, if each of five individuals were known to possess a dominant gene, and yet only four of the five exhibited the trait controlled by the gene (the fifth being normal), this gene would be exhibiting 80 per cent penetrance. Retinoblastoma (p. 152) is an example of an inherited condition that is governed by a dominant autosomal gene with incomplete penetrance.

The concept of expressivity can be likened to that of clinical severity. Many genetic disorders are characterized by a number of different abnormalities in a given individual. Not all of these abnormalities, however, will be present in every affected person; thus, one can say that the gene involved is exhibiting variable expressivity. Marfan's syndrome (p. 222), inherited as an autosomal dominant, is a good example of a genetic disorder whose expression varies.

In *intermediate inheritance* the heterozygous individual differs from both the homozygous dominant and the homozygous recessive. This also can be roughly equated with clinical severity and thus can be likened to expressivity. A gene showing intermediate inheritance may exhibit a "dose response" curve; i.e., a homozygous recessive will not be expressed, the heterozygote will be partially expressed, and the homozygous dominant will be most completely expressed and also exhibit the most severe form of the disease. An excellent example of this phenomenon is seen in individuals with sickle cell disease (homozygous) and those with sickle cell trait (heterozygous).

Occasionally the clinical severity of an inherited disease or syndrome is so mild or insignificant as to be indistinguishable from a variation of normal. This extremely benign expression is known as a *forme fruste*.

In addition, it is now accepted that the expression or penetrance of a gene may be altered by interaction with a nonallelic gene. Moreover, the gene's expression or severity may be controlled to some extent by environment. For instance, the manifestations of galactosemia may never be expressed if the infant is kept on a galactose-free diet.

Dominant traits thus can be either inherited along classic Mendelian lines or modified. Table 4-3 lists the ocular and systemic abnormalities and disorders that exhibit classic or modified patterns of autosomal dominant inheritance.

Autosomal Recessive Inheritance

An individual who exhibits a trait that is strictly recessive is genotypically homozygous, having received a recessive gene from each parent. Because such genes are rare, it would be unusual for the parents of the affected individual to show any evidence of the trait. Each parent would be genetically heterozygous and phenotypically normal, and both would be carriers. Since genes are passed down through families, the appearance of a recessive trait (especially a rare one) in an individual suggests the possibility of parental consanguinity. The criteria then for diagnosing autosomal recessive inheritance are as follows:

1. An equal number of males and females are involved.

2. The parents of an affected individual do not exhibit the condition.

3. Approximately one fourth of the sibship will show involvement.

4. There is greater than usual chance that the parents are consanguineous.

5. Fifty per cent of the offspring will be carriers.

Occasionally both a parent and a child have a condition that is known to be an autosomal recessive. This is quasidominance or pseudodominance. The affected

TABLE 4-3 DISORDERS EXHIBITING REGULAR OR IRREGULAR PATTERNS OF
AUTOSOMAL DOMINANT INHERITANCE

I. Regular Autosomal Dominant Traits
  A. Ocular Abnormalities or Syndromes
     Absence of tears*
     Aniridia*
     Anisometropia*
     Anterior embryotoxon*
     Blepharochalasis
     Blepharophimosis
     Canaliculi absence or atresia
     Cataracts
        Acquired
        Congenital
     Choroidal sclerosis
     Corectopia
     Cornea plana
     Corneal dystrophies*
        Bückler's annular dystrophy
        Cornea guttata
        Fleischer's vortex dystrophy
        Groenouw's Type I (granular)
        Haab-Dimmer's lattice dystrophy
        Meesman's epithelial dystrophy
        Mottled dystrophy (Francois and Neetens)
        Posterior polymorphous degeneration
        Schnyder's crystalline dystrophy
     Ectopia lentis*
     Epiblepharon
     Epicanthus
     Entropion
     Esotropia*
     Exotropia
     External ophthalmoplegia (congenital)
     Fuchs' heterochromia
     Glaucoma*
        Narrow angle
        Open angle
     Hyperopia, mild
     Jaw-winking (Marcus Gunn)
     Keratoconus*
     Lenticonus*
     Macular degeneration*
        Best's vitelliform macular degeneration
        Doyne's honeycomb hyaline degeneration
        Mallatia leventinese
        Sorsby's inflammatory macular degeneration
        Stargardt's juvenile macular degeneration
        Tay's macular "choroiditis"
     Megalocornea*
     Megalopapilla
     Melanosis oculi*
     Microphthalmia*
     Myopia, mild and severe*
     Night blindness*
     Nystagmus*
     Optic atrophy*
        Congenital
        Infantile
     Polycoria
     Posterior embryotoxon (Axenfeld's)
     Pterygium
     Retinal detachment
     Retinitis pigmentosa*
     Retinoschisis*
     Rieger's anomaly*
  B. Systemic Disorders with Ocular Abnormalities
     1. Dermatological syndromes
          Peutz-Touraine syndrome
          Siemens' keratosis follicularis
     2. Hematological Disorders
          Familial hemorrhagic telangiectasia

*Asterisk designates disorders that have more than one type of inheritance pattern and appear in other tables.

TABLE 4-3   DISORDERS EXHIBITING REGULAR OR IRREGULAR PATTERNS OF AUTOSOMAL DOMINANT INHERITANCE *(Continued)*

3. Metabolic Disorders
   - Diabetes mellitus*
   - Primary amyloidosis
4. Musculoskeletal Disorders
   - Apert's syndrome*
   - Bonnevie-Ullrich syndrome
   - Congenital stippled epiphyses*
   - Crouzon's craniofacial dysostosis*
   - Hypertelorism*
   - Osteogenesis imperfecta
   - Osteopetrosis (Albers-Schönberg)*
   - Oxycephaly*
   - Paget's osteitis deformans
   - Pleonosteosis (Leri)
5. Neurological Disorders
   - Amyotrophic lateral sclerosis
   - Charcot-Marie-Tooth disease*
   - Huntington's chorea
   - Hypertrophic neuritis (Déjerine-Sottas)
   - Marie's cerebellar ataxia*
   - Myotonic dystrophy (Steinert's)
6. Unclassified Syndromes
   - Alport's syndrome
   - Ascher's syndrome
   - Nonne-Milroy-Meige hereditary lymphedema*

II. Irregular Autosomal Dominant Traits
   A. Ocular Abnormalities or Syndromes
      - Anisocoria
      - Ankyloblepharon
      - Astigmatism
      - Coloboma
         - Choroid
         - Iris
         - Lens
         - Optic nerve
         - Retina
   - Distichiasis
   - Fuchs' endoepithelial dystrophy
   - Iris flocculi
   - Macular degeneration*
      - Doyne's honeycomb macular degeneration
      - Sorsby's inflammatory macular degeneration
   - Microcornea
   - Optic atrophy* (Leber's)
   - Persistent pupillary membrane
   - Ptosis
   - Retinoblastoma
   - Retraction syndrome (Duane's)
   B. Systemic Disorders with Ocular Abnormalities
      1. Dermatological syndromes
         - Incontinentia pigmenti
      2. Hematological Disorders
         - Congenital hemolytic jaundice
      3. Metabolic Disorders
         - Familial hypercholesterolemia
         - Gaucher's disease*
         - Gout
      4. Musculoskeletal Disorders
         - Crouzon's craniofacial dysostosis*
         - Ehlers-Danlos syndrome
         - Klippel-Feil syndrome
         - Mandibulofacial dysostosis
         - Weil-Marchesani syndrome*
      5. Neurological Disorders
         - Marie's cerebellar ataxia*
         - Neurofibromatosis
         - Sturge-Weber syndrome
         - Tuberous sclerosis (Bourneville)
         - von Hippel-Lindau angiomatosis
      6. Unclassified syndromes
         - Waardenburg's syndrome

*Asterisk designates disorders that have more than one type of inheritance pattern and appear in other tables.

TABLE 4-4 DISORDERS EXHIBITING PATTERNS OF AUTOSOMAL RECESSIVE INHERITANCE

I. Ocular Abnormalities or Syndromes
    Absence of tears*
    Achromatopsia
    Aniridia*
    Anisometropia*
    Anophthalmia
    Anterior embryotoxon*
    Corneal dystrophies*
        Groenouw's Type II (macular)
        Kraupa's epithelial dystrophy
    Cryptophthalmia
    Ectopia lentis*
    Esotropia*
    Falciform fold of the retina
    Fuchs' gyrate atrophy of choroid and retina
    Fundus albipunctatus cum hemeralopia
    Glaucoma*
        Congenital
        Narrow angle
        Open angle
    Hyperopia, severe
    Keratoconus*
    Lenticonus*
    Macular degeneration*
        Favre-Goldmann's vitreotapetoretinal degeneration
        Stargardt's juvenile macular degeneration
    Melanosis oculi*
    Microphthalmia*
    Monochromatism*
    Myopia, severe*
    Night blindness*
    Nystagmus*
    Oguchi's disease
    Optic atrophy*
        Behr's syndrome
        Congenital or infantile
    Retinitis pigmentosa*
    Retinitis punctata albescens
    Retinoschisis*
    Rieger's anomaly*
    Spherophakia
II. Systemic Disorders with Ocular Abnormalities
  A. Dermatological syndromes
      Congenital icthyosis
      Cystic adenoid epithelioma (Brook's)
      Hereditary ectodermal dysplasia
      Keratosis palmoplantaris
      Progeria
      Rothmund's poikiloderma
      Sjögren-Larsson xerodermal idiocy
  B. Hematological disorders
      Acanthocytosis

      Chediak-Higashi disease
      Fanconi's aplastic anemia
  C. Metabolic disorders
      Albinism, complete general
      Alkaptonuria
      Batten-Mayou cerebromacular degeneration
      Cystinosis
      Diabetes mellitus*
      Essential familial hyperlipemia
      Galactosemia
      Gaucher's disease*
      Hepatolenticular degeneration (Wilson's)
      Homocystinuria
      Lipoid proteinosis (Urbach-Wiethe)
      Mucopolysaccharidoses*
        MPS I   (Hurler)
        MPS III (Sanfilippo)
        MPS IV (Morquio)
        MPS V (Scheie)
        MPS VI (Morateaux-Lamy)
      Niemann-Pick disease
      Phenylketonuria
      Porphyrinuria
      Tay-Sachs disease
      von Gierke's disease
  D. Musculoskeletal disorders
      Apert's syndrome*
      Hypertelorism*
      Osteopetrosis (Albers-Schonberg)*
      Oxycephaly*
      Progressive facial hemiatrophy (Romberg)
      Pseudoxanthoma elasticum
      Weil-Marchesani syndrome*
  E. Neurological disorders
      Aubineau-Lenoble (nystagmus-myoclonia)
      Behr's optic atrophy-ataxia
      Familial dysautonomia (Riley-Day)
      Friedreich's ataxia
      Hallgren's vestibulocerebellar ataxia
      Kloepfer's syndrome
      Lafora's disease
      Louis-Bar's ataxic telangiectasia
      Oligophrenia
      Pelizaeus-Merzbacher disease
      Refsum's syndrome
      Sjögren's syndrome
      Strumpell-Lorrain spasmodic paraplegia*
  F. Unclassified syndromes
      Cystic fibrosis
      Marinesco-Sjögren syndrome
      Pseudohypoparathyroidism

*Asterisk designates disorders that have more than one type of inheritance pattern and appear in other tables.

parent is genetically homozygous, but the unaffected one is phenotypically normal and genetically heterozygous, though a carrier for the recessive abnormal trait. Abnormalities and disorders that have exhibited simple autosomal recessiveness are shown in Table 4-4.

Sex-Linked Inheritance

When a gene is located on either the X or Y chromosome it is said to be *sex-linked*. Sex-linkage can be considered synonymous with X-linkage because the *Y-linked* traits, apart from sex determination, have not been recognized to any great extent. The only proven Y-linked gene is the "hairy pinna" trait, which shows *holandric* inheritance; i.e., it is passed on from an affected male to all his sons but never to his daughters, since the Y chromosome is normally found only in males.

Since the X chromosome appears as a homologous pair in the female, three genotypes are possible for X-linked traits in the female, regardless of whether the trait is recessive or dominant. Thus, in females, X-linked traits react much like autosomal traits, and the phenotype would depend on whether the trait is dominant or recessive. On the other hand, the male receives only one X chromosome and is therefore considered hemizygous for X-linked genes. Regardless of whether the trait is dominant or recessive, if it is present on the X chromosome in the male, it would be expressed because there is no corresponding locus on the Y chromosome for the homologous allele. Thus there are only two genotypes possible in the male (Table 4-5).

A sex-linked trait may be dominant, incompletely recessive, or completely reces-

TABLE 4-6 EXPECTED PROGENY FROM MATING A HETEROZYGOUS FEMALE CARRYING A RARE, ABNORMAL X-LINKED GENE WITH A NORMAL MALE*

Parental Genotypes	Possible Offspring
Mother $X_a X_o$	Daughters $X_a X_o$ $X_o X_o$
Father $X_o Y$	Sons $X_a Y$ $X_o Y$

Daughters: 50% normal, 50% carriers
Sons: 50% normal, 50% affected

*Sub-letter "a" designates *abnormal* X-linked gene; sub-letter "o" designates *normal* X-linked allele.

sive. When dominant, it is expressed in both the male and female; when incompletely recessive, it appears as a carrier state in the female and as a fully expressed trait in the male; when completely recessive, it tends to remain hidden in the female and appears only in the male. A rare, abnormal, sex-linked gene most commonly occurs as a hidden recessive in an otherwise normal-looking female. The progeny of this heterozygous female and a normal male is shown in Table 4-6.

Since X-linked disorders are inherited generally through completely or incompletely recessive genes, the criteria for diagnosing sex-linked recessive inheritance are the following:

1. The trait appears more often in males than in females.

2. An affected male must at least have a carrier mother.

3. A carrier mother will give birth to 50 per cent affected males and 50 per cent carrier females (Table 4-6).

4. An affected male will sire normal sons and 100 per cent carrier daughters. He *never* will transmit the trait to his son.

5. Consanguinity is suspected only when an affected female is born.

It has become increasingly obvious that recessive sex-linked traits may appear in the female in the heterozygous state. Thus, one occasionally sees no expression, inter-

TABLE 4-5 GENOTYPES OF X-LINKED INHERITED TRAITS *

X-linked Genes	Male Genotypes	Female Genotypes
		$X_A X_A$
X_A	$X_A Y$	$X_A X_a$
X_a	$X_a Y$	$X_a X_a$

*Sub-letters "A" and "a" designate dominant and recessive X-linked traits, respectively.

Chromosome	Barr Bodies
XO	0
XY	0
XXY	1
XXXY	2
XX	1
XXX	2
XXXX	3

mediate expression, or complete expression of a recessive X-linked gene that is presumed to be present in the female in only a single dose. This interesting phenomenon possibly can be explained by the Lyon hypothesis described subsequently.

In 1949, Dr. Murray Barr described a darkly staining body (Fig. 4-4) that is found just inside the nuclear membrane of most cells in a normal female. This mass of chromatin, known as the *Barr body*, is present whenever there are two or more X chromosomes in a given cell. The number of chromatin masses per cell now is recognized to be one less than the number of X chromosomes in that cell (Table 4-7).

Only one Barr body appears in normal females and is considered to be an inactive form of one of the X chromosomes of the cell. This led to the Lyon hypothesis proposed by Dr. Mary Lyon in 1961:

1. The sex chromatin appearing as a Barr body is an inactive X chromosome.

2. This inactive chromosome can be either the paternal or maternal X chromosome.

3. Inactivation occurs some time in embryonic life.

Apparently the selection of which X chromosome becomes inactivated (either the maternal or paternal X) is random, but once a particular inactivated X chromosome is established in a given cell, then all the daughter cells supposedly will have the same X inactivated. Therefore, a woman will be composed of a mosaic pattern with some cells containing an inactivated paternal X chromosome and others containing an inactivated maternal X chromosome.

The Lyon hypothesis explains several of the interesting phenomena that have been observed in sex-linked inheritance. It explains dosage compensation, in which a female homozygous for a recessive gene or trait is no more severely affected than the male who has only one of these recessive genes. It also explains the variability of expression in heterozygous females, from the telltale signs of a carrier state to the complete appearance of the full-blown syndrome in a woman who is heterozygous for a sex-linked recessive gene.

If one X chromosome with a normal gene becomes a Barr body, and the X chromosome carrying the recessive gene responsible for an abnormal trait is on the remaining, active chromosome, then the cell will exhibit the abnormal trait even though heterozygous. The earlier in embryonic life that this cell line is established, the more cells will be under the influence of the abnormal gene and the greater will be the systemic expression of the abnormal trait. At present, this concept is best applied in the explanation of the variable expression of albinism (from localized ocular involvement to a complete generalized affection) in heterozygous females. Table 4-8 lists the ocular and systemic disorders which show various types of X-linked hereditary patterns.

CHROMOSOMAL ABERRATIONS

The concept that human disorders can be caused by abnormalities in the number or the structure of chromosomes was removed

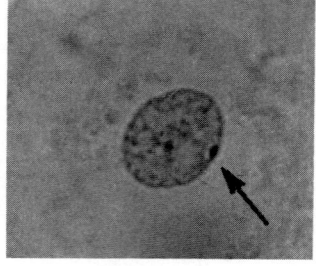

Figure 4-4 Single Barr body (arrow). It is evident as a darkly staining chromatin mass located on the nuclear membrane of a normal human female. (Courtesy of Genetics Laboratory, Children's Hospital of Philadelphia.)

TABLE 4-8   DISORDERS EXHIBITING PATTERNS OF X-LINKED INHERITANCE

   I. X-linked recessive inheritance
      A. Ocular abnormalities or syndromes
            Dyschromatopsia*
            Esotropia*
            Megalocornea*
            Monochromatism*
            Night blindness*
            Nystagmus*
            Optic atrophy (Leber's)*
            Retinitis pigmentosa*
            Retinoschisis*
            Rieger's anomaly*
      B. Systemic disorders with ocular abnormalities
            1. Dermatologic syndromes
                  Xeroderma pigmentosum*
            2. Hematologic disorders
                  Hemophilia
            3. Metabolic disorders
                  Glycolipid lipidosis (Fabry)
                  Mucopolysaccharidosis*
                   MPS II (Hunter)
            4. Musculoskeletal disorders
                  Congenital stippled epiphyses*
            5. Neurologic disorders
                  Charcot-Marie-Tooth disease*
                  Hydrocephaly
            6. Unclassified syndromes
                  Laurence-Moon-Biedl syndrome
                  Lowe's syndrome
                  Nonne-Milroy-Meige hereditary lymphedema*
                  Norrie's disease
  II. X-linked intermediate inheritance
      A. Ocular abnormalities or syndromes
            Albinism, ocular
            Choroideremia
            Dyschromatopsia*
            Retinitis pigmentosa*
      B. Systemic disorders with ocular abnormalities
            Anhidrotic ectodermal dysplasia
            Keratosis follicularis spinulosa decalvans
 III. X-linked dominant inheritance
      A. Ocular abnormalities or syndromes
            Nystagmus*
      B. Systemic disorders with ocular abnormalities
            Xeroderma pigmentosum*

*Asterisk designates disorders that have more than one type of inheritance pattern and appear in other tables.

from theoretical speculation in 1959 when Lejeune and Turpin demonstrated that mongolism was associated with 47 chromosomes instead of with the normal complement of 46. Since then other disorders involving abnormal numbers of either autosomes or sex chromosomes have been recognized.

Cell nuclei contain either extra complete sets of chromosomes or an extra single chromosome. When the number of chromosomes is greater than normal and a multiple of the haploid number, the condition is known as a *polyploidy*. Polyploid individuals usually do not live, but triploidy (69 chromosomes) and tetraploidy (92 chromosomes) have been reported in live, full-term neonates. If only one chromosome, however, is present or absent, the condition is called *aneuploidy*. The most common varieties of aneuploidy are those exhibiting 45, 47, or 48 chromosomes. When the extra chromosome is identifiable as to its classification number, the disorder usually is called a trisomy, as exemplified by trisomy 21, or mongolism. If the extra chromosome can only be identified according to its Denver group, the condition usually is named according to the letter corresponding to that group, such as the "D" and "E" trisomy syndromes.

Not only are autosomal chromosomes involved in aberrations of chromosomal number, but a number of disorders are known where there is aneuploidy of the sex chromosome. Moreover, certain individuals possess two distinct cell lines, some normal and some trisomic for either an autosomal or sex chromosome. These individuals, *mosaics*, may or may not be phenotypically abnormal.

Structural aberrations of chromosomes must also be considered, although most of the proved structural changes come from experimental research in lower animals, especially the fruit fly, Drosophila. These are described as deletions, duplications, inversions, translocations, and isochromosomes. In human genetics, deletions and translocations appear to be the only significant structural abnormalities that have been identified and studied.

Down's Syndrome (Trisomy 21; Mongolism). In this most common and best known of the chromosomal syndromes, the extra chromosome 21 may be found free within the cell nucleus (Fig. 4-5), translocated to the D group (13-15/21 translocation mongol), or translocated to the G group (21/22 translocation mongol) (Fig. 4-6).

There are no significant clinical differences between the trisomy 21 and the translocations; all the affected individuals show similar abnormalities. Systemic findings include mental retardation (IQ in 25 to 50 range), short stature, hypotonia, brachycephaly, saddle-shaped nose, and a large, protruding tongue. The skin usually is soft and the hair smooth. Abnormalities of the extremities include short, bent arms and legs, and short, broad hands with a simian crease. Cardiac abnormalities are present in about 35 per cent of cases.

Abnormalities of the eyes are common, with the infants frequently exhibiting hypertelorism, epicanthus, strabismus (usually convergent), and nystagmus. The fissures are small and oblique. In blue-eyed infants, small, white, iris speckles (Brushfield spots) are often seen, but some authors consider these insignificant. Cataracts, both lamellar and posterior polar, have been found in about 50 per cent of cases and may be progressive. Some 30 per cent have high myopia, and keratoconus has been reported in some series as frequently as 6 per cent of the time.

Trisomy 18 (E Syndrome; Edwards' Syndrome). Trisomy 18 was first described by Edwards in 1960. It is due to an extra chromosome present in the E group, probably number 18 (Fig. 4-7), and is more severe than Down's syndrome. Usually it is fatal by the time the individual is 6 months of age.

The systemic abnormalities consist of failure to thrive, mental retardation, low-set ears with malformed pinnae, hypertonicity, small mouth and mandible, flexion deformities of the fingers, "rocker bottom" foot deformity, renal anomalies, and congenital heart defects. Ocular defects thus far reported include ptosis, lenticular opacities, corneal opacities, congenital glaucoma, and optic atrophy.

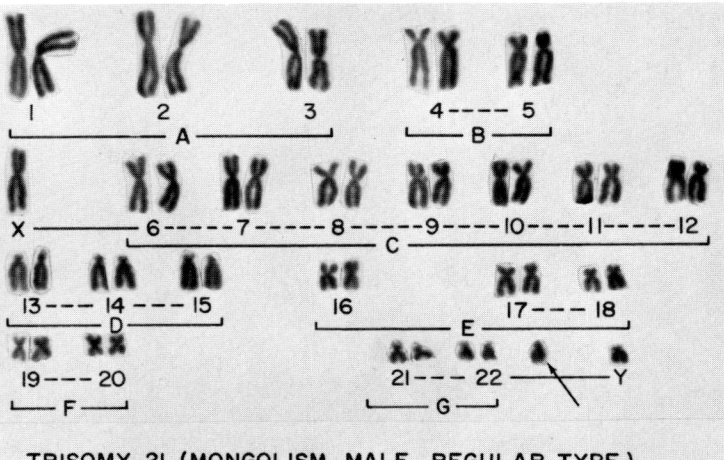

Figure 4-5 Karyotype of trisomy 21 showing an extra free chromosome (arrow). (Courtesy of Genetics Laboratory, Children's Hospital of Philadelphia.)

TRISOMY 21 (MONGOLISM, MALE, REGULAR TYPE)

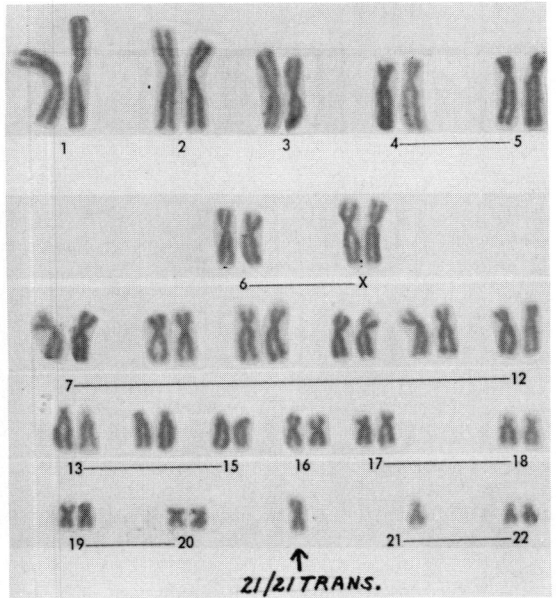

21/21 TRANS.

Figure 4-6 Karyotype of a 21/21 translocation mongol showing an extra chromosome attached to chromosome 21 (arrow). (Courtesy of Genetics Laboratory, Children's Hospital of Philadelphia.)

Figure 4-7 Karyotype of E syndrome showing extra chromosome 18 (arrow). (Courtesy of Genetics Laboratory, Children's Hospital of Philadelphia.)

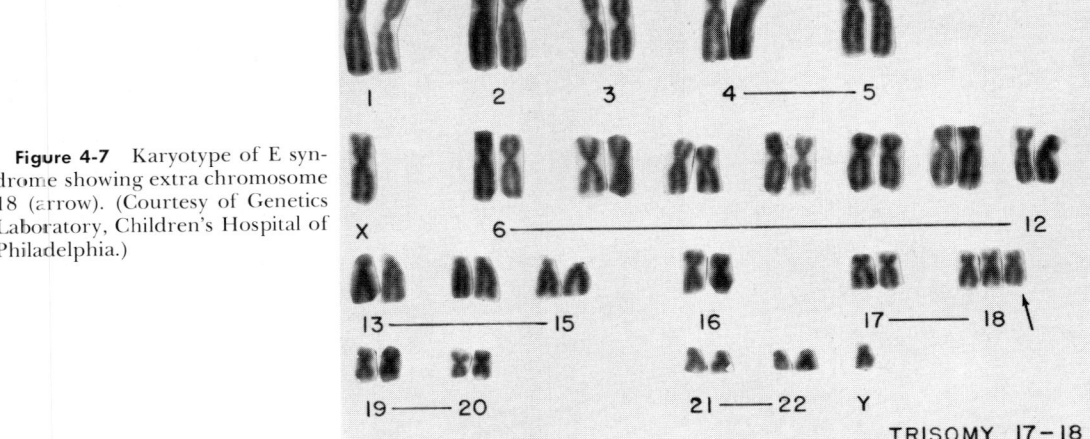

TRISOMY 17-18

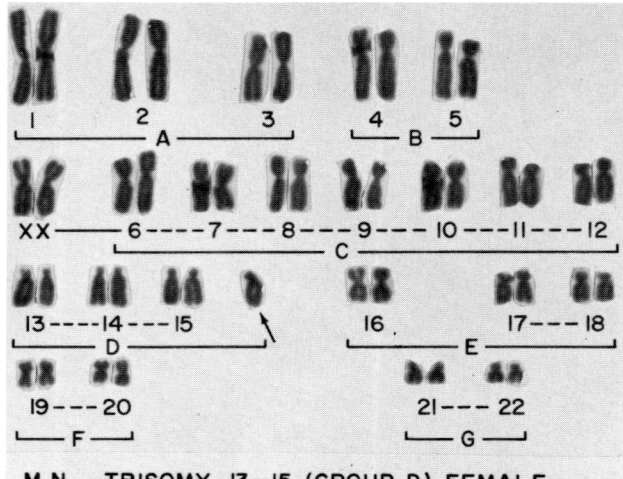

M.N. TRISOMY 13-15 (GROUP D) FEMALE

Figure 4-8   Karyotype of D syndrome showing an extra chromosome in the 13-15 group (arrow). (Courtesy of Genetics Laboratory, Children's Hospital of Philadelphia.)

Figure 4-9   Karyotype of Turner's syndrome. Note absence of Y chromosome and presence of only one X chromosome. (Courtesy of Genetics Laboratory, Children's Hospital of Philadelphia.)

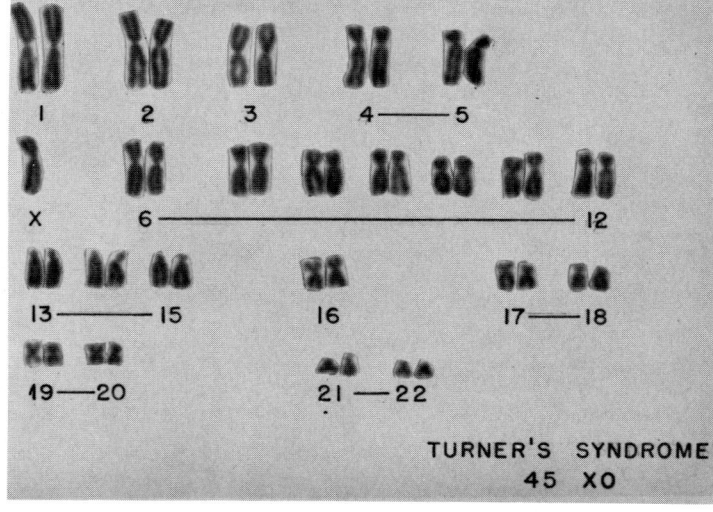

TURNER'S SYNDROME
45 XO

13-15 Trisomy (D Syndrome; Patau's Syndrome). The trisomy syndrome involving the D group of chromosomes is even rarer than trisomy 18, and the condition is more severe, with individuals exhibiting malformations of the brain, heart, and viscera (Fig. 4-8). Mental retardation, cleft palate and harelip, polydactyly, spina bifida, multiple hemangiomas of the skin, and congenital heart disease (especially intraventricular septal defects) have all been observed. The eyes may become glaucomatous from ocular changes that include anophthalmia or microphthalmia, retinal dysplasia, colobomata, cataract, and hypertelorism.

Turner's Syndrome (Gonadal Dysgenesis). This syndrome is characterized by females whose cells exhibit a male sex chromatin pattern (first example of Table 4-7). The karyotype reveals 44 autosomes but only one X chromosome (Fig. 4-9); the sex genotype is therefore XO, and the genetic result is believed to be due to the fertilization of a normal egg (carrying a normal X from the mother) by an abnormal sperm that is devoid of either the paternal X or Y chromosomes. In reality this type of female is hemizygous, as is a normal male, and she will exhibit X-linked recessive traits at a greater frequency than seen in normal (XX) females.

The systemic abnormalities include infantilism, pterygium colli, equinovarus, dwarfism, amenorrhea, and congenital heart defects. Epicanthus, strabismus, cataracts, corneal opacities, and congenital glaucoma have all been observed. About 8 per cent of individuals with Turner's syndrome are color blind, which is the same frequency of occurrence for this X-linked trait in the normal (XY) male population.

Other Chromosomal Abnormalities

Besides the specific syndromes mentioned previously, the literature is abounding recently with preliminary reports of new chromosomal disorders. One must be careful, however, not to relate a specific clinical abnormality with a specific chromosomal defect until enough cases justify the association.

The chromosomal abnormalities thus far reported include Klinefelter's syndrome (XXY), Sturge-Weber syndrome (partial trisomy 22), cri du chat syndrome (partial deletion of chromosome 5) (Fig. 4-10), and antimongolism (partial deletion of chromosome 21). Partial deletions involving chromosomes 6, 18, and 22 have also been noted.

BIBLIOGRAPHY

Barr, M. L.: Sex chromatin and phenotype in man. Science *130*:679, 1959.
De Grouchy, J., Veslot, J., Bonnette, J., and Roidot, M.: A case of ?6p-chromosomal aberration. Am. J. Dis. Child. *115*:93, 1968.

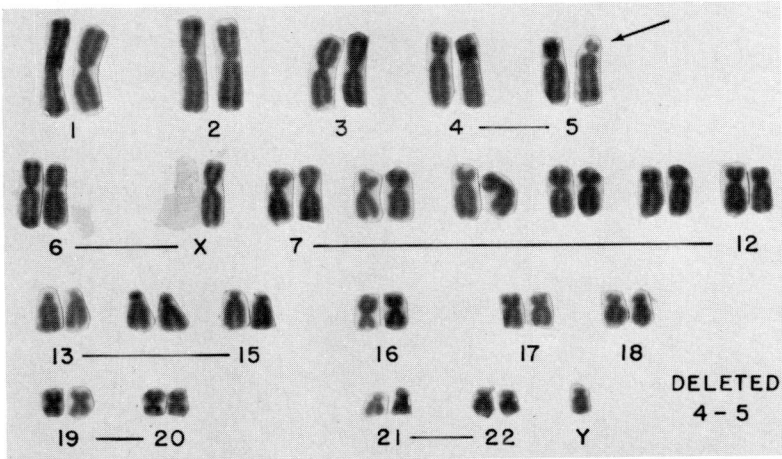

Figure 4-10 Karyotype of cri du chat syndrome showing partial deletion of chromosome 5 (arrow). (Courtesy of Genetics Laboratory, Children's Hospital of Philadelphia.)

Duke-Elder, S.: Normal and abnormal development. Part 2. Congenital deformities. *In* Duke-Elder, S. (ed.): System of Ophthalmology. Vol. 3. St. Louis, The C. V. Mosby Co., 1963.

Durham, R. H.: Encyclopedia of Medical Syndromes. New York, Paul B. Hoeber, Inc., 1960.

Falls, H. F.: A classification and clinical description of hereditary macular lesions. Tr. Am. Acad. Ophth. *70*:1034, 1967.

Falls, H. F.: Clinical detection of the genetic carrier state in ophthalmic pathology. Tr. Am. Acad. Ophth. *57*:858, 1953.

Falls, H. F.: The role of sex chromosome in hereditary ocular pathology. Tr. Am. Ophth. Soc. *50*:421, 1952.

Francois, J., and Matton-Van Leuven, M.: Chromosome abnormalities and ophthalmology. J. Pediat. Ophth. *1*:5, 1964.

Francois, J.: Congenital Cataracts. Assen, Netherlands, Charles C Thomas, 1963.

Francois, J.: Heredity in Ophthalmology. St. Louis, The C. V. Mosby Co., 1961.

Harrison, T. R.: Principles of Internal Medicine. Vols. 1 and 2. New York, McGraw-Hill Book Co., Inc., 1962.

Hayward, M. D., and Bower, B. D.: Trisomy associated with Sturge-Weber syndrome. Lancet *2*:844, 1960.

Human mitotic chromosomes: proposed standard system of nomenclature of Denver classification. Lancet *1*:1063, 1960.

Lejeune, J., and Turpin, R.: Chromosomal aberrations in man. Am. J. Human Genet. *13*:175, 1961.

Liebman, S. D., and Gellis, S. S.: The Pediatrician's Ophthalmology. St. Louis, The C. V. Mosby Co., 1966.

Lyon, M. F.: Sex chromatin and gene action in the mammalian x-chromosome. Am. J. Human Genet. *14*:135, 1962.

McKusick, V. A.: Heritable Disorders of Connective Tissue. St. Louis, The C. V. Mosby Co., 1966.

McKusick, V. A.: Human Genetics. Englewood Cliffs, New Jersey, Prentice-Hall, 1964.

Nelson, W. E.: Textbook of Pediatrics. Philadelphia, W. B. Saunders Co., 1964.

Newell, F. W.: Ophthalmology Principles and Concepts. St. Louis, The C. V. Mosby Co., 1965.

Riesman, L. E., Darnell, A., Murphy, J. W., Hall, B., and Kasara, S.: A child with partial deletion of a G-group autosome. Am. J. Dis. Child. *114*:336, 1967.

Smith, D. W., Patau, K., Therman, E.: Autosomal trisomy syndromes. Lancet *2*:211, 1961.

Stern, C.: Principles of Human Genetics. 2nd ed. San Francisco, W. H. Freeman, 1960.

Thompson, J. S., and Thompson, M. W.: Genetics in Medicine. Philadelphia, W. B. Saunders Co., 1966.

Thornton, S. P.: Ophthalmic Eponyms. Birmingham, Alabama, Aesculapius Publishing Co., 1967.

Waardenburg, P. J., Franceschetti, A., and Klein, D.: Genetics and Ophthalmology. Vols. 1 and 2. Springfield, Illinois, Charles C Thomas, 1961-62.

Walsh, F. B.: Clinical Neuro-ophthalmology. Baltimore, Williams & Wilkins Co., 1957.

Chapter Five

PEDIATRIC OPHTHALMOLOGY

Ocular abnormalities and diseases in children can occur from in utero to young adulthood, or even become manifest later in life. Not all of the myriad forms of childhood ocular diseases can be adequately covered or even included in this chapter.

NORMAL EYE IN INFANCY AND CHILDHOOD

The eye of the newborn infant differs from the eye of the adult more in size and functional capabilities than in structure. At birth, the eye is a fully functioning sensory organ that reacts with a normal, direct, and consensual pupillary reflex when stimulated by light. Experimental studies with the optokinetic nystagmus response indicate that the neonate has a visual acuity of 20/670 Snellen by one and one-half hours of life. Conjugate movements following slow moving, interesting objects appear in the fifth to sixth week of life. It should be remembered that testing for the presence or absence of vision by using a threatening gesture is not valid until the seventh to eighth week of life, since the protective blink reflex is not yet present.

The refractive power of the eye in a normal neonate usually ranges from one to three diopters of hyperopia. This may remain stable or increase one to two diopters up to 5 years of age. Physiologic hyperopia begins to decrease after the age of 7, and by maturity the normal eye has little refractive error. Accommodation, apparent by 6 months of age, can be detected simply by noting the child's ability to converge his eyes and constrict his pupils while observing an object held close to his face. This aspect of the near reflex increases in power until the age of 5. By 10 years of age, accommodation averages about 14 diopters. In other words, a 10 year old child with normal eyes should be able to focus clearly on an object held as near as 7 centimeters.

An infant's eyes are difficult to examine properly because most of the time they are closed. The child meets any attempt to separate the lids manually with a remarkably strong orbicularis oculi response. This results in eversion of the lids and a pronounced Bells' phenomenon, in which the pupil and cornea disappear underneath the superior lid even after being elevated. Furthermore, in infants the palpebral fissures are extremely narrow, and the pupil tends to be miotic. The examiner may use lid retractors, one or two assistants, a great deal of patience, perhaps sedation, or best of all a bottle containing formula. If, in spite of this effort, a truly adequate examination is not possible, general anesthesia should be considered.

For an older child, a simple toy that moves may maintain his interest and go a long way in persuading him to keep his eyes open or to look in the desired direction while his eyes are being observed. Simple games make the examination fun for the child. One of the simplest is to have the child look at a small flashlight and tell him to blow out the light "like the candles on a birthday cake." As he blows, the holder flicks off the light. Since most children find this a source of delight, it will maintain their interest surprisingly long if skillfully maneuvered with variations. Another useful aid is a lollipop.

An infant's orbits tend to be round and close together. A flat nasal bridge with relatively prominent epicanthal folds separates the orbits, making the infant look cross-eyed (pseudostrabismus). At birth, the palpebral fissure is about 18 mm. long and increases to about 30 mm. by maturity. The tear ducts should be patent and provide adequate drainage. Reflex tearing to noxious stimuli should be present at or shortly after birth. Psychic or emotional tearing usually does not appear until several weeks later, but it has been reported present as early as the first week of life.

The eyes should be mostly straight in the primary position during the first six months of life, and rotations should be conjugate, i.e., the eyes should rotate together. Persistent crossing or divergence is abnormal. The infant's eyes cross intermittently, but when the accommodative convergence reflex appears at the age of 6 months, this phenomenon should disappear.

At first the sclera appears slightly blue, turning glossy white as it thickens and becomes hydrated. The cornea is mildly hazy, but soon clears. The horizontal diameter of the cornea, which at birth is approximately 10 mm., increases rather rapidly during the first year of life, reaching 12 mm. by 1 year of age. In Caucasians, the iris tends to be blue for the first six months of life, and, as pigmentation increases, it becomes progressively hazel, then brown. Several small blood vessels normally may be seen through the transparent, nonpigmented iris stroma. The pupil tends to be miotic, and the dilator fibers do not reach their maximum strength until about 5 years of age. For this reason, good pupillary dilatation for funduscopic examination is obtained more adequately with the parasympathetic blocking agents than with the sympathetic stimulating agents.

Although it may appear shallow, the anterior chamber of the eye of the neonate is well formed. The pupil, therefore, may be dilated safely because narrow-angle glaucoma has not been known to occur in the normal eye of an infant. On ophthalmoscopic observation, the media (cornea, aqueous, lens, and vitreous) should be clear, and a red reflex should be seen. The optic disc appears paler than that of an adult, especially if the child has a fair complexion. In fact, differentiating between the normally pale disc of the neonate and optic atrophy may be difficult if not impossible. The macula appears redder than the remainder of the retina, but the foveal reflex is not visualized until the child is about 4 months of age, when the foveal pit is fully developed. Since there is a lack of pigment in the newborn fundus, the choroidal pattern stands out everywhere except in the macular region. As choroidal pigmentation develops, the fundus appears diffusely granular, and by 6 months of age it appears identical to the adult fundus.

DEVELOPMENTAL ABNORMALITIES

During fetal development, many normal growth patterns may be altered, resulting in mild to gross abnormalities. Developmental defects are produced by multiple mechanisms, not all of which are understood. The most common cause is genetic. An individual may inherit a gene that gives rise to abnormal structure, or a genetic mutation may arise in utero, resulting in the same defect occurring sporadically. These mutations usually are spontaneous, but they can also be produced by such exogenous agents as ionizing radiation and by certain drugs (chemotherapeutic agents, antimetabolites, LSD). In addition to the abnormal development caused by single genes, chromosomal aberrations, such as nondisjunctions, translocations, and deletions or eliminations, must also be considered. These abnormalities are discussed in the chapter on genetics (p. 98).

A second mechanism is the so-called transplacental effect. For example, maternal infections, especially early in pregnancy, may cross the placenta to cause multiple defects in the fetus (p. 136). Many drugs, dietary deficiencies or excesses (especially vitamins and minerals), and some hormonal imbalances have also been implicated as causal agents.

Intrauterine structures, such as fibrous bands and umbilical cords, as well as uterine shape, must also be considered, along with injury to the mother during pregnancy. Some of these have been shown to cause some of the defects in congenitally deformed children, but there is no clear causal relationship between these abnormal mechanical factors and specific ocular abnormalities. Generally, the earlier the insult, regardless of type, the grosser the defect in the product of gestation.

Abnormal Skull and Face Formation

ANENCEPHALY

This is the most severe malformation involving the brain. The whole brain fails to develop above the medulla, and the cranial vault is absent. The eyes may be proptotic, but grossly appear normal. Microscopic examination, however, reveals the absence of the nerve fiber layer of the retina, a partially developed optic nerve, and imperfect development of the ganglion cell layer of the retina. The infant lives at most only a few hours after birth.

CONGENITAL FAILURE OF THE ORBITS

This cranial defect is characterized by normal development of the eyes and lids and by extremely shallow orbital cavities. The globes are proptosed, and the lids are difficult to close. The children are often microcephalic and fail to thrive. A milder and insignificant variation may be the shallow orbital formation commonly seen in Negroes.

CRANIOFACIAL DYSOSTOSES

Oxycephaly (Tower Skull). Premature union of the coronary and lambdoidal

sutures arrests the growth of the skull in its anterior-posterior and lateral planes. The skull thus expands only in height. The abnormality, seemingly more common in males than in females, exhibits an autosomal dominant inheritance pattern with relatively weak penetration. Neurologic, hematologic, and skeletal (especially digital) anomalies may also be present. The ocular findings are probably caused by the abnormal growth of the cranial vault and by associated increased intracranial pressure. They consist of exophthalmia, extraocular muscle problems (including ptosis), papilledema, and eventual optic atrophy. Zonular cataracts have also been reported.

A number of less common craniostenoses have been reported, the differences in appearance depending on which cranial suture has become stenosed prematurely. These include *scaphocephaly*, in which the head is long and narrow in its anterior-posterior direction and has a keel-shaped vault from early closure of the sagittal suture; *hemicraniosis*, in which enlargement, limited to one side of the skull, is probably caused by the premature closure of the sutures on the side opposite the deformity; and *trigonocephaly*, in which a high, retreating forehead is caused by the premature synostosis of the coronal suture. The variable ocular findings are similar to those of oxycephaly.

Craniofacial Dysostosis of Crouzon (Crouzon's Disease). This is a dominantly inherited disorder that results in a marked froglike facies (Fig. 5-1), occasional hearing loss, neurologic abnormalities (including subnormal mentality), and prognathism (Fig. 5-2). The ocular defects consist of exophthalmia (Fig. 5-3) (occasionally so severe that the globes prolapse) (Figs. 5-4, 5-5), divergent strabismus (Fig. 5-6), nystagmus, and optic atrophy. The eyes tend to be oblique, with the outer canthus slanting downward. Occasionally cataracts are present.

Acrocephalosyndactylia of Apert (Apert's Syndrome). Similar to Crouzon's disease, with varying degrees of syndactylism (Figs. 5-7, 5-8), this syndrome usually is inherited as an autosomal recessive trait.

Figure 5-1 Crouzon's disease. Typical froglike facies and downward slant of lateral canthus.

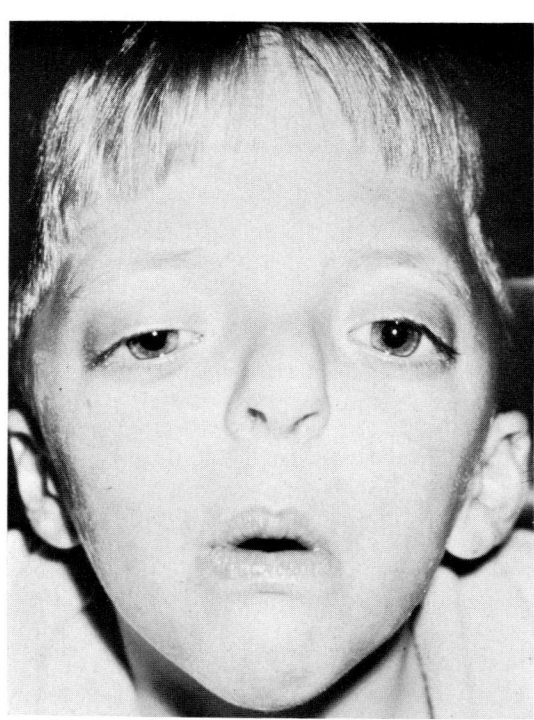

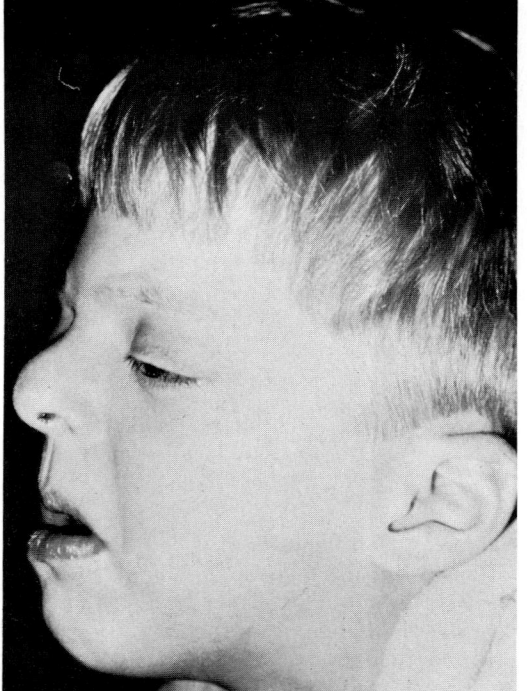

Figure 5-2 Crouzon's disease. Lateral view of same patient as in Figure 5-1 showing slight proptosis and prognathism.

Figure 5-3 Crouzon's disease. Exophthalmia and divergent strabismus.

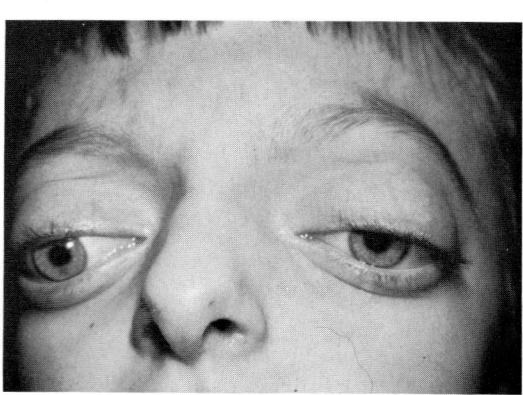

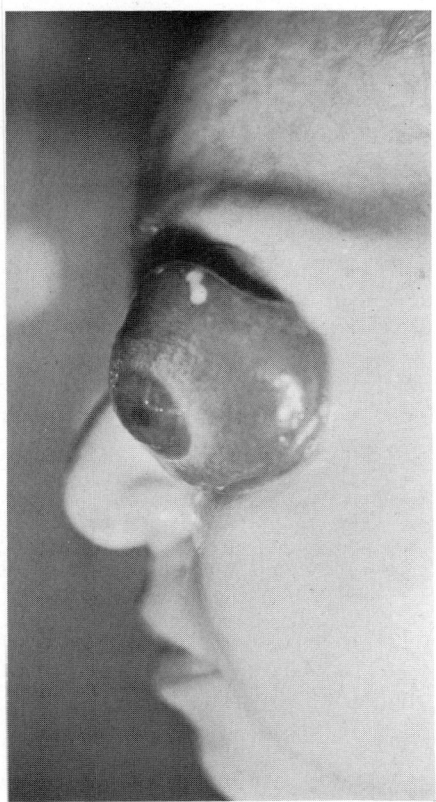

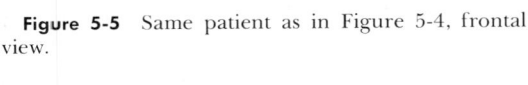

Figure 5-5 Same patient as in Figure 5-4, frontal view.

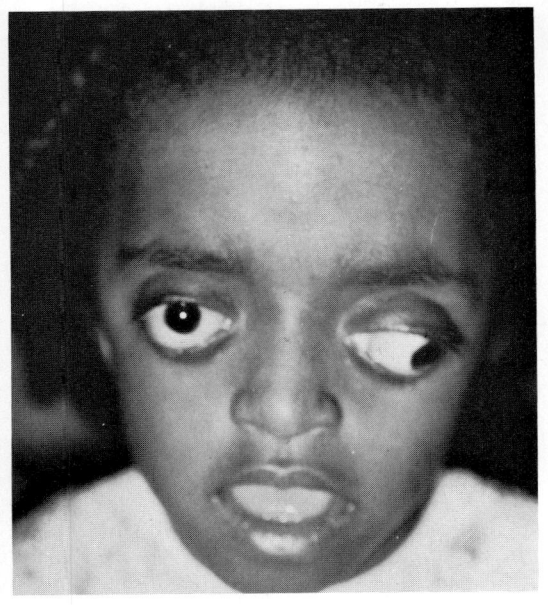

Figure 5-4 Crouzon's disease. The abnormally shallow orbits may result in severe proptosis during labor and delivery.

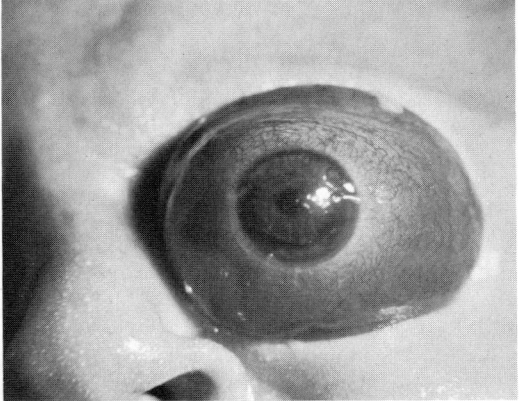

Figure 5-6 Crouzon's disease. Marked divergent strabismus and proptosis.

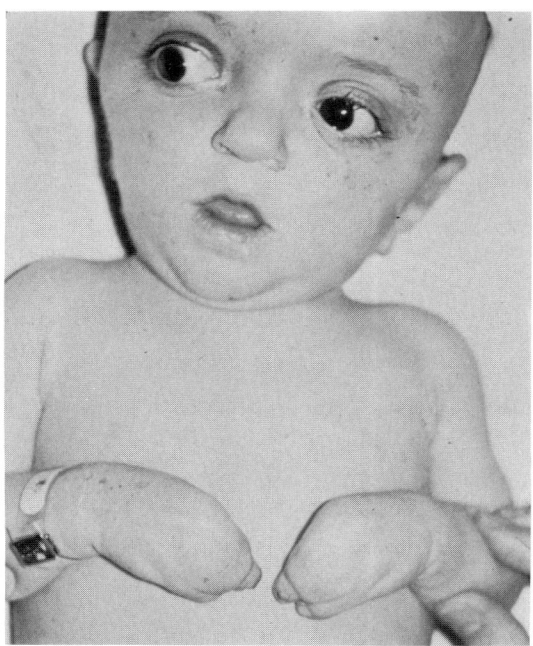

Figure 5-7 Apert's syndrome. Syndactyly of fingers.

Hypertelorism. An excessive distance between the two orbits characterizes this abnormality. Normally the distance between the two caruncles is 30 to 33 mm., but in this autosomal defect (dominant or recessive), the distance can reach 50 mm. In addition, the lacrimal puncta are displaced laterally, so that when the eye is in the primary posi-

tion, a vertical line drawn through the inferior punctum will cross the cornea. In a healthy child, such a line crosses the eye nasal to the limbus. Associated anomalies include renal hypoplasia, and ocular findings such as ptosis, inverse epicanthus, divergent strabismus, and optic atrophy. When Axenfeld's posterior embryotoxon (p. 120) is present, it should warn the physician of the possibility of congenital glaucoma. The more severe varieties appear to be associated with recessive inheritance patterns.

Finding hypertelorism should alert the physician to the possibility of the following two clinical syndromes:

WAARDENBURG'S SYNDROME. This condition follows an autosomal dominant inheritance pattern. In addition to hypertelorism and laterally displaced puncta, there is heterochromia irides, a growing together of the eyebrows, a white forelock, and congenital deafness of varying degree.

CORNELIA DELANGE SYNDROME. This condition, transmitted as an autosomal recessive disorder, is marked by mental and growth retardation; varying degrees of skeletal abnormalities ranging from syndactyly to phocomelia; a feeble, raucous cry; multiple ocular anomalies; and distinctive facies. The facial characteristics include a low hairline, hypertrichotic eyebrows joined in the midline, long eyelashes, hypertelorism, and a small, upturned nose. In addition, reported eye findings include antimongoloid slant, strabismus, nystagmus, ptosis, pupillary abnormalities, high myopia, and pallor of the optic discs.

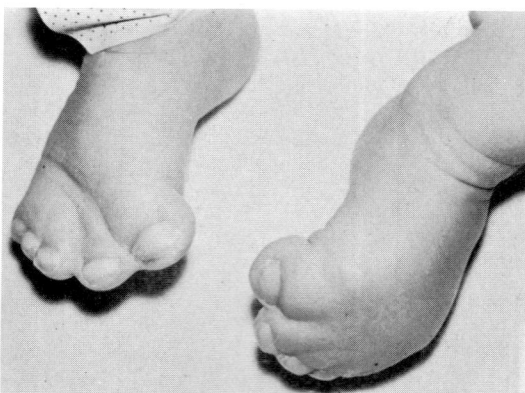

Figure 5-8 Apert's syndrome. Syndactyly of toes.

MANDIBULOFACIAL DYSOSTOSES

Franceschetti's Syndrome. This facial dysplasia is inherited as an autosomal dominant trait with weak penetrance. It is characterized by hypoplasia of the malar and mandibular bones, macrostomia, atresia of the external ear and auditory meatus, and mental retardation. The ocular abnormalities include antimongoloid slant, atypical coloboma of the lower eyelids, and abnormal positioning of the eyelashes. This disorder, as well as other mandibulofacial syndromes mentioned below, is believed to arise from some compromise to the normal development of the first branchial arch. When the ears are not malformed, the condition is known as the *Treacher-Collins syndrome*.

Pierre Robin Syndrome. This congenital disorder is characterized by micrognathia, glossoptosis, cleft palate, dysphagia, and a birdlike facies. The ocular pathology includes high myopia, retinal detachment, glaucoma, cataracts, and microphthalmia.

Goldenhar's Syndrome. This oculoauriculovertebral disorder consists of epibulbar dermoids and/or lipodermoids (Fig. 5-9), colobomas of the upper lids, preauricular appendages (Fig. 5-10), micrognathia and macrostomia, facial microsomia, and multiple vertebral anomalies that are usually diagnosed by X-ray. Other reported ocular abnormalities include microphthalmia, microcornea, colobomas of the iris and choroid, and polar cataracts. The etiology is unknown.

Hallerman-Streiff Syndrome. Known also as oculomandibulofacial dyscephalia, this syndrome is characterized by dyscephalia, a "parrot-beak" nose, and a hypoplastic mandible. These result in a birdlike facies (Fig. 5-11), localized hypotrichosis and localized atrophy of the skin. Bilateral microphthalmia is present with an associated, severe, congenital glaucoma. Congenital cataracts also are common.

Similar to this condition is *Seckel's syndrome (bird-headed dwarf)*, in which the head is extremely small (nanocephalia), the nose is

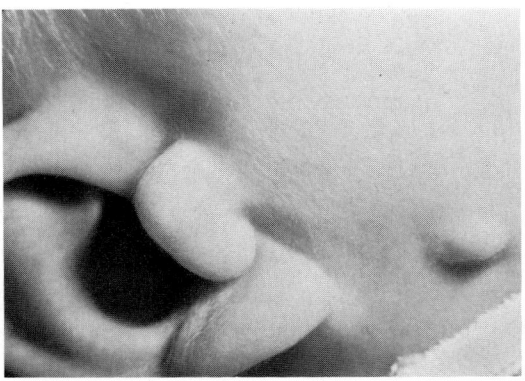

Figure 5-10 Goldenhar's syndrome. Abnormal tragus and preauricular appendage in same patient as in Figure 5-9.

long and prominent, and the child is mentally retarded and of small stature. Microphthalmia and congenital glaucoma can be present.

Rubenstein-Taybi Syndrome. This relatively new entity is characterized by mental

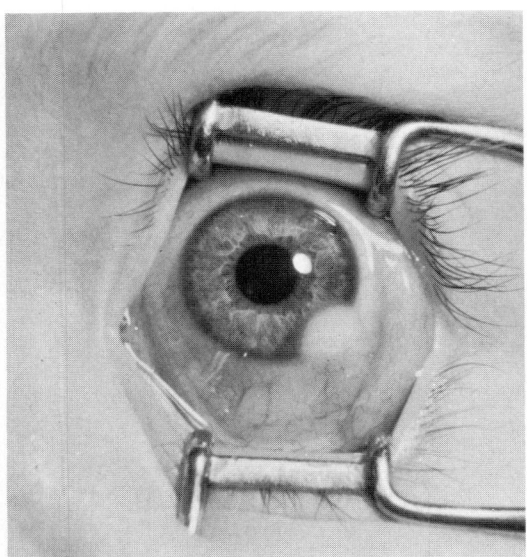

Figure 5-9 Goldenhar's syndrome. Corneoscleral dermoid associated with a dermolipoma laterally.

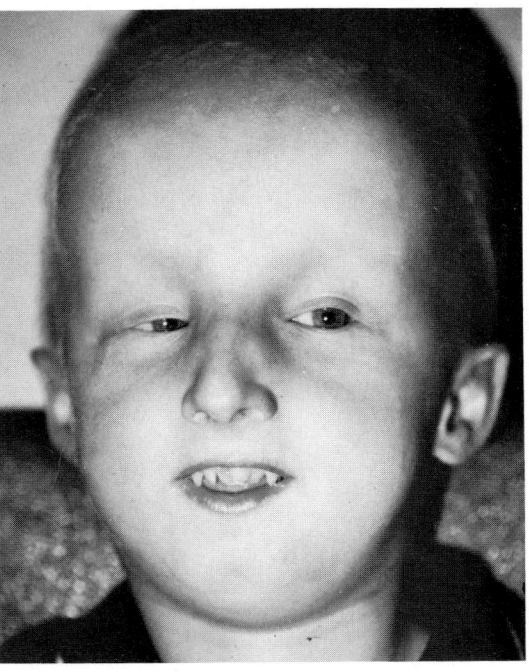

Figure 5-11 Hallerman-Streiff syndrome. Birdlike facies with "parrot-beak" nose, hypoplastic mandible, and bilateral microphthalmia.

and motor retardation; a prominent, beak-like nose; elfin facies; high arched palate; broad, flat thumbs and great toes; generally small stature; and ocular defects. In addition, many of these children are microcephalic and have cardiac abnormalities, hirsutism, and multiple deformities of the axial skeleton.

The more common ocular anomalies include antimongoloid fissures, strabismus, epicanthus, and significant refractive errors. Less frequently, these infants exhibit hypertrichosis, cataracts, colobomas, blepharoptosis, obstruction of the nasolacrimal canals, enophthalmia, and optic atrophy.

The differential diagnosis, mainly because of the characteristic facies, includes the syndromes of Hallerman-Streiff, Franceschetti, Seckel, and the chromosomal deletion known as cri du chat.

Oculodentodigital Dysplasia (Meyer-Schwickerath Syndrome). Microphthalmia, congenital glaucoma, iris abnormalities, hypotrichosis, syndactyly, and flexion deformities of the fingers characterize this condition. The children's nasal bridges appear broad and high, and their teeth have a brown tint from lack of enamel formation.

Dyscraniopygophalangea (Ullrich's Syndrome). In this syndrome, an arched forehead, broad nose, hypoplastic mandible, polydactyly, and spina bifida are characteristic. The ocular defects range from bilateral anophthalmia to such abnormalities as microphthalmia, chorioretinal coloboma, complete aniridia, congenital glaucoma, and gross mesodermal abnormalities of the anterior chamber.

MENINGOENCEPHALOCELE

During development the meninges and cerebral substance sometimes protrude through a bony defect in the skull. A protuberance containing only the meninges is known as a *meningocele*. This appears as a round, soft, and often pulsatile mass that usually is noted at birth or shortly thereafter. Encephaloceles are most frequently found in the occipital region. Another common site of great interest to the ophthal-

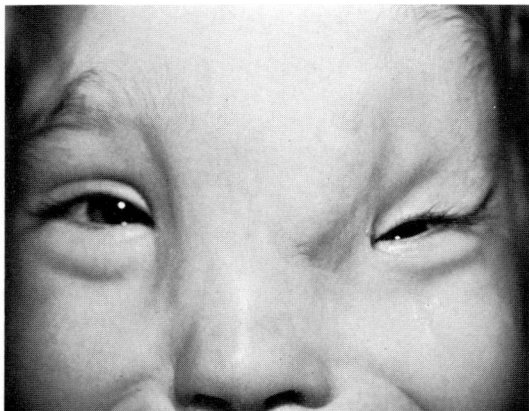

Figure 5-12 Encephalocele presenting at the supero-medial wall on the left orbit.

mologist is the root of the nose (Fig. 5-12). Subsequently the orbit becomes involved. Frequent associated defects include mental deficiency, hydrocephaly, spina bifida, clubfoot, harelip, and cleft palate.

Finding any naso-orbital mass in the newborn should suggest the possibility of such a lesion. Ocular involvement depends entirely on the position of the encephalocele. The mass can cause exophthalmos, lateral displacement of the eye, and varying defects of ocular motility ranging from specific muscle palsies to defective mechanical movements. When the lesion involves the superior orbital fissure, more severe ocular abnormalities occur, including microphthalmia and even apparent anophthalmia (Fig. 5-13).

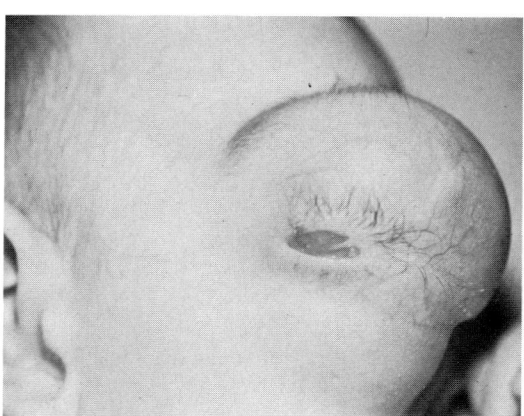

Figure 5-13 Large meningoencephalocele involving the entire orbit and resulting in apparent anophthalmia. The palpebral fissure can be seen on the protruding mass.

The mass can be either excised or replaced within the cranial vault. Meningitis and meningoencephalitis are commonly encountered in both the preoperative and postoperative periods, especially when the mass is closely associated with the nasopharyngeal passages. Although little brain damage occurs from the procedure itself, the prognosis is poor. Recurrences of the protruding masses are not uncommon when the defect in the bony cranium is large.

Abnormalities of the Lids and Lacrimal Apparatus

Cryptophthalmia or Ablepharia. This is an autosomal recessive genetic trait in which the palpebral fissures are absent. Lashes may or may not be present. The eye may be normal except for the absence of a true cornea caused by the fusion of the overlying skin and cornea into one structure. In other cases, however, the eye is severely disorganized, with iris adherent to the back of the cornea, loss of the lens, vitreous in the anterior chamber, and a low-grade, chronic, inflammatory infiltrate in the choroid. The severe cases suggest that the condition was the result of an intrauterine inflammatory process causing perforation of the globe and loss of intraocular contents.

Palpebral Colobomas. Palpebral colobomas are gaps or triangular notches occurring in either the upper or lower lids. They may be unilateral or bilateral. The genetic

pattern and etiology are unclear. The bands of skin and conjunctiva that run from the gap to the conjunctiva or cornea suggest a mechanical, intrauterine cause. Colobomas of the upper lid usually occur at the junction of the inner and middle third of the lid (Fig. 5-14). In the lower lid they are found at the junction of the middle and lateral third of the lid.

Other ocular abnormalities associated with lid colobomas include corneal opacities, microphthalmia, and defects of the iris and pupil. The presence of dermoids or lipodermoids in the upper lid suggests Goldenhar's syndrome; atypical colobomas in the lower lids suggest the mandibulo-facial dysostosis syndrome (p. 110).

Epicanthus. This is a dominantly inherited autosomal trait, consisting of a crescent-shaped, redundant fold of skin that begins in the upper lid and runs medially to cover the normal inner canthus of the palpebral fissure. It is a racial characteristic of the Mongol and is also a consistent finding in Down's syndrome. Epicanthus is often associated with ptosis.

Inverse epicanthus, also known to occur through simple, dominant inheritance, is characterized by a redundant skin fold running from the lower lid medially toward the nose and covering the inner palpebral angle.

Entropion and Ectropion. In entropion the lid margins turn in, causing the cilia to rub against the globe. It is much more common in the lower than in the upper lid, and is frequently associated with epicanthus. The inheritance pattern for entropion appears to be an autosomal dominant trait.

In ectropion the lid margins turn out so that they do not ride against the globe. It is more common in the upper lids, but it has been reported also in the lower. Congenital ectropion is even rarer than congenital entropion, and its inheritance pattern has not been established.

Both entropion and ectropion may be corrected surgically. In entropion, surgery would be required if the lashes were scratching and damaging the cornea; in ectropion, it would be performed either for persistent conjunctivitis from lack of adequate drain-

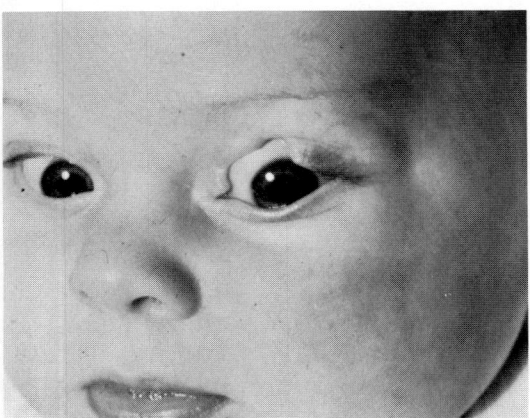

Figure 5-14 Palpebral coloboma of left upper lid.

age of tears and conjunctival excretions or for cosmetic reasons.

Blepharochalasis. Congenital or juvenile blepharochalasis is an autosomal dominant trait involving the upper lids. The dermis atrophies and the underlying subcutaneous tissue relaxes. Consequently, the orbital fat protrudes through the weak orbital septum and forms a large, loose, skin fold that hangs down over the lid margin. When severe, the condition can be treated surgically by excising the loose skin and the underlying fatty tissue through a horizontal incision at the level of the superior lid fold.

Epiblepharon. This autosomal dominant trait consists of a horizontal fold of skin in the lower lid that runs parallel to the lid margin across the length of the palpebral fissure. It is of no significance unless it is associated with an entropion, at which time it may be corrected surgically.

Ankyloblepharon and Blepharophimosis. Ankyloblepharon is an irregular, autosomal dominant trait in which the superior and inferior lid margins do not completely separate, usually in the lateral aspects. Occasionally, medial ankyloblepharon gives the child an appearance of pseudostrabismus. Treatment is surgical, depending on the severity of the condition.

Blepharophimosis is a simple, autosomal dominant trait that consists of a symmetrical decrease in the size of the palpebral fissure, but with the lids structurally normal. It is not uncommonly associated with an inverse epicanthus (Fig. 5-15). The diagnosis of Waardenburg's syndrome should be considered, since blepharophimosis is a defect of that syndrome.

Ptosis. Congenital ptosis, an inherited, irregular, autosomal dominant trait, consists of a drooping upper lid. In most instances it is bilateral (Fig. 5-16). It usually is due to failure of the levator muscle to develop completely. In unilateral cases an intracranial third nerve lesion or birth trauma could be involved. Hereditary ptosis usually is present at birth and either remains constant or increases as the child grows older. Late onset, between the fifth and twentieth years of life, also has been reported. Associated weakness of the superior rectus muscle on the same side as the ptosis is not unusual because both muscles arise from the same mesodermal anlage. Horizontal strabismus may be present as well as the previously discussed lid abnormalities. A careful check for the jaw-winking phenomenon always should be made.

The treatment of congenital ptosis is

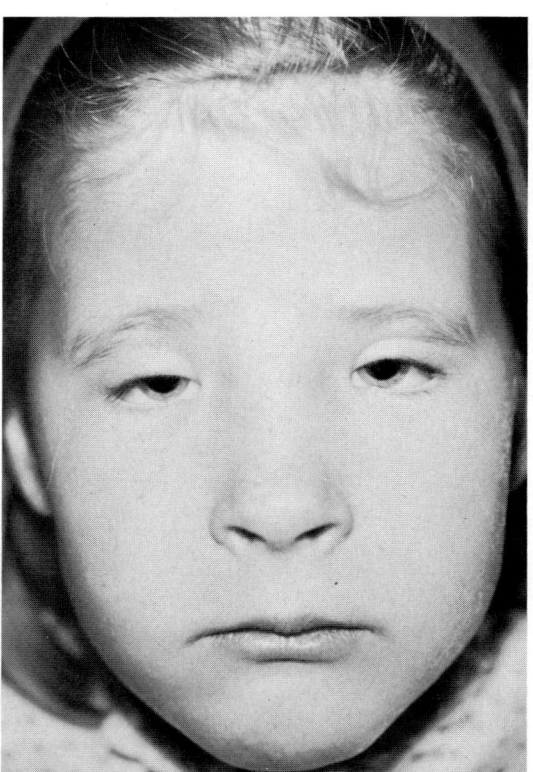

Figure 5-16 Bilateral congenital ptosis.

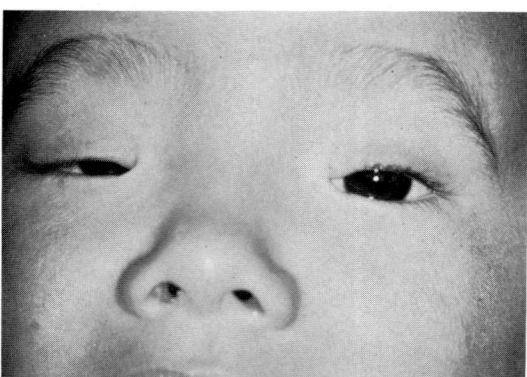

Figure 5-15 Blepharophimosis associated with ptosis, inverse epicanthal folds, and strabismus.

surgical. It usually is performed when the child is 3 or 4 years old, but may have to be performed earlier if the ptosis is severe enough to cause the child to tilt his head in order to see out beneath the drooping lids. Early surgery also may be indicated when the ptosis is unilateral and complete, and when the prolonged occlusion of one eye may lead to an amblyopic situation.

The various operations can be classified into three basic groups. The first consists of suspending the weak lid from the brow, usually by means of a strip of fascia lata, to make use of the frontalis muscle for lifting power. In the second group, the superior rectus muscle is attached to the lid for elevation. However, this procedure frequently results in abnormal blinking and in the patient's inability to close the eye completely when asleep, thus leading to exposure keratitis. A third group, probably the procedure of choice, is the resection of the weak levator muscle itself. When properly performed, the shortening of this muscle allows for a normal blinking reflex, a cosmetically acceptable result, and less chance for exposure keratitis. The surgeon should forewarn the parents that, with any of these procedures, the likelihood of perfect bilateral symmetry is highly improbable.

An interesting and rare variety of con-

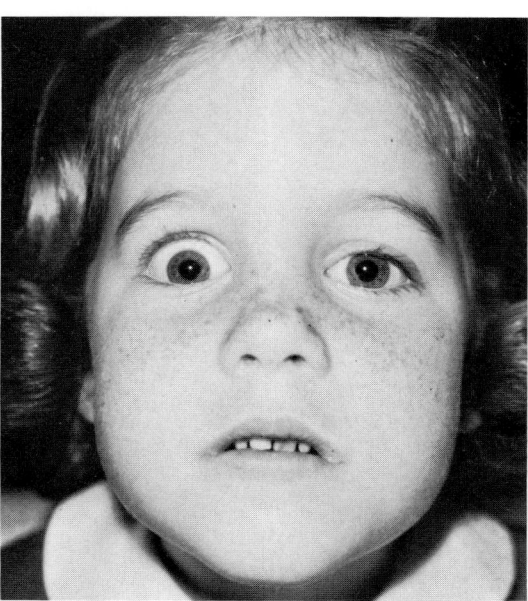

Figure 5-18   Marcus Gunn phenomenon. Note elevation of the right upper lid as the jaw is moved to the left.

genital ptosis is known as the *Marcus Gunn, or jaw-winking, phenomenon* inherited as a simple, autosomal dominant trait (Fig. 5-17). It is characterized by the elevation of the ptotic lid when the patient opens his mouth or moves his jaw laterally to the side opposite the ptosis (Fig. 5-18). The lid droops again if the jaw maintains its new position or is closed. Since the external pterygoid muscle contracts in both movements, the etiology usually is attributed to an anomalous connection between the nerves to the external pterygoid and the levator muscles. The usual complaint is social embarrassment.

Treatment consists of tenotomy of the levator. Next, the lid is attached to either the superior rectus muscle or to the frontalis muscle by means of a fascia lata sling.

Distichiasis.   In this autosomal dominant condition, the meibomian glands are absent or poorly developed and replaced with an abnormal second row of lashes. The abnormal row is directed backward towards the eyeball and is a constant source of irritation, abrasion, and eventual ulceration of the cornea. Treatment consists of surgical

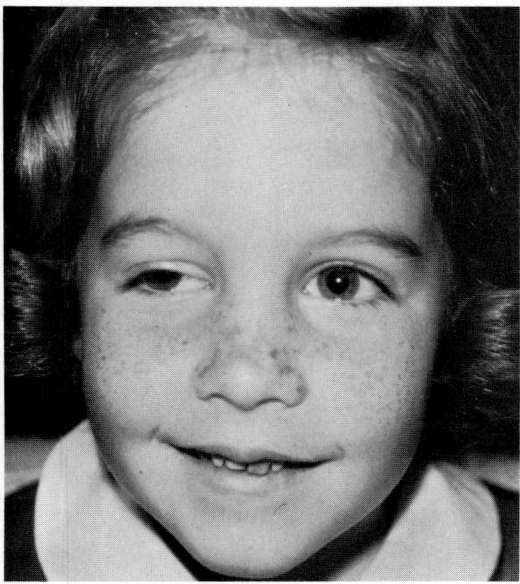

Figure 5-17   Marcus Gunn phenomenon. Ptosis of the right upper lid.

excision of the abnormal row of lashes or galvanic electrolysis of each individual hair follicle.

Defects of the Lacrimal Apparatus. For the most part, congenital defects of both the lacrimal gland and the drainage system are rare. Disorders of the gland itself include complete absence, forward dislocation (so that it is readily apparent under the lateral aspect of the upper lid), and the presence of accessory lacrimal gland tissue, especially in the caruncle. The puncta and canaliculi also may be absent, laterally displaced, or fistulized.

By far the most common problem in infants is obstruction of the nasolacrimal duct. This usually is caused by epithelial debris in the lower portion of the duct or by lack of spontaneous absorption of the epithelial membrane that separates the inferior portion of the duct from its opening into the nose underneath the inferior turbinate. Symptoms include excessive tearing, frequently recurrent or persistent conjunctivitis, and dacryocystitis. In the infant the obstruction may open spontaneously within the first six months, which may be assisted by mechanical massage downward over the lacrimal sac and canal, by warm compresses, and by the instillation of an antibiotic ointment if infection is present. At 6 months of age, probing and irrigation of the nasolacrimal ducts should be successful, although it may have to be repeated one or more times in order to secure permanent drainage.

Abnormalities of the Eye as a Whole

Cyclopia. Only one eye is present in this condition, usually at the midline. Cyclopia is associated with many severe cranial and systemic abnormalities. It is inherited through a simple, recessive, autosomal gene that is lethal. The midline structures of the brain and skull lack formation, resulting in a single median eye or varying degrees of fusion of two abnormal eyes.

Anophthalmos. Anophthalmos (absence of the eye) seldom, if ever, is total. It can be inherited as an autosomal recessive trait or drug induced (Thalidomide). Occasionally it has been reported with the 13-15 trisomy syndrome. Usually it is associated with multiple abnormalities and only rarely exists as an isolated entity.

Congenital Cystic Eyeball. This condition of unknown etiology represents an arrest in the outgrowth of the optic vesicle. The lids and fissures are present. They can be normal or cryptophthalmic. A thin, blue-walled cyst, probably scleral tissue, is in the orbit, and contains remnants of varying degrees of abnormal retinal and uveal tissue. There is no evidence of a cornea.

Microphthalmos

PURE MICROPHTHALMOS. Inherited as either a dominant or recessive autosomal trait, pure microphthalmia is characterized by a normal-appearing eye that is about two thirds of its proper size. It can be unilateral (Fig. 5-19), but usually is bilateral. The abnormality is frequently associated with other ocular defects, such as severe hyperopia, spherophakia, microphakia, cataract, and hypoplastic macula. The small, abnormal globes show a marked disposition to glaucoma.

Systemic abnormalities should be searched for carefully, especially in unilateral microphthalmia. Besides its genetic origin, microphthalmia occurs with multiple syndromes (p. 110) of unknown etiology, as well as with congenital toxoplasmosis or rubella and other prenatal intrauterine infections.

COLOBOMATOUS MICROPHTHALMOS. This

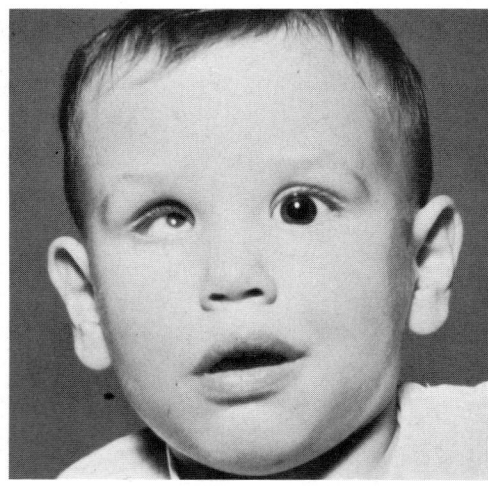

Figure 5-19 Unilateral pure microphthalmia.

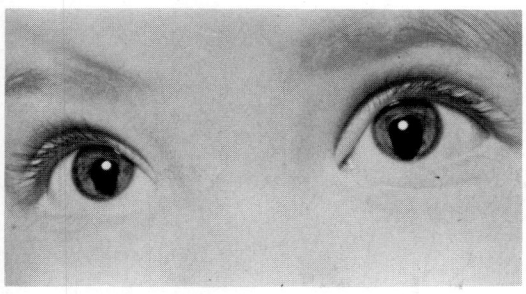

Figure 5-20 Colobomatous microphthalmia with bilateral iris defects.

condition appears to be a distinct entity that is inherited as either an irregular or regular dominant trait. Besides a microphthalmic eye, varying degrees of colobomatous defects of the iris, choroid, or optic nerve are present (Fig. 5-20).

A more severe variant of the condition is *microphthalmia with cyst*. The cyst usually extends inferiorly through the unclosed fetal fissure and can be palpated through the lower lid. The cyst wall usually is scleral in origin and lined with abnormal retina, frequently exhibiting a rosette formation.

Coloboma of the Eye. A coloboma is a congenital abnormality resulting from failure of some portion of the fetal fissure to close. The various types of colobomas are inherited as irregular autosomal dominant traits; they are usually bilateral and they may involve the choroid, retina, optic nerve, ciliary body, and iris. Any or all of these structures may be involved in a single patient.

Posterior colobomas of the choroid and retina are found below the disc (Plate 2A) and may extend far out to the ora serrata (Plate 2B). On funduscopic examination the coloboma appears as a white, oval area with its apex toward the disc and its base extending down beyond the limit of direct ophthalmoscopy. The edges of colobomas usually are clear-cut and may be pigmented (Plate 2C). Visual acuity commonly is decreased, often strabismus and nystagmus are associated, and the eyes may be microphthalmic.

Anterior colobomas of the ciliary body and the iris can occur as a forward extension of a posterior coloboma or they can exist as a separate entity. When they involve the ciliary body, the lens zonules are absent in this region and the lens itself

appears notched (or colobomatous). The defect is inferior and slightly nasal, representing the failure of the fetal fissure to close either partially or completely.

Colobomas of the optic nerve (Plate 3A) can exist separately or within large, choroidal colobomas (Plate 2D). When present as a separate entity, a coloboma can be of minor significance and merely appear as physiologic cupping. More commonly, however, the defect is two to four times the size of the disc, and the vessels emerge separately around the edge of the coloboma. When the defect involves the entire disc, it looks almost as though the nerve head has been avulsed. The defect, however, may involve just the inferior aspect of the disc. Cystic changes of the retina may be an associated finding. In more severe optic nerve colobomatous defects, visual acuity is diminished seriously.

Colobomatous defects of the macula are uncommon and are inherited as irregular, autosomal dominant traits. They cannot be explained, however, by failure of the fetal fissure to close. The defect usually appears as round or horizontally oval ranging from 1 to 10 disc diameters in size. Because of the location, the most important differential diagnosis will be a necrotizing chorioretinitis, such as seen with toxoplasmosis. At times, however, they may be impossible to differentiate, and many ophthalmologists feel that macular colobomas represent an inflammatory, rather than a developmental, defect.

Buphthalmia. Buphthalmia, or primary infantile glaucoma, is inherited through an autosomal recessive gene, and accounts for 5 to 13 per cent of the children in schools for the blind throughout the world. The most important way to reduce this percentage is to diagnose and recognize congenital glaucoma early. This is discussed in Chapter 8, Glaucoma (p. 354).

Prompt recognition of infantile glaucoma is important because proper surgical management can control the pressure in at least 80 per cent of the victims. Typical signs are present at birth in about 33 per cent, by 6 months of age in about 67 per cent, and by the end of the first year of age in 80 to 90 per cent. The remainder occur before the child is three years of age.

The findings, in order of their occurrence and increasing severity, are:

1. Photophobia, lacrimation, and blepharospasm
2. Corneal haziness
3. Corneal enlargement
4. Ruptures in Descemet's membrane
5. Glaucomatous cupping of the optic nerve.

Once the elevated intraocular pressure has caused the cornea to become cloudy, with or without the subsequent findings, the diagnosis is suspected readily. It is extremely important, however, to realize that, frequently, excessive tearing and photophobia are the first indications of infantile glaucoma. Because many of these children undergo probings for nasolacrimal duct obstruction before the proper diagnosis is made, the intraocular pressure is taken routinely in any infant who is anesthetized for a preoperative diagnosis of the obstruction, regardless of how classic the history and physical findings are.

Abnormalities of the Cornea

Microcornea. This condition is inherited as either a regular or irregular autosomal dominant trait. It is characterized by a horizontal corneal diameter of less than 11 mm. after 1 year of age. A small cornea can exist in an otherwise normal eye, in an eye that is elongated, in microphthalmia, and in the presence of hydrophthalmia. Frequently it is associated with a variety of other ocular abnormalities, including multiple anterior chamber defects, colobomas, cataract, nystagmus, and strabismus. About 20 per cent of eyes with microcornea are complicated by glaucoma.

Cornea Plana. Cornea plana is characterized by a flattened cornea, an indistinct limbus, and a diffuse, stromal opacification in the deeper layers of the cornea. The visual acuity generally is diminished because other ocular abnormalities of the retina, iris, and choroid coexist. The condi-

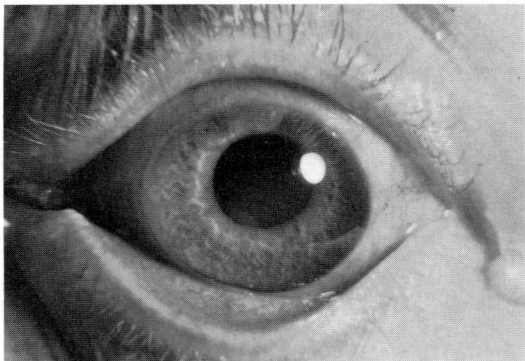

Figure 5-21 Congenital megalocornea. Note the clear cornea.

tion is inherited as an autosomal recessive trait.

Megalocornea. True megalocornea is characterized by a congenital, stationary enlargement of the cornea whose diameter varies between 12 and 16 mm. (Fig. 5-21). This enlargement is not accompanied by glaucoma, nor by any abnormality in the iridocorneal angle (Fig. 5-22). The functional integrity of the eye is unimpaired. Megalocornea is inherited as a sex-linked recessive, but rarely as an autosomal dominant, trait. Occasionally it is found in Marfan's syndrome along with ectopia lentis. It must be differentiated from the enlarged cornea of infantile glaucoma.

Keratoconus. This corneal ectasia (p. 280), usually begins about the tenth year of life and probably is inherited through a recessive gene, although there is some evi-

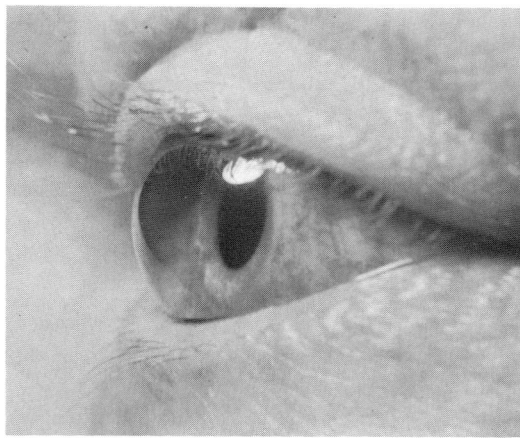

Figure 5-22 Congenital megalocornea, lateral view. Note the deep anterior chamber and normal angle.

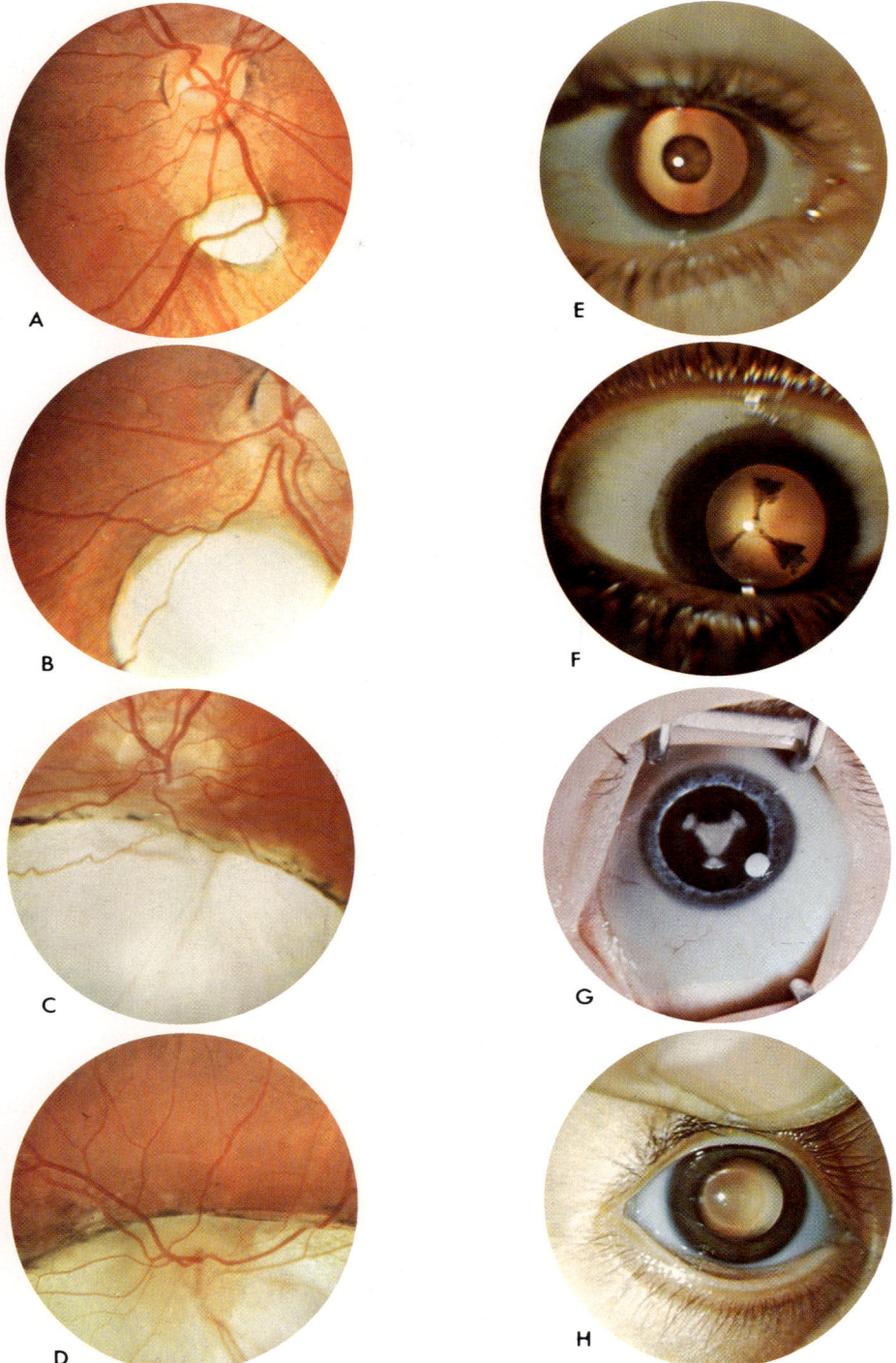

Plate 2 *(A)* Partial coloboma of choroid below disc.   *(B)* Coloboma of choroid extending far out to periphery. *(C)* Coloboma of choroid and retina with sharp, pigmented edge.   *(D)* Massive coloboma of entire fetal fissure that extends posteriorly and involves the optic nerve.   *(E)* Congenital nuclear cataract.   *(F)* Congenital zonular cataract.   *(G)* Congenital nuclear and sutural cataract.   *(H)* Galactosemia. Note "oil-droplet" appearance of nucleus of lens; it is seen best with dilated pupil and reflected light.

119

dence that it may require two separate dominant genes at different loci.

Hereditary Familial Corneal Dystrophies. Of the variety of corneal dystrophies or degenerations that are known, the great majority are hereditary in nature (p. 279). They usually are bilateral, have their onset at various ages, and cause corneal opacification in specific layers or patterns. These corneal dystrophies cause a loss of visual acuity of varying extent. In their severest forms, they must be treated by corneal transplantation.

Abnormalities of the Anterior Segment

An extensive group of ocular abnormalities involving the structures and differentiation of the anterior segment of the eye have recently been reclassified by Reese. They are collectively named *anterior chamber cleavage syndromes.*

Posterior Embryotoxon of Axenfeld. Axenfeld's syndrome, inherited as an autosomal dominant trait, is characterized by the anterior displacement of Schwalbe's line, which can be seen by gross inspection or by slit lamp examination. Prominent processes traverse the anterior chamber angle from this line to the base of the iris. Glaucoma, hypertelorism, and any of the anomalies noted below can be associated findings.

Mesodermal Dysgenesis of Rieger. Rieger's syndrome, inherited as an autosomal dominant trait, consists of posterior embryotoxon in association with iridotrabecular adhesions and hypoplasia of the anterior stromal leaf of the iris. It is frequently complicated by glaucoma.

Posterior Keratoconus. Known also as von Hippel's posterior corneal ulcer, this syndrome is characterized by the absence of Descemet's membrane centrally with subsequent corneal edema. Iris adhesions to the "ulcer" and corneal opacification may be present. Glaucoma and any other anterior chamber abnormality may coexist.

Besides the entities described previously, conditions such as sclerocornea, dyscoria, corectopia, slit pupil, polycoria, and iris

dehiscences and diastases have all been described. Several investigators have pointed out that any combination of these anterior segment abnormalities may exist together as well as separately, and they probably represent a continuum. Their major importance is that glaucoma may be associated with any of them.

Abnormalities of the Iris

Aniridia. Absence of the iris is never complete. A rudimentary iris can always be observed by gonioscopic examination. The disorder follows an autosomal dominant pattern. Although usually bilateral, an occasional unilateral case has been reported. Particularly severe congenital glaucoma is present in greater than 50 per cent of the cases. Frequent associated findings include corneal opacities, cataract, ectopia lentis (Fig. 5-23), aplasia of the macula, retinal photophobia, nystagmus, strabismus, and poor vision.

Aniridia occurs in about one of 100,000 individuals, and one of every 73 of these also may have a congenital neoplasm of the kidney (Wilms' tumor). The increased incidence of this condition becomes even more obvious in view of the fact that Wilms' tumor occurs in only one of every 50,000 individuals.

Persistent Pupillary Membrane. During the intrauterine growth and differentiation of the human eye, a vascular network surrounds the fetal lens. These vascular arcades cross the pupil anteriorly and con-

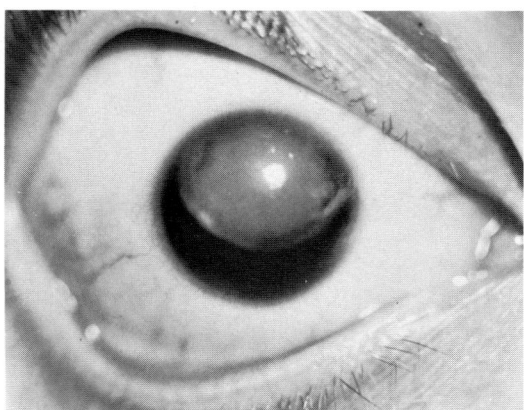

Figure 5-23 Marked aniridia with cataractous, subluxated lens.

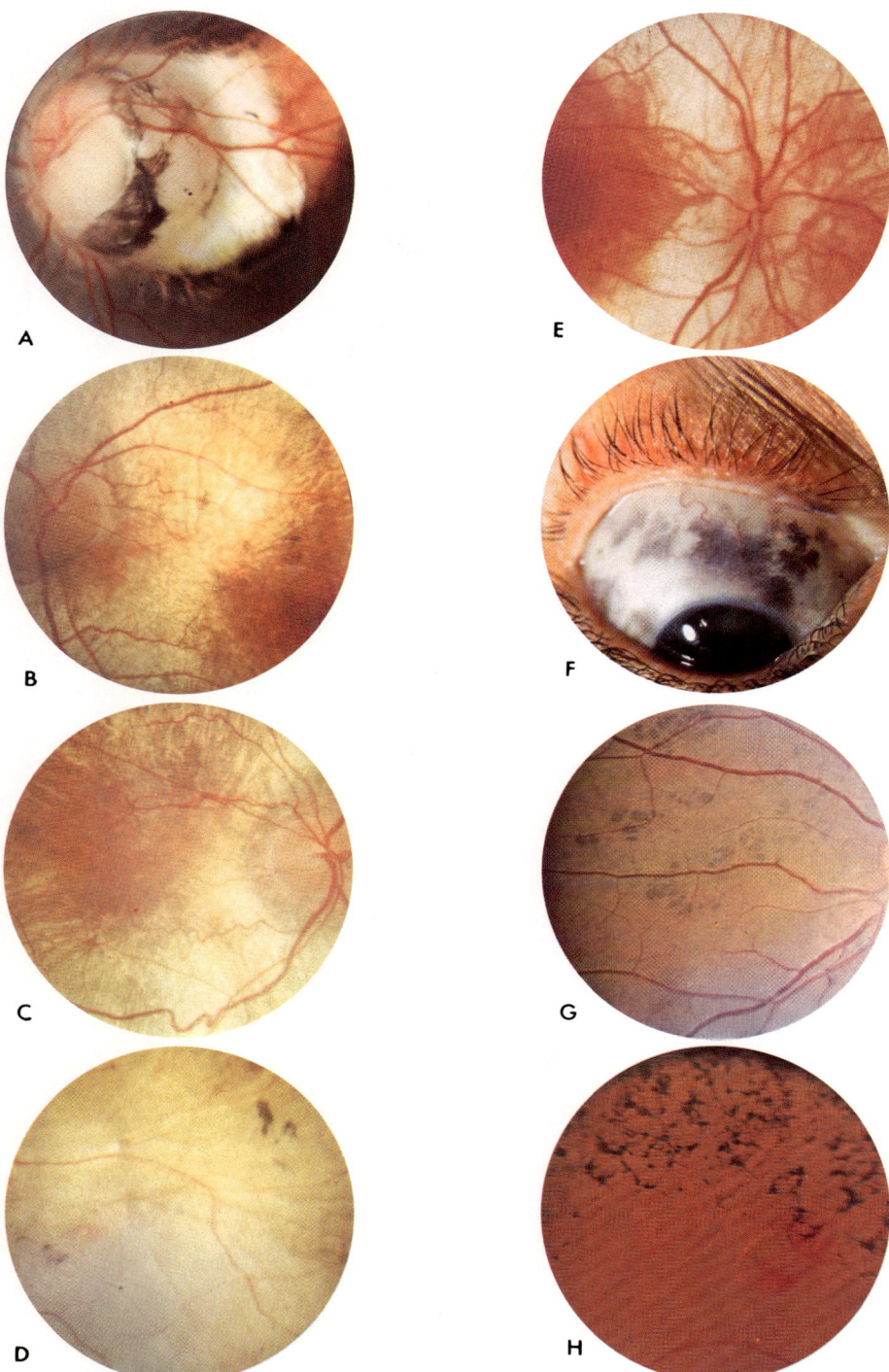

Plate 3 *(A)* Large coloboma of the optic disc.   *(B)* Choroideremia. Yellow-white atrophy and choroidal sclerosis in posterior pole.   *(C)* Same as shown in 3B.   *(D)* Peripheral fundus appearance of choroideremia in end stages.   *(E)* Choroideremia in earlier stage than shown in 3B and 3C, revealing less vascular attenuation and choroidal sclerosis.   *(F)* Congenital melanosis oculi and surrounding skin pigmentation, known as a nevus of Ota.   *(G)* Congenital, grouped pigmentation (bear tracks) of the upper nasal quadrant.   *(H)* Primary retinitis pigmentosa. Peripheral "bony spicule" distribution of degenerating retinal pigment epithelium.

nect the various meridians of the lesser arterial circle of the iris. As the eye develops, these arcades atrophy and regress back to the iris collarette, leaving a clear pupil. This regression of the anterior portion of the vascular cover of the lens may abort at any stage, which accounts for the various degrees of persistent pupillary membranes seen in many individuals. Remnants have been reported in up to 80 per cent of individuals examined carefully by biomicroscopy. The hereditary pattern suggests irregular autosomal dominance.

Persistent membranes of such magnitude as to interfere with vision are rare, but minor remnants of insignificant nature are rather frequent. The more severe variety not infrequently is associated with an anterior polar cataract. Perhaps of greatest diagnostic importance is the ability to differentiate these developmental membranes from the fibrous adhesions that result from inflammatory conditions in the anterior chamber. Although persistent pupillary membranes extend from one portion of the iris collarette (the lesser arterial circle) to another, inflammatory strands may attach to any structure in the anterior chamber.

Anisocoria. Unequal pupils, or anisocoria, is a condition inherited as an autosomal dominant trait. It must be differentiated from the multiple neurological causes for unequal pupils (p. 327). About 25 per cent of normal individuals exhibit pupillary inequality to some extent.

Heterochromia. A difference in the color of the two irides is, in its simplest form,

inherited as an autosomal dominant trait. A number of disorders, however, can give rise to this difference in iris color, the differential diagnosis being shown in Table 5-1. Each condition is described more completely elsewhere in this book.

Abnormalities of the Lens

Defects in Size, Shape, and Position. Although cataract formation is the most common developmental lenticular abnormality, other less frequent lens abnormalities occur. Like cataracts, they frequently are inherited, may be unique findings or associated with other ocular and/or systemic disorders, and may cause severe visual distortion. Although the lens may be clear, its abnormal size, shape, or position may alter its refractive properties to such an extent as to require surgical extraction for visual improvement alone. Moreover, several of these lenticular defects may give rise to secondary glaucoma, necessitating surgical removal to protect the eye.

Microphakia (spherophakia) can be inherited as an autosomal recessive trait and is characterized by a small, spherical lens that is prone to cause pupillary block glaucoma. The condition may be suspected when the lens border and the zonular fibers are easily visible through a properly dilated pupil, when the iris is tremulous, and when a marked myopia is present from the increased curvature of the lens. Not infrequently, subluxation occurs.

Lenticonus, lenticular umbilication, and lens colobomas are all abnormalities in the shape of the lens. *Lenticonus* may be either an autosomal dominant or recessive trait and is characterized by a conical protrusion of the anterior or the posterior surface of the lens in its axial portion. The opposite of lenticonus is *umbilication* (the indentation of the central lens axis so that the lens appears dumbbell-shaped in cross section). The narrow central portion of the lens frequently is opaque and may even be membranous. The center is never completely absent, however, and the anterior and posterior chambers do not communicate. *Lens colobomas* occur as irregular, autosomal dominant traits, separately or in conjunction with colobomas of the ciliary body. They are situated inferonasally. The lens is

(*Text continues on page 126.*)

TABLE 5-1   DIFFERENTIAL DIAGNOSIS
OF HETEROCHROMIA

1. Inherited variation from the normal
2. Congenital Horner's syndrome
3. Fuchs' heterochromic iridocyclitis
4. Iris atrophy, particularly secondary to iritis
5. Melanosis
6. Hemosiderosis
7. Diffuse melanoma
8. Hemifacial atrophy of Romberg
9. Waardenburg's syndrome
10. Status dysraphicus

TABLE 5-2 ETIOLOGY OF CATARACTS IN CHILDREN

   I. Hereditary
  II. Intrauterine Infections
     A. Rubella (Plates 5*C*, 7*E*)
     B. Toxoplasmosis
     C. Cytomegalic inclusion disease
 III. Chromosomal Aberrations
     A. Down's syndrome (mongolism)
     B. Trisomy 18
     C. 13-15 Trisomy
     D. Turner's syndrome
  IV. Prematurity
   V. Drug-Induced (Toxic) Cataracts
     A. Systemic steroids
     B. Triparanol (MER/29)
     C. Chlorpromazine (Thorazine)
  VI. Ocular Disease (Secondary Cataracts)
     A. Multiple ocular developmental defects
     B. Trauma
     C. Glaucoma
     D. Retinoblastoma
     E. Retrolental fibroplasia
     F. Uveitis
     G. Endophthalmitis
     H. Retinitis pigmentosa
     I. Retinal detachment
 VII. Ionizing radiation
VIII. Inborn Metabolic Disturbances
     A. Galactosemia (Plate 2*H*)
     B. Diabetes mellitus
     C. Hypoparathyroidism
     D. Aminoaciduria (Lowe's syndrome)
     E. Homocystinuria
     F. Cretinism
     G. Hepatolenticular degeneration (Wilson's disease)
  IX. Associated with Systemic Disorders
     A. Rheumatoid arthritis
     B. Congenital hemolytic icterus
     C. Laurence-Moon-Biedl syndrome
     D. Albers-Schönberg syndrome
     E. Congenital stippled epiphysis (Conradi's syndrome)
     F. Mandibulofacial dysostoses
     G. Craniofacial dysostoses
     H. Oxycephaly
     I. Bonnevie-Ullrich syndrome
     J. Marfan's syndrome
     K. Marchesani's syndrome
     L. Myotonic dystrophy
     M. Oligophrenia
        1. Sjögren's syndrome
        2. Marinesco-Sjögren's syndrome
     N. Dermatoses (syndermatotic cataracts)
        1. Atopic dermatitis
        2. Werner's syndrome (scleropoikiloderma)
        3. Rothmund's syndrome (infantile poikiloderma)
        4. Incontinentia pigmenti
        5. Congenital dyskeratosis (Schäfer)
        6. Congenital ichthyosiform erythroderma
        7. Siemens' syndrome
        8. Ectodermal dysplasia

TABLE 5-3   CLASSIFICATION OF CONGENITAL CATARACTS*

I. Anterior Axial Embryonal	Multiple, fine, irregular opacities lying close to the anterior embryonal suture, usually at its exact level; most common form of congenital cataract; like most congenital cataracts, these are stationary.
II. Sutural or Stellate	Opacities involving the regions of the fetal sutures (Plate 2G).
A. Cataracta cerulea (Blue dot cataract)	Small, punctate opacities; blue tint on slit lamp examination; may also be scattered irregularly throughout nucleus and cortex.
III. Congenital Opacities at the Anterior Pole of the Lens	
A. Anterior polar or pyramidal cataract	Sharply circumscribed opacity at the anterior lens capsule; one of the most common forms of congenital cataract; may affect anterior subcapsular lens fibers and project forward into the aqueous humor, forming a pyramid.
B. White flakelike opacities at the anterior lens capsule	
C. Circular capsular or subcapsular cataract	
D. Reduplication cataract	Localized opacity of the anterior capsule, with a similar opacity under it but separated from it by normal lens fibers; presence indicates intrauterine or postnatal inflammation or injury.
IV. Posterior Lens Changes	
A. Posterior polar cataract	May interfere with vision because of its posterior central location; may be stationary or give rise to postnatal progression.
B. Mittendorf dot and posterior lenticonus	
V. Zonular (Lamellar) Cataract (Plate 2F)	A circumscribed layer of lens fibers lying in the fetal nucleus is affected; characteristically extends over about two thirds of the central portion of the lens with the peripheral portions clear; surrounded by clear lens material and associated with U-shaped opacities called riders; usually is a dominantly inherited defect, but may result from local disease or trauma; may be associated with tetany.

*After Cordes, F. C.: Cataract types. Home Study Courses. 4th ed. Am. Acad. Ophth. 1961.

TABLE 5-3   CLASSIFICATION OF CONGENITAL CATARACTS* *(Continued)*

VI. Embryonal Nuclear Cataract (Cataracta centralis pulverulenta) (Plate 2E)	A fine, gray-white opacity located in the embryonal nucleus between the anterior and posterior Y sutures.
VII. Total Congenital Cataract	Complete opacification of the lens; cataract may be shrunken or may degenerate to the point of liquefaction.
VIII. Membranous Cataract	Absorption of the lens parenchyma with residual, folded, white membrane.
IX. Other Types of Congenital Cataracts A. Punctate cataract	Small gray or light blue opacities scattered throughout the lens without involving the embryonal nucleus.
B. Coronary cataract	Arrangement of opacities in a ring or crown; center and extreme periphery of lens remain transparent; opacities are club-shaped or have an oil-droplet appearance with rounded ends pointing to center of lens; present in 25 per cent of normal persons.
C. Spindle cataract (Axial fusiform cataract)	Anterior and posterior polar cataracts united or connected by threadlike opacities extending axially through the lens.
D. Spirochete-like opacities	Corklike opacities in the region of the posterior adult nucleus associated with irregular gray streaks or bands.
E. Coralliform cataract	Opacity resembling a piece of coral located near the center of the lens.
F. Spear cataract	Spiky, branching opacities running through the axial portion of the lens.
G. Disc-shaped or ring cataract	A ring-shaped opacity resembling a life preserver surrounded by clear lens.

*After Cordes, F. C.: Cataract types. Home Study Courses. 4th ed. Am. Acad. Ophth. 1961.

flattened or notched in this area when the pupil is dilated. Zonular fibers are absent in the coloboma.

Ectopia lentis, in the form of subluxation or complete dislocation of the lens, may be inherited as a separate entity through either a dominant or recessive autosomal gene. Characteristically, iridodonesis is present, and the equatorial rim of the lens crosses the dilated pupil. The subluxation most commonly occurs posteriorly into the superior nasal quadrant, although complete dislocation into the anterior chamber may occur and give rise to a severe, reverse, pupillary-block glaucoma. In addition to its occurrence as a separate entity, subluxation of the lens occurs commonly with megalocornea, spherophakia, Marfan's syndrome, Marchesani's syndrome, and homocystinuria.

Defects in Clarity (Cataracts). Cataracts (Plate *2E* to *H*) in the pediatric age group represent a major ocular problem and account for some 11.5 per cent of blindness in preschool children. They can arise from many causes and can occur at any age. Like so many ocular abnormalities, cataracts can be unique, or associated with other ocular problems or with systemic disorders. A cataract may be obvious and appear as a white pupil (Plate *7E*), but its presence should be considered whenever a child presents with strabismus, decreased visual acuity, a positive family history, other ocular abnormalities, multiple systemic defects, and any of the syndromes with which cataracts are associated.

Although a detailed discussion of the multiple etiologies for congenital and acquired cataracts goes beyond the scope of this text, several aspects should be considered. Both congenital and acquired cataracts can be inherited as autosomal dominant traits. About 25 per cent of cataracts are inherited. It is important to note that regardless of etiology, any congenital cataract, including the inherited variety, can either remain stationary or increase in severity as the child grows older. This also is true of acquired cataracts. An etiologic classification of cataracts in children is given in Table 5-2, and a classification according to the appearance of the cataract is given in Table 5-3.

Treatment of cataracts must be conservative, because indications for surgery depend on several factors, including the degree of visual impairment. Associated anomalies, especially the presence of other ocular defects or of mental retardation, usually cause operative treatment to be delayed. Even in the presence of anomalies, however, dense congenital cataracts can be removed surgically at any time after 6 months of age or when it is agreed that the child has a marked visual impairment from the cataracts. An exception to this rule should be made in congenital rubella cataracts (discussed later in the chapter). It may be wise to allow the child to reach nursery or early grade school levels to be sure that the cataracts are interfering with his development or education.

The visual prognosis (20/70 vision or better) is best when cataracts are bilateral, when the eyes are otherwise normally developed, when the child is of good intelligence, and when nystagmus is absent. If these prerequisites are lacking, the prognosis should be guarded. A unilateral congenital cataract, with or without microphthalmia, usually is associated with such profound amblyopia that functional rehabilitation through surgery is practically impossible. Surgery for unilateral congenital cataracts usually is not justified at a young age unless there is need for fundus examination. Surgery may be performed in older children for cosmetic reasons when appearance becomes an important psychologic factor.

Abnormalities of the Hyaloid System

Mittendorf Dot. During the fetal development of the human eye, the hyaloid artery breaks up spontaneously near its center around the seventh month of gestation. The anterior half of the vessel can be seen attached to the posterior capsule of the lens and extending back into the vitreous in a coil-like fashion. The anterior attachment to the lens may remain as a black dot throughout life within the dilated pupil and can be seen by direct ophthalmoscopy (Fig. 5-24). In the direct light of bio-

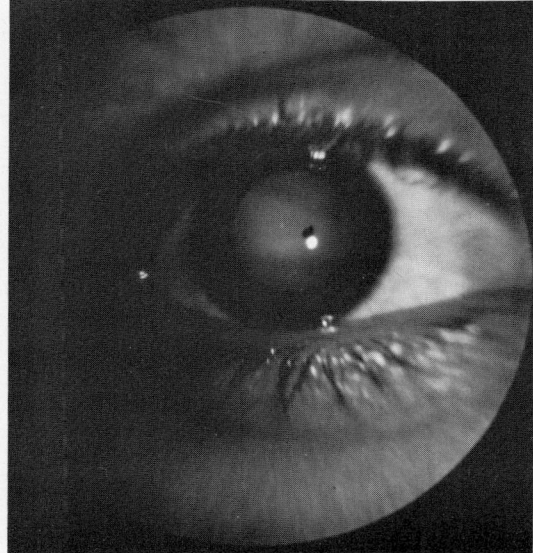

Figure 5-24 Mittendorf dot as seen by reflected light on the nasal aspect of the posterior lens capsule.

microscopy, the dot will be white. Known as a Mittendorf dot, it is situated just inferonasally to the center of the lens, is extremely small, and is of no visual consequence.

Persistent Hyaloid Artery. If the embryonic hyaloid artery should fail to atrophy, the Mittendorf dot can be seen to extend posteriorly into the vitreous, attaching to the optic disc. This persistent hyaloid artery can be nonpatent and appear as a white cord, or it may be open and seen as a healthy red blood vessel. In the more severe forms, varying degrees of persistence of the posterior vascular capsule of the lens may cause a partially or completely opaque pupil, and the fundus is difficult to examine. In these more severe cases, the eye is not infrequently microphthalmic.

Persistence of the *posterior* aspect of the hyaloid system may occur as a separate entity and be seen as a cystlike body in the vitreous, situated over the optic disc. The cysts exist in various sizes, are extremely rare, and may or may not be associated with persistence of the anterior portion of the hyaloid system. Persistence of the posterior hyaloid artery also can be seen as a small white bud over the central retinal artery as it emerges from the disc. It appears either as a strand of tissue or as a patent, vascular loop extending into the vitreous from the disc. This vessel frequently is twisted like a corkscrew and can often be seen to pulsate

freely. The vascular loops usually are arterial, rarely venous, and are formed within the absorbing Bergmeister's papilla, which usually regresses and leaves the loops floating free in the vitreous.

Persistent Hyperplastic Primary Vitreous (PHPV). This usually is found in full term infants. It is unilateral in over 90 per cent of the cases and results from the failure of spontaneous regression of the hyaloid vascular system and of the tunica vasculosis lentis, both of which are part of the primary vitreous.

Characteristically, PHPV is present at birth and presents as a white pupil (leukokoria). The involved eye may be microphthalmic, although this can be of minimal degree. The anterior chamber often is shallow, and the iris stroma exhibits prominent blood vessels that may extend into the pupillary space or onto the lens surface (Plate 7G). An extremely important diagnostic feature that is seen with the pupil dilated is elongated ciliary processes (Plate 7F) attached to the persistent, contracting, retrolental fibrovascular mass that pulls the processes centrally by traction. If the pupil is not completely occluded, remnants of the hyaloid may be seen behind the white membrane. Although clear initially, the lens may become completely opaque as the fibrovascular tissue extends into the lens through a defect in the posterior lens capsule.

Glaucoma may result from associated malformations of the anterior chamber angle, from swelling of the lens as the cataract develops, from posterior synechiae, or from recurrent hemorrhages. Organization of the hemorrhages may cause a total retinal detachment. The changing, progressive nature of PHPV may make it extremely difficult to differentiate from retinoblastoma.

Abnormalities of the Optic Disc

Bergmeister's Papilla. When the embryonic fetal fissure is closing, the axons of the retinal ganglion cells begin to make their way toward the primitive optic disc.

These axons run along the retina until the region of the optic stalk where they turn at right angles, pass through the retina, and out into the stalk. When the axons make the right angle turn, retinal elements are isolated from the remainder of the retina. This primitive epithelial papilla, which is composed of glial tissue from the retina, is pushed anteriorly by the steadily increasing number of axons turning posteriorly to form the optic nerve. The mass of tissue forms a cone known as Bergmeister's papilla. The cone is vascularized by the hyaloidal system, and as this artery atrophies, so does the glial sheath. Frequently the regression of Bergmeister's papilla is incomplete, resulting in varying degrees of congenital gliosis of the disc, prepapillary membranes, and glial veils. On the other hand, atrophy of this glial cone posterior to the retinal plane results in physiologic cupping of the optic disc.

Crescents. The apparent circular shape of the disc often varies; usually the retinal pigment epithelium falls short of the edge of the optic nerve head. This allows the sclera to appear as a white crescent-shaped area encircling part of the normal disc. The crescent, most frequently located inferiorly when congenital, is called a Fuchs' coloboma. Stationary throughout life, this should not be confused with the increasing crescent that is seen in myopic eyes; the latter most often is situated temporally and seems to represent the abnormal growth of the temporal retina in large eyes.

Situs Inversus. Situs inversus is a rare anomaly of the disc that is characterized by a tilting of the nerve head so that the vessels enter onto the *nasal* retina before fanning out. Variations of this 180 degree inversion of the disc can occur, and the nerve head is occasionally seen entering obliquely from any direction. All these anomalies of insertion may be associated with defects of vision secondary to an abnormal macula or high refractive errors, especially myopia and astigmatism.

Aplasia and Hypoplasia. Complete absence of the optic nerve (aplasia) is rare. The choroid is continuous over the posterior pole, and the nerve and central retinal vessels are absent. Occasionally a narrow opening appears (the stalk), which when normal contains the nerve and the retinal vessels.

Hypoplasia of the disc is the incomplete formation of the optic nerve (p. 299). Clinically, the nerve may appear small or a portion may be absent, but the retinal vessels are present, even though they may appear attenuated. Hypoplasia may be unilateral or bilateral and is associated frequently with other ocular or central nervous system deformities. The optic foramen on the involved side may be abnormally small. Usually vision is compromised severely, even when the eye and central nervous system are otherwise normally developed.

Both the oblique disc and the half-formed, hypoplastic nerve must be differentiated from the apparently oblique or oblong disc caused by a pronounced astigmatic refractive error.

Colobomas and Optic Pits. Colobomas (Plate 3A), crater-like holes, and small pits in the optic nerve may represent varying degrees of severity of a similar condition. Apparently they result from imperfect closing of the fetal fissure (p. 80). They tend to be located more temporally than true colobomas. Clinically, the small defects are purely asymptomatic, incidental findings. They are more often associated, however, with various field defects, especially central or paracentral scotomas, and visual acuity often is defective. There may be cystic retinal changes, macular abnormalities, and central serous retinopathy, especially with optic pits. Both physiologic and glaucomatous cupping of the optic disc must be considered in the differential diagnosis.

Congenital Pigmentation. Aside from the normal pigmented border of the disc, congenital pigmentation of the disc is uncommon. The occasional patient has papillae that show dense, black plaques covering a sector of the disc and even extending onto the retina. Others may have fine, linear strands or lacelike veils of pigment associated with the vasculature. The pigment can be mesodermal (choroidal) or ectodermal (retinal) in origin and appears to have no pathologic significance. The more denselike collections should not be mistaken for melanomas.

Miscellaneous Abnormalities of the Optic Disc. Drusen of the optic nerve (Plate 9*D*), myelinated nerve fibers, and pseudopapillitis may occur as congenital or inherited abnormalities. Since they must be considered in the differential diagnosis of a pathologically "choked" disc, they, as well as congenital and hereditary optic atrophies, are discussed in the chapter on neuro-ophthalmology (p. 299).

Abnormalities of the Choroid and Retina

Choroideremia. Inherited as a sex-linked intermediate trait, choroideremia although rare (Plate 3*B, C, D, E*) represents the most commonly seen primary choroidal degeneration. It is a progressive chorioretinal abiotrophy that begins in the first decade of life, usually presenting with the chief complaint of night blindness, and is indistinguishable from an atypical retinitis pigmentosa. Examination reveals a normal visual acuity, but the visual fields usually are constricted. Ophthalmoscopy reveals a diffuse, peripheral pigmentary ("salt and pepper") degeneration. Both the electro-oculogram (EOG) and the electroretinogram (ERG) are abnormal.

As the pigment epithelium of the retina progressively atrophies, the choroidal vessels slowly sclerose and eventually disappear. The fundus begins to appear yellow-white and the choroidal vascular pattern is completely lost. The retinal vessels attenuate, and the pigmentary deposits scatter at random, particularly in the periphery. Initially the changes are most marked in the midperiphery, spreading both peripherally and centrally. The macular region often is spared until late in the disease, and good visual acuity may be maintained for 50 years or more. More commonly, blindness occurs around 40 years of age.

Besides the chief complaint of nyctalopia (night blindness) in the male child and the physical findings of a constricted visual field, atypical pigmentary retinopathy, and abnormal electrophysiologic retinal responses, the diagnosis can be further suggested by an examination of the patient's mother. Since choroideremia is a sex-linked intermediate trait, she will present minor abnormalities. Functionally, she usually will be normal, but she will

often exhibit an atypical pigmentary retinopathy, possibly the salt and pepper variety, which may extend into the posterior pole. Peripapillary atrophy is present occasionally. In fact, the complete syndrome as it appears in a male has been reported in a 2 month old female. Conceivably this case report conforms to the Mary Lyon's hypothesis, although additional reports are needed to substantiate this viewpoint.

Fuchs' Chorioretinal Gyrate Atrophy. Like choroideremia, Fuchs' gyrate atrophy begins with night blindness and progresses with constriction of the visual fields, loss of the ERG response, and eventual marked loss of vision. Clinically, there is progressive atrophy of the choroid and retina with large yellow-white, confluent, doughnut-shaped areas appearing first in the periphery. The lesions spread centrally, leaving only the macula and, occasionally, the peripapillary regions looking normal. Both the optic disc and the retinal vessels remain within normal limits. Throughout the involved areas, there is an irregular, coarse clumping of pigment and, in a majority of cases, marked myopia. Gyrate atrophy usually is inherited as a simple autosomal recessive trait, and rarely through a sex-linked recessive pattern.

Choroidal Sclerosis. Both the generalized (autosomal dominant) and central (autosomal recessive) varieties of this disorder can begin late in the second decade of life, and commonly do not occur before age 20. They cause field defects and the loss of central vision, but without night blindness.

Functional Retinal Abnormalities

Night Blindness (Nyctalopia). There are two main types. In *essential night blindness*, an inherited functional defect of the retina, the fundus is not visibly abnormal. It can be inherited as an autosomal dominant, X-linked recessive, or autosomal recessive trait. Both recessive varieties are associated with a significant amount of myopia, with the sex-linked form occasionally revealing nystagmus.

Oguchi's disease, a rare type of nyctalopia, is an autosomal recessive trait that is characterized by a diffusely yellow or gray discoloration of the fundus that otherwise is within normal limits. Complete darkness for two to three hours will cause the return of normal coloration; this is known as *Mizuo's phenomenon*. Occasionally, dyschromatopsia is an associated finding. Although the disease is seen more frequently in Japanese than in other people, it is not limited to the Japanese.

Color Blindness. There are two main types of color blindness. *Achromatopsia*, complete loss of color vision, is inherited as an autosomal recessive factor characterized by the additional findings of poor vision (about 20/200 Snellen), photophobia, and nystagmus. Both the photophobia and nystagmus commonly decrease or disappear completely in the mid-teens. Amblyopia may or may not be present, and the achromatopsia may be complete or partial. Characteristically, colors are seen as shades of gray.

Several ocular abnormalities have been associated with achromatopsia: subtle macular changes, minimal peripapillary atrophy, and severe corneal astigmatism. A variety of systemic deformities also have been reported, especially otological defects, apical malformations, and dwarfism.

Congenital dyschromatopsias, incomplete color blindness, occur in about 8 per cent of males and ½ per cent of females. The three known types are the more common protanopia and deuteranopia, both inherited as sex-linked recessives, and the very rare tritanopia, inherited as an autosomal dominant defect.

In protanopia and deuteranopia the patient confuses reds and greens. Their differentiation lies in protanopes being insensitive to red light, whereas deuteranopes are sensitive to it. Tritanopes do not confuse red and green, but are blind to yellow and blue.

Pigmentary Abnormalities

Congenital Melanosis Oculi. Usually unilateral, this disorder most frequently is inherited as an autosomal dominant defect with weak penetrance, although recessive transmission is also known. Characteristically, hyperpigmentation of the conjunctiva and sclera is patchy, and pigment of the entire uveal tract may be increased. Heterochromia irides are present, with the involved eye being darker. The fundus in an affected Caucasian may resemble the normal fundus of a Negro, and often the disc has spotty pigmentation. About 10 to 20 per cent of patients with ocular melanosis may exhibit increased pigmentation of the periorbital skin. This blemish resembles the so-called mongolian spot, but in the periorbital location is known as a *nevus of Ota* (Plate 3*F*). Melanosis oculi is not associated with any functional defect or systemic abnormality, but the disorder is prone to degenerate into malignant melanomas.

Congenital, Grouped Pigmentation. Localized patches of pigment may occur throughout the retina. Frequently the lesions appear in a pie-shaped sector, the apex toward the disc. The pigmented groups look like animal footprints and often are referred to as "bear tracks" (Plate 3*G*). The finding usually is unilateral, with unimpaired function. No hereditary pattern has been shown.

Choroidal Nevus. Benign melanomas (nevi) can be seen in any region of the fundus and can be flat or slightly elevated. Situated in the choroid, they represent a localized increase in the size and number of pigment-bearing cells. A nevus usually is round or oval and may be larger than the diameter of the disc. Although choroidal nevi usually do not cause decreased vision, they should be followed periodically because of the suggested tendency to transform into malignant melanomas. Occasionally they may be confused with a choroidal hemorrhage.

Hereditary Pigmentary Degenerations (Tapetoretinal Degenerations)

Retinitis Pigmentosa. A generalized retinal pigment degeneration of unknown etiology, this condition exhibits a variety of inheritance patterns. Most frequently it is seen as a simple recessive trait in which it generally exhibits the most severe symptoms, the fastest progression, and the most associated defects. Less severe symptoms and slower progression are seen in the sex-linked recessive and the sex-linked intermediate types. The least severe is an autosomal dominant variety.

Typically, the condition begins in the early teens with night blindness. There may be no physical findings at this stage. Functional tests, however, will show a markedly decreased or absent ERG response, and tangent screen testing may reveal a ring scotoma. As the disorder progresses, the visual field further constricts with ultimate loss of visual acuity.

Physical findings may be absent at the onset of symptoms, but they soon become obvious. At first, the retinal pigment epithelium degenerates and appears as "bony spicules" scattered throughout the midperiphery (Plate 3H) and especially distributed along blood vessels. The process spreads both centrally and peripherally (Plate 4A), the retinal arterioles become attenuated, and the disc atrophies with a dirty yellow or gray appearance (Plate 4B). In the final stages there are posterior subcapsular cataracts, choroidal sclerosis, and, occasionally, macular degeneration. Associated ocular abnormalities may include glaucoma, microphthalmia, keratoconus, and ectopia lentis. A rarer variety exhibits all the functional and physical findings of retinitis pigmentosa with the exception of pigment clumping. This form has been called *retinitis pigmentosa sine pigmento*.

DIFFERENTIAL DIAGNOSIS OF RETINITIS PIGMENTOSA. True or atypical varieties of retinitis pigmentosa have been found in a number of diseases and syndromes.

1. *Usher's syndrome:* retinitis pigmentosa, labyrinthian deafness, and, occasionally, mutism.

2. *Laurence-Moon-Biedl syndrome:* an autosomal recessive disorder characterized by retinitis pigmentosa, polydactyly (Fig. 5-25), mental deficiency, obesity, and hypogonadism.

3. *Status dysraphicus (syringomyelia):* retinitis pigmentosa, heterochromia, kyphoscoliosis, cervical ribs, and syringomyelia or syringobulbia. The disorder is believed to be secondary to a defective closure of the primitive neural tube.

4. *Acanthrocytosis (Bassen-Kornzweig):* an autosomal recessive disorder that shows a predilection for Jewish people and is charac-

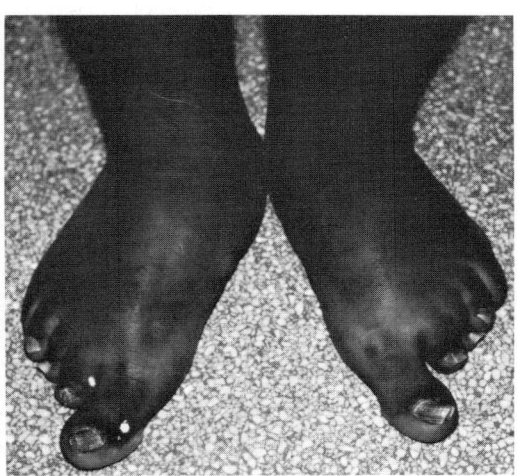

Figure 5-25 Abnormal feet of a child with Laurence-Moon-Biedl syndrome.

terized by crenated red blood cells, spinocerebellar degeneration, absence of serum beta-lipoprotein, and atypical retinitis pigmentosa. Celiac disease may be an associated finding.

5. *Friedreich's ataxia:* an hereditary ataxia with cerebellar degeneration, profound sensory abnormalities, secondary skeletal changes, frequent cardiac arrhythmias, nystagmus, and occasional retinitis pigmentosa.

6. *Refsum's disease:* hypertrophic polyneuritis, deafness, ataxia, increased cerebral spinal fluid protein, atypical retinitis pigmentosa, cataract, and corneal opacities.

7. *Leber's congenital amaurosis:* an autosomal recessive disorder beginning with decreased vision and eventually associated with an atypical retinitis pigmentosa with vascular attenuation, atrophic disc changes, and cataracts. The disorder begins before the age of 7, and these children frequently exhibit the oculodigital reflex that consists of constantly rubbing or pressing on their eyes with their fists or fingers.

8. *Other systemic disorders:* both myotonic dystrophy and Hurler's syndrome may also have an associated retinitis pigmentosa.

9. *Secondary pigmentary degenerations of the retina (pseudoretinitis pigmentosa):* pigmentary degenerations simulating the inherited dis-

orders can also arise from vascular lesions such as arteriolar occlusions, or from intra-uterine viral infections such as rubella or cytomegalic inclusion disease. In addition, it has been seen also in children following an attack of measles (rubeola). Disseminated chorioretinitis (Plate 4C), especially a syphilitic neuroretinitis, may cause an identical picture. Toxic factors, such as phenothiazine derivatives and antimalarial drugs, must also be considered.

Retinitis Punctata Albescens. This is an autosomal recessive trait characterized by progressive nyctalopia and a fundus covered with tiny white dots. The visual fields become constricted, and central vision diminishes. Eventually, vascular attenuation, optic atrophy, and pigment clumping may occur. Associated defects include choroidal sclerosis, macular degeneration, loss of the ERG response, and various forms of dyschromatopsia.

Fundus Albipunctatus. This appears to be a stationary form of albipunctate dystrophy and is an autosomal recessive disorder. Occasionally it is referred to as Lauber's disease.

The condition is characterized by a congenital night blindness and gray or white mottling of the fundus. Visual acuity, central fields, color vision, and the ERG response remain within normal limits. The retinal vasculature and optic discs are unchanged.

Fundus Flavimaculatus. A final variety of the "flecked retina" (Plate 4D), the familial occurrence of this syndrome suggests autosomal recessive inheritance. This usually appears about the age of 25, but it has been reported in 10 year old children. The condition may present with decreased vision, or it may be an incidental finding during a routine examination. The lesions range from yellow to white. They are usually irregular and deep in the retina, often appear to be outlining the choroidal vessels, and are usually located in the midperiphery or perimacular region (Plate 4E). Patients having impaired vision also may have an associated macular degeneration, a small central scotoma, and an abnormal ERG response.

Vitelliform Degeneration of Best. This macular degeneration is an autosomal dominant disorder that can be congenital or have an onset as late as 7 years of age. It is usually bilateral and begins with cyst-like changes in the macula. The lesion quickly takes on a "sunny-side-up" egg appearance (yellow-red) which is still compatible with adequate visual acuity (Plate 4F). The yolklike material eventually absorbs, leaving an atrophic, pigmented, disoriented macula in its place (Plate 4G). Once the pigment epithelium is disrupted, the visual acuity suffers accordingly. In the early "fried egg" stages, the diagnosis is relatively easy. The end stage, however, looks like many of the macular degenerations, and the diagnosis often depends on a reliable family history and on examination of siblings and other immediate relatives.

Juvenile Macular Dystrophy of Stargardt. This dystrophy occurs between the ages of 6 and 20, and usually exhibits autosomal recessive inheritance, although dominant patterns also are known. Unlike Best's degeneration, juvenile macular dystrophy begins with a rapid loss of acuity without ophthalmoscopic changes. Within a year, however, the foveal reflex is lost, and the macula begins to show pigment clumping surrounded by a *peau d'orange* or hammered metal appearance. This may progress to a circular or ovoid area of degeneration extending up to 3 disc diameters in size. Peripheral vision usually is retained, but an occasional patient may have a fundus not unlike that found in retinitis pigmentosa, with the associated functional abnormalities.

Late Onset Macular Degenerations. These can be inherited, familial, or acquired, and include the macular degenerations of Sorsby and Behr, mallatia leventinese, Doyne's honeycomb hyaline degeneration, Tay's macular choroiditis, and Khunt-Junius disciform macular degeneration (p. 284).

MACULAR DEGENERATIONS ASSOCIATED WITH SYSTEMIC DISEASES

A variety of systemic diseases whose major ocular finding consists of macular degeneration occur in children.

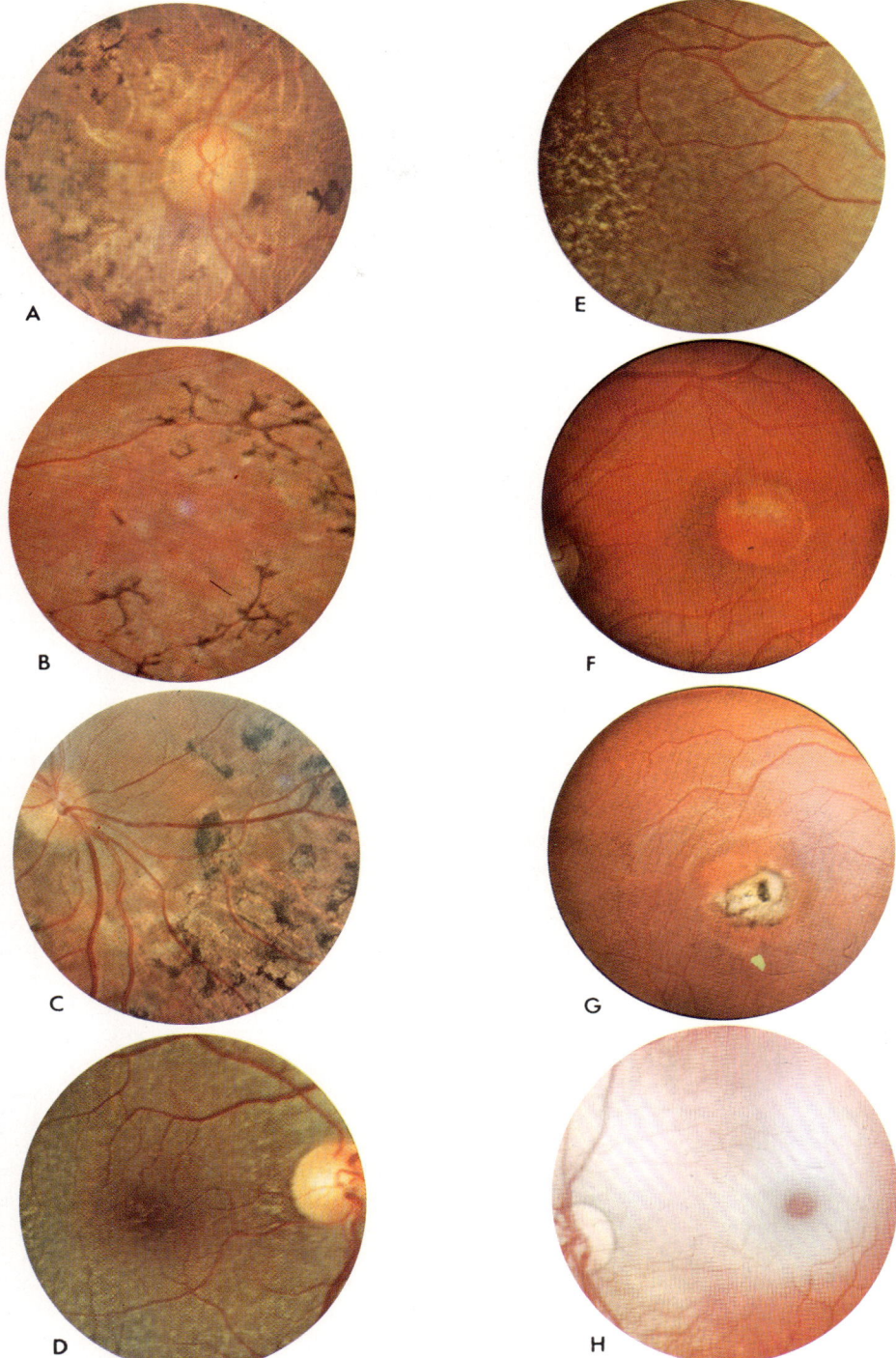

Plate 4 *(A)* Primary retinitis pigmentosa with attenuated vasculature, optic atrophy, choroidal sclerosis, and pigmentary clumping. *(B)* Peripheral fundus of 4A. *(C)* Pseudoretinitis pigmentosa. Pigmentary degeneration following a diffuse chorioretinitis. Note the lack of vascular attenuation. *(D)* Fundus flavimaculatus. Abnormal macular pigmentation and yellow-white lesions in posterior pole. *(E)* Fundus flavimaculatus. Same as shown in 4D, temporal to macula. Note typical "flecked" retina. *(F)* Best's macular degeneration. Early, "sunny-side-up" egg appearance. *(G)* Best's macular degeneration. Atrophic, pigmented, disoriented macula in the end stages of Best's disease. *(H)* Tay-Sachs disease. Characteristic cherry-red spot of the macula.

133

Von Gierke's Disease. This glycogen storage disease (Type I) is an autosomal recessive disorder characterized by the absence of the enzyme, glucose-6-phosphatase. This results in short stature, hepatosplenomegaly, hypoglycemia, lactic acidosis, and hyperlipemia. Retinal changes recently have been reported that consist of discrete, nonelevated, round, yellow flecks in the paramacular and macular regions. They are not associated with impaired vision or visual field defects.

Gaucher's Disease. This systemic lipidosis is inherited as either a dominant or recessive autosomal trait. The cerebroside, kerasin, accumulates in the reticuloendothelial cells of the liver, spleen, and bones. It can be rapidly fatal in infants. The retina may exhibit a ring-shaped, perimacular degenerative change that has been likened to a cherry red spot. Other ocular findings include corneal opacities, conjunctival infiltrates, and, commonly, strabismus.

Fabry's Angiokeratoma. Known as angiokeratoma corporis diffusum, this sex-linked recessive disorder of lipid metabolism is characterized by azotemia, maculopapular skin eruptions, proteinuria, febrile crises, and death from heart or renal failure in early adulthood. Dilated, tortuous, varicose vessels are seen in the retina and on the conjunctiva, and the cornea exhibits opacification in the deeper layers of the epithelium. Retinal hemorrhages, peripheral cystoid degeneration, and perimacular edema also have been described. This latter finding may result in a cherry red spot in the macula.

Amaurotic Familial Idiocy. This group of inherited cerebroretinal degenerations is presumed to be the result of an inborn error of lipid metabolism. The lipid is mainly ganglioside, and the conditions exhibit autosomal recessive inheritance. They can be divided by their age of onset into a rare congenital variety, an infantile form (Tay-Sachs), a late infantile form (Jansky-Bielschowsky), a juvenile form (Batten-Mayou), and the adult form (Kufs). A discussion of the first three forms follows.

TAY-SACHS DISEASE. This is the most common variety of amaurotic familial idiocy and begins between 6 and 12 months of age. Although it is most frequently seen in Jewish infants, it is not limited to them. After a normal initial period of development, the condition appears with hypotonia, hyperacusis, lack of interest in surroundings and the characteristic cherry red spot in the macula (Plate 4*H*). The condition progresses with increasing dementia, spastic paralysis, and blindness. It ends fatally when the child is 2½ to 3 years of age. Recent laboratory studies have shown a decrease or absence of fructose-1-phosphate aldolase in both the affected infants and their parents.

JANSKY-BIELSCHOWSKY DISEASE. This variety begins between 2 and 4 years of age and may run three to seven years before its fatal outcome. The child initially loses his intelligence, becomes ataxic, develops seizures, and loses sight. He becomes spastic, demented, and comatose prior to death. The fundus abnormalities begin with a cherry red spot in the macula, which, however, is not as striking as that seen in Tay-Sachs disease. This progresses to degeneration of the pigment epithelium in the macula, optic atrophy, attenuation of the vessels, and a peripheral retina degeneration somewhat like retinitis pigmentosa.

BATTEN-MAYOU DISEASE. This juvenile form of amaurotic idiocy is known also as Spielmeyer-Vogt-Stock disease and has its onset between 5 and 15 years of age, most commonly beginning around 8 years. Since the child is of school age, the *initial* symptom may likely be decreased vision. Seizures, mental deterioration, and extrapyramidal signs appear early. Blindness results in six to seven years from the onset, and the disorder progresses to death at 18 to 20 years of age.

The ocular findings begin with a macular degeneration characterized by irregular pigmented mottling or clumping. In rare cases a cherry red spot has been seen. The degenerative changes extend peripherally, and the fundus eventually looks like that described in the late infantile disease, with optic atrophy, vascular attenuation, and diffuse retinal atrophy. In this final stage, the ERG is markedly irregular or absent.

An additional laboratory finding, which is not pathognomonic, is vacuolated lymphocytes (Alder's anomaly) in the peripheral blood and conjunctival scrapings.

The cells have been found in infectious diseases, Niemann-Pick disease, occasionally in Tay-Sachs disease, and in the unaffected heterozygous relatives of children with Batten-Mayou disease.

Niemann-Pick Disease. Known as essential lipid histiocytosis, this is an autosomal recessive inborn error of lipid metabolism that has a predilection for Jewish people. Usually it begins between the second and fifth month of life with hepatosplenomegaly and lymphadenopathy. Fever, anemia, mental retardation, convulsions, and spastic paralysis become apparent and progress to a fatal outcome by 2½ years. Occasionally, survival has been over 10 years.

An infiltration of sphingomyelin is found in the reticuloendothelial system, in parenchymatous organs, and in the central nervous system, including the retina. Like the familial amaurotic idiocies, this lipid infiltration in the multilayered ganglion cells of the macula causes the area around the fovea to appear yellow or white. The thin fovea, with an underlying vascular choroid, then appears as a cherry red spot in the center of the abnormally white macula. The disc also appears atrophic, and the patient becomes blind in the course of the disease. About 60 per cent of infants with Niemann-Pick disease will develop cherry red spots.

Disseminated Lipogranulomatosis. Known as Farber's disease, this condition appears to be a disseminated lipid, and, possibly, a carbohydrate disorder that begins early in infancy and is rapidly fatal. The infant has a weak cry, is irritable, develops subcutaneous swellings on his extremities, and fails to thrive. The eyes exhibit a fine pigmentary retinopathy in the periphery and a cherry red spot in the macula.

Leukodystrophies. These disorders represent a diffuse degeneration of the white matter of the central nervous system, are probably inherited, and usually have ocular findings that consist of extraocular muscle abnormalities and optic atrophy resulting from retrobulbar neuritis or papillitis. Two forms that are of interest because of the associated macular changes are described below:

1. *Metachromatic leukodystrophy.* The late infantile leukodystrophy of Greenfield occurs between 1 and 2½ years of age, and is now considered a sulfatide lipidosis. It begins with hypotonia, ataxia, and loss of vision. Occasionally, the macula may appear gray with a cherry red spot in the center.

2. *Orthochromatic sudanophilic leukodystrophy.* Clinically, this degenerative disorder is similar to Tay-Sachs disease. It is inherited as an autosomal recessive trait, and the ocular findings include nystagmus, ptosis, optic atrophy, and, occasionally, a cherry red spot in the macula.

In the differential diagnosis of central chorioretinal degenerations, inflammatory conditions, such as toxoplasmosis, histoplasmosis, and trauma, must be considered in addition to primary macular degenerations.

Gross Retinal Abnormalities

Retinal Detachments. Idiopathic retinal detachments in children are rare. They always follow the development of a retinal hole or vitreous degeneration. There appears to be an hereditary tendency that usually is autosomal dominant in nature, but occasionally this tendency shows an autosomal or sex-linked recessive pattern. More important than the idiopathic variety and more common in children are the multiple causes of *secondary* retinal detachments. These include trauma, tumor, inflammation, and vascular diseases. (See p. 376, secondary detachments, and p. 286, primary retinal detachments.)

Retinoschisis. Juvenile retinoschisis is a progressive, degenerative retinal disorder that is transmitted as a sex-linked recessive trait. The cystic changes are most often found in the inferior temporal quadrant, are frequently bilateral, and consist of a cleft developing in the retina in one of the layers internal to the rods and cones. The anterior layer of the schisis or cyst is thin and transparent, and the retinal vasculature can be seen to change color or become elevated as it passes over the involved area. If both the anterior and posterior walls of the cyst degenerate, an actual detachment can occur. Macular changes are not infrequently associated with the peripheral retinal findings. Eyes with juvenile retinoschisis are prone to exhibit massive vitreous hemorrhages.

Congenital Retinal Fold. This falciform fold of retinal tissue is inherited as an autosomal recessive entity and should not be confused with changes secondary to inflammation or to the proliferative membrane of retrolental fibroplasia. Falciform folds extend from the disc to the periphery and may even attach to the lens. They are usually found in the inferior temporal quadrant and may be associated with a number of ocular abnormalities including microphthalmia, coloboma, retinal rosettes, and macular changes.

Retinal Dysplasia. This is one of many causes of leukokoria. It occurs in full-term infants and is usually bilateral. The eyes are microphthalmic, with a shallow anterior chamber, and long ciliary processes. Abnormalities of the central nervous system, cardiovascular system, and skeleton may also be present. When bilateral and associated with multiple systemic abnormalities, the diagnosis of 13-15 trisomy should be considered.

Bilateral retinal dysplasia has been found in children with the 13-15 trisomy syndrome and also as a sex-linked recessive trait in one family that did not exhibit any systemic abnormalities. Frequently, unilateral retinal dysplasia is not associated with any syndrome or systemic defects. Histologic examination of these abnormal eyes reveals that in 13-15 trisomy the dysplastic retina contains cartilage; by contrast, in the unilateral retinal dysplasia that is not associated with systemic defects, cartilage is absent.

Besides occurring in full-term infants, retinal dysplasia is associated with microphthalmia, and a pink-white membrane is visible behind a clear lens. The lens may quickly become cataractous, and both vitreous hemorrhage and secondary glaucoma are not uncommon. The condition must be differentiated from all the other causes of leukokoria, especially retinoblastoma.

CONGENITAL INFECTIONS

Developmental ocular defects can be produced by congenital infections as well as by hereditary and other causes. Such infections, which are usually transmitted hematogenously through the placenta, may seriously damage all of the developing systems, including the eyes. The extent of fetal damage is governed mostly by random distribution of the infectious agent; the age of the fetus at the time of the maternal infection; and, in part, by the tissue predilection of the specific infectious agent. The earlier in pregnancy the infection occurs, the more extensive the injury to the fetus. Congenital infections can result in abortion or stillbirth; multiple teratogenic abnormalities; or active, inflammatory disease that simulates the adult disorder.

Congenital Syphilis

Caused by the transplacental transmission of the *Treponema pallidum* organism from the mother to the fetus, syphilis usually occurs after the fourth gestational month. In untreated syphilitic mothers, about 30 per cent of the pregnancies will result in a stillborn infant, and 70 per cent of the infants born alive will be affected. In its early stages, congenital syphilis is somewhat comparable to secondary syphilis in adults, whereas its final stages are comparable to tertiary syphilis.

Early congenital syphilis can present a variety of systemic signs and symptoms. The infant may exhibit a slightly elevated, maculopapular rash over his entire body, particularly on the palms of his hands and soles of his feet (Fig. 5-26). Involvement of the mucous membranes causes rhinitis, or "snuffles" (Fig. 5-27), which is characterized by a mucopurulent discharge from the nose. The skeletal system changes may include osteochondritis and even multiple fractures. Periostitis and true osteomyelitis are not infrequent. Central nervous system manifestations in the form of meningitis and subsequent hydrocephaly may occur. Other common systemic findings include fever, anemia, edema, jaundice, hepatosplenomegaly, lymphadenopathy, pneumonitis, nephritis, and hemorrhaging, especially from the nose or periumbilical region.

The ocular findings include acute iritis, interstitial keratitis, chronic iridocyclitis, chorioretinitis, retinal periphlebitis, optic neuritis, vitreous opacities, and secondary cataracts. Pupillary abnormalities and optic atrophy may occur if neurosyphilis results.

Acute iritis may be present at birth, but it more commonly begins around 6 months of age. Chorioretinitis with a "salt and pepper" retinopathy, frequently referred to as pseudoretinitis pigmentosa, also may be present at birth. The posterior lesions may appear as a focal choroiditis or, less commonly, as large atrophic chorioretinal scars with circumscribed pigmentation that simulate the lesions of toxoplasmosis.

The classic ocular finding of congenital syphilis, however, is interstitial keratitis, which occurs in about 10 to 15 per cent of the cases. It rarely appears before two years of age and may not begin until as late as 20 years, but most commonly appears between the sixth and twelfth year of life. It may be unilateral at first, but usually becomes bilateral. Its onset is heralded by lacrimation and photophobia. Corneal edema, infiltrates, and vascularization of the deep layers of the cornea are characteristic.

Vessel formation may be so marked as to give the cornea a pink or "salmon patch"

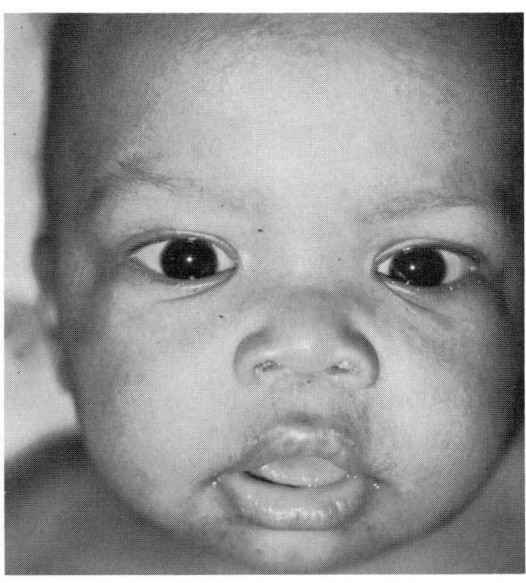

Figure 5-27 Congenital syphilis. Involvement of nasal mucous membranes causing rhinitis or "snuffles."

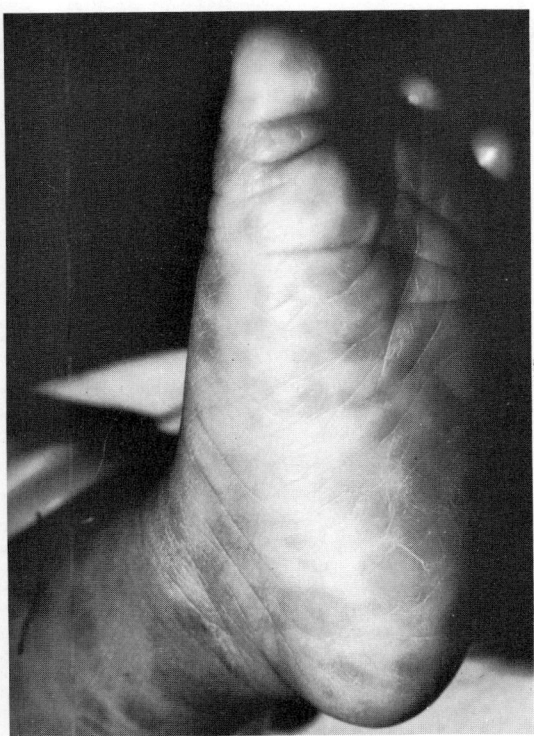

Figure 5-26 Congenital syphilis. Elevated maculopapular rash on sole of foot.

appearance (Plate 5A). Usually the overlying epithelium becomes hazy, and anterior uveitis nearly always is present, leaving peripheral, pigmented scars. These scars and residual ghost vessels, which are seen with a slit lamp biomicroscope at the level of Descemet's membrane in the cornea, persist throughout life, and are diagnostic signs of congenital lues. The process may remain active for one week to several years. The cornea may be grossly clear with good vision or may be grossly scarred and nearly opaque.

Therapy consists in treating the systemic disease with penicillin, and the active ocular involvement with local cycloplegics and steroids. If the ocular inflammation is refractory to local medications, systemic steroids may be necessary.

Congenital Rubella

The syndrome originally was described by an Australian ophthalmologist, Sir Norman Gregg, in 1941. The full significance of the disease was not appreciated, however, until 1962, when the virus was isolated and identified by Weller and Neva and, independently, by Parkman and Buescher. Like congenital syphilis, rubella is transmitted to the fetus via the placenta when a viremia occurs in the mother. In the United States today, about 15 per cent of women in their childbearing years have not had rubella, as evidenced by their lack of serum neutralizing antibody. The risk to the fetus varies according to the week of gestation in which the maternal infection occurs. The overall results show that one of five infants born to women who have contracted rubella in the first trimester will be abnormal in some way. If the mother contracts rubella during the first four weeks of gestation, there is a 50 per cent chance that the infant will be damaged.

The effects to the fetus are multiple and include many teratogenic anomalies as well as active inflammatory disease. Why this occurs is not known precisely, but it has been shown that the virus can inhibit mitosis and cellular multiplication, and cause an increase in nonspecific chromosomal breaks. It may persist in viable cells for a long time, even when the serum neutralizing antibody level is adequate. Moreover, rubella can spread through a developing organ or entire fetus without being exposed to this antibody because the viral particles are passed directly from parent to daughter cell during cellular division.

Clinically, the rubella virus is capable of causing spontaneous stillbirth or abortion in 15 per cent of infected mothers, usually within two weeks after the infection appears. If the pregnancy continues to term, the infant is commonly of low birth weight, fails to thrive, and shows poor growth and development.

The classic congenital rubella syndrome, as originally described by Gregg, consists of a triad of eye, ear, and heart defects. Other systems, however, are now known to be involved just as frequently.

The congenitally infected rubella infant shows a severe loss of hearing secondary to the viral destruction of the organ of Corti. Auditory defects may not be found in many of the infants, however, until they are older and more subtle testing can be done. The

most common heart anomalies caused by rubella are patent ductus arteriosis, pulmonary stenosis, and ventricular septal and endocardial cushion defects. The infant tends to be microcephalic, although hydrocephaly has been reported. Central nervous system involvement includes meningoceles and spina bifida. A viral encephalomyelitis is not infrequent.

If the liver, spleen, and bone marrow are involved, the result is hepatosplenomegaly, jaundice, anemia, thrombocytopenia, and dermal erythropoiesis (Plate 5B). The classic morbilliform rash seen in adult rubella infections occurs in about 15 per cent of the infants. The long bones may exhibit an irregular and thin trabecular pattern that resolves spontaneously by eight weeks of age. Oral anomalies, pneumonitis, and genitourinary defects are found less frequently.

Microphthalmia and cataracts are the most common ocular abnormalities. In 75 per cent of the cases, the cataracts are likely to be bilateral if the maternal infection has occurred within the first nine weeks of gestation. Typically, the cataracts are nuclear (Plate 7E), although they may be complete with all layers of the lens involved (Plate 5C). They also may become denser as the child grows older.

Opaque corneas can occur from the absence of Descemet's membrane centrally, resulting in a picture identical to von Hippel's posterior corneal ulcer. Cloudy corneas also can result from the congenital glaucoma.

Cataracts tend to be caused by early infection, and glaucoma commonly results when the maternal involvement occurs after the hyaline lens capsule has formed. Earlier infection, however, can cause both cataract and glaucoma in the same eye (Plate 5D), and the two conditions are not mutually exclusive.

Anterior uveitis or iridocyclitis is frequent. The iris stroma may be severely atrophic and even transilluminates. Both the dilator and sphincter muscles are poorly developed. The pupil tends to be small and cannot be widely dilated.

Another major ocular finding in over 40 per cent of the involved neonates is an atypical retinitis pigmentosa, which, as in syphilitics, is referred to as "salt and pepper" retinopathy (Plate 5E, F). The find-

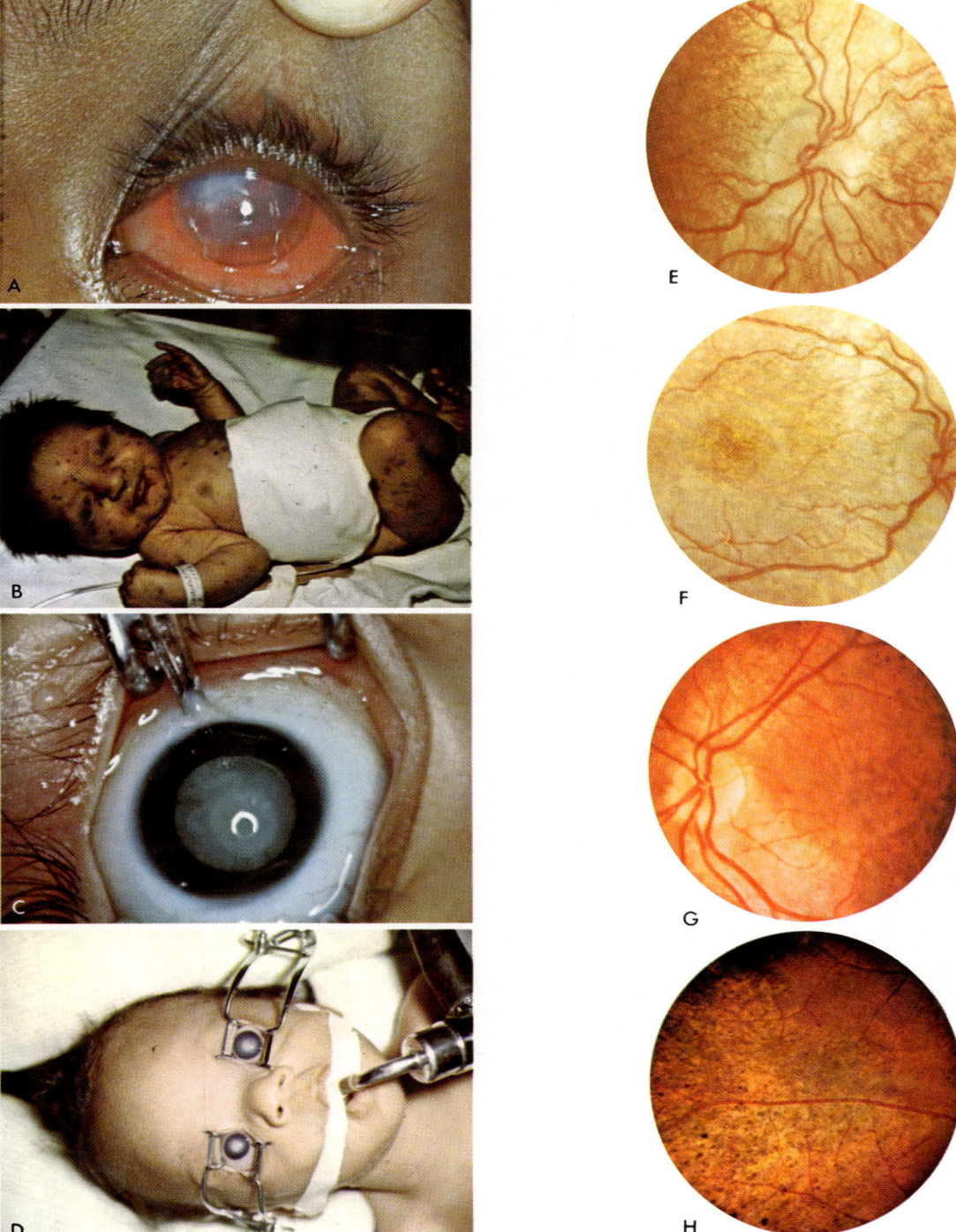

Plate 5 *(A)* Congenital syphilis. Typical "salmon patch" of acute interstitial keratitis. *(B)* Congenital rubella. Thrombocytopenic purpura of face, trunk, and extremities. *(C)* Congenital rubella cataract showing opacification of both the nucleus and cortex. *(D)* Congenital rubella. Bilateral congenital glaucoma and cataracts. *(E)* Congenital rubella. Fine peripapillary "salt and pepper" retinopathy. *(F)* Same as shown in 5E. Fine pigmentary stippling in macula of 4 year old child. *(G)* Congenital rubella. Macular pseudoretinitis pigmentosa in a 12 year old child. *(H)* Periphery of 5G. Compare with 5E and 5F, and note lack of progression of the retinopathy.

139

ing represents alternating areas of hypertrophy and atrophy of the pigment epithelium, which can be peripheral, central, segmental, or diffuse. At present, the chorioretinitis of congenital rubella is felt to be nonprogressive (Plate 5G, H) and is associated with good visual acuity and a normal ERG. The retinopathy can be unilateral or bilateral.

Other ocular findings include obstructed nasolacrimal canals, viral dacryoadenitis, strabismus, and nystagmus.

An adequate vaccination is the only treatment to prevent maternal infection during pregnancy. One vaccine became available in 1969. When natural or induced immunity is absent, there is no sure way to prevent viremia in the pregnant mother. The use of gamma globulin or hyperimmune serums has proved to be only of sporadic and nonpredictable benefit.

The management of children who have had a congenital rubella infection is discouraging. Cataracts and glaucoma are treated surgically, but the prognosis is poor. Unfortunately, the virus persists within the eye, especially within the lens itself, and probably leads to poor surgical results. Normally a rubella infant stops excreting the virus from his nasopharynx by 12 months of age, but it can be found in the lens of the same infant as late as 3 years of age. It is likely to be released at the time of cataract surgery and causes a uveitis. This explains why severe complications occur in 35 per cent of rubella eyes after cataract extraction. It has been recommended, therefore, that congenital cataract surgery be delayed in affected children until they are at least two years of age. Preliminary sector iridectomies can be performed safely in younger children and often improve vision.

Congenital Cytomegalic Inclusion Disease (CID)

Originally described by Ribbert in 1882, CID is another transplacental viral infection that has received renewed interest in the past few years. The cytomegalovirus (CMV), a DNA virus that produces both intranuclear and intracytoplasmic inclusion bodies, was first isolated from the human salivary gland in 1956, by Smith. Shortly thereafter. Rowe isolated the virus from the urine of infected infants and made possible the ante mortem diagnosis.

In the adult the virus can produce a subclinical infection, a flulike respiratory disease, or a mononucleosis-like syndrome. Since 30 to 40 per cent of women in their maximum childbearing years show no antibody levels to CMV, they presumably are susceptible to a new infection. Since the number of adults susceptible to cytomegalic inclusion disease is greater than those susceptible to rubella, and since CMV is constantly present and not epidemic in nature, CMV may prove to be more important than rubella virus as a cause of congenital disease. Although the risk to the infant is undetermined at this writing, the finding that about 40 per cent of microcephalic infants are seropositive for CMV (as compared with 4 per cent of normocephalic infants) suggests an alarming frequency of previously unsuspected congenital involvement. From 1 to 2 per cent of newborns are presently suspected of showing serologic evidence of CMV infection.

The virus seems to have a predilection for both the central nervous and the reticuloendothelial systems. The congenital syndrome is characterized especially by microcephaly, mental retardation, and spastic diplegia. The infants involved frequently have low birth weights, encephalomyelitis, jaundice and thrombocytopenia, hepatosplenomegaly, pneumonitis, and chorioretinitis.

Diagnosis can be made by the virus being cultured from urine, tears, conjunctival scrapings, cerebrospinal fluid, or liver biopsy. The inclusion bodies also may be found in urine sediment, conjunctiva, and liver. Serologic studies may show elevated immunoglobulin M levels, usually over 18 milligrams per cent. A finding of intracranial calcifications (Fig. 5-28) by X-ray is not uncommon, and the distribution of the lesions in the periventricular regions suggests cytomegalic inclusion disease (Fig. 5-29), but this is definitely not as characteristic as once thought. The calcium deposits can be both randomly distributed and periventricular.

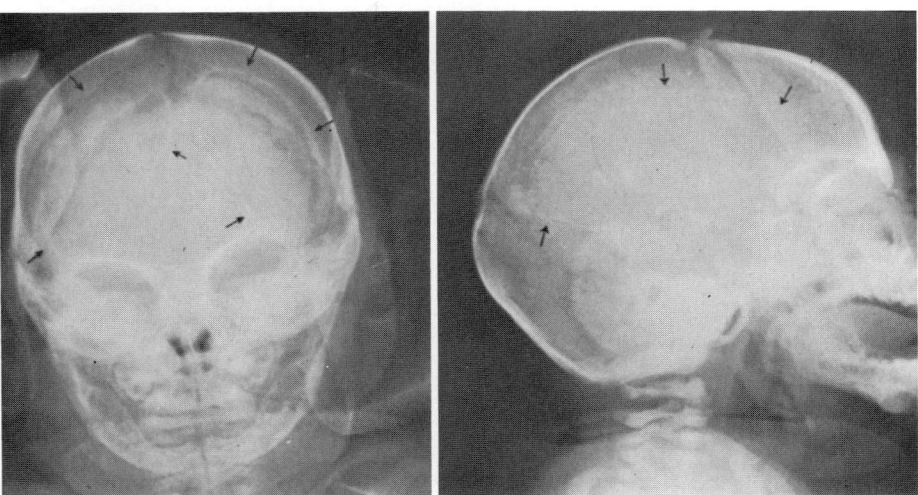

Figure 5-28   Congenital cytomegalic inclusion disease with intracranial calcifications (arrows).

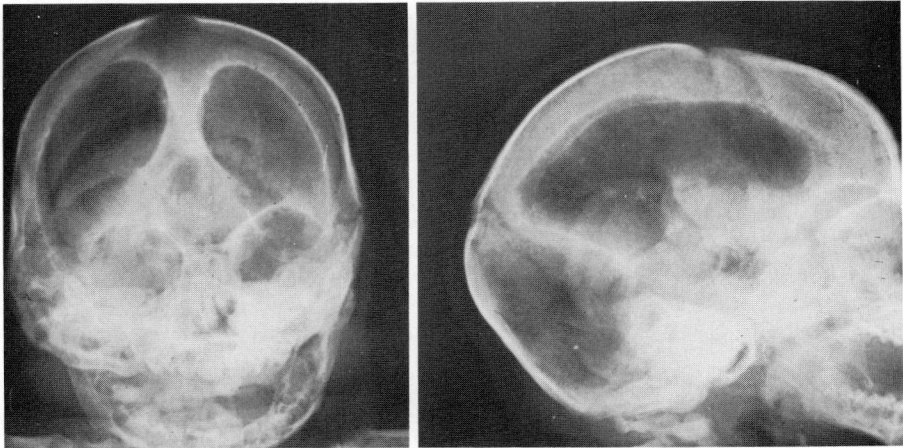

Figure 5-29   Congenital cytomegalic inclusion disease. Pneumoencephalogram reveals intracranial calcifications that appear to outline ventricles.

The most consistent ocular finding secondary to CID appears to be a retinochoroiditis, with the retina primarily involved and the choroid affected secondarily. The lesions usually are described as multiple, small, and in the periphery. However, increased interest in CID has made it obvious that the retinochoroiditis can be expressed in many forms (Plate 6A). These lesions may be scattered throughout the entire posterior pole and may coalesce as activity continues, resulting in one large necrotic area similar to that of toxoplasmosis. Solitary macular lesions also can occur. New areas of involvement can arise in previously normal fundi, so the infants should be followed as long as they excrete the virus in their urine. Cytomegalic inclusion disease less frequently has been reported to cause anterior uveitis, cataract, and optic atrophy.

At present, there is no treatment for the disease, although steroids have been tried with varying success, and antiviral agents, such as fluorodeoxyuridine, with inconclusive results. The use of hyperimmune serum taken from the infant's mother has been suggested. No vaccination is available at present.

Congenital Toxoplasmosis

This disease first was described in 1923 by Janku, some 15 years after the organism originally was discovered in animals by Nicolle and Manceaux. It was not until 1952, however, that it actually was found within the eye by Wilder, proving conclusively that ocular toxoplasmosis was a definite entity.

The organism, *Toxoplasma gondii,* is an incompletely classified and poorly understood protozoan that is widespread throughout the animal kingdom. It is believed to be transmitted to man through ingestion of raw meat and possibly through contact with domestic animals that excrete the encysted forms in their feces. The organism also infects nematode eggs, especially those of *Toxocara cati,* suggesting another possible source of human infection.

Congenital toxoplasmosis was thought to occur only from transmission across the placenta during parasitemia in the mother. In 1962, however, Werner showed that the toxoplasma organism could be found in menstrual blood and uterine muscle of women who were chronic aborters. A year later, Langer confirmed this finding in a separate study and showed that the organisms could be found in the milk of a lactating woman. This implies that congenital toxoplasmosis could result from direct invasion of an involved uterus by the developing trophoblast. Moreover, Langer's finding of *Toxoplasma gondii* in maternal milk suggests the possibility that some of the cases of "congenital" toxoplasmosis that went unnoticed at birth were, in reality, acquired anew by the infant during neonatal life.

Clinically, congenital toxoplasmosis is characterized classically by a hydrocephalic infant with massive retinochoroiditis and randomly distributed intracranial calcifications (Fig. 5-30). As with many congenital infections, prematurity and low birth weights are more frequent, and common findings include neonatal jaundice, failure to thrive, fever, hepatosplenomegaly, and lymphadenopathy. Variations of the disease include microcephaly, meningoencephalitis, convulsions, and a maculopapular rash.

Often the manifestations of the disease are subclinical in the newborn period and may not present until sometime during the first decade. In this more subtle variety of congenital toxoplasmosis the first symptom may be a convulsion, and the associated findings may include slight retardation, intracranial calcifications, and old chorioretinitis. As mentioned previously, this tetrad (convulsions, retardation, intracranial calcifications, and chorioretinitis) could be explained by the infection occurring either late in gestation or even in the neonatal period.

The classic ocular involvement is a large, yellow-white, atrophic, chorioretinal scar that is surrounded by dense pigmentation (Plate 6B). The lesions may have a predilection for the macular areas and the involvement may be unilateral or bilateral (Plate 6C).

Not infrequently more severe involvement is seen, with the infant revealing microphthalmia and leukokoria from sec-

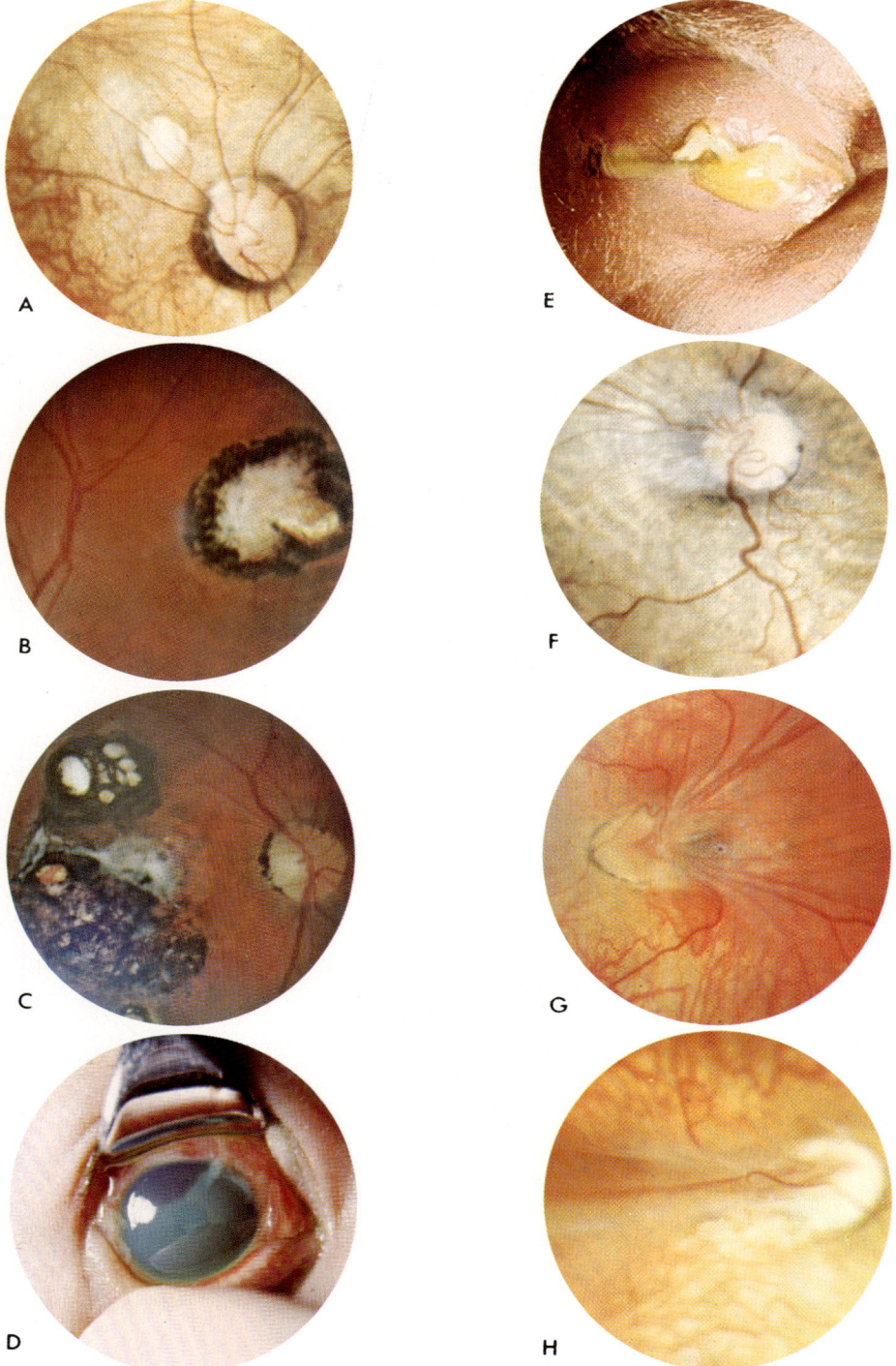

Plate 6 (A) Congenital cytomegalic inclusion disease. Chorioretinal lesion involving the posterior pole. (B) Congenital toxoplasmosis. Large yellow-white chorioretinal scar in macula, surrounded by marked pigmentation. (C) Congenital toxoplasmosis. Massive, old inactive chorioretinal scar exhibiting gliosis, atrophy, and pigmentary hypertrophy. Notice the occurrence of several smaller satellite lesions. (D) Ophthalmia neonatorum. Corneal staining and keratoconjunctivitis of newborn infant following instillation of silver nitrate solution. (E) Ophthalmia neonatorum. Heavy, purulent discharge and swollen lids of gonorrheal conjunctivitis in the newborn. (F) Retrolental fibroplasia. Cicatricial grade 2. (G) Retrolental fibroplasia. Cicatricial grade 2, more advanced. (H) Retrolental fibroplasia. Cicatricial grade 3, with retinal fold extending to temporal periphery.

ondary cataract or from massive retinal destruction or vitreous organization. Active retinitis may appear as elevated, yellow masses that are hazy from the overlying vitreous reaction. Both strabismus and nystagmus may result from either decreased vision or from central nervous system involvement.

The diagnosis of congenital toxoplasmosis can be indicated strongly by the clinical findings, and can be confirmed by the Sabin-Feldman dye test and by the complement fixation titer. A more rapid diagnosis can be obtained by use of the immunoglobulin M assay and fluorescent antibody technique as described by Remington in 1967. This should be employed when possible because many of these infants exhibit an active inflammatory process against which specific therapy might be of value if started early.

Treatment of toxoplasmosis consists of pyrimethamine (Daraprim), sulfadiazine, steroids, and folinic acid in various combinations, but it is still unsatisfactory. None of the therapeutic regimens are of pre-

dictable definite value, and Daraprim and steroids are not without serious side effects. An ophthalmologist should follow surviving children for the rest of their lives for evidence of reactivation of the posterior uveitis.

Parents of these children often raise the question of repeated, multiple sibling involvement. Contrary to most of the present literature, it may be unwise to inform them that congenital toxoplasmosis is a one-time occurrence, especially if there is a history of spontaneous abortion. Several factors now point with validity toward the concept of repeated congenital toxoplasmosis within a family. They are:

1. Atypical colobomas of the macula have been reported to repeat within a family, and, therefore, have been considered to be an hereditary developmental abnormality. Many investigators, however, point out that the lesions appear inflammatory and that there is no embryologic reason for macular colobomas to develop.

2. Animal experimentation and human hysterectomy specimens have revealed that the toxoplasma organism is capable of encysting within the uterus and producing an endometritis. If the endometritis is in the area of the developing trophoblast, there is reason to suspect that the fetus may be involved.

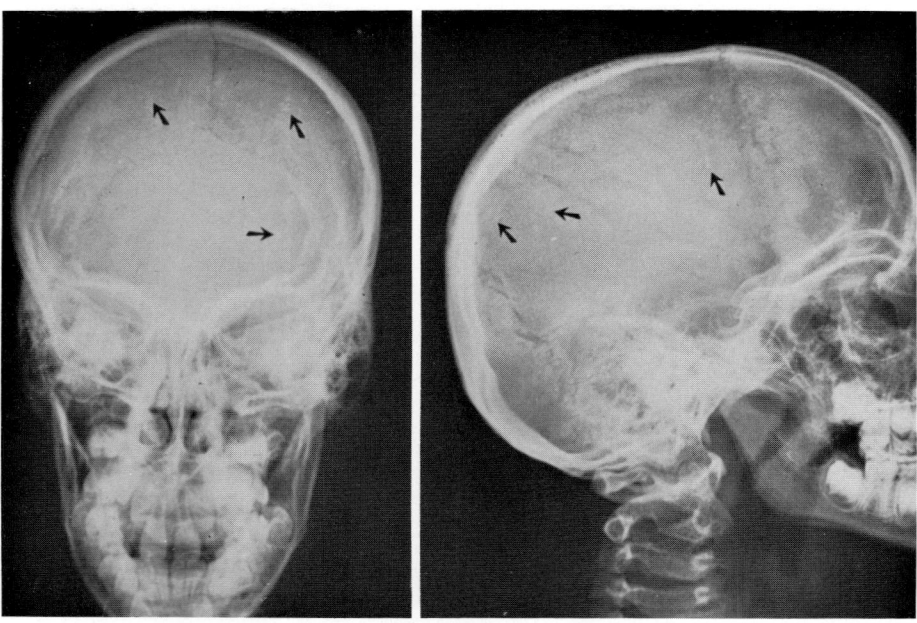

Figure 5-30 Congenital toxoplasmosis. Randomly distributed intracranial calcifications (arrows).

TABLE 5-4 ORGANISMS IMPLICATED IN CONGENITAL INFECTIONS

1. Rubella virus
2. Cytomegalovirus
3. *Toxoplasma gondii*
4. *Treponema pallidum*
5. Newcastle disease virus
6. Herpes simplex virus
7. Mumps virus
8. Coxsackie B virus
9. Influenza A virus
10. St. Louis encephalitis virus

3. Isolation of *Toxoplasma gondii* from fetal or maternal tissues in habitual or repeated miscarriages, premature births, and stillbirths has been reported in two separate studies (Werner, 1962; Langer, 1963). These authors obtained the toxoplasma organism from about 35 per cent of the involved individuals. The organisms were cultured from fetal tissues, placenta, uterine muscle, uterine scrapings, menstrual blood, and maternal milk.

4. In 1963, Langer reported a proven instance of successive, congenital toxoplasmosis-infected infants born to one mother. Both infants had the classic syndrome and the diagnosis was proved by isolation of the organism. It would appear, therefore, that congenital toxoplasmosis will prove to be a repeating disease within a given family, and will simulate an hereditary disorder.

OTHER CONGENITAL INFECTIONS

There is reason to believe that in time other infectious agents will prove to be etiologies of congenital disease. The list of implicated organisms is growing (Table 5-4). Cataracts alone have been produced in humans or in animals by intrauterine infection with the viruses of rubella, St. Louis encephalitis, mumps, Newcastle disease, and influenza A.

NEONATAL OPHTHALMOLOGY

Besides the many disorders already discussed that are present at birth and must be considered in the diagnosis of ocular diseases in the neonatal period, a number of ophthalmologic problems exist that are related to birth but not associated directly either with genetic or intrauterine factors. Specifically, they are the ocular problems arising from birth trauma, conjunctivitis of the newborn period, and abnormalities resulting from premature delivery.

Birth Trauma

Ocular injuries at birth can occur from the pressures applied directly to the infant's head by the narrow birth canal, from the forces of labor, and by the inappropriate application of forceps during delivery.

Injuries to Orbit, Lids, and Extraocular Muscles. Lid edema and petechiae are common companions of birth, especially with vertex presentations and even more often in forceps delivery. Moreover, proptosis may result from retrobulbar hemorrhage or from orbital fractures. Occasionally, especially when the orbits are shallow, a complete prolapse of the globe may result (Figs. 5-4 and 5-5) and an emergency tarsorrhaphy may have to be performed. Severe, rapid proptosis of this type may also be associated with avulsion of the optic nerve.

Both local orbital trauma and intracranial hemorrhages, especially subdural hematomas, can lead to damage of any cranial nerve and result in "congenital" ptosis, anisocoria, and various types of paralytic strabismus. These are all rare, but they should be suspected when there is a history of difficult delivery.

Rupture of Descemet's Membrane. This corneal injury is due to the application of a forceps over the eye and the direct compression of the globe between the forceps and the orbital roof. The left eye is involved most frequently because the most common fetal presentation is left occipitoanterior, which brings the left eye into a posterior position where the forceps is applied.

The cornea is cloudy and clears slowly with residual, fine, corneal striae (tears in Descemet's membrane). These can be seen by magnification and reflex illumination. They usually run diagonally across the term effect of retinal hemorrhages at birth has not been proved.

pupillary space. As the cornea eventually clears, the ruptures in Descemet's membrane result in high astigmatic errors and often a refractive amblyopia.

Of greatest importance is the differentiation of this injury from congenital glaucoma, interstitial keratitis, and the cloudy cornea of some rare metabolic diseases. Characteristically, ruptures of Descemet's membrane usually are unilateral, are associated with other evidence of orbital injury or with a history of traumatic labor, and clear with time.

Other Ocular Trauma. Besides retrobulbar hemorrhages, subconjunctival and intraocular hemorrhages also are reported, the latter being a fairly frequent neonatal finding. Intraocular bleeding may occur in the anterior chamber, in the vitreous body, and most commonly in the retina.

Both anterior chamber and vitreous hemorrhages usually are a result of deliveries with maladjusted forceps and may or may not be associated with tears in Descemet's membrane. They are treated no differently from those that occur in adults. Both must be differentiated from other conditions, especially retinoblastoma, that cause intraocular hemorrhage at birth.

Retinal hemorrhages, on the other hand, are not associated with forceps delivery and occur in up to one half of all normal vertex deliveries. They probably are of no more significance than the dermal petechiae of the presenting structure normally seen in infants, except that the former have possible long-term effects. The hemorrhages usually are multiple, scattered throughout the posterior pole, and have a round configuration.

Although the presence of these retinal hemorrhages does not mean that a systemic or intracranial problem is present, they may be responsible for some cases of absolute amblyopia and strabismus seen in childhood. It is possible that a hemorrhage located in the macula could result in subtle anatomical changes, such as disorientation of the cones, that would lead to a permanent decrease in visual acuity in the involved eye and subsequently to secondary strabismus. Although suspected, this long-

Ophthalmia Neonatorum

This name once was reserved for ocular gonorrheal infections in the newborn. Now, however, it often is used to describe any hyperacute, purulent conjunctivitis occurring in the first 10 days of life. Several specific entities exist that can be differentiated partially by the day of onset and absolutely by appropriate bacteriologic and microscopic studies.

Chemical Conjunctivitis. Since prophylaxis for neonatal ocular gonorrhea, originally introduced by Credé in 1880, is now a procedure required by law, almost every newborn infant has 1 per cent silver nitrate instilled into his eyes within minutes after birth. As a result, gonorrhea ophthalmia rarely is seen. Today the most common cause for ophthalmia neonatorum is iatrogenic, consisting of a chemical conjunctivitis secondary to silver nitrate. It is estimated to occur in about 6 per cent of all neonates.

The injury usually is produced by allowing the silver nitrate to remain too long in contact with the eye before neutralizing the chemical with normal saline. In addition, chemical burns have resulted from using too concentrated a solution, either from a mistake in preparation or from an outdated solution that has evaporated, and even from instilling the wrong solution.

Silver nitrate irritation is present from the first day and usually is unilateral. The lids are slightly swollen and the conjunctiva is congested and chemotic. In more severe cases, corneal staining and cloudiness can be present, but these are uncommon (Plate 6D). The reaction will clear spontaneously in three to four days if no complications occur. Secondary bacterial infection, however, is common, and causes marked persistence and increased severity of the conjunctivitis. If the secondary invader is Pseudomonas, a hypopyon ulcer may occur rapidly. The discharge, at first serous, becomes mucopurulent, and an increase in injection occurs with the palpebral conjunctiva often becoming friable and hemorrhagic.

Silver nitrate irritation should be treated

like any chemical injury. Antibiotics can be used locally to prevent secondary infection. Rarely is there any permanent residual damage, although scarring and vascularization of the cornea has been seen in the most extreme cases.

Gonococcal Conjunctivitis. Because of the Credé prophylaxis just discussed, neonatal conjunctivitis due to *Neisseria gonorrhoeae* occurs in less than 0.03 per cent of infants born in the United States today. The infection, which is contracted from the birth canal at delivery, usually becomes obvious at 24 to 48 hours of life. In rare cases onset can be as late as the fifth day, and although at first it often is unilateral, it quickly becomes bilateral.

The lids are swollen, and the conjunctiva may be so chemotic as to protrude through the closed fissures. There usually is beefy red injection and a serosanguineous exudate (Fig. 5-31) that quickly becomes purulent (Plate 6E). If untreated the disease remains acute for about five days and slowly abates in four to six weeks. In these neglected cases corneal involvement is common and usually results in a perforated cornea with loss of the eye.

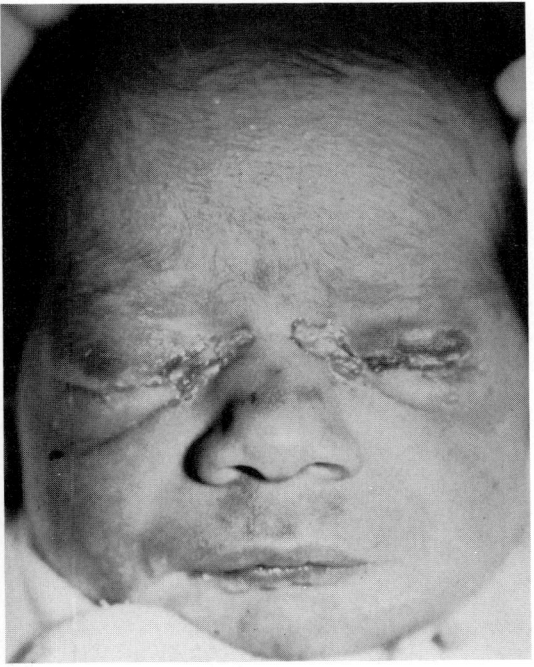

Figure 5-31 Ophthalmia neonatorum. Acute gonococcal conjunctivitis with swollen, erythematous lids and a purulent discharge bilaterally.

Diagnosis is made by examining conjunctival scrapings and finding intraepithelial gram-negative diplococci. This must then be confirmed by appropriate cultures in order to rule out the other *Neisseria* diplococci as causal agents.

Culture specimens should be fresh and the sample should be taken to the laboratory immediately for inoculation. Since *Neisseria* organisms do not grow on routine agars, the laboratory should be forewarned to be sure that the proper growth media is used. Treatment, however, should be started at once if the smear of conjunctival scrapings is positive. Strict infectious precautions should be instituted.

Treatment of gonococcal conjunctivitis should include systemic penicillin and frequent local application of broad spectrum antibiotics. Cycloplegics are indicated when corneal involvement has begun. One should be aware, however, of the possible presence of a penicillin resistant strain of gonococcus. Such infants should be watched carefully and treatment adjusted if severity increases, or if the results of the culture and sensitivity tests reveal such a strain.

Nongonococcal, Bacterial Conjunctivitis. Hyperacute, purulent conjunctivitis, having its onset in a newborn by the fifth day of life, can be caused by a number of other bacterial pathogens. Clinically they are indistinguishable from gonococcal infections except that there is less tendency for corneal involvement. The bacteria most commonly found are staphylococci, streptococci, *Hemophilus influenzae*, pneumococci, and coliform organisms.

Diagnosis should be made by examination and culture of conjunctival scrapings. Broad spectrum, local antibiotic treatment should be started immediately. Once sensitivities are known, therapy can be adjusted.

Inclusion Blennorrhea. Inclusion conjunctivitis is caused by a large atypical virus belonging to the psittacosis-lymphogranuloma venereum-trachoma group that causes "swimming pool" conjunctivitis in adults. Since the virus inhabits the genitourinary tract, it primarily causes disease in newborns. The conjunctivitis is bilateral, with onset between the fifth to tenth day. It begins as an acute purulent conjunctivitis and develops papillary hypertrophy of the palpebral conjunctiva, especially in the lower fornix. If there is no secondary bacterial invasion, the untreated disease may run an acute course for up to three weeks and then resolve into a chronic follicular conjunctivitis that lasts for several months. Follicles are not present in the early phases of the disease since infants do not develop conjunctival lymphoid tissue until they are 4 to 6 weeks old.

Giemsa-stained smears of conjunctival scrapings taken from the lower lid will reveal diagnostic basophilic inclusion bodies in epithelial cells. The predominant inflammatory cells in the exudate will be polymorphonuclear leukocytes.

Although the long-term effects of inclusion blenorrhea in newborns usually is of no significance, the disease can be cleared in about one week with appropriate treatment. Like other atypical viruses in this group, inclusion blenorrhea responds well to sulfonamides and broad spectrum antibiotics, either of which can be given locally with adequate results.

Obstructed Nasolacrimal Duct. An obstructed nasolacrimal duct, previously discussed, may be either unilateral or bilateral and may be the cause of a recurrent or persistent conjunctivitis that has been present from the first day of life. The conjunctivitis may be associated with a medially located mass that is the enlarged lacrimal duct or sac. Both diagnosis and treatment have been mentioned previously.

Prematurity as Related to Ocular Abnormalities

Myopia of Prematurity. A fluctuating myopia of 10 to 20 diopters, changing rapidly in the first few weeks, occasionally is found in infants with birth weights of 1250 grams or less. No etiologies have been proved for this condition, but some authors feel it is a result of the fluctuation of the corneal curvature, the medial refractive index, and the axial length of the globe. Often there is a residual myopia of 2 to 6 diopters present at 6 months of age, but this disappears at about 1 year. The eyes are otherwise normal, and no pathologic changes associated with myopia can be seen in the fundi.

Cataracts of Prematurity. In several large series of infants with congenital cataracts, no etiologic factor other than prematurity was found in 5 to 8 per cent. These cataracts are bilateral and usually begin to appear between the fifth and tenth weeks of life. They start as nuclear opacities which can rapidly become complete, sometimes in less than four weeks. No associated ocular anomalies are present, and the visual outlook is good with surgical correction. With the new techniques in virologic diagnosis, it is possible that many of these so-called cataracts of prematurity will be shown to be caused by a mild, congenital, virus infection, such as rubella.

Retrolental Fibroplasia. This disease, now referred to as retinopathy of prematurity, was virtually unknown prior to 1940. At about that time it became the vogue to treat irregular respiration in premature infants with high concentrations of oxygen. Shortly thereafter, in 1942, Terry reported a series of infants, all premature, who exhibited gray-white opaque membranes behind their lenses. The finding usually was bilateral and considered to be a result of prematurity. Over the next 10 years, the frequency of these retrolental membranes increased alarmingly, and in 1953 it was estimated that 50 per cent of all blindness in institutionalized children up to the age of 7 was a result of retinopathy of prematurity.

The implication that high concentrations of oxygen given to premature infants was in some way responsible for the retinopathy was first suggested by Gordon at the University of Colorado in 1950 and further elaborated by Kinsey in a massive study. In 1951, Patz performed a controlled study by placing alternate neonates weighing less than 3.5 pounds into either low (40 per cent) or high (60 to 70 per cent) oxygen atmospheres. The low oxygen group showed a significantly decreased frequency of retrolental fibroplasia. The relationship of this disease to both the level and duration of oxygen therapy was further confirmed by Campbell in Australia and Crose in England, both in 1952. It is now well understood and accepted that the incidence of retrolental fibroplasia will increase with any one of three factors, each of which may act independently:

1. *Oxygen concentration.* The higher the concentration of the oxygen, the greater the chance of retrolental fibroplasia developing within a given time period. In humans, administration of 60 to 70 per cent oxygen can cause vasoconstriction of retinal arterioles in one to two hours. This vascular spasm can become irreversible after three weeks of continuous treatment at this oxygen level. The accepted "safe" oxygen concentration has been less than 40 per cent, but this must be modified when one considers the variables mentioned below.

2. *Duration of oxygen treatment.* The longer the continuous oxygen treatment, the greater the chance for retinopathy of prematurity to develop for any fixed oxygen concentration. Thus, six to eight weeks of 40 per cent oxygen therapy may be just as dangerous as three weeks of 60 to 70 per cent.

3. *Prematurity of the infant.* If both the above variables are held constant, the degree of prematurity becomes important; the smaller the infant, the greater the chance for retrolental fibroplasia.

The effect of oxygen on the immature retina has been studied extensively. For some unknown reason, the incompletely vascularized retina is sensitive to hyperoxia, whereas the fully vascularized retina is resistant. In the developing human retina, the vessels arise at the disc from the central retinal artery at about 4 months gestational age and grow both nasally and temporally at the same time. By about 8 months gestation, the nasal retina is completely vascularized. Temporally, the retinal vasculature becomes complete at term or shortly thereafter. This explains the third variable mentioned above and also why the pathology is seen most frequently in the temporal retina. It has even been stated that retrolental fibroplasia occasionally appears in full-term infants, since a reasonable amount of variation can be expected in the development of human retinal vasculature.

The clinical course of retinopathy of prematurity was classified into active stages and those of regression and cicatrization by Owens in 1955. Activity usually begins during the first month after birth, but rarely onset may be as late as the tenth week of life.

ACTIVE STAGES OF RETROLENTAL FIBROPLASIA

Stage 1 — Vascular. The initial finding is vasoconstriction, which, as mentioned previously, can occur after one or two hours and becomes irreversible in three weeks. There is a paucity of vessels, especially in the temporal portion of the retina, which is accentuated by a general lack of vessel branching. In addition, there is pallor of the disc. These changes probably represent the earliest stage and pass unnoticed.

After approximately three weeks or sooner, signs of tortuosity and dilatation of the vessels are seen and the veins become three to four times their normal size. The arteries also are extremely tortuous, and fine, twiglike, delicate neovascularization occurs in the periphery at the end of the most dilated vessels.

Stage 2 — Retinal. Vitreous haze develops and the neovascularization becomes more profuse, with elevated gray areas of edema appearing in the periphery of the retina. Vessels that pass through these regions become obscure, and multiple, small, retinal hemorrhages appear peripheral to the equator.

Stage 3 — Early proliferation. Fine strands of newly formed vessels with their supporting tissue extend into the vitreous from areas of retinal elevation and form veils of neovascular tissue, at first in the equatorial regions. Localized areas of retinal detachment also begin in the periphery.

Stage 4 — Moderate proliferation. This stage is associated with detachment of one half or more of the retina. This may be one side of the globe in a hemispheric fashion, or the entire periphery (360 degrees) may be involved. The other half of the retina may not be detached, but areas of activity are present.

Stage 5 — Advanced proliferation. The entire retina may become detached, and occasionally massive intraocular hemorrhage occurs, filling the entire vitreous.

THE REGRESSIVE PHASE OF RETROLENTAL FIBROPLASIA. By definition this phase is no more than a stabilization of activity. Although spontaneous regression is characteristic of retrolental fibroplasia, once the activity has begun there is no way to predict at what stage it will stop, even though the child has been removed from oxygen. Regression is diagnosed when the active stage reveals no further signs of progression after one or two weeks.

In general, infants with milder degrees of activity recover with little damage. About one third do not progress beyond stage 1, and an additional one fourth do not progress beyond stage 2. Cicatricial changes, however, now occur, and usually are proportionate to the extent of the active stage. Indeed, about one fourth of those cases that show activity go on to the cicatricial grades 4 and 5 (see the following section), and an additional one third of the active stages result in the lesser degrees of residual damage.

CICATRICIAL PHASES OF RETROLENTAL FIBROPLASIA

Grade 1 — Minor changes. The fundus may be generally pale, or a slight decrease in vessel diameter is noted. Areas of irregular pigmentation occur, and occasionally a small opaque mass representing a tuft of neovascular tissue may be present in the periphery. Myopia is common.

Grade 2 — Disc distortion. The optic nerve is pale, and the vessels are pulled to one side (Plate 6F). Opposite to this pull of the vessels, a pigmented crescent commonly is present at the disc margin. In the periphery a small mass of opaque tissue can be seen toward which the vessels and disc seem to be pulled (Plate 6G).

Grade 3 — Retinal fold. The peripheral mass of opaque tissue, now more obvious and usually lying in the temporal periphery, exerts traction on the retina and optic nerve, and a retinal fold is seen extending from the nerve to the peripheral mass of scar tissue (Plate 6H). Retinal vessels can be seen incorporated in this fold.

Grade 4 — Incomplete retinal mass. Where proliferation has been marked, a portion of the retina becomes detached and forms a partial retrolental mass. A red reflex may be present through the remaining portion of the uninvolved pupil.

Grade 5 — Complete retrolental mass. The entire retrolental space is filled with a mass of fibrous tissue containing the disorganized retina (Plate 7A). Elongated ciliary processes may be present in the periphery of the pupil, and the anterior chamber is not infrequently shallow. Anterior and posterior synechiae are present, and the cornea may be cloudy if secondary glaucoma occurs or if synechiae are extensive. Microphthalmia is not uncommonly present when this degree of damage has occurred, and the eye may appear to be enophthalmic. This grade of complete retrolental fibroplasia takes about five months to develop.

PROGNOSIS. The prognosis for visual result must be extremely guarded once activity has occurred. The final cicatricial stage cannot be predicted with assurance, although there is a tendency for the lesser degrees of activity to result in the lower phases of cicatrization. In general, the visual results of the scarring phases can be summarized as follows:

Grades 1 and 2; commonly resulting in myopia.

Grade 3; visual acuity of 3/200 to 10/200 when the fold is on the temporal side, but vision may be better if the fold does not involve the macula.

Grades 4 and 5; not infrequently, light perception or blindness.

A number of other complications can result from retrolental fibroplasia. The most common is a secondary glaucoma that is present in 25 to 33 per cent of the severe cases and is due to peripheral anterior synechiae and occasionally to a closed angle of the anterior chamber. This usually occurs in blind eyes and is transient. It may be treated by miotics if symptoms are present or by surgery when there is residual vision. In addition to secondary glaucoma, corneal opacification, cataracts, and enophthalmos may result. Strabismus is not an infrequent finding and may consist of exotropia when there is a temporal pull on the macula, or an esotropia when one eye is more involved than the other. A secondary nystagmus from decreased visual acuity also is not infrequent. Moreover, in older children who have experienced lesser degrees of scarring, vitreoretinal traction may result and cause various findings such

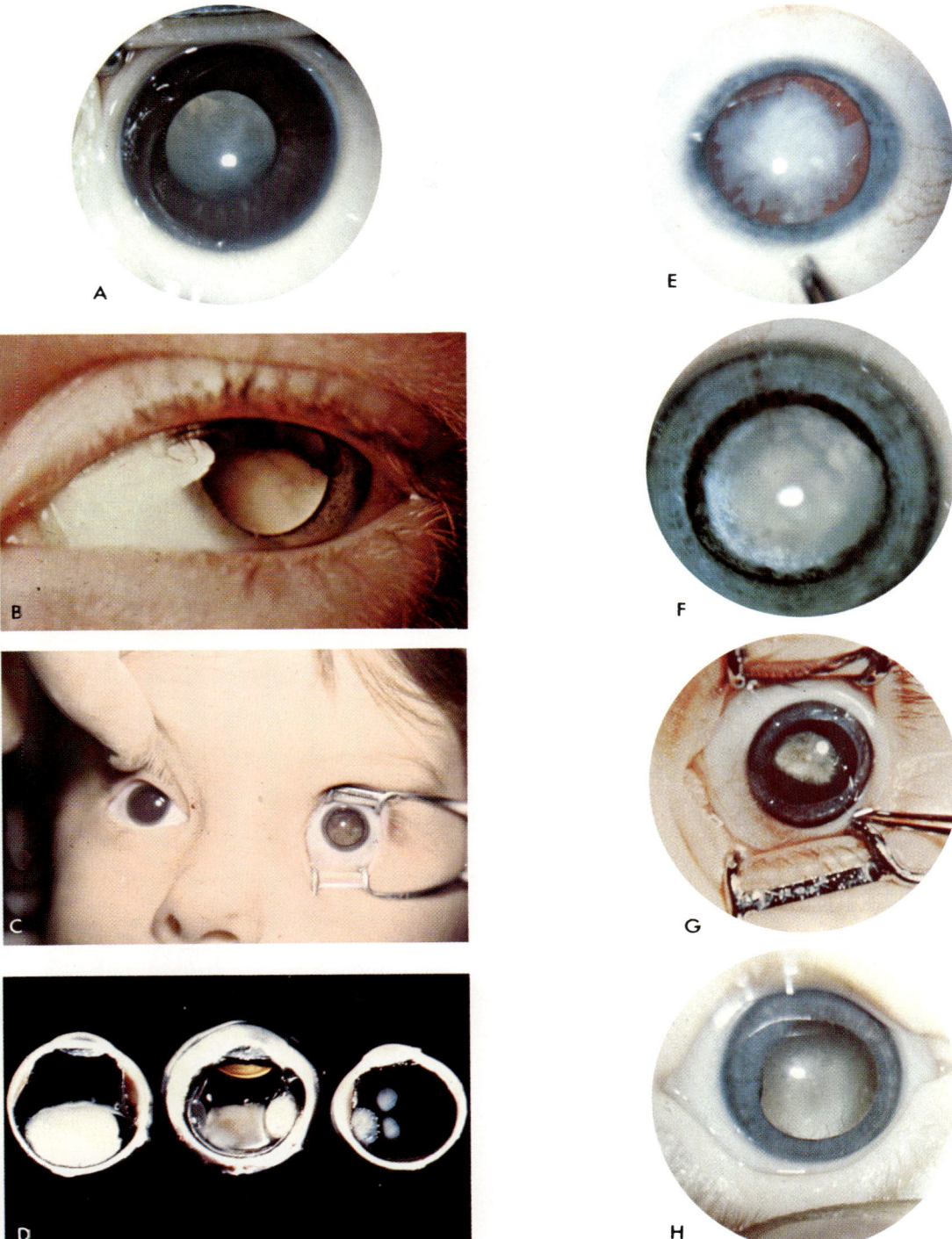

Plate 7 *(A)* Retrolental fibroplasia. Cicatricial grade 5. Leukokoria indicates development of total retrolental membrane. *(B)* Retinoblastoma filling the vitreous and resulting in the so-called amaurotic cat's eye. *(C)* Retinoblastoma causing a unilateral white pupil. *(D)* Retinoblastoma. Cross-section of an involved eye showing development of tumors from multiple foci. (Courtesy of Armed Forces Institute of Pathology.) *(E)* Leukokoria secondary to congenital rubella cataract. *(F)* Persistent hyperplastic primary vitreous resulting in leukokoria. Note prominence of ciliary processes in pupillary space. *(G)* Persistent hyperplastic primary vitreous. Leukokoria with vascularization of retrolental mass. *(H)* Leukokoria resulting from severe nematode endophthalmitis (visceral larva migrans).

151

as lattice degeneration, retinoschisis, retinal breaks, and retinal detachment.

Until recently, retrolental fibroplasia was a disease of the past. Pediatricians have now realized, however, that since premature infants, especially those suffering from the respiratory distress syndrome, have an increased survival rate when treated with high concentrations of oxygen, retinopathy of prematurity is occurring with increased frequency. Such infants differ from "normal" premature infants in that sustained high ambient oxygen levels in the incubator do not necessarily mean that toxic levels of oxygen are reaching the infant's retina. Indeed, these infants need excessively high oxygen levels to raise the arterial pO_2 to that of a normal infant. Unfortunately, the pulmonary alveolar block may disappear at any time rather abruptly, and abnormally high arterial pO_2's may quickly result. These children should be monitored carefully, and arterial gas levels should be taken frequently. At present, the arterial pO_2 which is safe for the immature retina is not known.

In addition to monitoring blood oxygen levels, an ophthalmoscopic examination should be done at least twice a week to discover the early stages of vasoconstriction (Patz, 1967). Once it is noted, the child should be removed from oxygen treatment and observed for 10 to 15 minutes. If the vasoconstriction does not disappear within that time, one should suspect that retrolental fibroplasia will develop after oxygen therapy. If the vasoconstriction does resolve, however, an adjustment in oxygen therapy can be made. The most important consideration, therefore, is the blood oxygen tension and not the ambient oxygen concentrations in the incubator. Since there is no treatment for this disease once activity has begun, the physician's major concern must be toward prevention.

Because of its onset in early life, retrolental fibroplasia is particularly important in the differential diagnosis of white pupil (leukokoria). The characteristics that help to differentiate retrolental fibroplasia from other causes of leukokoria, especially retinoblastoma, are as follows: the eye is of normal size initially; the white pupil does not occur until some months after birth; the condition tends strongly to be bilateral and involves both eyes to the same degree; the infant is premature, usually under 3 pounds; oxygen therapy was administered in the neonatal period.

WHITE PUPIL

The presence of a white pupillary reflex (leukokoria) is one of the most disturbing ocular problems in the pediatric age group (Plate 7A). The diagnosis may be extremely difficult, but it is of utmost importance because of the ever-present danger of retinoblastoma, a highly malignant ocular neoplasm that can be cured if treated early.

When a light is shone into the eyes of normal children, a red reflex should be produced, indicating that the media is clear and the light is being reflected properly from the vascular retina and choroid. When the media is sufficiently opaque due to cataract, massive vitreous opacity, or retinal separation from the choroid by a liquid or solid mass, or when the choroid and retina are absent (coloboma) or destroyed by inflammation or degeneration, the red reflex is lost and leukokoria, or white pupillary reflex (the so-called amaurotic cat's eye) results (Plate 7B). Many conditions can cause white pupil, but because of the possibility of neoplasm, the differential diagnosis is primarily between retinoblastoma and the group of diseases simulating it.

Retinoblastoma

This is an inherited, highly malignant, congenital neoplasm arising from the nuclear layers of the retina (Plate 7C). It occurs in about one of every 23,000 to 34,000 births, has no predilection for race or sex, and is the most frequent ocular malignancy in childhood. Involvement is bilateral in about 25 to 35 per cent of patients. The neoplasm develops from one or more foci in one or both eyes (Plate 7D). Although the disease is congenital, the average age at the time of diagnosis is 13 months. Retinoblastomas have been reported as early as 3 weeks of age and as late as 52 years. However, the diagnosis is made in 72 per cent of patients before the age of 3, and in 90 per cent by the age of 4 years.

The tumor arises spontaneously through a gene mutation or is inherited through a rare, autosomal dominant gene that exhibits 80 to 95 per cent penetrance. Sporadic occurrence is the more common, although the inherited variety appears to be slowly increasing in frequency, which probably reflects the increased rate of cures. In the familial variety, the percentage of cases with bilateral involvement is significantly higher, and bilaterality seems to increase in successive generations, a fact that has been attributed to increased penetrance.

Knowledge of the type of tumor (sporadic versus familial) is extremely important, since it helps to guide the physician in counseling parents on the risk of transmitting the malignancy to other children. The eugenic considerations can be summarized as follows:

1. Normal parents having one affected child have only a 4 to 6 per cent chance of producing another affected child.

2. Phenotypically normal parents with two affected children run a 50 per cent risk for each additional child being at least a carrier, and there will be a 40 to 50 per cent chance that each child will exhibit the tumor.

3. An affected individual who has survived a proved hereditary retinoblastoma will have a 50 per cent risk that each of his offspring will be affected.

4. An individual surviving the sporadic variety of tumor will have at least a 25 per cent chance of producing affected offspring.

5. The parents and all siblings of an affected child should be examined carefully and followed.

The clinical characteristics of retinoblastomas vary considerably and depend on the severity of the condition at the time it presents. When the lesions are minimal, the presenting complaint usually is decreased vision or strabismus. At this stage leukokoria may be absent, but there will be one or more white, elevated, retinal masses with indistinct borders. As the tumor progresses, it may grow from the retina into the vitreous (endophytic) or into the choroid (exophytic), in which instance it causes a solid, retinal detachment. In either situation, a white pupillary reflex results. With further enlargement of the tumor, secondary glaucoma may result. The patient becomes photophobic and develops a steamy, enlarged cornea identical to that seen in congenital glaucoma. Although retinoblastoma does not cause microphthalmia, it is important to realize that tumors have been reported in eyes which are microphthalmic to begin with.

In the advanced stages, retinoblastomas are prone to necrose and may present as a severe uveitis or endophthalmitis. Hypopyons may be present from intraocular inflammation or from seeding of the anterior chamber by the tumor. Moreover, neoplasms frequently hemorrhage, and a diagnosis of retinoblastoma should be suspected in any young child who develops a spontaneous hyphema. Rarely, in ignored cases the child presents with proptosis and metastatic disease.

The diagnosis of retinoblastoma can be further confirmed by finding intraocular calcifications with radiologic studies. Optic foramen views may reveal enlargement from extension of the tumor into the optic nerve. Moreover, ultrasonography can indicate the presence of a solid mass when opaque media makes ophthalmoscopic visualization impossible. Prior to removal of the eye by surgery, transillumination of the globe may help to differentiate between solid and cystic masses. Even with these additional tests, however, histologic examination of an eye with leukokoria may still be needed to rule out the presence of tumor.

Treatment of retinoblastoma consists of enucleation of the involved eye when the condition is unilateral, with removal of as much of the optic nerve as possible. The fellow eye should be examined under general anesthesia every three to four months for three years following surgery, and at less frequent intervals thereafter throughout childhood.

When the tumor is bilateral, the eye with the more advanced lesions should be enucleated to establish the diagnosis. The fellow eye may then be treated with radiation and/or chemotherapy, such as triethylene melamine (TEM) or cyclophosphamide (Cytoxan), if less than one third of

TABLE 5-5 ETIOLOGY OF LEUKOKORIA

1. Cataract
2. Persistent hyperplastic primary vitreous
3. Retrolental fibroplasia
4. Retinal dysplasia
5. Retinoblastoma
6. Chorioretinal colobomas
7. Congenital retinal folds
8. Retinoschisis
9. Retinal detachment
10. Persistent pupillary membrane
11. Hyaloid cyst
12. Uveitis
13. Nematode endophthalmitis
14. Panophthalmitis
15. Coats' disease
16. Norrie's disease
17. Juvenile xanthogranuloma
18. Ocular tumors
19. Trauma
20. Vitreous hemorrhages
21. Medullated nerve fibers
22. Chorioretinal degenerations
23. Incontinentia pigmenti

the retina is involved. If the tumor is advanced, bilateral enucleation may be necessary to save the child's life. To destroy small, discrete lesions, light coagulation and local implantation of radon seeds have been employed with varying degrees of success.

The prognosis for patients with retinoblastoma has become increasingly favorable over the past 20 years. If the lesion is unilateral, diagnosed early, and treated promptly by adequate enucleation, there is a 90 per cent chance for survival. This high rate of cure is markedly reduced when the disease is bilateral, when the pathologic specimen reveals tumor in the vortex veins, when the tumor extends beyond the end of the sectioned optic nerve, or when there is evidence of intracranial spread or distant metastases at the time of diagnosis.

Differential Diagnosis of Leukokoria

Although retinoblastoma is the most important cause of leukokoria, it is not the most frequent one. Depending on the series reported, the two commonest are either cataract (Plate 7E) or persistent hyperplastic primary vitreous. Table 5-5 lists the etiology of leukokoria. Many of the conditions listed have been discussed previously in this chapter and only those not mentioned before are considered now.

Coats' Disease. Exudative retinitis of Coats usually is a unilateral retinal disorder characterized by hemorrhagic and exudative retinal lesions (Plate 8B) that occurs most commonly in males between the ages of 8 months and 8 years. The condition begins with an abrupt decrease in visual acuity that often is indicated by strabismus in a young child. The fundus reveals an exudative, retinal detachment associated with telangiectatic blood vessels and multiple hemorrhages. A total retinal detachment may result (Plate 8A), and the disease may terminate with complications such as retinitis proliferans, cataract, iritis, glaucoma, and phthisis bulbi. The etiology is unknown.

Toxocara (Visceral Larva Migrans). Toxocara is a nematode acquired from dogs and cats. It is capable of producing a larval granulomatosis involving the eye. It usually is unilateral, occurs in children ranging from 3 to 12 years of age, and often is associated with a history of pica, especially for dirt. Beginning insidiously, the ocular lesions result in a slow loss of vision. The fundus usually reveals an elevated, yellow mass with an overlying vitreous reaction. This may result in total disorganization of the vitreous and retina (Plate 7H). Toxocara is further discussed in Medical Ophthalmology (p. 201).

Other Ocular Inflammatory Conditions. Severe uveitis, especially toxoplasmosis and tuberculosis, and endophthalmitis and panophthalmitis from any cause, can result in leukokoria. The white pupillary reflex may be the result of a vitreous abscess, or it can be secondary to a complicated cataract, vitreous organization, retinal detachment, or severe chorioretinal inflammation.

Trauma. Traumatic ocular injuries can result in a number of lesions, all of which can appear as leukokoria. Trauma can cause cataracts, vitreous hemorrhages, retinal detachments, or severe chorioretinal degeneration. Any of these can give a white pupillary reflex. The insults can occur at any time in childhood and may even be a result of labor and delivery. Whenever trauma is suspected in a child, a careful history should be taken and a radiologic

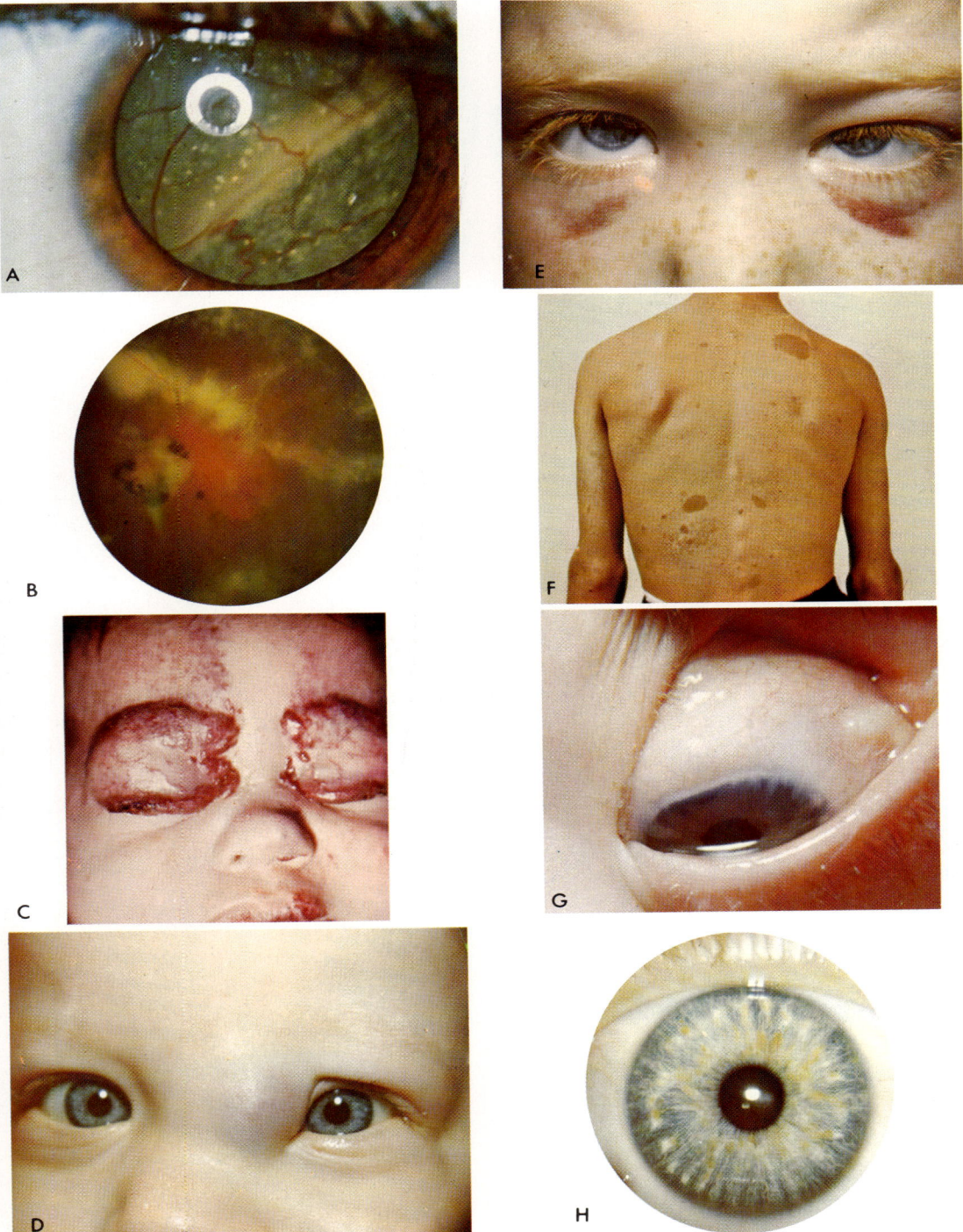

Plate 8 *(A)* Coats' disease resulting in total retinal detachment and leukokoria. The retinal exudates still can be seen on the detached retina within the pupil.   *(B)* Exudative chorioretinitis of Coats.   *(C)* Marked hemangiomatous involvement of both upper lids and forehead.   *(D)* Hemangioma presenting as a red-blue mass at the superior nasal wall of the left orbit.   *(E)* Neuroblastoma. Bilateral orbital involvement presenting with characteristic ecchymoses and hematomas.   *(F)* Neurofibromatosis. Multiple café au lait spots.   *(G)* Neurofibromatosis. Neurofibromas of the conjunctiva and cornea.   *(H)* Neurofibromatosis. Iris neurofibromas can be seen as diffuse nodules and thickening of the stroma, and resemble poorly pigmented nevi.

survey performed of the skeletal system. Any evidence of old or new fractures, in addition to the traumatic ocular lesions, should arouse suspicions of the battered child syndrome.

Norrie's Disease. First described in 1933 by Norrie, the disease appears to be a recessive, sex-linked disorder and is found only in males. It is characterized by the presence of bilateral blindness from massive retinal detachments, deafness, and mental retardation.

Juvenile Xanthogranuloma (Nevoxantho-endothelioma). This condition (JXG) is a self-limited condition that usually affects only the skin. It is classified in the group of diseases known as histiocytoses. Ocular juvenile xanthogranuloma affects the iris and usually is heralded by a spontaneous anterior chamber hemorrhage or by an attack of glaucoma. The iris lesion that has caused the hemorrhage is salmon pink, raised, and demarcated from the surface of the iris. The onset may be slow or fast. The presence of skin lesions helps to confirm the diagnosis.

Viewed grossly, the xanthogranuloma is an orange raised nodule, which under the microscope appears to be an infiltrate of histiocytes. The histiocytes contain sudanophilic material, and giant cells are present in the lesions. The normal clinical course is spontaneous resolution of the lesions, but this may occur after the eye has been destroyed by hemorrhage and secondary glaucoma. Radiation, steroids, and surgical excision of the iris lesions have all been claimed by some to help resolve the ocular disease.

Other Tumors. Ocular tumors, other than retinoblastomas, are extremely rare causes of leukokoria. Hemangiomas (von Hippel-Lindau disease), astrocytomas, and intra-ocular extensions of meningiomas occasionally have resulted in white pupil (Plate 9H).

Dictyomas (tumors of the pars ciliaris retinae) are rare ocular malignancies that begin in infancy and are always unilateral. Clinically they cannot always be differentiated from retinoblastoma. Microscopic examination sometimes reveals areas of cartilage, pigment epithelium, embryonic retina, and neuroglial elements. Ocular melanomas also have caused white pupils in children, although the tumor is far more common in adults.

Chorioretinal Atrophy. Any severe, chorioretinal, degenerative disorder may give a white pupillary reflex. This includes inflammatory degenerations of the choroid and retina, choroideremia, and severe myopic degeneration.

Medullated Nerve Fibers. Extensive medullation of the fibers of the optic nerve extending from the disc may cause such a large white area that leukokoria may result.

Incontinentia Pigmenti. This condition, known as the Bloch-Sulzberger syndrome, is a pigmentary dermatosis that is inherited as either an autosomal or sex-linked dominant. It is present at birth or begins shortly thereafter. The condition is characterized by swirling patterns of slate gray, cutaneous pigmentation that often begin like herpetiform dermatitis. Associated anomalies include multiple skeletal defects, dental anomalies, alopecia, mental retardation, seizures, and cardiac malformation. The ocular abnormalities include strabismus, nystagmus, optic atrophy, congenital cataracts, and pseudoglioma, with the latter two conditions sometimes causing leukokoria.

STRABISMUS AND AMBLYOPIA

Strabismus

For the visual axes of the two eyes to be aligned perfectly at all times requires fine motor and sensory adjustment that rarely is found. Yet only about 2 per cent of all children demonstrate overt deviations. Many important factors must exert an influence to permit both eyes to work together comfortably. When any one of these adjustment facilities is disrupted, strabismus (squint) results.

Of primary importance is the resting position of the eyes. This depends upon normal development of the bony orbits and a balance between tonic convergence and divergence. Orbital maldevelopment, such as that seen in both craniofacial and mandibulofacial dysostoses, can cause such poor ocular positioning that proper alignment of the visual axes is impossible. If the orbital anatomy is normal, the basic resting position (when all the extraocular muscles are receiving equal impulses) is the result of tonic convergence and divergence impulses which are supranuclear in origin. Since convergence prevails in infants and children, the resting position normally tends to be inward. Past puberty, divergence prevails. These differences help to explain why a child with poor vision in one or both eyes tends to develop convergent strabismus, whereas an adult develops divergent strabismus.

A further prerequisite for orthophoria (straight eyes) is the normal development and strength of the individual extraocular muscles and their tendon and fascial attachments. If the muscles are paretic or fibrotic, or if restrictive bands are present, the tonic impulses have difficulty holding the eyes in a normal basic resting position. Furthermore, rotations are inhibited so that strabismus increases or occurs when the eyes move in a particular direction.

As previously noted, a child's eye normally is hyperopic and requires accommodation (focusing) to see clearly. Since a convergence reflex accompanies this accommodative effort, a fine balance must exist between accommodation and convergence for the visual axes to remain together. In children who are excessively farsighted, the amount of accommodation required for clear vision is enormous and can result in too great a simultaneous convergence reflex. This overaction of the accommodative-convergence relationship may then produce crossed eyes.

In myopic (nearsighted) children, the situation may be reversed. The nearsighted child need not accommodate to see clearly. This may result in a weak or absent convergence reflex, and the eyes tend to diverge.

From the relative infrequency of strabismus, however, it is apparent that most of the above disrupting factors normally are overcome. In the great majority of children this is accomplished through the innate desire of the child for *fusion* (perception of an object as a single entity with two eyes) and by his *fusional amplitude* (the ability to overcome any tendency for ocular deviation). If imperfect motor or sensory factors unduly weaken or obstruct either the desire or the ability for binocular single vision, then strabismus can result. For an infant to develop the desire for fusion requires relatively equal vision in each eye. Moreover, the power (accommodation) expended to obtain clear vision also must be fairly equal. This equality of vision is extremely important, for a child whose vision is equal, even if it is poor, does not tend to develop strabismus as easily as a child whose vision is poor or distorted in one eye only. Retinoblastoma, chorioretinitis, cataracts, glaucoma, and high refractive errors all can be unilateral and cause monocular loss of vision and strabismus in children. Therefore, a child who develops strabismus should be examined immediately by an ophthalmologist so that such disorders may be treated early.

Even when vision is not decreased, strabismus may result from any of a number of anatomical problems, from an imbalance of the convergence-divergence mechanism, or from poor fusional amplitudes. These, in turn, are either idiopathic or hereditary. Strabismus also occurs more commonly in brain-damaged children. Since about 50 per cent of all children with strabismus have a positive family history, the siblings of an affected child also should be examined.

When strabismus occurs in a child with otherwise normal eyes, a chain of events may lead to the permanent loss of vision from one eye if treatment is not instituted promptly. The first symptom that a child experiences is diplopia or double vision. In young infants this often goes unnoticed or presents with the chief report from the parents that their child is "awkward" or that "he tends to keep one eye closed."

The child does not tolerate double vision and begins to suppress the image received by one eye. If the same eye is suppressed continually, amblyopia (loss of vision) or the so-called "lazy eye" results. The younger the child at the onset of strabismus, the easier and more rapid the onset of suppression. The earlier suppression starts, and the longer it is allowed to persist, the more profound and permanent the loss of vision. In infants, amblyopia can become deep within one week.

Amblyopia

A discussion of amblyopia is mandatory when considering strabismus, for either may give rise to the other. Amblyopia is defined as a reduction in visual acuity (with the proper correction in place) in an eye that is ophthalmoscopically normal. It is present in 1.5 to 2.0 per cent of the young adult population in the United States today, and about half of the cases can be related to strabismus in cause or result. Many authors feel that amblyopia may be diagnosed when the visual acuity in each eye differs by two or more lines on the Snellen chart. The existence of several types of amblyopia is suspected, and the classification as suggested by von Noorden (discussed in the following sections) appears to be the most useful to keep in mind.

Strabismic Amblyopia. This is a result of strabismus and appears to occur readily in children, 4 years of age or younger, who develop ocular malalignment and constant preference for one eye in an effort to avoid confusion or diplopia. The earlier the onset the more rapidly it can occur; the longer it remains the harder it is to overcome. Parks and Friendly feel that true strabismic amblyopia can be cured always if treatment is begun before 4 years of age. Therapy at this age consists of constant occlusion of the preferred eye. Although there is great individual variation, the cure of strabismic amblyopia is considered to be virtually impossible after the child has reached 8 or 9 years of age.

Amblyopia Ex Anopsia. By strict definition, amblyopia ex anopsia refers to visual loss from disuse, and in von Noorden's classification is restricted to amblyopia resulting from some type of occlusion. The causes of this type of amblyopia include tarsorrhaphy, ptosis, cataract, and occlusion therapy for strabismic amblyopia.

Occlusion amblyopia may have an actual organic basis. Wiesel and Hubel deprived newborn cats of vision in one eye by suturing the lids together at birth. They found that after two to three months this form of sensory deprivation produced atrophy of neurons in the lateral geniculate body. The atrophy did not occur, however, if the tarsorrhaphy was performed after the third month of life, or if the lids remained open and a surgical strabismus was induced.

In other work chimpanzees were raised in total darkness, and after several months the eyes were removed. Degeneration of the retinal ganglion cell layer could be identified histopathologically. These organic changes, however, have not been confirmed in man.

That occlusion amblyopia occurs in humans is evidenced by the temporary amblyopia that can result in a preferred eye when it is patched for treatment of strabismic amblyopia. For this reason, any child undergoing treatment for amblyopia must be watched carefully for decreased vision in the patched eye. In very young children occlusion can produce amblyopia in the patched eye in less than two weeks. Frequent follow-up examinations at short intervals are therefore necessary. Once the eyes are equal, alternate patching may be required to maintain good visual acuity in each eye until the visual axes are properly aligned, or until the child is old enough so that amblyopia will no longer result (usually around the age of 6 years).

Anisometropic Amblyopia. Anisometropia refers to dissimilar refractive errors in the eyes of an individual. This type of visual loss is considered a refractive amblyopia. Refractive inequalities can result in such great differences in size or sharpness of the two images that fusion is impossible. Approximately 1 diopter difference in hyperopia or astigmatism, and slightly higher differences in myopia, may cause amblyopia. There appears to be no relationship between the degree of anisometropia and the depth of the amblyopia. Since this type of amblyopia also can be prevented if discovered early, ophthalmologists feel that every child should have a thorough ocular examination at the preschool (4 to 5 years) age.

Organic Amblyopia. Organic, or congenital, amblyopia is suspected when the visual acuity remains below normal, even after adequate therapy. It may be from cone malalignment resulting from a macular hemorrhage at birth, from latent or micronystagmus, from achromatopsia, or from any subclinical anatomic changes in the macula. This type of amblyopia varies in degree, is untreatable, and therefore is permanent.

Regardless of the cause or type of amblyopia, all physicians who deal with children should realize that the only way to prevent amblyopia is to recognize and treat it early. The functional amblyopias (resulting from strabismus, occlusion, or refractive errors) will result in *permanent* visual loss that is unidentifiable from, and as untreatable as, the loss of vision secondary to organic amblyopia. Moreover, since strabismus can cause permanent visual loss and since visual loss can result in strabismus, the diagnosis of either condition should be sufficient to require consultation with an ophthalmologist *at the time the diagnosis is made*. The belief that strabismus will disappear without treatment, or without any residual sensory deficit if given enough time, is no more than an old wives' tale. Again, the earlier the diagnosis and the earlier the treatment, the greater the chance for a functional as well as a cosmetic cure.

Classification and Diagnosis of Strabismus

Incomitant Strabismus. This is present when the angle of deviation varies in different directions of gaze. It usually is synonymous with paralytic strabismus, in which there is a paresis or paralysis of one or more of the extraocular muscles. The deviation always is manifest and is in a direction away from the field of action of the involved muscle. Conversely, the angle of strabismus is greatest in the field of action of the involved muscle, because the involved eye cannot move in that direction.

Double vision often is a symptom, but it may not be present if the onset of the strabismus either was at a young enough age for suppression to occur or if compensatory head positioning is present. If diplopia is present or can be elicited, it usually is helpful in identifying the particular extraocular muscle that is involved. This is determined by placing a red glass over one eye (by convention, the right eye) and having the patient fixate on a white light; he then will perceive two lights, one red and the other white. The patient is asked to follow the light as it is moved through the cardinal fields of gaze, observing in which

position the lights are farthest apart, and which light (red or white) is farther from his body, As a rule, diplopia is greatest in the field of action of the affected muscle, and the false image (always the distal image) belongs to the eye with the paralytic muscle (Table 5-6).

Another characteristic of incomitant strabismus is the phenomenon of primary and secondary deviations in the angle of strabismus. In primary deviation the patient is fixating with the eye that has normal muscles. In secondary deviation, always greater than primary, the patient fixates with the eye that has the paretic muscle. Regardless of which eye fixates, however, the deviation still is greatest in the field of action of the paretic muscle.

Compensatory head posturing is another sign more commonly associated with incomitant than with comitant squints. In general the patient will turn or tilt his head in the direction of the field of action of the paretic muscle. This allows the eyes to be moved away from this position, thereby decreasing or overcoming the angle of deviation and diplopia. Head turning usually indicates a horizontal muscle weakness, especially of the lateral rectus. Tilting usually occurs with a cyclovertical (p. 166) muscle, and most commonly is seen with a superior oblique palsy.

All the preceding characteristics are typical, but not pathognomonic, of a paralytic squint. Moreover, the rules are valid only for diagnosing a weakness of recent onset. In time, secondary anatomical changes, such as hypertrophy of the yoke muscle or contracture of the direct antagonist, tend to make the deviations similar in all fields of

TABLE 5-6 PARALYTIC STRABISMUS*

Muscle	Normal Function	Ocular Deviation When Involved	False Image
Superior rectus	Elevates Intorts Adducts	Down Extorted Out	Elevated Intorted Crossed

*Note the similarity between the normal functions of the muscle and the positions of the false image when the muscle is paretic.

gaze, and the offending muscle is not so easily found. Many of the nonparalytic deviations also simulate some of the characteristics of incomitant strabismus, and appear paretic in nature, although they may be due to muscular fibrosis, restrictive fascial bands, and congenital or familial strabismus that otherwise is idiopathic. This is true especially of the cyclovertical muscle problems and the "A-V" patterns discussed later. Physicians should keep in mind that not all incomitant squints are paralytic and that incomitant paralytic squints tend to become comitant in time.

Comitant Strabismus. This is present when the angle of deviation is identical in all the cardinal positions of gaze. It can vary, however, when distant (6 meters) fixation measurements are compared with near (1/3 meter) fixation measurements. The deviation remains the same regardless of which eye fixates, providing that good alternation is present. Anisometropia or amblyopia may complicate the picture and simulate primary and secondary deviations. Motion is not limited.

Diplopia usually is absent, but it may be induced when the strabismus is intermittent or partially latent. Either present or induced diplopia, however, will be equidistant in all fields of gaze. Since diplopia symptoms usually are absent, compensatory head posturing is not necessary, and thus is a rare finding.

Measuring Strabismus. The discovery and measurement of either comitant or incomitant strabismus in a child requires careful observation and a few relatively simple tests. Careful observation begins the moment the child enters the examining room, particularly noting any constant head turn or tilt. An obvious ocular deviation should be watched to see if it is intermittent or constant, variable in degree, and constantly involving the same eye. If no obvious strabismus is present, the physician should question the parents about the occurrence of any of the above signs.

In older children if the difference in the visual acuity of each eye is two or more lines on the reading chart, it may mean only anisometropia; the possibility of stra-

bismus with secondary amblyopia, however, should be considered. In younger children monocular fixation should be noted. Any child who constantly fights the occlusion of one eye, yet does not seem to mind occlusion of the other, should be suspected of having decreased visual acuity and possibly strabismus.

After visual acuity is ascertained, *the cover-uncover test* is performed with the child fixating on a target. The fixation target usually depends on the age of the patient, and may be a light, a small bright picture, a toy, or a Snellen number or letter. The right eye is covered first while the examiner watches the left eye. If no movement is noted, the left probably was being used properly; that is, the image was centered on the fovea. Then the cover is removed from the right eye, and after several seconds is placed over the left eye. The observer now watches for any compensatory shift of the right eye. If neither eye moves, it usually indicates that both were fixating simultaneously and that no strabismus is present. Conversely, if either exposed eye has to shift to see the target, then malalignment exists. For instance, if, when the right eye is covered, the left eye makes an inward movement to fixate on the target, then the left eye must have been displaced laterally and a divergent squint was present.

To expose latent or intermittent deviations, the *alternate cover test* should be attempted after the cover-uncover test. The patient continues to watch the fixation target as the examiner alternately covers first the right, then the left eye. This alternating occlusion is continued in a smooth, pendulum-like manner, inhibiting the use (fusion) of both eyes together. The examiner observes for motion in the eye being *uncovered.* Any movement indicates the eyes are not aligned when fusion is interrupted. As with manifest deviations, the direction of the movement is opposite the direction of the deviation. Ideally, in both tests the patient should fixate first at a distant (6 meters) and then at a near (1/3 meter) target. Although the tests may reveal that the eyes are orthophoric (straight) in the primary position of gaze, ocular rotations should be carefully observed for the presence of one of the incomitant squints.

The amount of deviation can be estimated from the position of the corneal light reflexes. A small light is held in front of the patient so that the light reflex from the cornea of the fixating eye is centered in the pupil. The location of the light's reflection from the cornea of the deviating eye then is observed, and its position is noted in relation to the iris or corneoscleral junction. A reflex at the pupillary border indicates about 15 degrees deviation; over the middle of the iris, about 25 degrees; at the limbus, 45 to 60 degrees; and beyond the limbus, over 60 degrees. Each millimeter of deviation is equal roughly to an angle of about 7 degrees when the light is one third meter from the patient. A more accurate evaluation and measurement of the strabismus should be made by an ophthalmologist.

TYPES OF STRABISMUS

Pseudostrabismus. The intermittent crossing of an infant's eyes is one of two conditions referred to as pseudostrabismus. During the first four months of life an infant often exercises convergence and thereby appears cross-eyed. This intermittent crossing should disappear by 6 months of age, when he begins to accommodate. A second type of pseudostrabismus is the cross-eyed *appearance* of infants and young children who have broad, flat noses and prominent epicanthal folds (Fig. 5-32). The extra skin between the eyes often hides part of the nasal sclera, whereas the lateral sclera is readily exposed making the child appear as if his eyes are crossed. This pseudostrabismus is readily diagnosed by observing the position of the corneal light reflection, which will be in the same position on each eye. The phenomenon of pseudostrabismus is responsible for the myth that strabismus can be cured spontaneously.

Latent Strabismus. When an individual exhibits an ocular deviation only after fusional impulses have been totally or partially removed, he is said to have a *heterophoria.* This type of deviation usually remains latent under normal, everyday conditions. Heterophoria of some degree and type exists in almost every individual, and the so-called "normal" or orthophoric (straight eyes even with fusion disrupted) person is a rarity. Because latent deviations are so common, they should not be considered abnormal

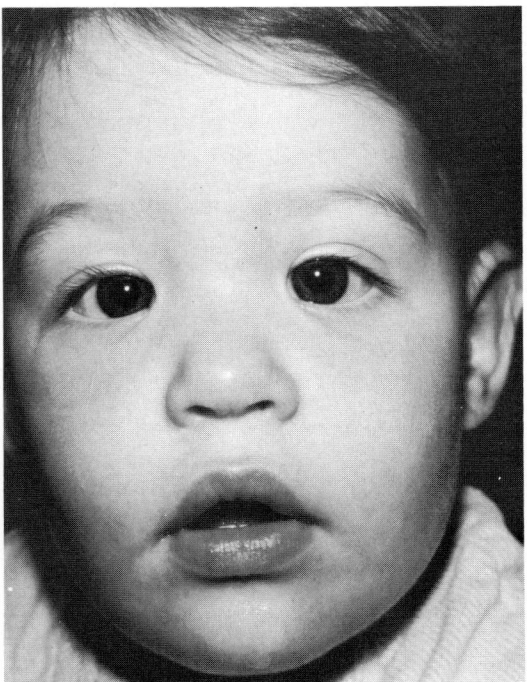

Figure 5-32 Pseudostrabismus. Marked epicanthal folds cover the medial sclera and give the false impression of esotropia. However, the light reflexes from both corneas can be seen to be in identical positions.

unless they are great enough to produce symptoms. The symptoms attributable to large phorias are all included under the term asthenopia (eyestrain) and usually occur after prolonged visual activity such as that seen with driving, watching movies, and especially reading. Sleepiness, blurred vision, diplopia, and headache are the more common complaints, and they tend to occur more readily when the individual is nervous, tired, or ill than when he is rested and healthy.

Latent strabismus can be subclassified, depending on the direction of the deviation that occurs when fusion is broken. *Esophoria* refers to the visual axes turning in; *exophoria,* to divergence; and right or left *hyperphoria,* to vertical deviations resulting when one eye is higher than the other.

The etiology of heterophorias is poorly understood. That they are related to refractive errors seems clear, since esophorias are more commonly seen with hyperopic errors, whereas exophorias are associated with myopia. Not all horizontal phorias can be based on refractive errors, however, and latent vertical deviations must have an entirely different etiology. Improper tonic convergence-divergence impulses and weak amplitudes of fusion may play some role. The horizontal phorias usually do not produce symptoms unless the angle of deviation is large. On the other hand, minimal degrees of hyperphorias readily cause difficulty.

Treatment of a heterophoria is necessary only when it is symptomatic. Some patients will be relieved by wearing simple spectacles, whereas others may require special prisms. Occasionally, especially in exophorias, exercising may be of some value. In rare instances extraocular muscle surgery may have to be employed.

Manifest Strabismus. Ocular deviations that remain present even when individuals are allowed to use both their desire and ability for fusion are referred to as *heterotropias,* or squints. They may be congenital, acquired, intermittent, constant, comitant, or incomitant. Like phorias, tropias are subdivided according to the direction of deviation.

ESOTROPIA. A deviation resulting in the crossing of the visual axes is referred to as esotropia, convergent strabismus, or, more simply, "crossed-eyes." *Accommodative esotropia* (Fig. 5-33), by far the most common esodeviation, results from a breakdown of the accommodative-convergence reflex. Characteristically, accommodative esotropia usually begins between the ages of 18 months and 4 years, although it can occur any time in the second half year of life or as late as 7 years of age. The onset is concurrent with either the beginning or an increase in a child's accommodative abilities, and usually is associated with an uncorrected hyperopia ranging from 2 to 5 diopters. Because of this farsightedness and the constant need for focusing to see clearly, the child has to learn to accommodate without converging. The greater the hyperopic error, the more difficult is this dissociation, and eventually the child's

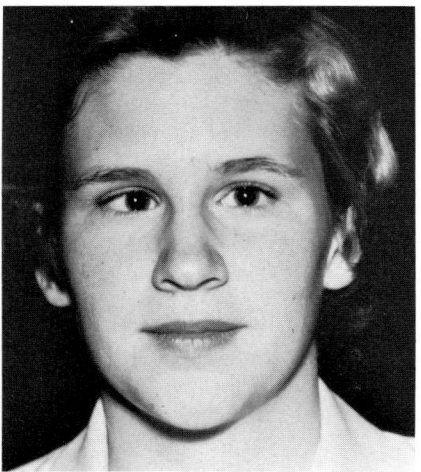

Figure 5-33 Manifest accommodative esotropia, uncorrected.

fusional mechanisms are overcome. Once this breakdown develops, the child is presented with an unsatisfactory choice: either he can have blurred, single, binocular vision, or he can clear the image by accommodating. The accommodative effort causes excessive convergence, and diplopia results. Both conditions, either blurred or double (but clear) vision, are intolerable. In young children, this problem is readily solved by his ability to suppress the image from one eye. He therefore develops into a preferred pattern of crossed-eyes, clear vision, and monocular suppression. Initially the suppression alternates between the two eyes. However, anisometropia, which is not an infrequent finding, results in preference for the more normal eye, and continued disuse of the eye with the higher refractive error results in amblyopia.

Early in its onset accommodative esotropia usually is alternating and intermittent, occurring at only near fixation targets toward the end of the day, or when the child is tired or ill. In time, crossing begins to occur at distant fixation as well as near, although the latter usually reveals a greater angle of deviation. In addition, secondary muscular changes (hypertrophy of the medial recti) and poor fusional amplitudes tend to make the esodeviation constant. Finally, continued use of a preferred eye inhibits the original alternating pattern. A constant monocular esotropia results. In these final stages the crossing

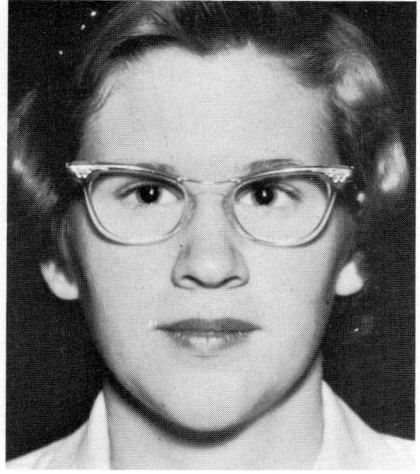

Figure 5-34 Same patient shown in Figure 5-33. Accommodative esotropia is completely corrected with glasses in place.

ceases to become strictly accommodative, and amblyopia of the constantly deviating eye commonly is found.

In its pure form, accommodative esotropia responds completely to corrective lenses (Fig. 5-34). This usually has to be ascertained by a full cycloplegic (atropine) refraction. The first sign of a decompensated state is the need for bifocals. These correct the residual esodeviation remaining at near fixation, even after the proper cycloplegic refraction has straightened out the amount of crossing that was present at distant fixation.

If allowed to go untreated, accommodative esotropias develop nonaccommodative aspects. Even with the proper spectacles in place, crossing of the visual axes remains constant both for distant as well as for near fixation targets. If this amount of decompensated crossing is cosmetically displeasing, surgery may have to be utilized to make the child socially acceptable. Prior to surgical correction, amblyopia should be reversed by occluding the preferred eye until true alternation, or equal visual acuity, indicates that a preference pattern no longer exists.

Accommodative-nonaccommodative esotropia can arise either from the decompensation of true accommodative squint or from the superimposition of an accommodative element over a congenital esotropia. Decompensation occurs if treatment is not instituted early because constant excessive convergence leads to hypertrophy of the medial recti. In time, a purely accommodative squint can become completely nonaccommodative and treatable only by surgery.

On the other hand, a congenital, nonaccommodative esotropia also can have an accommodative element. This is evidenced by an increase in the angle of deviation occurring after the sixth month of life. It is at this age that accommodation begins to develop, and as it increases in strength it may cause a greater esodeviation.

Any esotropia that has mixed accommodative and nonaccommodative elements can be diagnosed by the finding of a residual esodeviation after the cycloplegic refraction has been worn for an adequate length of time. This nonaccommodative element, if large enough to be noticeable, can be overcome only through surgical correction. The parent should be forewarned that a child with this type of problem most likely still will need glasses after surgery.

Nonaccommodative esotropia can be congenital or secondary to bilateral sixth nerve palsies. It may result from total decompensation of an accommodative esotropia and from the unilateral loss of vision at an early age. Congenital esotropia, the most common of this group, usually is hereditary and has its onset during the first year of life. It even may be present from birth, but goes unnoticed because of the infant's tendency to keep his eyes closed. Characteristically the child tends to alternate freely and does not develop amblyopia.

The refractive error generally is low and bilaterally equal. The angle of deviation often is huge (Fig. 5-35), and these children commonly look to the left with their right eye and to the right with their left. This phenomenon of cross-fixation makes the child appear as if his lateral recti muscles are paralyzed. In fact, differentiating between bilateral sixth nerve palsies and congenital esotropia may be difficult. Proper diagnosis can be made by causing a forced, rapid, tonic-neck reflex, or by stimulating the labyrinths by spinning the child. When the neuromuscular mechanism is intact, the eyes deviate opposite the direction of head

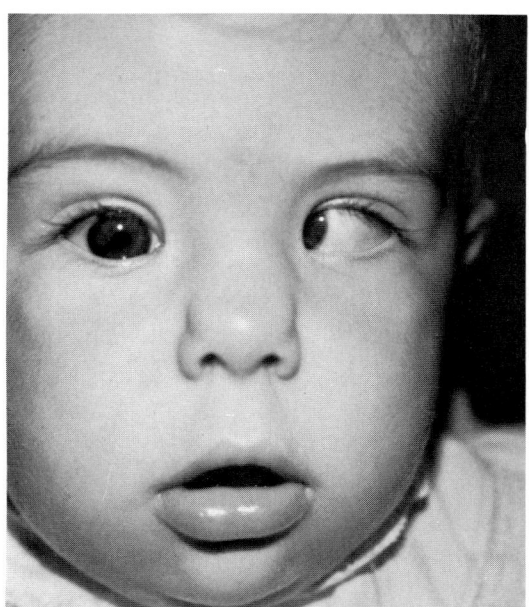

Figure 5-35 Marked nonaccommodative congenital esotropia.

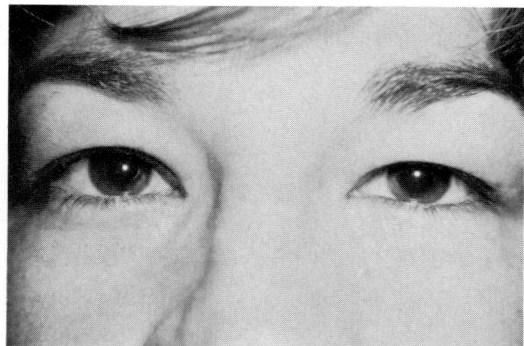

Figure 5-36 Duane's retraction syndrome. Eyes straight in primary position.

turn or spinning. For example, a forced, rapid, head turn to the left causes both eyes to turn to the right, and the abduction of the right eye reveals a normal sixth nerve on that side. If doubt still persists, the eyes may need patching alternately for several days to reveal the status of the lateral recti.

Since congenital esotropia must be differentiated from bilateral sixth nerve palsies and from organic ocular disease (e.g., retinoblastoma) causing monocular loss of vision, an examination should be performed immediately upon diagnosis. If the eyes are otherwise normal and visual acuity is judged to be equal, surgical correction of the strabismus usually is performed before the child is 2 years of age.

Duane's retraction syndrome is an incomitant strabismus that usually presents as an esotropia during the first decade of life. It is characterized by the inability to abduct the involved eye along with the retraction of this eye into the orbit when adduction is attempted (Figs. 5-36, 5-37). The palpebral fissure, also on the involved side, widens upon attempted abduction and narrows on adduction (Fig. 5-38). Although esotropia is the most common deviation, the eyes may be straight or exotropic in the primary position. Occasionally a vertical deviation has been noted. Bilateral involvement occurs rarely.

Some authors feel that the retraction syndrome is a result of a lateral rectus muscle being replaced by inelastic fibrous tissue, but other investigators suggest that this fibrosis is a secondary and not a primary change. Some electromyographic (EMG) studies have revealed activation of both the lateral and medial recti on adduction, with inhibitional medial rectus activity and no lateral rectus activity on abduction. In addition, aplasia of the sixth cranial nerve and normal extraocular muscles have been found at autopsy. Both the EMG and autopsy findings could be explained by aberrant growth of the third nerve and absence of the sixth nerve.

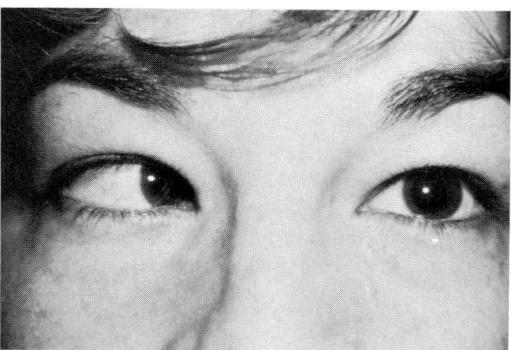

Figure 5-37 Duane's retraction syndrome (same patient as in Figure 5-36). Inability to abduct left eye during an attempted left lateral gaze.

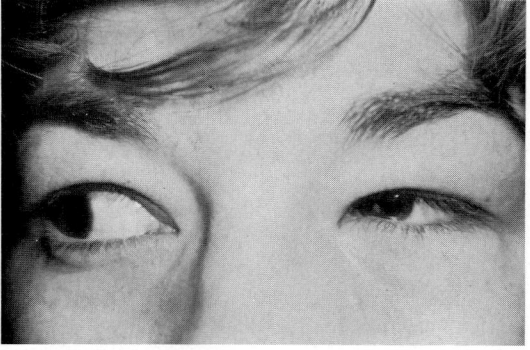

Figure 5-38 Duane's retraction syndrome (same patient as in Figure 5-36). Retraction of the left eye and narrowing of the left palpebral fissure on adduction of the left eye.

EXOTROPIA. Divergent deviation (exotropia) of the visual axes commonly is referred to as "wall-eyes." *Intermittent exotropia (exophoria-tropia)* shows a strong hereditary tendency and most commonly begins between 1 and 4 years of age. At first the strabismus alternates between phoria and tropia with the manifest element being present only for distant fixation. Fatigue, illness, visual inattention, and bright sunlight all tend to shift the balance from phoria to tropia, or increase the amount of tropia if the exodeviation already is manifest. Because of this latent nature, intermittent exotropia may be overlooked even by the ophthalmologist early in its course. A small examining room and a rested, attentive child both help to hide the phoria as well as the tropia. The diagnosis still should be suspected when the history reveals that the child constantly closes or rubs one eye when he is tired, when he is watching television, or when he is exposed to bright sunlight. Repeated examinations at different hours of the day eventually should reveal the strabismus to the physician.

Clinically, the exodeviation tends to be greater for distant than near vision. These patients commonly have small, bilaterally equal, refractive errors, tend to alternate the fixating eye easily, and do not develop amblyopia. Suppression occurs only when the strabismus is manifest, and diplopia may be present during the confusing moments when the phoria breaks into a tropia. Fusion, depth perception, and near points of convergence often are exceptionally good and help to give a favorable prognosis.

Treatment consists of optical correction of refractive errors, especially when myopia or astigmatism are present. Occasionally convergence exercises may help overcome a small deviation. However, intermittent exotropias most frequently are corrected by surgery. If left untreated, they tend to decompensate into constant, manifest strabismus with equal degrees of exotropia for both distant and near fixation targets.

Constant exotropia (Fig. 5-39) can be either congenital or acquired. It is much less common than intermittent exotropia. Regardless of the etiology, constant exodeviations do not produce symptoms of blurred or double vision, and usually do not vary with the physical status of the patient. Frequently the deviation is monocular, the deviating eye often being organically or functionally amblyopic, and the angle of deviation often being greater at near than at distant fixation targets.

Congenital, constant exotropia usually is inherited and is rare. Acquired exotropias usually are secondary to abnormal anatomy of the bony orbits (hypertelorism, facial dysostoses, and so forth). They also may result from deterioration of intermittent exotropias or from impaired vision in one eye. The latter are more likely to occur after 6 years of age, and can arise from

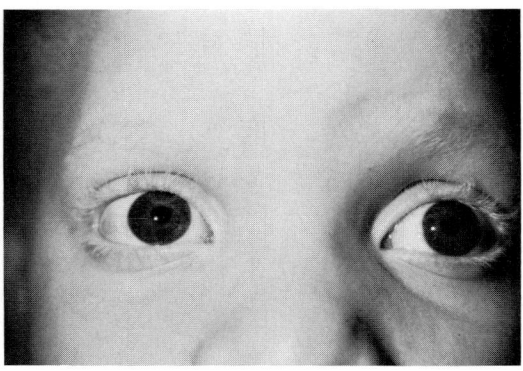

Figure 5-39 Exotropia. Note the lateral deviation of the left eye while the child is fixating with her right eye.

anisometropia or organic disease involving central vision.

Treatment of any constant exotropia is surgical, usually only for cosmetic reasons; even when the visual acuity is bilaterally equal, functional restoration of single binocular vision is rare.

"A-V" PATTERNS. Significant differences in the horizontal deviation of the eyes in midline up-and-down gaze are referred to as "A-V" syndromes or patterns. An "A" pattern reveals more divergence in down gaze or more convergence in up gaze. "V" syndromes show a reverse pattern, that is more divergence in up than in down gaze. Either pattern may occur in a patient who is orthophoric in the primary position, with a mild "V" tendency being physiologically normal. However, about 10 per cent of people with horizontal squints exhibit significant "A" or "V" phenomena. These are named according to the horizontal deviation existing in the primary position (e.g., "A" or "V" esotropia, and "A" or "V" exotropia).

In order to discover an associated "A-V" pattern, all horizontal deviations should be measured with the eyes 30 degrees above and below the horizontal plane as well as in the primary position. All measurements are taken while the patient fixates on a distant target. Moreover, the visual acuity should be bilaterally equal, as "A-V" syndromes tend to disappear when one eye is amblyopic. Therefore, deviations should be properly reevaluated after patching has overcome any amblyopic situation.

The etiology of the "A-V" patterns is highly controversial. One school of thought says they occur from overacting oblique muscles. Another theory claims the vertical recti. A third group of investigators blames the horizontal recti. These differences of opinion have naturally resulted in conflicting thoughts on the significance as well as the treatment of the "A-V" syndromes.

VERTICAL DEVIATIONS. Malalignment of the visual axes, resulting in one eye being higher than the other, is by convention referred to as a *hypertropia* of the elevated eye, even if the pathology exists in the lower eye. For example, weakness of the left superior rectus might cause the left eye to be depressed, but it would be called a right hypertropia.

Hypertropias usually result from some abnormality of the superior and inferior recti or obliques. These four muscles function primarily in both torsional and vertical movements, and therefore often are referred to as *cyclovertical muscles*. The action of a particular cyclovertical muscle depends upon the horizontal position of the globe. In abduction, the recti are pure elevators and depressors, and the obliques are responsible for torsional motion; in adduction, the obliques move the eye in a vertical plane and the recti are rotators. In the primary position all four recti exert combined cyclovertical actions, with the recti having a slightly stronger vertical element and the obliques more torsional. Weakness or overaction of a cyclovertical muscle results in both vertical and torsional deviations, with the vertical element increasing toward one side and the torsional deviation more obvious in the opposite lateral gaze field.

Vertical deviations may be either congenital or acquired. Because of the variation in the angle of strabismus, hypertropias generally are incomitant and appear paralytic. Since diplopia may be a symptom, *ocular torticollis* (compensatory head tilting) often is an associated finding. As a rule the tilt is away from an *underacting* intorter (superior oblique or superior rectus), or toward an *underacting* extorter (inferior oblique or inferior rectus). Conversely, the tilt would be toward the side of an *overacting* intorter and away from an *overacting* extorter.

Incomitant vertical squints frequently are associated with secondary muscular changes that tend to cause comitancy, and the discovery of the offending muscle in a longstanding hypertrophy may be difficult. The torsional aspect of cyclovertical muscle problems, however, provides a valuable diagnostic adjunct, the Bielschowsky (forced head tilt) test. It is based on the principle that the two intorters or the two extorters of each eye have opposite vertical functions; one of each pair depresses and the other elevates. Under normal circumstances these opposite actions counterbalance each other, and when the head is tilted the eyes rotate properly around an anterior-posterior axis.

If one muscle is underacting, however, forced tilting of the head can expose this weakness because the normal, torsional partner appears overactive. For example, forcible tilting of the head *toward* the side of a paretic *superior oblique* increases the vertical deviation, because the homolateral, normal superior rectus is the only intorter remaining. As it produces an inward rotary motion, its unopposed vertical action allows the eye to elevate as well as rotate. This increases the vertical deviation. In contrast, tilting the head *away* from the side of a paretic *inferior oblique* also increases the vertical strabismus through the unopposed depressor action of the inferior rectus that extorts against a weak inferior oblique. As a rule, weakness of an intorter causes a compensatory head tilt away from the involved muscle and an increase in vertical deviation when the head is tilted toward the weak muscle. The reverse holds true for a weak extorter. The Bielschowsky test can be of value in either congenital or acquired, isolated cyclovertical muscle problems.

In the pediatric age group, the most common causes for vertical deviations are overacting inferior obliques, weakness of a superior oblique, and the superior oblique tendon sheath syndrome.

Inferior oblique overaction, either unilateral or bilateral, results in the elevation of the involved eye when it is in a position of adduction (Fig. 5-40*A, B*). The overaction often, but not always, is associated with a horizontal strabismus (especially esotropia). Besides causing a hypertropia in an attempted lateral gaze, it may lead to a "V" pattern. When unilateral, inferior oblique overaction can present with a head tilt toward the opposite shoulder. Surgery usually corrects both the hypertropia and head tilt.

Superior oblique weakness is the most common, acquired, isolated cyclovertical muscle problem. It usually results from a lesion of the fourth nerve or from direct trauma to the muscle at the medial wall of the orbit. The paresis results in hypertropia and extorsion of the involved eye, and frequently in a compensatory head tilt toward the opposite shoulder. The involved eye cannot be depressed when it is in an adducted position and cannot be intorted in abduction.

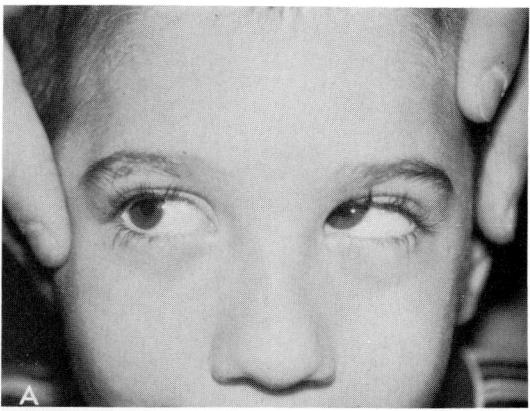

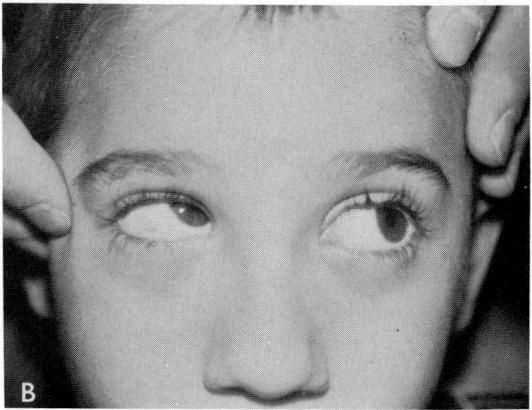

Figure 5-40 (*A*), (*B*) Bilateral overaction of the inferior oblique muscles. Note the marked hypertropia of the adducted eye.

Brown's superior oblique tendon sheath syndrome, reported in 1950, seems to result from a shortening of the superior oblique tendon sheath and may be congenital or acquired. The shortened fibrous sheath acts as a check ligament for the homolateral inferior oblique, and elevation is grossly limited when the affected eye is in the adducted position (Fig. 5-41*A, B*). The condition, commonly unilateral, often is overlooked because the eyes may be orthophoric in the primary position. Not infrequently, however, the involved eye is depressed in the primary position as well as in adduction. This usually results in the head being slightly elevated and turned to the opposite shoulder. Such posturing allows the

EXOPHTHALMOS AND ORBITAL TUMORS

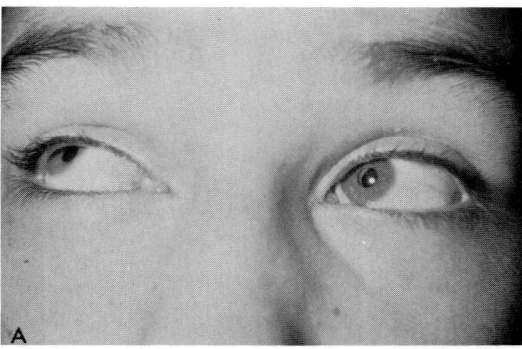

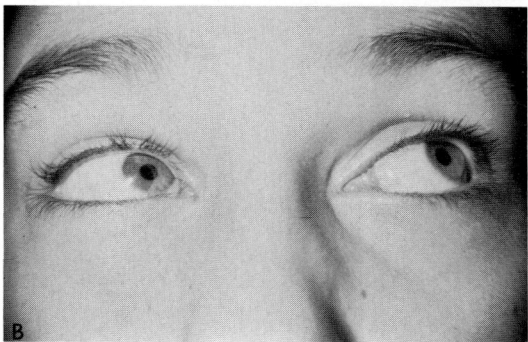

Figure 5-41 (A), (B) Bilateral superior oblique tendon sheath syndrome. Note the inability to elevate the adducted eye.

Since the bony orbit is a rigid, enclosed space except for its anterior opening, any increase in the volume of tissue housed inside results in a forward protrusion of the globe. This is known as exophthalmos or proptosis. Protrusion can be confirmed by measuring with an exophthalmometer the position of the front of the cornea in relation to the anterior rim of the lateral orbital wall. Normally the cornea may extend some 11 to 18 mm. anterior to this wall. Early proptosis is best found by comparing the exophthalmometry readings obtained from each eye. A difference of more than 4 mm. is considered significant. The palpebral fissure is usually wider on the affected side and ocular rotations may be limited in one or more directions.

Benign tumors most frequently cause exophthalmos in children. Primary malignant lesions, metastatic disease, inflammatory conditions simulating tumors, the reticuloendothelioses, and developmental orbital anomalies resulting in proptosis are all less common. Specifically, the most common, primary, space-occupying lesions resulting in exophthalmos in children are, in order of decreasing frequency, hemangiomas (Plate 8C, D), dermoids, rhabdo-

affected eye to be placed into a position of depression and abduction, or out of the field of the restriction.

Brown's syndrome should be distinguished from a true paralysis of an inferior oblique muscle because both appear clinically identical. The differentiation usually is made by a forced duction test under anesthesia. The physician adducts the eye with a forceps and then attempts to elevate it while the eye is in the adducted position. If a restricting superior oblique tendon sheath is present, the eye cannot be elevated by force. No restriction occurs in true paralysis of the inferior oblique muscle.

The type of treatment is controversial, for even surgically removing the fibrous tendon sheath of the superior oblique muscle does not always produce a cure. Moreover, since spontaneous regression has been reported, many authorities do not feel surgery is indicated.

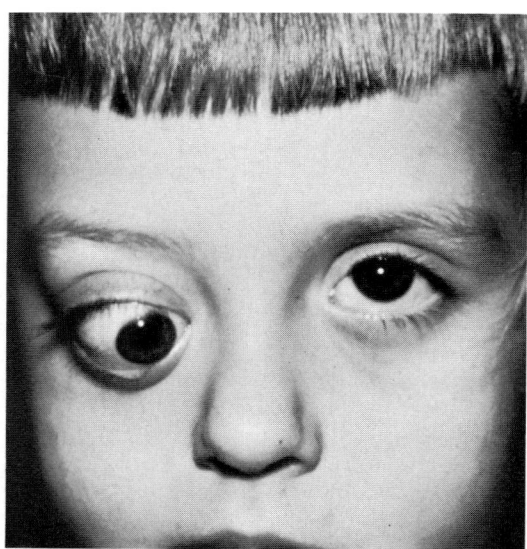

Figure 5-42 Rhabdomyosarcoma of the right orbit resulting in marked proptosis.

myosarcomas (Fig. 5-42), and gliomas of the optic nerve.

Secondary or metastatic malignancies that most commonly involve the orbit in children are neuroblastoma and leukemia. Neuroblastomas usually arise from the adrenal gland or retroperitoneal ganglia, but not infrequently either long bone or orbital metastases appear before the primary tumor is detected. In the orbit, neuroblastomas tend to cause pain, and they frequently undergo necrosis that produces characteristic ecchymosis and hematomas in the periorbital tissues (Plate 8E). The growth of the tumor may be so rapid that its appearance and course resemble the abrupt onset of inflammatory disease. Resistance to antibiotic treatment, radiologic evidence of bony destruction, and eventual biopsy confirm the diagnosis. The prognosis is poor.

Leukemic infiltrates into the orbit less commonly cause exophthalmos than neuroblastoma, but like the neurogenic tumor, they occasionally may represent the initial manifestation of the disease. Diagnosis usually is made by biopsy. Treatment is palliative, consisting of either radiation or chemotherapy.

Orbital cellulitis is the most frequent inflammatory disease causing exophthalmos in children. It results from extension of an infection originating in the sinuses, lids, teeth, or face. Proptosis, lid edema and erythema, conjunctival chemosis, pain, and limitation of ocular motility may be present and usually are associated with fever. Intravenous administration of antibiotics is the treatment of choice, and this usually prevents the one time complications of corneal ulcer, optic nerve atrophy, and posterior extension of the infection into cavernous sinuses with subsequent thrombosis. Prolonged persistence of the symptoms after adequate treatment may be an initial clue that the disease is not due to infection, and malignancy or a reticuloendotheliosis should be suspected.

The reticuloendothelioses are a group of disorders arising from proliferating cells of the reticuloendothelial system. The conditions commonly classified as reticuloendothelioses include the rapidly fatal Letterer-Siwe disease, the more chronic Hand-Schüller-Christian disease, and the relatively benign eosinophilic granuloma. Many investigators consider these disorders as variants of a single, underlying defect, and, in addition, believe that juvenile xanthogranuloma (discussed previously) is a fourth disease belonging to this group. Only in Letterer-Siwe disease are there no ocular findings.

Hand-Schüller-Christian disease classically is described as a triad of findings that include diabetes insipidus, exophthalmos, and multiple defects in the membranous bones of the head. Granulomatous involvement of the viscera now also is recognized as part of this syndrome. Occasionally, unilateral exophthalmos is the presenting symptom.

Eosinophilic granuloma is the most benign of the reticuloendothelioses and usually begins as a solitary, radiolucent lesion of the long bones, ribs, vertebrae, or bony orbit that can cause pain, pathologic fractures, swelling, and inflammation. About the orbit the eosinophilic granuloma may occur so rapidly that often it is mistaken for cellulitis, rhabdomyosarcoma, or neuroblastoma. Diagnosis is made by biopsy, and the lesions often regress after this subtotal surgical excision. The tumors also respond to radiation and chemotherapeutic agents. The prognosis usually is good, but solitary granulomas tend to recur and occasionally they may disseminate.

Developmental abnormalities of the orbit are the final cause of exophthalmos that is seen more commonly in children than in adults. Congenitally shallow orbits and maldevelopment associated with the various cranial or facial dysostoses have been mentioned previously. Absence of the posterior wall of the orbit, resulting in a pulsating exophthalmos, most commonly is associated with neurofibromatosis.

PHAKOMATOSES

Four neuroectodermal syndromes comprise the group of diseases known as the phakomatoses (Greek, meaning "mother spot"). They are neurofibromatosis, tuberous sclerosis, encephalotrigeminal angiomatosis, and cerebroretinal angiomatosis.

All show a strong hereditary or familial tendency and are characterized by disseminated hamartomas that commonly involve the eye, skin, and brain.

Neurofibromatosis

Also called von Recklinghausen's disease, this congenital disorder is characterized by dermal pigmentation and tumors of various tissues. It is inherited through a regular or irregular dominant gene that varies markedly in its expression. Although congenital and capable of appearing at birth or in early childhood, the disease more commonly becomes manifest at puberty, during pregnancy, or at menopause. The most common systemic manifestations of the disease are flat, light brown (café au lait) spots, varying in size and with irregular borders, which usually are best seen on the trunk (Plate 8F). Since they are invariably present, finding even one spot should alert the physician to the possibility of neurofibromatosis.

In addition to these characteristic spots, the skin also often is involved with a variety of subcutaneous tumors. These are plexiform neurofibromas that probably arise from the Schwann cells of peripheral nerves (Fig. 5-43). The tumors may be so diffuse and plexiform in one area as to cause hypertrophy of the skin so that it hangs in folds (elephantiasis neuromatosis) (Fig. 5-44). In contrast, the neuromas can be small and pedunculated, and can appear as subcutaneous nodules over the entire body (fibroma molluscum) (Fig. 5-45).

In addition to the dermal involvement, the skeletal system also may show many changes. Both the axial skeleton and appendages can be involved, with bony hypertrophy or erosion occurring. The eroded lesions appear radiologically and microscopically like the lesions of osteitis fibrosa cystica. They commonly are found about the orbit, where they may cause pulsating exophthalmos, in the cranial vault, and in vertebral bodies or in the extremities.

Less frequently, systemic findings include neuropsychiatric abnormalities such as mental retardation, various endocrinopathies, and multiple congenital anomalies. There also is an increased frequency of pheochromocytomas associated with neurofibromatosis.

Besides these systemic manifestations of von Recklinghausen's disease, neurologic

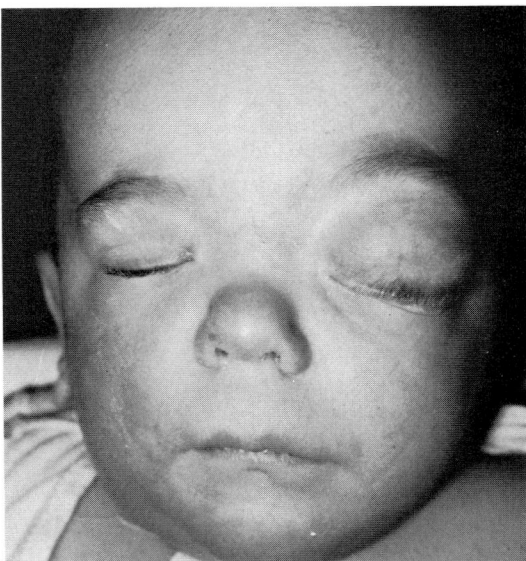

Figure 5-43 Neurofibromatosis. Large plexiform neurofibroma of the left upper lid.

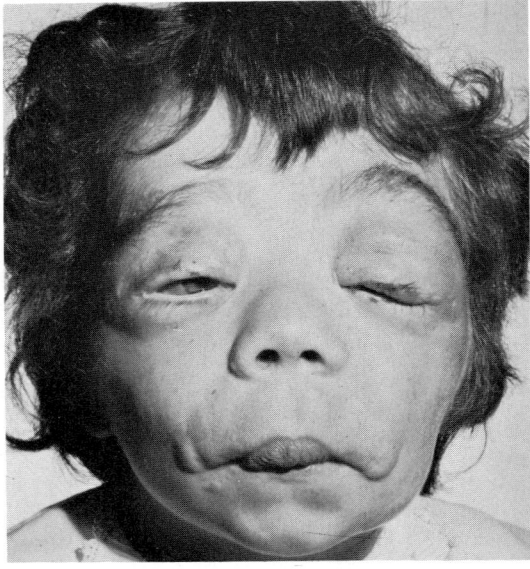

Figure 5-44 Neurofibromatosis. Elephantiasis neuromatosis.

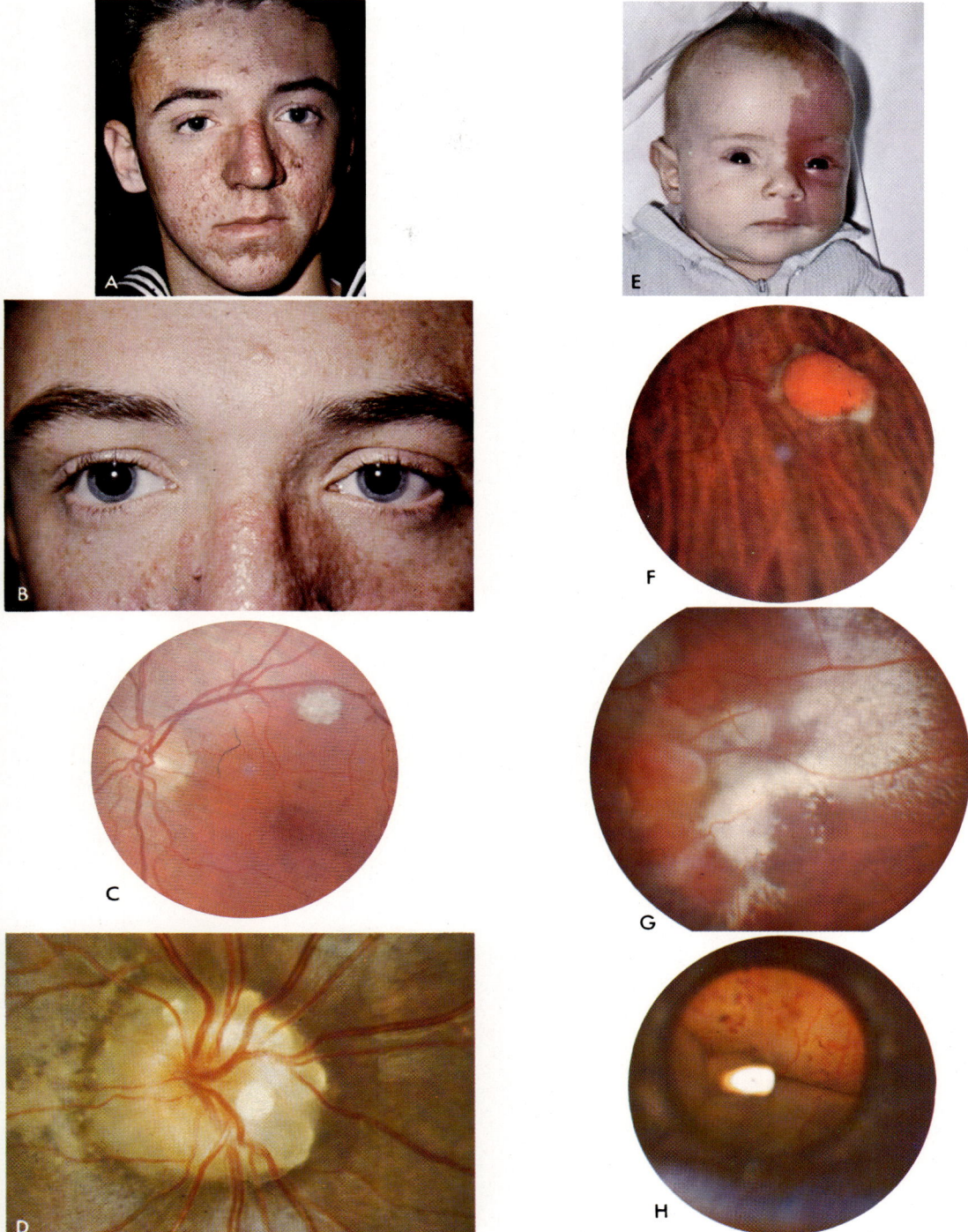

Plate 9 *(A)* Tuberous sclerosis. Adenoma sebaceum of face. *(B)* Tuberous sclerosis. Close-up of 9*A*. Note lesions distributed across nose and on face in butterfly pattern. *(C)* Tuberous sclerosis. White retinal mass (mulberry nodule) situated just above macula. *(D)* Tuberous sclerosis. Multiple large drusen of the optic disc. *(E)* Sturge-Weber disease. Nevus flammeus of left side of face with associated congenital glaucoma. *(F)* von Hippel-Lindau disease. Elevated hemangioma of the peripheral retina. *(G)* von Hippel-Lindau disease. The hemangioma has resulted in a marked exudative and hemorrhagic retinopathy. *(H)* von Hippel-Lindau disease. Total retinal detachment and white pupil resulting from untreated retinal hemangioma.

171

and ocular signs and symptoms are of extreme importance. The disease frequently is complicated by intracranial tumors, especially meningiomas and gliomas. These tumors can give rise to any of the signs or symptoms of intracranial mass lesions, such as increased intracranial pressure, seizures, and motor and sensory deficits including visual field defects. There is a high incidence of bilateral, acoustic neurofibromas. These will produce symptoms of a pontine angle tumor.

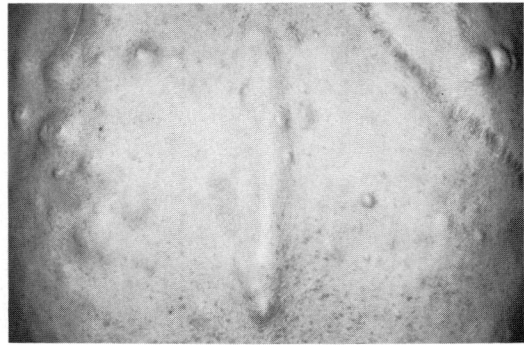

Figure 5-45 Neurofibromatosis. Scattered subcutaneous nodules (fibroma molluscum).

Besides the ocular manifestations of intracranial tumors, neurofibromatosis can present as localized lesions in the eye or periorbital tissue. Most commonly, the lids are affected by either diffuse plexiform or localized pedunculated neurofibromas. The lesions may be so marked as to cause complete ptosis of an eyelid. The neurofibromas also can be found in the conjunctiva and cornea (Plate 8G), where they are seen especially well with the slit lamp biomicroscope. Neurofibromas of the iris are not an infrequent finding. They appear as either localized tan nodules hanging from the fine iris stroma, or as diffuse, tan, thickened areas resembling poorly pigmented nevi (Plate 8H). These lesions of the lids, con-

junctiva, cornea, and iris all represent localized tumors of the nerves of these structures. Choroidal and retinal neurofibromas also have been reported, with the latter appearing similar to the retinal tumors of tuberous sclerosis.

Congenital glaucoma of a very severe type also is associated with von Recklinghausen's disease. The glaucoma may be present at birth or appear at any time thereafter, is commonly of the open-angle variety, and often is unilateral. Several authors feel that the finding of unilateral glaucoma in an infant should alert the physician to the possibility of one of the phakomatoses. Early onset produces all the findings of congenital glaucoma, whereas later onset

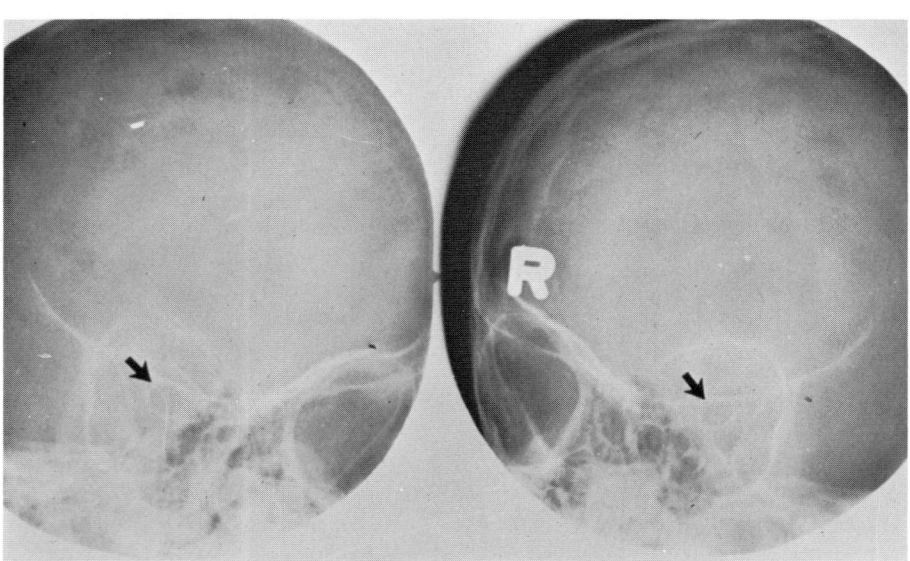

Figure 5-46 Neurofibromatosis. Bilateral optic foramen enlargement indicating optic nerve gliomas (arrows).

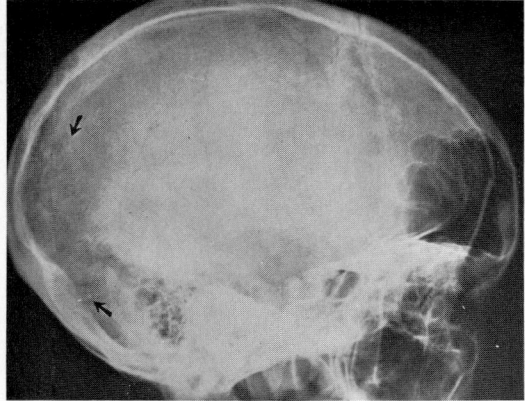

Figure 5-47 Tuberous sclerosis. Intracranial calcifications (arrows).

may lead to the findings seen in adult, open-angle glaucoma.

Loss of vision, in addition to resulting from intracranial tumors or from the development of glaucoma, may result from optic nerve gliomas. These are present in about 15 per cent of patients. Often the diagnosis of an optic nerve glioma can be confirmed from an enlarged optic nerve foramen (Fig. 5-46). Thus the optic foramen of patients with neurofibromatosis should be compared by roentgenography.

The disease also may present with exophthalmos resulting from hyperostosis of the orbital bones or from an erosion of the posterior orbital wall. The latter causes a pulsating exophthalmos. No *bruit* will be heard since the pulsations are secondary to the transmission of the carotid pulsation through the brain.

The prognosis is not invariably unfavorable, although the treatment for any of the tumors is purely palliative. The glaucoma can be handled as any open-angle glaucoma, and the tumors must be excised. Usually, however, the tumors regrow slowly, and malignant degeneration is not infrequent. Optic nerve gliomas may respond to radiotherapy. The most common cause of death appears to be intracranial expansion of one of the tumors.

Tuberous Sclerosis

Also known as Bourneville's disease, and sometimes epiloia, tuberous sclerosis is inherited as an irregular dominant trait with high penetrance and variable expres-

sivity. The disease classically is characterized by adenoma sebaceum, mental retardation, epilepsy, and ocular lesions. Tuberous sclerosis may appear in either childhood or adulthood.

The skin lesions, referred to as Pringle's disease, are sebaceous adenomas (Plate 9*A*) that usually begin about the fifth year of life. They start as pale, pink, slightly raised lesions usually distributed in a butterfly pattern around the nasolabial fold (Plate 9*B*). Recently a new and apparently reliable initial finding has been described. In the early stages of tuberous sclerosis, a white, ash leaf–shaped skin lesion can be detected with the use of a Wood light. These lesions occur on the trunk and seem to be pathognomonic of this phakomatosis.

Mental deficiency usually becomes apparent within the first decade of life and may be so severe as to cause complete idiocy. Convulsions start shortly after the disease appears, are grand mal, petite mal, or jacksonian in nature, and may proceed to status epilepticus. X-rays of the skull often show intracranial calcifications (Fig. 5-47), especially situated about the third and lateral ventricles.

Besides involvement of the skin and brain, tumors of other tissues may occur. Rhabdomyomas, tumors of the thyroid gland, and mixed tumors of the kidneys are frequent, but rarely are diagnosed clinically.

Ocular involvement in tuberous sclerosis consists of white retinal tumors (Plate 9*C*). They may be single or multiple, flat and smooth or raised with a cobblestone appearance (mulberry nodules). The retinal vessels appear to pass underneath the tumor. In time, both retinal tumors and intracranial lesions calcify. Also, drusen of the optic nerve (Plate 9*D*) are found with increased frequency. The prognosis is very poor, for these patients often require institutional care and treatment of the convulsive disorder. They usually die between 5 and 15 years of age.

Encephalotrigeminal Angiomatosis

Also called Sturge-Weber disease, this syndrome is characterized by intracranial
(*Text continues on page 179.*)

TABLE 5-7 EYE FINDINGS IN OTHER PEDIATRIC SYSTEMIC DISEASES

Systemic Disease	Ocular Findings
Acne rosacea	Keratoconjunctivitis and corneal vascularization.
Acrodynia	Photophobia, proptosis, keratoconjunctivitis.
Albinism	Photophobia, nystagmus, transillumination of the irides, macular hypoplasia, high refractive errors, poor vision.
Alkaptonuria	Accumulation of melanin in sclera, especially just anterior to the insertions of the horizontal recti.
Alport's syndrome	Anterior lenticonus, cataracts, spherophakia.
Amyloidosis	Vitreous veils, Argyll Robertson pupils, extraocular muscle palsies.
Amyotonia congenita (Oppenheim's disease)	Extraocular muscle palsies, nystagmus, ptosis, optic atrophy.
Anemia	Pale fundi, retinal hemorrhages and exudates, papilledema.
Anhidrotic ectodermal dysplasia	Deficient tearing, keratoconjunctivitis, corneal opacities, iris atrophy, cataract, pigmentary retinopathy.
Ankylosing spondylitis (Marie-Strümpell's disease)	Severe anterior uveitis, less commonly, scleritis and scleromalacia perforans.
Ataxia telangiectasia (Louis-Bar syndrome)	Bulbar and conjunctival telangiectasia, nystagmus, partial ophthalmoplegia.
Atopic dermatitis	Cataracts, keratoconus.
Battered child syndrome	Subconjunctival hemorrhages, hyphemas, subluxation of the lens, vitreous and retinal hemorrhages, commotio retinae, cataracts, retinal detachments, papilledema.
Bonnevie-Ullrich syndrome	Paralytic strabismus, ptosis, hypertelorism, epicanthus, coloboma, cloudy cornea, cataract.
Canavan's spongy degeneration	Nystagmus, optic atrophy.
Cerebral diplegia (Little's disease)	Nystagmus, strabismus, cataracts, optic atrophy.
Cerebral sclerosis	
Krabbe's form	Nystagmus, optic atrophy.
Pelizaeus-Merzbacher's form	Nystagmus, strabismus, pupillomotor abnormalities, optic atrophy.
Scholz's form	Nystagmus, strabismus, decreased corneal sensation, optic atrophy.
Cerebrotendinous xanthomatosis (van Bogaert-Scherer-Epstein syndrome)	Xanthelasma, cataracts.
Chediak-Higashi syndrome	Ocular albinism with photophobia and decreased vision; papilledema.
Chloramphenicol intoxication	Optic neuritis.
Chloroquine intoxication	Keratopathy, retinopathy.
Chronic polyarthritis (Still's disease)	Band keratopathy, iridocyclitis, secondary cataracts. Secondary glaucoma or phthisis bulbi occurs in terminal stages.
Cockayne's syndrome	Photophobia, loss of orbital fat, cataracts, pigmentary retinopathy, optic atrophy.
Congenital dyskeratosis (Shäfer's syndrome)	Corneal dystrophy, cataracts.
Congenital hemolytic icterus (congenital spherocytosis)	Microphthalmia, heterochromia, mongoloid palpebral fissures, cataracts, myopia, dyschromatopsia.
Congenital ichthyosiform erythroderma	Cataracts.
Congenital lymphedema (Nonne-Milroy-Meige disease)	Thickened, ptotic lids; strabismus; distichiasis.
Congenital stippled epiphysis (Conradi's disease)	Cataracts.

Systemic Disease	Ocular Findings
Cretinism (congenital hypothyroidism)	Wide-set eyes with narrowed fissures, myxedematous lids, strabismus, hyperopia, and occasionally, lens opacities.
Cystic fibrosis	Retinal venous dilatation, retinal hemorrhages, papilledema.
Cystinosis (Fanconi's syndrome)	Cystine crystals in cornea, conjunctiva, and sclera; pigmentary retinopathy.
Dandy-Walker syndrome (atresia of the foramen magnum)	Ptosis, sixth nerve paralysis, papilledema.
Dermatomyositis	Periorbital edema; exophthalmos; extraocular muscle palsies; scleritis; iritis; large, white, fluffy exudates scattered around the optic nerve. Occlusive vascular phenomena can occur.
Diabetes mellitus	Extraocular muscle palsies, rapidly changing refractive error, cataracts, and the vascular and exudative retinopathy of adult diabetes mellitus (p. 255).
Disseminated lupus erythematosus	Keratoconjunctivitis, interstitial keratitis, band keratopathy, iridocyclitis, secondary cataracts, retinal hemorrhages and exudates, papilledema.
Epidermolysis bullosa	Blepharitis, conjunctivitis, keratitis, symblepharon, corneal scarring.
Erythroblastosis fetalis (kernicterus)	Nystagmus, strabismus, retinal hemorrhages, optic atrophy.
Facial hemiatrophy (Romberg's syndrome)	Ptosis, strabismus, Horner's syndrome, iridocyclitis, heterochromia, optic atrophy.
Familial dysautonomia (Riley-Day syndrome)	Decreased lacrimation, corneal hypesthesia, sleeping with eyes open. Frequently results in superficial punctate corneal staining, exposure keratitis, recurrent corneal ulcers.
Fanconi's aplastic anemia	Strabismus (especially esotropia), band keratopathy, retrobulbar hemorrhages.
Foster-Kennedy syndrome	Optic atrophy on the side of the intracranial lesion with contralateral papilledema.
Friedreich's ataxia	Ptosis, nystagmus, strabismus, Argyll Robertson pupils, pigmentary retinopathy, optic atrophy.
Fröhlich's syndrome (dystrophia adiposogenitalis)	Visual field defects, papilledema, poor dark adaptation.
Galactosemia	"Oil droplet" appearance of lens nucleus which becomes irreversibly opaque if treatment not instituted.
Glomerulonephritis	Periorbital edema, hypertensive retinopathy.
Guillain-Barré syndrome	Facial nerve paralysis, extraocular muscle palsies, mydriasis, papilledema, optic atrophy.
Hartnup disease	Photophobia, nystagmus, double vision.
Hemoglobinopathies (SS and SC disease)	Multiple vascular abnormalities in the conjunctiva, anterior uveitis, rubeosis iridis, secondary cataract, multiple retinal vascular abnormalities secondary to occlusive vascular phenomena, angioid streaks, papilledema, retinal detachment.
Hemophilia	Retrobulbar and subconjunctival hemorrhages; hyphemas and vitreous or retinal hemorrhages are rare.
Hepatolenticular degeneration (Wilson's disease)	Kayser-Fleischer ring of cornea and, rarely, copper cataracts (chalcosis lentis).

Table continues on following page.

Systemic Disease	Ocular Findings
Hereditary hemorrhagic telangiectasia (Rendu-Osler disease)	Conjunctival telangiectasias, subconjunctival hemorrhages, retinal telangiectasias and hemorrhages.
Homocystinuria	Ectopia lentis and its complications, cataracts, cystic degeneration of the retina, myopia, optic atrophy.
Hydrocephaly	Strabismus, papilledema, optic atrophy.
Hyperlipemia	Xanthelasma, arcus juvenilis, lipemia retinalis.
Hyperparathyroidism	Band keratopathy, optic atrophy.
Hyperthyroidism	Multiple lid motor abnormalities, exophthalmos, pupillomotor abnormalities, extraocular muscle palsies, papilledema.
Hypoglycemia	Nasal lacrimal duct obstructions, strabismus, congenital glaucoma, and occasionally, cataracts.
Hypoparathyroidism	Blepharospasm, keratoconjunctivitis, tetany, cataracts, papilledema.
Idiopathic thrombocytopenic purpura	Ecchymosis of eyelids, subconjunctival hemorrhages, retinal hemorrhages, papilledema, optic atrophy, transient extraocular muscle palsies.
Infantile cortical hyperostosis (Caffey's disease)	Periorbital soft tissue swelling and tenderness, proptosis, conjunctivitis.
Keratosis follicularis (Siemen's disease)	Follicular keratosis of lids and eyelashes, blepharitis, corneal scarring, cataracts.
Keratosis palmaris et plantaris	Corneal opacities.
Kiloh Nevin's syndrome	Ptosis, progressive external ophthalmoplegia.
Klippel-Feil syndrome	Paralytic strabismus, Duane's retraction syndrome.
Lead poisoning	Paralytic strabismus, pupillomotor abnormalities, papilledema, optic atrophy.
Leukemia	Conjunctival, lid, and orbital infiltrates; retinal hemorrhages, frequently resembling Roth spots; sheathing of retinal vessels; retinal infiltrates; papilledema and optic neuritis.
Lipid proteinosis (Urbach-Wiethe syndrome)	Small fatty nodules on the lids, moniliform blepharitis, loss of lashes.
Macroglobulinemias	Marked venous engorgement, papilledema, retinal hemorrhages and exudates, venous occlusions.
Marchesani's syndrome	Ectopia lentis, aniridia, anterior chamber abnormalities, cataracts, secondary glaucoma.
Marfan's syndrome	Blue sclera, megalocornea, ectopia lentis, iridodonesis, cataracts, secondary glaucoma, myopia, retinal detachment.
Meniere's disease	Vestibular nystagmus, diplopia.
Moebius' syndrome	Facial nerve paralysis, congenital paralytic strabismus, exposure keratitis.
Monilethrix	Broken lashes, blepharitis, conjunctivitis, cataracts.
Mucopolysaccharidoses	
MPS I (Hurler's disease)	Cloudy cornea, buphthalmia, pigmentary retinopathy, optic atrophy.
MPS II (Hunter's disease)	Cloudy cornea, pigmentary retinopathy, optic atrophy.
MPS III (Sanfilippo's disease)	None.

Systemic Disease	Ocular Findings
MPS IV (Morquio's disease)	Hypertelorism, cloudy cornea.
MPS V (Scheie's disease)	Cloudy cornea, pigmentary retinopathy.
MPS VI (Mauriteaux Lamy's disease)	Corneal clouding.
Multiple sclerosis	Paralytic strabismus, retrobulbar neuritis, optic atrophy.
Myasthenia gravis	Ptosis, extraocular muscle palsies.
Myotonic dystrophy (Steinert's disease)	Cataract, ptosis, pigmentary retinopathy.
Oculocerebrorenal syndrome (Lowe's syndrome)	Cataracts, glaucoma, nystagmus, strabismus, anophthalmia.
Oligophrenia (Marinesco-Sjögren syndrome)	Cataracts, aniridia.
Osteitis fibrosa desseminata (McCune-Albright's syndrome)	Proptosis, papilledema, optic atrophy.
Osteogenesis imperfecta	Blue sclera, arcus juvenilis, keratoconus, megalocornea, ectopia lentis, glaucoma.
Osteopetrosis (Marble bones; Albers-Schönberg disease)	Ptosis, extraocular muscle palsies, optic atrophy.
Otitis media (Gradenigo's syndrome)	Sudden onset of the sixth nerve paralysis from the extension of a middle ear infection into the petrous bone.
Peroneal muscular atrophy (Charcot-Marie-Tooth disease)	Nystagmus, pupillomotor abnormalities, optic atrophy, pigmentary retinopathy.
Phenylketonuria	Photophobia, decreased ocular pigmentation.
Platybasia (Arnold-Chiari deformity)	Nystagmus, extraocular muscle palsies, papilledema.
Pleonosteosis (Leri's disease)	Thickening of lids, corneal haziness, strabismus.
Polyarteritis nodosa	Anterior uveitis, choroiditis, perivascular infiltrates, retinal hemorrhages and exudates, optic atrophy, papilledema, vascular occlusive and hypertensive retinopathies.
Polycythemia (primary or secondary)	Dilated tortuous veins and arterioles, cyanosis retinae, retinal hemorrhages, hyperemic discs, papilledema.
Porphyria	Photophobia, corneal opacities, cataracts, keratomalacia, xerophthalmia.
Progressive spinomuscular atrophy (Werdnig-Hoffmann disease)	Nystagmus, extraocular muscle palsies, optic atrophy.
Pseudohypoparathyroidism (Albright's disease)	Same as true hypoparathyroidism, with a slightly decreased incidence of cataracts.
Rheumatic fever	Iritis, papillitis, ocular findings of subacute bacterial endocarditis (see table entry).
Rothmund's syndrome (poikiloderma atrophicans vasculare)	Corneal dystrophy, congenital cataracts.
Rud's disease (ichthyosis)	Pigmentary retinopathy, ectropion, exposure keratitis, corneal dystrophy.
Sarcoidosis	Ptosis, extraocular muscle palsies, keratoconjunctivitis sicca, interstitial keratitis, granulomatous iridocyclitis, band keratopathy, chorioretinitis, perivasculitis, optic neuritis.
Schilder's disease (periaxialis diffusa)	Extraocular muscle palsies, nystagmus, optic atrophy, papilledema, cortical blindness.
Schönlein-Henoch purpura	Retinal hemorrhages and, rarely, iritis.
Scleroderma	Tightening and thickening of the lids, extraocular muscle palsies, and rarely, retinal changes similar to disseminated lupus erythematosus.

Table continues on following page.   177

TABLE 5-7 EYE FINDINGS IN OTHER PEDIATRIC SYSTEMIC DISEASES *(Continued)*

Systemic Disease	Ocular Findings
Serum sickness	Conjunctival chemosis, iridocyclitis, retinal hemorrhages and exudates.
Sinusitis	Orbital cellulitis, mucocele, pyocele, orbital abscess, exophthalmos, cavernous sinus thrombosis.
Steroid intoxication	
Systemic treatment	Cataracts, papilledema from pseudotumor cerebri.
Local treatment	Exacerbation of herpes simplex keratitis; glaucoma.
Stevens-Johnson syndrome	Purulent pseudomembranous conjunctivitis, keratitis, secondary iritis. Often results in trichiasis, symblepharon, corneal opacification or perforation.
Subacute bacterial endocarditis	Conjunctival hemorrhages, retinal hemorrhages, Roth spots, papilledema, optic neuritis, perivasculitis, embolic chorioretinitis; occasionally, panophthalmitis.
Subacute sclerosing leukoencephalopathy (Dawson's disease)	Diffuse chorioretinal degeneration.
Subdural hematoma	Retinal hemorrhages, extraocular muscle palsies, papilledema.
Tetracycline intoxication	Papilledema, sixth nerve palsy from pseudotumor cerebri.
Ulcerative collitis	Anterior uveitis.
Vitamin A deficiency	Xerophthalmia, Bitot's spots, keratomalacia, poor dark adaptation, nyctalopia.
Vitamin A intoxication	Retinal hemorrhages, exophthalmos, papilledema from pseudotumor cerebri.
Vitamin B deficiencies	
Beri-beri (thiamine deficiency)	Optic atrophy, ptosis, nystagmus, extraocular muscle palsies.
Pellagra (nicotinic acid deficiency)	Optic neuritis, optic atrophy.
Riboflavin deficiency	Photophobia, keratoconjunctivitis, superficial interstitial keratitis.
Vitamin C deficiency (scurvy)	Proptosis secondary to retrobulbar hemorrhages, periorbital ecchymosis, subconjunctival hemorrhages, and rarely, hyphemas, retinal hemorrhages. Roth's spots.
Vitamin D deficiency (rickets and tetany)	Hypocalcemic cataracts, excessive lacrimation, papilledema (see hypoparathyroidism).
Werner's syndrome (scleropoikiloderma)	Hypotrichosis, corneal scarring, cataracts.
Wilms' tumor	Aniridia.
Xeroderma pigmentosum	Chronic conjunctivitis, ectropion, lid and conjunctival papillomas, which often undergo malignant degeneration.

angioma, facial angioma, and choroidal angioma, all homolateral and present from birth. In rare cases the disorder may be bilateral. There is no clear evidence that the disease is inherited, and at least one authority suggests that the disorder is due to a chromosomal aberration.

The intracranial hemangioma involves the meninges on one side of the brain and may become calcified, appearing on radiologic examination as fine parallel lines ("tram tracks"), which outline the walls of the involved blood vessels (Fig. 5-48). The intracranial lesion is associated with atrophy of both cerebral and cerebellar cortex on the homolateral side. It can give rise to grand mal or contralateral jacksonian seizures, visual field defects, and mental deficiency.

The cutaneous angioma is known as a nevus flammeus and involves the face in the area of the first or second division of the fifth cranial nerve on the same side as the intracranial lesion. The lesion almost invariably involves the skin of the lid. It may involve both the palpebral and bulbar conjunctiva. Facial hemihypertrophy of the involved side is not infrequent.

The most important ocular abnormality is congenital glaucoma, which also is homolateral to the facial nevus (Plate 9E). Occasionally the glaucoma may be bilateral. The conjunctival vessels may appear dilated and tortuous; there is heterochromia iridis; and the involved choroid appears darker due to

a choroidal hemangioma. The prognosis is good, although the individuals may need treatment for seizures and surgery is necessary for the glaucoma.

Cerebroretinal Angiomatosis

Known as von Hippel-Lindau disease, angiomatosis of the retina and cerebellum often is inherited as an irregular dominant, with incomplete penetration and variable expression.

The retinal lesion, first described by von Hippel, presents in its earliest stages as an elevated red mass (hemangioma) in the periphery of the retina (Plate 9F). The lesion usually is discovered because the artery and vein leading to and from the hemangioma are extremely tortuous and markedly dilated. These vessels can be two or three times their normal diameter. The hemangiomas are bilateral in about 50 per cent of the patients. If the hemangioma has gone unnoticed or untreated, secondary changes occur and result in transudation, exudation, hemorrhage (Plate 9G), organization, retinal detachment (Plate 9H), and secondary glaucoma. The ophthalmoscopic picture, therefore, varies according to the stage at which the disorder is discovered.

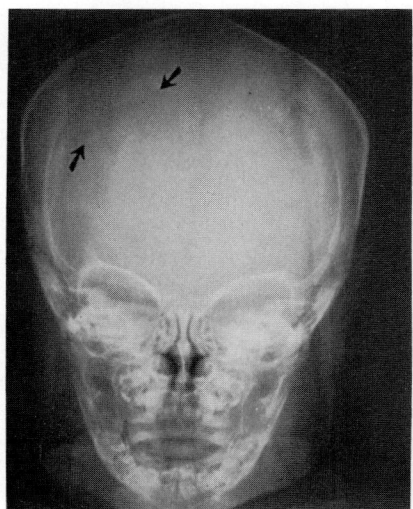 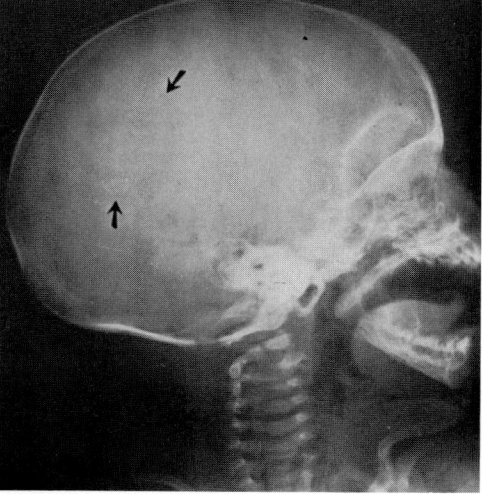

Figure 5-48 Sturge-Weber disease. Intracranial calcifications outlining the vessels of the intracranial hemangioma (arrows).

The association of cerebellar hemangiomas with the retinal hemangiomas was first noted by Lindau. Hemangiomatous cysts can be found in the cerebellum and spinal cord. They can produce symptoms similar to those produced by lesions of the posterior fossa or spinal cord. Neuropsychiatric symptoms, seizures, and mental retardation also may be present.

Variability in expression of the disease allows for independent occurrence of either the retinal or central nervous system lesions. They are found concomitantly, however, in about 25 per cent of patients. In addition to the cerebroretinal lesions, hemangiomas also have been reported in the pancreas, kidneys, ovaries, adrenals, liver, and spleen. Any of the extraocular lesions, and especially cerebral lesions, may undergo malignant degeneration.

If the disorder is limited to the eye and diagnosed early, the prognosis is fairly good. In its early stages the retinal hemangiomas can be treated with photocoagulation. When intracranial lesions are present, however, the prognosis is poor.

EYE FINDINGS IN OTHER PEDIATRIC SYSTEMIC DISEASES

The accompanying Table 5-7 summarizes, alphabetically, the ocular findings of a wide variety of other systemic diseases of pediatric interest.

BIBLIOGRAPHY

Normal Eye in Infancy and Childhood

Duke-Elder, S.: Normal and abnormal development. Part 1. Embryology. In Duke-Elder, S., (ed.): System of Ophthalmology, Vol. 3. St. Louis, The C. V. Mosby Co., 1963.

Kiff, R. D., and Lepard, C.: Visual response of premature infants. Arch. Ophth. 75:631, 1966.

Liebman, S. D., and Gellis, S. S.: The Pediatrician's Ophthalmology. St. Louis, The C. V. Mosby Co., 1966.

Tyner, G. S.: Ophthalmoscopic findings in normal premature infants. Arch. Ophth. 45:627, 1951.

Wolff, E.: The Anatomy of the Eye and Orbit. 4th ed. New York, Blakiston Division, McGraw-Hill Book Co., Inc., 1954.

Developmental Abnormalities

Blodi, F. C.: Developmental anomalies of the skull affecting the eye. Arch. Ophth. 57:593, 1957.

Cogan, D. G., and Kuwabara, T.: The sphingolipidoses and the eye. Arch. Ophth. 79:437, 1968.

Duke-Elder, S.: Normal and abnormal development. Part 2. Congenital deformities. In Duke-Elder, S. (ed.): System of Ophthalmology, Vol. 3. St. Louis, The C. V. Mosby Co., 1963.

Falls, H. F.: A classification and clinical description of hereditary macular lesions. Tr. Am. Acad. Ophth. 70:1034, 1966.

Fine, R. N., Wilson, W. A., and Donnell, G. N.: Retinal changes in glycogen storage disease Type 1. Am. J. Dis. Child., 115:328, 1968.

Francois, J.: Congenital Cataracts. Springfield, Illinois, Charles C Thomas, 1963.

Francois, J.: Heredity in Ophthalmology. St. Louis, The C. V. Mosby Co., 1961.

Goodman, G., Ripps, H., and Siegel, I. M.: Sex-linked ocular disorders: trait expressivity in males and carrier females. Arch. Ophth. 73:387, 1965.

Keitel, H.: Peculiar versus diagnostic facies in pediatrics. Med. Sc. 17/6:47, 1966.

Krill, A. E., and Klien, B. A.: Flecked retina syndrome. Arch. Ophth. 74:496, 1965.

Linksz, A.: A short primer on color vision and its defects. J. Ped. Ophth. 5:183, 1968.

Mann, I.: Developmental Abnormalities of the Eye. Philadelphia, J. B. Lippincott Co., 1958.

Reese, A. B., and Ellsworth, R. M.: The anterior chamber cleavage syndrome. Arch. Ophth. 75:307, 1966.

Rubin, M. L., Fishman, R. S., and McKay, R. A.: Choroideremia. Arch. Ophth. 76:563, 1966.

Sabates, F. N.: Juvenile retinoschisis. Am. J. Ophth. 62:683, 1966.

Shaffer, R. N., et al.: Symposium on congenital anomalies of the eye associated with glaucoma. Invest. Ophth. 7:123, 1968.

Sugar, H. S.: Heterochromia iridis. Am. J. Ophth. 60:1, 1965.

Symposium on Surgical and Medical Management of Congenital Anomalies. New Orleans Academy of Ophth. St. Louis, The C. V. Mosby Co., 1968.

Tasman, W.: Juvenile retinal detachment. J. Ped. Ophth. 5:160, 1968.

Veirs, E. R.: Disorders of the nasolacrimal apparatus in infants and children. J. Ped. Ophth. 3:32, 1966.

Congenital Infections

Alford, C. A.: Congenital syphilis, a problem again. Reported at symposium on intrauterine infections, New York, Jan. 10, 1968.

Hanna, C., Jarman, R. V., Keatts, J. G., and Duffy, C. E.: Virus-induced cataracts. Arch. Ophth. 79:59, 1968.

Hanshaw, J. B.: Congenital cytomegalo-virus infection. Reported at symposium on intrauterine infections, New York, Jan. 10, 1968.

Hogan, M. J., Kimura, S. J., and O'Connor, G. R.: Ocular toxoplasmosis. Arch. Ophth. 72:592, 1964.

Langer, H.: Repeated congenital infection with toxoplasma gondii. Obs. Gyn. 21:318, 1963.

Maumenee, A. E.: Toxoplasmosis. Baltimore, Williams & Wilkins Co., 1962.

Remington, J. S.: Detection of congenital toxoplasmosis. Reported at symposium on intrauterine infections, New York, Jan. 10, 1968.

Scheie, H. G., Schaffer, D. B., Plotkin, S. A., and Kertesz, E.: Congenital rubella cataracts. Arch. Ophth. 77:440, 1967.

Smith, M. E., Zimmerman, L. E., and Harley, R. D.: Ocular involvement in congenital cytomegalic inclusion disease. Arch. Ophth. 76:696, 1966.

Weller, T. H., and Hanshaw, J. B.: Virologic and clinical observations on cytomegalic inclusion disease. New England J. Med. 266:1233, 1962.

Yanoff, M., Schaffer, D. B., and Scheie, H. G.: Rubella ocular syndrome — correlation of clinical, viral, and pathologic studies. Tr. Am. Acad. Ophth. 72:896, 1968.

Zimmerman, L. E.: Histopathologic basis for ocular manifestations of congenital rubella syndrome. Am. J. Ophth. 65:837, 1968.

Zimmerman, L. E.: Toxoplasma gondii from toxocara cati. Arch. Ophth. 76:159, 1966.

Neonatal Ophthalmology

Fedukowicz, H. B.: External Infections of the Eye. New York, Appleton-Century-Crofts, 1963.

New Orleans Academy of Ophthalmology: Infectious Diseases of the Conjunctiva and Cornea. St. Louis, The C. V. Mosby Co., 1963.

Patz, A.: New role of the ophthalmologist in prevention of retrolental fibroplasia. Arch. Ophth. 78:565, 1967.

Patz, A.: The effect of oxygen on immature retinal vessels. Invest. Ophth. 4:988, 1965.

Reese, A. B., Owens, W. C., Friedenwald, J. S., Silverman, W. A., Kinsey, V. E., Hemphill, F. M., and Patz, A.: Symposium: retrolental fibroplasia (retinopathy of prematurity). Am. J. Ophth. 40:159, 1955.

White Pupil

Hansen, A. C.: Norrie's disease. Am. J. Ophth. 66:328, 1958.

Hogan, M. J., and Zimmerman, L. E.: Ophthalmic Pathology: An Atlas and Textbook. 1st ed. Philadelphia, W. B. Saunders Co., 1962.

Howard, G. M., and Ellsworth, R. M.: Differential diagnosis of retinoblastoma: a statistical survey of 500 children. I. Relative frequency of the lesions which simulate retinoblastoma. Am. J. Ophth. 60:610, 1965.

Morales, A. G.: Coats' disease: natural history and results of treatment. Am. J. Ophth. 60:855, 1965.

Reese, A. B.: Tumors of the Eye. 2nd ed. New York, Hoeber Medical Division, Harper & Row, 1963.

Unsworth, A. C., Fox, J. C., Rosenthal, E., and Shelton, P. A.: Larval granulomatosis of the retina due to nematode. Am. J. Ophth. 60:127, 1965.

Zimmerman, L. E.: The ocular manifestations of juvenile xanthogranuloma (nevoxanthoendothelioma). Tr. Am. Acad. Ophth. 69:412, 1965.

Strabismus

Adler, F. H.: Physiology of the Eye. 3rd ed. St. Louis, The C. V. Mosby Co., 1959.

Burian, H. M.: Exodeviations: their classification, diagnosis, and treatment. Am. J. Ophth. 62:1161, 1966.

Chow, K. L., Riesen, A. H., and Newell, F. W.: Degeneration of retinal ganglion cells in infant chimpanzees reared in darkness. J. Comp. Neurol. 107:27, 1957.

Cogan, D. G.: Neurology of the Ocular Muscles. 2nd ed. Springfield, Illinois, Charles C Thomas, 1956.

Haik, G. M., (ed.): Strabismus Symposium of the New Orleans Academy of Ophthalmology. St. Louis, The C. V. Mosby Co., 1962.

Hardesty, H. H.: Diagnosis and surgical treatment of paretic vertical muscles. Arch. Ophth. 77:147, 1967.

Linksz, A.: Pathophysiology of amblyopia. J. Ped. Ophth. 1:19, 1964.

von Noorden, G. K.: Classification of amblyopia. Am. J. Ophth. 63:238, 1967.

von Noorden, G. K., and Maumenee, A. E.: Atlas of Strabismus. St. Louis, The C. V. Mosby Co., 1967.

Wiesel, T. N., and Hubel, D. H.: Effects of visual deprivation on morphology and physiology of cells in the cat's lateral geniculate body. J. Neurophysiol. 26:973, 1963.

Exophthalmos and Orbital Tumors

Albert, D. M., Rubenstein, R. A., and Scheie, H. G.: Tumor metastasis to the eye: II. Clinical study in infants and children. Am. J. Ophth. 63:727, 1967.

Iliff, C. E., and Ossofsky, H. J.: Tumors of the eye and adnexa in infancy and childhood. Springfield, Illinois, Charles C Thomas, 1962.

Oberman, H. A.: Idiopathic histiocytosis: a correlative review of eosinophilic granuloma, Hand-Schüller-Christian disease and Letterer-Siwe disease. J. Ped. Ophth. 5:86, May 1968.

Reese, A. B.: Tumors of the Eye. 2nd ed. New York, Paul B. Hoeber, Inc., 1963.

Silva, D.: Orbital tumors. Am. J. Ophth. 65:318, 1968.

Phakomatoses

Grant, W. M., and Walton, D. S.: Distinctive gonioscopic findings in glaucoma due to neurofibromatosis. Arch. Ophth. 79:127, 1968.

Hayward, M. D., and Bower, B. D.: Trisomy associated with Sturge-Weber syndrome. Lancet 2:844, 1960.

Joe, S., and Spencer, W. H.: Von Hippel-Lindau disease. Arch. Ophth. 71:508, 1964.

Saran, N., and Winter, F. C.: Bilateral gliomas of the optic discs: associated with neurofibromatosis. Am. J. Ophth. 64:607, 1967.

Eye Findings in Pediatric Systemic Diseases

Anderson, B.: Ocular lesions in relapsing polychondritis and other rheumatoid syndromes. Am. J. Ophth. 64:35, 1967.

Cogan, D. G., and Kuwabara, T.: Ocular pathology of cystinosis. Arch. Ophth. 63:51, 1960.

Day, R. M.: Ocular manifestations of thyroid disease. Current concepts. Arch. Ophth. 64:324, 1960.

Dow, D. S.: Ocular sarcoidosis. Am. J. Ophth. 59:93, 1965.

Fisher, N. F., Hallett, J., and Carpenter, G.: Oculocerebrorenal syndrome of Lowe. Arch. Ophth. 77:642, 1967.

Frenkel, M.: Myasthenia gravis: current trends. Am. J. Ophth. 61:522, 1966.

Goldberg, M. F., and von Noorden, G. K.: Ophthalmologic findings in Wilson's hepatolenticular degeneration. Arch. Ophth. 25:162, 1966.

Greaves, D. P.: Symposium on metabolic diseases of the eye: galactosemia. Proc. Roy. Soc. Med. 56:24, 1963.

Hanno, H. A., and Weiss, D. I.: Hypoparathyroidism, pseudohypoparathyroidism, and pseudo-pseudohypoparathyroidism. Arch. Ophth. 65:238, 1961.

Hyams, S. W., Reisner, S. H., and Neumann, E.: The eye signs in ataxia-telangiectasia. Am. J. Ophth. 62:1118, 1966.

Maumenee, A. E.: Ocular manifestations of collagen diseases. Arch. Ophth. 56:557, 1956.

McKusick, V. A.: Heritable Disorders of Connective Tissue. 2nd ed. St. Louis, The C. V. Mosby Co., 1960.

McLaren, D. S.: Malnutrition and the Eye. New York, Academic Press Inc., 1963.

Moses, L., and Heller, G. L.: Ocular myopathy. Am. J. Ophth. 59:1051, 1965.

Muller, S. A., and Brunsting, L. A.: Cataracts associated with dermatologic disorders. Arch. Derm. 88:330, 1963.

Safir, A., Paulsen, E. P., Klayman, J., and Gerstenfeld, J.: Ocular abnormalities in juvenile diabetics. Arch. Ophth. 76:557, 1966.

Shafey, S.: The diffuse scleroses. In Smith, J. L. (ed.): The University of Miami and the Bascom Palmer Eye Institute Neuro-Ophthalmology Symposium, Vol. III, St. Louis, The C. V. Mosby Co., 1967, pp. 218-254.

Thornton, S. P.: Ophthalmic Eponyms. Birmingham, Ala., Aesculapius Publishing Co., 1967.

Walsh, F. B.: Clinical Neuro-Ophthalmology. Baltimore, Williams & Wilkins Co., 1957.

Welch, R. B., and Goldberg, M. F.: Sickle-cell hemoglobin and its relation to fundus abnormality. Arch. Ophth. 75:353, 1966.

Chapter Six

MEDICAL OPHTHALMOLOGY

ALLERGIC STATES AFFECTING THE EYE

General Concepts

Allergy or hypersensitivity is an altered inflammatory reaction by an animal host to the reintroduction of a foreign substance into the external environment. Allergy, the result of an antigen-antibody reaction, should be distinguished from purely toxic, idiosyncratic, and hyperreactive responses. The tendency to develop allergies is influenced by hereditary factors. The predisposition to acquire certain types of allergies, such as hay fever and asthma, is referred to as atopy. Allergic reactions can be of the immediate or delayed type. This depends on the time elapsed between exposure to the allergen and the first signs of reaction.

Immediate allergy occurs within seconds or minutes after re-exposure to the antigen. It includes such forms of allergy as anaphylactic shock, the Arthus reaction, urticaria, and atopic allergy. Circulating antibody to the antigen usually can be found. Tissue damage is thought to result from antigen-antibody complexes attaching themselves to certain cells, especially the vascular endothelium. Reactivity to a particular antigen may be transferred temporarily to another host by transfusion of

serum from the individual with the immediate type of allergy.

Delayed type allergy (cellular; tuberculin) is not manifest until several hours or days after exposure to the antigen. Certain cells, particularly lymphoid cells, are thought to be the site of the antigen-specific reaction. Circulating antibodies are absent, and hypersensitivity cannot be transferred by means of serum. The two principal forms are contact and microbial ("microbiallergic") allergy. The former is a result of body surface contact with the antigen, from which dermatitis or conjunctivitis occurs. Microbial allergy results from hypersensitivity to viruses, bacteria, fungi, or helminths.

In addition to these types of allergies, immunization to antigens of one's own tissues (autoimmunity) plays an important role in certain ocular diseases. Frequently it is not clear which specific type of allergy is responsible for a particular ophthalmic reaction. All of the allergic mechanisms described can affect the eye.

Allergies of the Conjunctiva, Lids, and Adjacent Skin

IMMEDIATE ALLERGY OF THE LIDS AND CONJUNCTIVA

Allergic reactions of this type usually occur in patients with a strong personal and

183

family history of other allergic disorders, such as infantile eczema, asthma, hay fever, and urticaria. Within a few minutes after contact with the antigen, there may be a generalized systemic reaction, including ocular changes. The response may be limited to the lids, conjunctiva, or both.

Lid involvement commonly occurs in response to generalized drug reactions, serum sickness, foods, insect bites, inhalants, local drugs, and other contactants. The principal symptom is itching. In acute cases the appearance may range from frank urticaria or angioneurotic edema to swollen, weeping skin, or only to slight wrinkling of the skin. When the problem is chronic, the skin appears dry, red, and scaly (Plate 10*A*). This type of allergy, particularly when chronic, must be differentiated from seborrheic dermatitis, microbiallergic dermatitis, and contact dermatitis. Treatment consists of avoiding the allergen and using mild astringents, bland creams, and corticosteroid preparations.

Allergic conjunctivitis of the immediate type is caused by airborne allergens such as pollens, dusts, moldspores, and animal hairs and feathers. In acute cases edema of the conjunctiva forms a swelling around the cornea (chemosis), and there is a profuse, watery discharge. In severe cases, a mucopurulent discharge may be seen. In more chronic cases edema and congestion are slight, and the conjunctiva has a "glassy" appearance. In both acute and chronic cases a conjunctival smear shows eosinophils. Papillary hypertrophy of the conjunctiva, a nonspecific vascular reaction, and follicles from an accumulation of lymphocytes may both develop in acute and chronic forms. Patients complain of itching, burning, and photophobia. This condition may be confused with other forms of conjunctivitis, particularly virus infection, microbiallergic conjunctivitis, and drug irritation of the conjunctiva. If the allergen can be determined and avoided, permanent relief may be obtained, although patients may develop new allergies and suffer a recurrence of symptoms. Vasoconstrictors, antihistamines, and topical corticosteroid preparations are helpful in treatment.

Contact Allergy. Contact dermatoconjunctivitis does not depend on a personal or family history of atopy. Among the allergens responsible are locally applied drugs (Table 6-1), cosmetics, industrial chemicals, plastics, articles of clothing, jewelry, and other animal or vegetable products. The patient complains of severe itching. Symptoms develop one or two days after exposure. If the allergen is instilled in the eye, the allergic reaction generally begins as a conjunctivitis. The adjacent eyelids and skin are soon involved in an eczematous dermatitis whose appearance overshadows the reaction of the conjunctiva and cornea. Conjunctival scrapings typically show eosinophils and basophils after several days or weeks. When the skin surrounding the eye is the site of primary contact, there may be no conjunctivitis (Plate 10*B*). The appearance of the skin may vary from a dry wrinkling to a weeping eczema. If the allergy is

TABLE 6-1 ALLERGENIC DRUGS WHICH MAY CAUSE ALLERGIC DERMATOCONJUNCTIVITIS*

1. Local anesthetics, particularly Metycaine, Tetracaine, Butyn, Nupercaine, Larocaine
2. Antibiotics
     Neomycin
     Streptomycin
     Bacitracin
     Tetracyclines
     Chloromycetin
     Erythromycin
3. Sulfonamides
4. Mydriatic and miotic alkaloids
     Atropine
     Hyoscine
     Homatropine
5. Other ophthalmic drugs
     Mercurials
     Dionin
     Boric acid
     Zinc salts
     Argyrol
     Privine
     Furacin
     Quaternary ammonium compounds
       (Zephiran)
     Phenylephrine
6. Ophthalmic Vehicles
     Preservatives
     Ointment bases including lanolin and
       petrolatum

*From Theodore, F. H., and Schlossman, A.: Ocular Allergy. Williams & Wilkins, 1958.

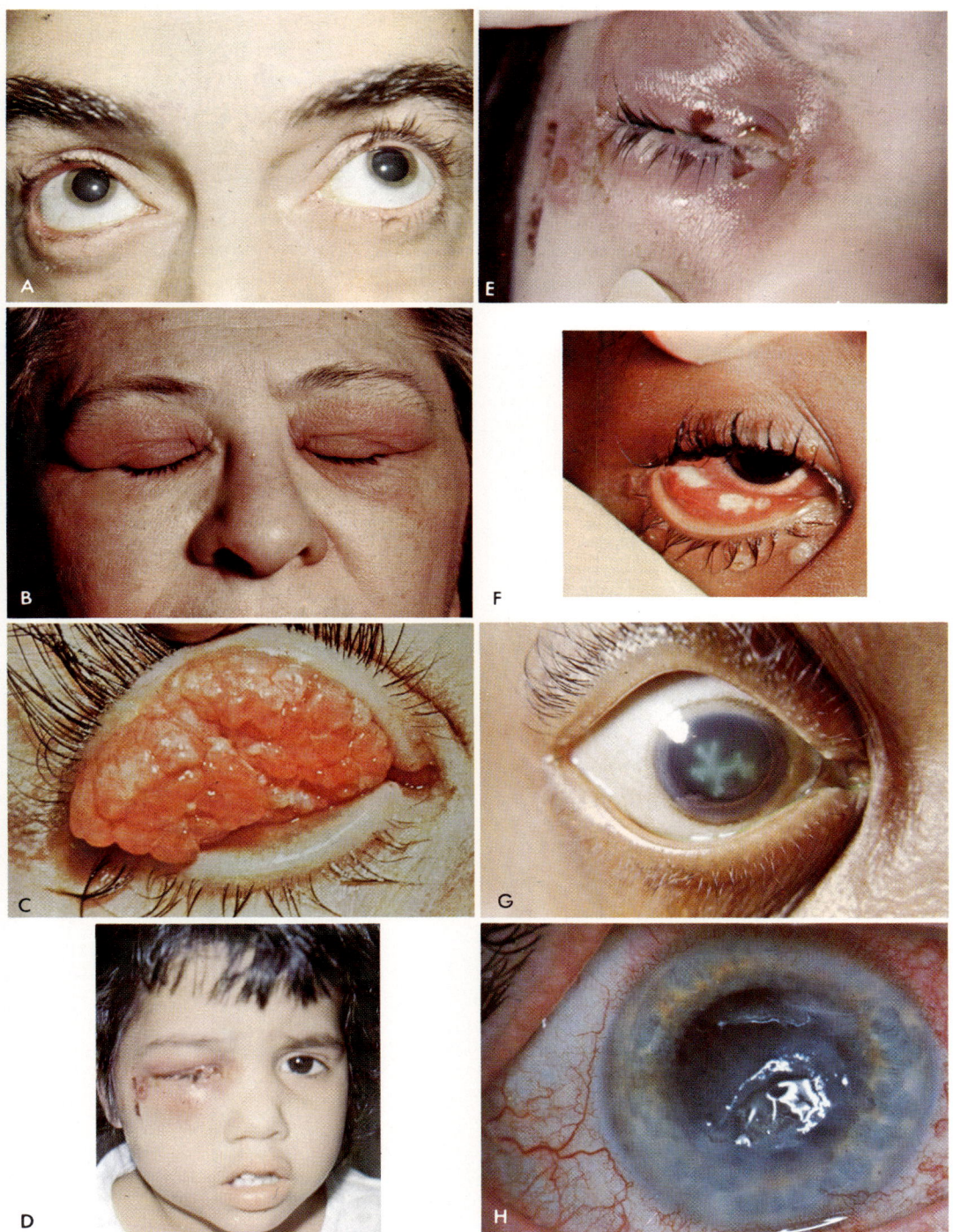

Plate 10 (*A*) Chronic blepharoconjunctivitis (common etiologies are seborrhea, infection, and allergy). (*B*) Allergic blepharitis (contact). (*C*) Vernal catarrh (palpebral type). (*D*) Ocular vaccinia with lid involvement. (*E*) Ocular vaccinia with lid involvement. (*F*) Ocular vaccinia with conjunctival involvement. (*G*) Herpes simplex (dendritic keratitis). (*H*) Herpes simplex (metaherpetical keratitis).

long-lasting, conjunctival follicles may form. This condition must be differentiated from an infectious eczematoid dermatitis due to staphylococci and also from blepharo-conjunctivitis due to drug irritation. Treatment depends upon eliminating the allergen. The local instillation of corticosteroids is helpful.

Conjunctivitis Due to Drug Irritation. Certain substances are primary irritants to the skin and conjunctiva or are degraded into end products that are irritants. The resultant clinical picture is a nonspecific, watery conjunctivitis with the lower lid and adjacent bulbar conjunctiva showing the most involvement. Follicles occur if the irritation is chronic. Epithelial scrapings show mononuclear phagocytes but no eosinophils or basophils. Results of skin patch tests with the irritants are negative. Notable offenders are atropine, eserine, pilocarpine, and synthetic miotics such as DFP, prostigmine, mecholyl, and carbachol.

Microbial Allergies of the Conjunctiva and Lids (Microbiallergic Reactions). Certain chronic infections of the conjunctiva and lids are accompanied by an allergic reaction to exotoxins or other antigens produced by bacteria, fungi, and helminths. The most important such agent is the staphylococcus. The eyelid margins are inflamed, swollen, and may show scaling and ulcers. Inflammation of the meibomian glands is also common. Frequently there is a secondary superficial punctate keratitis of the inferior half of the cornea. Cultures of the lid margins occasionally are positive for *Staphylococcus aureus*; a positive culture, however, is not necessary for diagnosis. Conjunctival scrapings are negative for eosinophils. Patients complain of dryness, burning, and crusting; itching is not a prominent symptom. Intradermal tests with staphylococcal exotoxin or staphylococcal toxoid give a strongly positive, delayed response. Treatment is difficult. Local infection should be eradicated with topical antibiotics; local corticosteroids are of value. Vasoconstrictors and antihistamines afford little relief of symptoms. Staphylococcal allergy may play a role in hordeolum (stye), chalazion, and meibomitis.

Allergies to other bacteria (including various pneumococci, streptococci, colibacillus, and pyocyaneus), fungi (Alternaria, Cladosporium, Trichophyton, and Candida), and helminths (Oxyuris) causing inflammation of the lids and conjunctiva are uncommon but have been described.

Vernal Conjunctivitis. Vernal conjunctivitis is a severe bilateral inflammation of the conjunctiva. It is a childhood disease that occurs every spring and summer, usually for several years. Warm weather triggers it, but whether or not it is an allergy to pollens or other dusts is not clear. Over 50 per cent of patients with vernal conjunctivitis have other allergic diseases of an atopic nature. Clinically there are two forms of this disease. In the *palpebral* type, large granulations occur on the upper tarsus (Plate 10C). In contrast to the round, red papillae of trachoma, they are flattened on their conjunctival surface and are packed together in angular shapes so as to resemble a cobblestone pavement. Their characteristic coloring is pale pink to gray. The conjunctiva of the lower lid has few or no granulations. Characteristically, a milky-appearing film clings to the upper tarsus and conjunctival folds. Conjunctival smears contain numerous eosinophils.

Limbal vernal conjunctivitis is less common than palpebral. It is characterized by a peculiar hypertrophy of the conjunctiva at the limbus but not on the lids. It presents the same pink or gray color as the palpebral conjunctiva. Grossly visible papillae do not occur, but the tissue is elevated over the limbal area.

It may surround the entire cornea or appear at only one sector of the border. The characteristic symptom of both forms is itching. Severe corneal ulceration, and even loss of the eye, may occur. Occasionally the palpebral form is mistaken for trachoma. The limbal type must be differentiated from phlyctenulosis. Healing is spontaneous without cicatrization or other complications. Although antibodies to grass pollen and certain other antigens are found regularly in the blood serum, symptomatic treatment with topical steroids usually will suffice; desensitization should be reserved for severe cases. Antihistamines may be of some help. Dramatic relief may be obtained by the use of air conditioning and filtered air.

IMMEDIATE ALLERGY OF THE CORNEA

Keratitis is an occasional complication of atopic blepharitis and conjunctivitis caused by pollens, dusts and certain foods. Usually this is a superficial keratitis that is recognizable on examination with slit lamp biomicroscope following fluorescein staining. Instances of deep keratitis, consisting of gray, vascularized opacities within the cornea, have been attributed to immediate allergy.

DELAYED ALLERGY OF THE CORNEA

Contact Keratitis. A superficial keratitis frequently accompanies contact allergy of the lids and conjunctiva. More severe reactions of deep keratitis and deep ulceration have been reported. In most instances treatment by local corticosteroids is effective.

Certain microorganisms are associated with specific corneal changes based on allergy. These include (1) interstitial keratitis associated with congenital syphilis and, less frequently, tuberculosis and other infections; (2) phlyctenular keratoconjunctivitis, thought to be due to sensitization to the human tubercle bacillus and, less commonly, the staphylococcus and other microbic agents; (3) disciform edema of the corneal stroma; and (4) marginal ulcers and infiltrates probably related to an allergy to bacterial exotoxins.

Interstitial Keratitis. This disease usually is a late manifestation of congenital syphilis. Its clinical features are described elsewhere (p. 193). There is considerable evidence for an allergic mechanism: similar lesions can be produced experimentally by allergic techniques; antiluetic therapy is ineffective, whereas corticosteroid treatment frequently is followed by improvement; and the lesion occasionally occurs following a Herxheimer reaction during the course of systemic antiluetic therapy. It is postulated that spirochetal material enters the cornea during the intrauterine infection. Subsequently antigenic material from the blood enters the cornea and produces a local allergic response that results in the clinical picture of interstitial keratitis. It has also been suggested that prenatal syphilitic infection alters the cornea, causing it to be sensitive to antigens that normally do not cause an allergic reaction.

Phlyctenular Keratoconjunctivitis (Phlyctenulosis). This disease often is the result of sensitization to the human tubercle bacillus; less commonly it arises from allergy to the staphylococcus. Also, there are well documented cases of phlyctenular disease associated with gonococcus, coccidioidomycosis, moniliasis, leishmaniasis, trypanosomiasis, ascariosis, and helminthiasis. Phlyctenules have been produced experimentally in animals by numerous allergic methods in which many different antigens were used.

Phlyctenular keratitis may develop in the cornea primarily, although usually it spreads to the cornea from the conjunctiva. The limbus is the favorite site of the phlycten, a small, gray nodule elevated above the surface of the superficial layers of the cornea (Fig. 6-1). The epithelium over a phlycten breaks down, forming a shallow ulcer that may clear up without scar formation. Usually, however, as the peripheral portion heals, the ulcer migrates toward the center of the cornea. As it does, it carries with it a leash of blood vessels from the conjunctiva across the limbus. This is often termed a *fascicular keratitis*. Nodular corneal scars may occasionally result, and are referred to in the literature as Salzmann's nodular dystrophy.

When numerous phlyctenules have af-

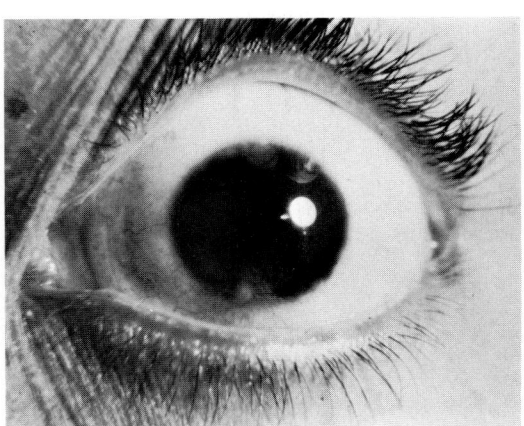

Figure 6-1 Phlyctenular keratoconjunctivitis.

fected the cornea, vascularization may be seen around the entire periphery of the cornea and extending toward the center. This condition is known as a *phlyctenular pannus*. It is distinguished from trachomatous pannus in that it shows no predilection for the upper segment of the cornea. At any time secondary infection of the ulcer possibly may result in loss of the eye. Phlyctenular conjunctivitis usually responds to treatment with local corticosteroids. The patient's general physical condition should be evaluated and tuberculosis looked for. In most cases antituberculous treatment does not improve the phlyctenular disease. Attention should be directed also to nutrition, especially to possible vitamin deficiency.

Disciform Edema of the Corneal Stroma. Many investigators consider this lesion to be a hypersensitivity phenomenon in which herpes simplex antigen from the epithelium unites with an antibody from the limbal vessels to produce a toxic antigen-antibody complex. Herpes simplex keratitis is discussed in detail elsewhere (p. 195). Hypersensitivity is manifested also in the subepithelial opacity of epidemic keratoconjunctivitis and other types of subepithelial opacities.

Marginal Ulcers and Infiltrates. Frequently manifestations of bacterial allergy, these often are conditions associated with chronic conjunctivitis and blepharitis. Less frequently they are the result of systemic allergy or contact sensitization. These lesions and phlyctens have many similarities. Corneal infiltrates and ulceration may result from drug allergies, especially Pontocaine hydrochloride and Butyn sulfate.

Sclera, Episclera, and Tenon's Capsule

The various types of scleritis and episcleritis have been enumerated elsewhere (p. 14). The etiology of these disorders is often difficult to determine, but attacks frequently occur in patients with an atopic history. Many types respond dramatically to local corticosteroid therapy. These factors suggest an allergic basis. Episcleritis has been reported in patients with inhalant and food allergies, especially seafood, that represent an immediate (atopic) allergy. More commonly, episcleritis and scleritis are examples of delayed types of bacterial (microbial) allergy. Chronic, severe cases often are associated with rheumatoid arthritis. They may be related to the streptococcus. Allergy associated with staphylococcus, tubercle bacillus, and other microorganisms is also a cause of scleritis and episcleritis. These disorders are frequently associated with collagen diseases (p. 226). Inflammation of Tenon's capsule is now rarely seen, but once it was a common complication of gonococcal arthritis.

Uveal Tract

ROLE OF ALLERGY IN UVEITIS

The uvea contains a high concentration of proteins, antibodies, and antigens originating elsewhere in the body. In certain experimental conditions the uvea may be seeded with immunologically competent cells. Upon later exposure to antigenic challenge, local antibody production then can occur within the uvea. Consequently the uvea may be involved in immediate allergic reactions, including antiphylaxis and the Arthus phenomenon, and in delayed allergic reactions, including hypersensitivity due to microbial allergy. Although it is generally accepted that allergy is an important factor in many cases of uveitis, the mechanisms of uveal allergy are extremely complex and, in most clinical situations, not well understood.

Immediate Allergy Causing Uveitis. Immediate allergy of the uvea (anaphylactic and atopic reactions) is rare. When it does occur, it results in a nongranulomatous uveitis, usually an iritis. An example of this is acute iridocyclitis occurring with serum sickness: a bilateral, thick, fibrinous exudate is seen in the anterior chamber within 24 hours after the injection. Angioneurotic edema of the eye may also be accompanied by severe iritis. In addition, there have been reports of uveal inflammation from pollen and other inhalants and foods.

Delayed Allergy in Nongranulomatous Uveitis. In considering the role of microorganisms in uveitis, it must be kept in mind that these organisms may produce disease both by their primary cytopathogenic effects and by serving as a source of sensitizing antigens. The importance of streptococcal allergy as a cause of acute iritis has received much attention. The incidence and significance of elevated antistreptolysin titers and of intradermal streptococci sensitivity in patients with nongranulomatous uveitis is a matter of considerable dispute. Also open to question is the usefulness of desensitization injections with specific streptococcal antigen in the treatment of nongranulomatous uveitis. Delayed allergy, however, does appear to be a factor in the severe iritis seen in gonorrhea. Bacteria have been reported as acting as antigens in allergic iritis. Among them are *Bacillus pyocyaneus,* pneumococcus, staphylococcus, and *Bacillus coli.* It also has been suggested that delayed allergy is a factor in glaucomato-cyclitic crises (p. 358).

Delayed Allergy in Granulomatous Uveitis. In earlier years tuberculous infection was cited as the major cause of granulomatous uveitis. This diagnosis is made less frequently now. It is well established that tuberculous infection of the eye may cause granulomatous uveitis and that the allergic reaction in the ocular tissues is an important cause of the pathologic changes that ensue. Desensitization with tuberculin has been stated by some authors as beneficial and by others as dangerous to patients with supposed tuberculosis-related uveitis.

In ocular toxoplasmosis the infecting parasites are contained in pseudocysts within the retina. A relapse causes an acute edematous reaction over a large area of the retina. This is thought to be the result of a hypersensitive tissue reaction to the antigenic products escaping from ruptured pseudocysts (pp. 142 and 200).

Sympathetic Uveitis. Sympathetic uveitis is a bilateral, granulomatous inflammation that occurs after perforating trauma to the eyes. Its precise etiology is unknown. Most authors presently feel that it is at least partly an allergic phenomenon, and possibly an autoallergic condition against uveal pigment (p. 373).

Phacoanaphylactic Endophthalmitis. This condition is considered to be a form of autosensitivity to lens protein. The patient is sensitized to lens protein by rupture of the lens capsule and escape of lens material into the aqueous. After a latent period ranging from several weeks to months, a severe inflammation occurs around the lens matter in the anterior chamber. In some cases the patient is sensitized to lens protein as the result of an operation or injury to one eye, and phacoanaphylactic endophthalmitis occurs after subsequent surgery or trauma to the other eye. When this condition is diagnosed, the lens in the inflamed eye should be completely removed. Phacoanaphylactic endophthalmitis has been produced experimentally. The condition bears many similarities to sympathetic uveitis and frequently coexists with it.

Allergy of the Retina and Optic Nerve

Well documented instances of allergic reactions of the retina and optic nerve are rare. Edema of the retina and optic nerve have been described in serum sickness. Retinal edema, superficial and deep retinal hemorrhages, and blurring of the optic disc have been attributed to anaphylactic and atopic reactions caused by food, pollens, and drugs, including sulfonamide and local anesthetics. Edema of the retina with hemorrhages, sheathing of vessels, and retinal bulbar neuritis have been described after injection of tuberculin and rabies vaccination.

OCULAR MANIFESTATIONS OF SYSTEMIC INFECTIONS

The orbital contents are vulnerable to numerous infections. This section first describes ocular changes in systemic infections. Then discussed in detail are the primarily localized eye infections that were introduced in the chapter on ophthalmic entities.

Systemic Bacterial Infections

Mycobacteria ("Acid-Fast" Bacilli). This group of rod-shaped bacteria includes

M. tuberculosis and *M. leprae,* species causing chronic granulomatous disease. Other agents that cause granulomatous inflammation include syphilis, sarcoidosis, brucellosis, yaws, lymphogranuloma inguinale, blastomycosis, sporotrichosis, histoplasmosis, toxoplasmosis, and certain virus infections.

TUBERCULOSIS. Ocular involvement usually is related to pulmonary or generalized tuberculosis. Primary tuberculosis of the eye and adnexa is rare. Tuberculosis involving the lids may occur as *lupus vulgaris.* Usually this is an extension of infection on the face. The lesions characteristically are nodules with ulcerated scars in the center. Lupus vulgaris usually begins early in childhood, becomes chronic, and leads to severe ectropion and damage to the cornea.

The lacrimal sac also is involved by spread of infection from adjacent structures. Drainage is impaired and fistulas may form. Primary infection of the conjunctiva results in small, indolent ulcers, usually on the tarsus or in the fornix. Nodules are less commonly seen. Interstitial keratitis, usually the result of congenital syphilis, may be caused by tuberculosis. Phlyctenular keratoconjunctivitis is believed to be an allergic response of the cornea to tuberculoprotein and other foreign proteins.

Granulomatous uveitis is the ocular lesion most frequently attributed to tuberculosis. Authorities once thought that uveitis resulted from metastasis of the organism to the eye from an involved hilar gland or some other reservoir of infection. This now seems unlikely. First, tuberculous uveitis is rare in patients with active pulmonary disease. Presumptive tuberculous uveitis usually is found in apparently healthy individuals for whom there is no history of active pulmonary disease, but in whom there is x-ray evidence of healed pulmonary tuberculous lesions. Second, in many enucleated eyes clinically diagnosed to have tuberculous uveitis, no acid-fast organisms were found. Some of these eyes contained toxoplasma and nematodes.

Some authorities now believe that hypersensitivity may be the principal mechanism of tuberculous uveitis. It seems certain that tuberculosis is not as important a cause of chronic uveitis as previously claimed.

Tuberculous iridocyclitis is characterized by yellow or white, fatty deposits on the posterior surface of the cornea (called mutton-fat keratic precipitates); small, white nodules in the iris stroma or at the pupillary margin (Koeppe's nodules); and extensive posterior synechiae. Diffuse tuberculous involvement of the choroid is seen in association with the iridocyclitis. Initially a fine haze of vitreous opacities may be present; later this may progress to a dense cloud, obscuring the fundus. One or more exudative patches develop, frequently with satellite lesions around them. After necrosis and healing, the final picture appears as a severe pigmentary disturbance, with gliosis and exposed choroidal vessels. A secondary cataract frequently is present. A solitary tubercle of the choroid, appearing as a sharply outlined, elevated, white or gray mass is more rare. In the terminal stages of generalized miliary tuberculosis, multiple tubercles may be seen in the choroid as well as in the iris and ciliary body. In all forms of tuberculous choroiditis the retina is involved.

Eales' disease is a syndrome characterized by recurrent retinal and vitreous hemorrhages, and abnormalities of vessels such as perivascular sheathing. Possible causes are tuberculosis, sickle cell disease, obscure vasculitis, and others. Optic neuritis is sometimes seen as a result of tuberculous meningitis. Optic atrophy may occur after adhesive arachnoiditis and internal hydrocephalus.

The following findings, in addition to the clinical picture, would support the diagnosis of ocular tuberculosis: isolation of *M. tuberculosis* from the sputum, gastric washings, or urine; x-ray evidence of current or past infection with tuberculosis; and a strongly positive tuberculin test. The disease is treated by chemotherapy, including streptomycin, aminosalicylic acid and isoniazid. If iritis is present, topical mydriatics and corticosteroids are useful. Systemic steroids must be used with extreme caution because of the danger of reactivating pulmonary tuberculosis. Desensitization with tuberculin, once the principal therapy for uveitis that was suspected to be of tuberculous origin, is used infrequently.

LEPROSY. The two types of this disease

are lepromatous and tuberculoid. About 90 per cent of lepromatous lepers have some ocular complications and about 30 per cent are blind. In contrast, eye involvement is rare in the tuberculoid type. Characteristically in lepromatous leprosy, red, elevated nodules of various sizes affect the brow and upper lid, and the hair is lost from these sites. Conjunctival lesions may be seen. Interstitial or superficial keratitis may be accompanied with invasion of the cornea by blood vessels and subsequent scarring. Large granulomas (lepromas) eventually may cover the entire cornea and parts of the sclera. White, chalklike nodules may be found on the iris surface. In addition to the various systemic drugs used to treat this disease, the keratitis and uveitis should be treated by local therapy.

Brucellosis. Brucellosis (undulant fever) is caused by small, aerobic, gram-negative coccobacilli. Clinically an acute septicemic phase is followed by a chronic stage associated with intermittent, low grade fever, lassitude, fatigue, and pain in the muscles and joints. An infrequent complication is a nodular iritis with lesions at the pupillary border of the iris and mutton-fat deposits on the posterior surface of the cornea. The diagnosis should be suspected when there is a history of raw milk ingestion. Nummular keratitis, consisting of discrete stromal infiltrates, has been attributed to brucellosis.

The Pasteurellae. These are short, gram-negative rods that show bipolar staining by special methods. Those that produce serious disease in man are *P. tularensis* (tularemia) and *P. pestis* (plague).

TULAREMIA. Parinaud's oculoglandular syndrome is one of the main clinical types of tularemia and results from the infecting organism contaminating the conjunctiva. After an incubation period of from one day to two weeks, single or multiple necrotic papules appear, usually in the lower cul-de-sac. A generalized conjunctivitis follows, lasting about four weeks, with associated enlargement and tenderness of the ipsilateral preauricular lymph nodes. The lids commonly are swollen and reddened. The disease usually is confined to the eye for about one week before systemic symptoms occur. Streptomycin and the broad spectrum antibiotics are effective in treatment. Parinaud's oculoglandular syndrome may be produced by other agents (pp. 8 to 9).

PLAGUE. The rare instances of ocular involvement in this disease probably result from bacterial metastasis. Conjunctivitis, keratitis, corneal ulceration, and uveitis have been described.

The Clostridia. These are anaerobic, gram-positive rods found in the soil and in the feces of animals. The types that cause disease in man are *C. botulinum* (botulism), *C. tetani* (tetanus), and several others that cause gas gangrene and enterotoxemias. Secondary infection of the eye and adnexa by anaerobic organisms following injury is rare because of the rich blood supply in these areas.

BOTULISM. Ocular signs may be one of the first indications of this disease. These include loss of accommodation, extraocular muscle palsies accompanied by diplopia, paralytic mydriasis, nystagmus, loss of light reflex, and ptosis of the lid.

TETANUS. Instances of a cephalic local tetanus after penetrating wounds of the lid or eyeball have been described. The first symptoms are spasms of the ocular muscles, particularly the orbicularis muscle.

Streptococci. These are gram-positive microorganisms characteristically arranged in chains. A number of distinct disease processes are associated with streptococci infections: *erysipelas* is an acute, recurrent infection of the skin with massive edema and a rapidly advancing margin. When the lids are involved, they become extremely swollen, and the skin is shiny, red, and raised, with sharply defined borders. Suppurative vesicles may form on the surface and gangrene of the lid may develop. During this disease a conjunctivitis is common, and the cornea may become involved as well. Penicillin is the antibiotic of choice in treatment, but streptomycin and tetracycline also are effective.

In *scarlet fever*, as in most febrile conditions, a mild catarrhal conjunctivitis is usual. In patients with *glomerulonephritis* the retina may later show hypertensive retinopathy. *Streptococcus* viridans accounts for approximately 50 per cent of *subacute* or *chronic bacterial endocarditis*. Numerous petechial conjunctival hemorrhages are common. Flame-shaped retinal hemorrhages, extravasations with white centers (Roth's spots), and similar white spots scattered over the retina may occur. Papilledema and occlusion of the central retinal artery by emboli are additional complications.

Neisseriae. These are gram-negative cocci containing two important human pathogens: *N. gonorrhoeae* (gonococcus) and *N. meningitidis* (meningococcus).

GONOCOCCUS. A description of gonorrheal conjunctivitis is given elsewhere in this book (p. 147). In addition to exogenous infection, gonococci may affect the eye through hypersensitivity phenomenon from other sites of infection or conceivably through metastatic infection. In gonorrheal iritis the anterior chamber characteristically fills rapidly with exudate that coagulates and obscures the iris. A history of a previous attack of gonorrhea with a subsequent migratory arthritis that affects the knees, wrists, or ankles usually can be obtained from infected individuals, most of whom are males. The treatment of acute iritis should be employed along with systemic antigonococcal therapy, particularly penicillin.

Reiter's disease (syndrome) is characterized by the simultaneous inflammation of the eyes (usually with conjunctivitis or keratitis), joints, and urogenital tract, similar to the complications of gonorrhea. During the active disease, however, there is an absence of gonococci in the urethral discharge and no increase in the gonococcal complement fixation titer. Reiter's disease may be of viral etiology, but this has not been confirmed.

MENINGOCOCCUS. A conjunctivitis with petechiae and ecchymosis is a common complication of meningococcal meningitis. Endophthalmitis and panophthalmitis resulting from intraocular invasion have been described. The sulfonamides are particularly effective.

Pertussis. Severe paroxysms of coughing may cause hemorrhages in the lids and subconjunctiva. Occasionally orbital hemorrhages result in unilateral exophthalmos. Other members of this genus of short, gram-negative bacilli are important causative agents of conjunctivitis. They include *Haemophilus aegyptius* (Koch-Weeks bacillus),

Moraxella lacunata (the diplobacillus of Morax-Axenfeld), and *Moraxella liquefaciens*.

Diphtheria. A gram-positive, nonmotile rod with a club-shaped end, *Corynebacterium diphtheriae*, causes this acute infectious disease. The bacilli may affect the conjunctiva in a patient suffering from throat infection, or ocular infection may occur as an isolated phenomenon. The eyelids are red, swollen, and painful. The preauricular and cervical nodes are enlarged. There is a profuse exudation from the cul-de-sac, and when the lids are everted, membranes are observed over the inner surfaces. Any attempt to remove these membranes usually results in raw, bleeding areas. The entire thickness of the lid may be involved, and necrosis may ensue. Extraocular muscle palsies are frequent, especially permanent paralysis of accommodation, which usually is the sole ocular residuum of the disease. The systemic disease generally is treated by large doses of diphtheria antitoxin. Antibiotics are effective against *C. diphtheriae*, but do not neutralize the toxin. Local antibiotics and antitoxin are advised in the treatment of the conjunctivitis.

Corynebacterium xerose is a nonpathogenic member of the same genus. It frequently is present in the normal conjunctival sac, but it has no pathologic significance.

Anthrax. Primarily a disease of sheep, cattle, and horses, anthrax is caused by *Bacillus anthracis*, a large, gram-positive rod occurring in chains. Infection usually results from spores entering injured skin or mucous membranes. The two clinical forms are a malignant pustule and edema caused by anthrax. The history usually reveals that the patient has handled animal hides. About one third of the cases are fatal. The absence of pain in anthrax associated with edema distinguishes it from swelling caused by cellulitis. Although anthrax sometimes is confused with an ordinary carbuncle, its pustule has a black center with surrounding vesicles, and a smear from the base of the ulcer will reveal the anthrax bacillus. The organism is sensitive to sulfonamides and antibiotics.

Other Bacterial Infections. In severe cases of typhoid fever, edema of the optic disc and surrounding retina, retinal hemorrhages, and Roth's spots occasionally are observed at the height of the disease. These changes commonly are seen in extremely toxic states resulting from other causes. Metastatic choroiditis, iritis, and paralysis of the sixth nerve also have been described in typhoid fever.

Glanders, primarily a disease of horses, is caused by *Malleomyces mallei.* When transmitted to man, granulomatous and ulcerative lesions result. Ocular involvement takes the form of a conjunctivitis which may resemble the oculoglandular syndrome of Parinaud or cellulitis. Abscesses of the lid and orbit may occur.

Systemic Spirochetal Infections

Syphilis. Ocular involvement may result from congenital syphilis (infection of the fetus in utero) or from acquired syphilis.

CONGENITAL SYPHILIS. About 70 per cent of children with congenital syphilis have ocular involvement. The most characteristic lesion is interstitial keratitis. This abnormality, together with typical changes in the teeth and deafness, form Hutchinson's triad. The keratitis, however, may be the only physical sign of the syphilitic condition.

Interstitial keratitis is a bilateral inflammation marked by edema, infiltration, and vascularization of the deep layers of the cornea. The first sign is a faint zone of opacity in the middle layers of the stroma ("salmon patch"). Usually only a part of the cornea, extending in from the limbus, is involved. Associated with this is a mild, limbal, ciliary flush. On examination with the slit lamp biomicroscope the corneal epithelium shows early edema (bedewing). Associated symptoms are pain, lacrimation, and photophobia. Within a few days, straight brushlike vessels grow from a sector of, or from the entire, limbus into the deepest layers of the cornea. The cornea becomes diffusely cloudy and may even become opaque. There is a coincident increase in the severity of the iridocyclitis that is evidenced by a marked ciliary flush, small pupil, congestion of the iris vessels, and cloudy aqueous. Sometimes secondary glaucoma develops. The active stage lasts from six weeks to a few months.

Subsequently the cornea slowly clears from the periphery toward the center. Vessels remain in the cornea throughout life.

They may become empty of blood and then are visible only with the slit lamp biomicroscope. Their presence can indicate a previous attack of interstitial keratitis in a patient who shows no other changes.

Interstitial keratitis usually is observed between the second year of life and puberty. Diagnosis is based on the eye findings and other stigmata of congenital syphilis together with positive serologic results from syphilis. Interstitial keratitis can occur from acquired syphilis or as a complication of tuberculosis, leprosy, and other diseases. Luetic interstitial keratitis is treated by the vigorous administration of penicillin or other antiluetic agents and corticosteroids, and mydriatics. The prognosis for useful vision generally is good. When there is severe residual corneal scarring, corneal transplantation may be indicated.

In addition to iridocyclitis, a choroiditis usually occurs in syphilis. Two forms are seen: the so-called "salt and pepper" fundus, having red or yellow spots with fine pigment granules scattered throughout the periphery, and, less commonly, circumscribed lesions in which clumps of choroidal pigment and heavy, white scars are seen throughout the fundus. The choroiditis probably is active very early in life, but usually the lesions are not observed until later in life when the inflammation has regressed.

Other ocular findings of congenital syphilis include periostitis of the orbital ridge, lesions deep in the orbit, swelling and redness of the lids, conjunctivitis, paresis of ocular muscles, chronic dacryoadenitis, retrobulbar neuritis, and optic atrophy. There may be pupillary abnormalities, but the Argyll Robertson phenomenon rarely is encountered in congenital syphilis.

ACQUIRED SYPHILIS. Before the era of serologic testing, syphilis was considered a major cause of disseminated choroiditis. Presently it is relatively infrequent that uveitis of any type can be demonstrated from this etiology.

A hyperemia (roseola) of the iris, unassociated with visual disturbance or other ocular inflammation, occurs in the early stage of secondary syphilis. More severe involvement of the uveal tract, particularly the iris, occurs in the late secondary and tertiary stages. In addition to the usual signs of acute iritis, an irregularly distributed hyperemia of the iris and the formation of fleshy, pink, inflammatory nodules in the sphincter region of the iris are characteristic. Disseminated choroiditis is commonly seen, usually with considerable retinal involvement; this results in a vasculitis with residual sheathing of the retinal vessels, particularly of the veins. Secondary pigmentary degeneration, an additional manifestation of acquired syphilis, probably is related to vascular inflammation. Optic atrophy occurs as a complication of tabes dorsalis (p. 311).

Macular, papular, or pustular lesions or gummas may affect the lids in syphilis. Interstitial keratitis occurs in fewer than 3 per cent of patients with acquired syphilis. Purulent, yellow infiltrates, deep in the cornea and associated with a hypopyon, also may develop. An episcleritis or scleritis may accompany other syphilitic ocular lesions.

Syphilis is diagnosed by clinical findings and positive serologic studies. The most sensitive of these is the fluorescent treponemal antibody absorption test (FTA-ABS). A recently developed technique whereby treponema can sometimes be identified in the aqueous by means of the fluorescent antibody technique may prove useful. Antisyphilitic agents should be used together with systemic and local corticosteroids and mydriatics, as indicated for ocular inflammation.

Other Spirochetal Diseases. Yaws, a chronic nonvenereal, spirochetal *(Treponema pertenue)* infection of tropical regions may be accompanied by granulomatous involvement of the eyelids, conjunctivitis, keratitis, and ocular muscle involvement. *Weil's disease* is caused by the *Leptospira icterohaemorrhagiae.* It produces an intense conjunctival dilatation of blood vessels with subconjunctival hemorrhages. Jaundice may discolor the sclera. *Relapsing fever,* which results from the *Borrelia recurrentis,* is associated with iridocyclitis, optic atrophy, and paralysis of the ocular muscles.

Variola and Vaccinia. These are two antigenically related but distinct viruses. Before smallpox vaccination was introduced, variola was an important cause of blindness. Ocular complications included involvement of the eyelids by cutaneous eruption, conjunctivitis, hypopyon ulcers, and, less commonly, iritis, choroiditis, and vitreous opacities.

Following smallpox vaccination, the eye sometimes is inoculated accidentally with vaccinia, which results in a pustular eruption on the lids (Plate 10D, E) that is frequently accompanied by enlarged preauricular glands and fever. Primary infection of the conjunctiva (Plate 10F) and cornea also may occur. In normal individuals, lesions of the lids and conjunctiva heal without sequelae, but corneal involvement may lead to loss of vision. In patients with agammaglobulinemia, vaccinia may be fatal. Patients are treated with topical antibiotics and sulfonamides (to prevent secondary infection), 5-iodo-deoxyuridine (IDU), together with vaccinia hyperimmune globulin.

The Herpesvirus Group. Three members of this group of viruses are pathogenic for man: *Herpesvirus hominis,* the virus of herpes simplex; varicella-herpes zoster virus, and *Herpesvirus simiae* (B virus). The last of these is found in "normal" monkeys, but when transmitted to man causes fatal central nervous system disease.

HERPES SIMPLEX. Primary infection with herpes simplex virus occurs in nonimmune individuals and usually results in a subclinical disease. Rarely acute keratoconjunctivitis occurs, with the initial infection frequently associated with multiple cold sores of the face. Ocular findings are a branching or dendritic ulcer on the cornea and an acute follicular conjunctivitis. Primary herpetic keratoconjunctivitis is self-limited, and the cornea usually heals without scarring.

Secondary or *recurrent* herpes simplex develops in patients who have neutralizing antibodies from a previous primary infection. About 90 per cent of adults have had herpes simplex infection and carry the virus in an inactive state. Recurrent infection may be precipitated by a wide range of

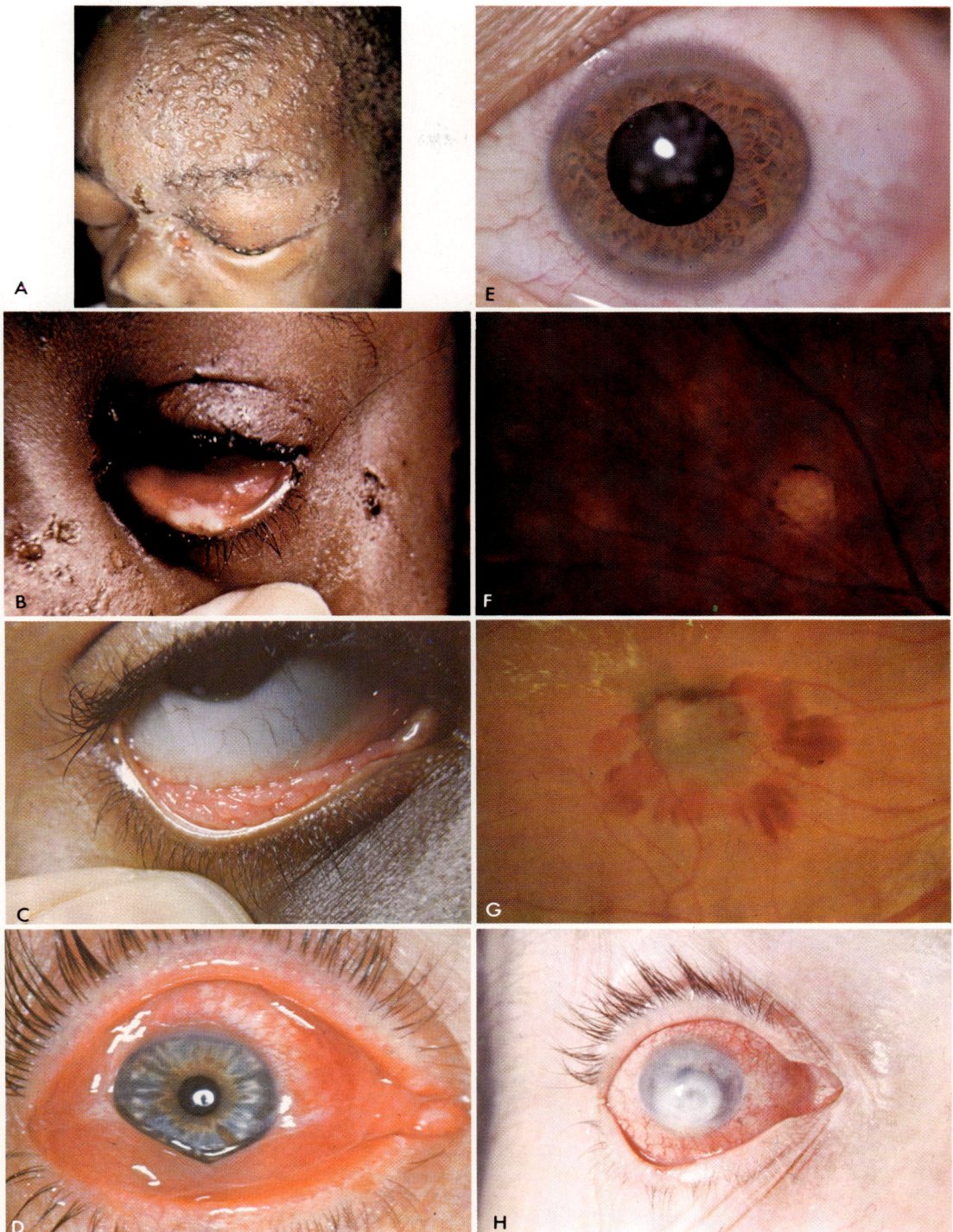

Plate 11 *(A)* Herpes zoster ophthalmicus (acute). *(B)* Varicella with ocular involvement. *(C)* Follicular conjunctivitis. *(D)* Acute epidemic keratoconjunctivitis showing conjunctival inflammation and corneal infiltrates. *(E)* Chronic epidemic keratoconjunctivitis showing corneal infiltrates. *(F)* Punched-out lesion in fundus of patient with presumed histoplasmosis chorioretinitis. *(G)* Active chorioretinitis presumed related to histoplasmosis. *(H)* Central corneal ulcer.

stimuli and usually takes the form of mild vesicular eruptions of the skin or mucous membranes. The skin of the lids, the conjunctiva, and the cornea may be affected; the corneal lesions are the most serious. The diagnosis usually can be made by the appearance of the corneal ulcer, a dendritic figure (Plate 10G). The lesions, however, are sometimes star-shaped, linear, or punctate. The patient usually complains of photophobia, tearing, and pain. A history of recent cold sores often can be obtained. Loss of corneal sensitivity is an important sign. Under the slit lamp biomicroscope the dendritic lesions appear to be composed of vesicles in the corneal epithelium. These subsequently rupture, whereupon the involved area stains with fluorescein. The dendritic figure may become more diffuse and assume a "geographic" pattern. A hypopyon occasionally develops.

The dendritic figure and corneal anesthesia are pathognomonic. The disease may be confirmed in the laboratory by isolating the virus in tissue culture or by staining scrapings from the ulcer with fluorescein-labeled antibody. For treatment, infected cells must be removed mechanically or cauterized chemically. Half strength tincture of iodine or ether has long been effectively used for this purpose. The topical use of anticancer chemotherapeutic agents (5-iododeoxyuridine, cytosine arabinoside, and 5-fluorouridine deoxyribose) may also be helpful. Corticosteroids are contraindicated in the therapy of dendritic lesions and may cause the virus to penetrate the corneal stroma with eventual loss of the eye. Dendritic keratitis runs an uncertain course and often heals without scars even when untreated.

However, the virus may, after repeated attacks, cause disciform keratitis, a localized chronic inflammation of the corneal stroma characterized by a discoid opacity. Loss of corneal stroma and corneal ulceration may result in perforation and loss of the eye. An eye with a perforated cornea may be saved with a conjunctival flap to cover the hole or with a keratoplasty. Chronic lesions or repeated attacks may leave a shallow ulcer in an anesthetic cornea (Plate 10H). This has been termed "trophic keratitis" and "metaherpes" by different authors. Persistent iridocyclitis or secondary glaucoma is often associated.

HERPES ZOSTER. When this infection involves the ophthalmic, or first division, of the trigeminal nerve, it is called herpes zoster ophthalmicus (Plate 11A). Typically a vesicular rash on an erythematous base occurs along the first division of the fifth nerve. The eruption usually does not cross the midline. Lancinating pain may precede the rash by 24 to 48 hours. The skin over the tip of the nose is supplied by the nasociliary branch of the fifth nerve, and lesions in this area frequently are followed by diffuse ocular inflammation.

The eye shows deep inflammation (iridocyclitis). Corneal involvement (keratitis) at times predominates. Typically the cornea is edematous, and subepithelial infiltrates are present. Deep stroma infiltrates may occur and coalesce to form a deep disciform keratitis. Corneal sensation is lost, never to recover fully. These changes leave the cornea vulnerable to secondary infection and sequelae such as ulceration with scarring, vascularization, and even perforation. The conjunctiva is hyperemic. Scleritis, and secondary glaucoma are frequent. Optic neuritis and ocular muscle paralysis also may occur.

The diagnosis is made from clinical findings. Systemic ACTH or corticosteroid therapy is beneficial. Local steroids also are of value. The disease usually occurs in older people and may be associated with systemic diseases such as tabes dorsalis, tuberculosis, or lymphoma. The course ranges from days to months. The patient should be followed carefully if the globe is involved.

Zoster and varicella may result from the same virus. Small papular lesions on the lid margin, conjunctiva, or limbus are sometimes seen in chickenpox (Plate 11B). Superficial punctate keratitis, as well as interstitial and disciform keratitis, also have been reported in this disease. Symptoms are treated.

Infectious Mononucleosis. This disease, recently proved to be of viral origin, usually affects young adults. Principal signs and symptoms are malaise, fever, lymphadenopathy, lymphocytosis, and an elevated titer of sheep cell agglutinins in the serum.

Conjunctivitis, edema of the eyelids, photophobia, and ocular pain frequently accompany its onset. An associated dacryocystitis and dacryoadenitis have been reported in some epidemics. Less frequent eye signs include mild, nongranulomatous uveitis, retinal periphlebitis, and a benign type of optic neuritis. Ocular involvement usually resolves without sequelae.

Lymphogranuloma Venereum. This viral infection is characterized by genital or anorectal lesions with involvement of the lymphatic system and late fibrotic changes. Among the ocular complications that occur occasionally, the most common is a conjunctivitis associated with preauricular adenopathy. The resulting clinical picture is indistinguishable from the oculoglandular syndrome of Parinaud. Keratitis, consisting of infiltrates localized within the upper, and less often the lower, limbus, may occur (Fig. 6-2). Superficial neovascularization of the cornea over the area of keratitis—dense and pink in appearance—is characteristic. It resembles an epaulet extending onto the cornea from the limbus. Diagnosis may be made by virus isolation, elementary body identification in infected material, Frei intradermal skin testing, and complement fixation testing. The virus may have some sensitivity to sulfonamides and broad spectrum antibiotics.

Cat-Scratch Fever. This infection, probably of viral etiology, results in enlargement of the regional lymph nodes in the area of a cat scratch. A droplet type of transmission

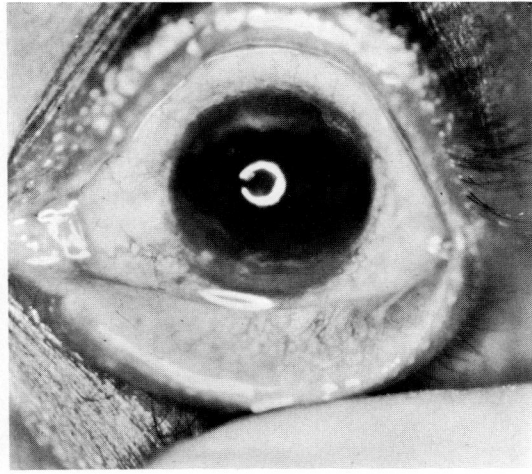

Figure 6-2 Lymphogranuloma venereum keratitis.

also has been described. Ocular involvement takes the form of Parinaud's oculoglandular syndrome, with monocular conjunctivitis and preauricular adenopathy. Inflammation of the lymph nodes may recede spontaneously or may progress to sterile suppuration. The disease is associated with malaise and moderate fever; in rare instances, encephalitis may occur. Diagnosis is made by skin testing with an antigen prepared from an infected lymph node. Primarily, symptoms are treated.

Adenovirus Conjunctivitis. Several types of adenovirus cause hyperemia and follicle formation of the bulbar and the palpebral conjunctiva (Plate 11C), serous exudation, excess lacrimation, and frequently edema of the conjunctiva of one or both eyes. Commonly, there is associated respiratory tract infection, fever, lymphadenopathy, headache, and malaise. The illness usually lasts from two to four weeks and recovery generally is complete. Antibacterial therapy may be used to prevent secondary infections. Two distinct types of adenovirus conjunctivitis, each with a distinct symptomatic complex, have been described: pharyngoconjunctival fever (PCF) and epidemic keratoconjunctivitis (EKC).

PHARYNGOCONJUNCTIVAL FEVER. This disorder is recognized by its characteristic triad of symptoms: pharyngitis, conjunctivitis, and fever. It is seen in both epidemic form and sporadic cases. Epidemics occur during the summer and early fall and involve children; transmission appears to be related to swimming pools. Secondary transmission to adults may occur. Sporadic cases involve all age groups. The conjunctivitis is an acute follicular type, with the follicles predominantly in the lower fornix and inferior tarsal conjunctiva. A transient and mild epithelial keratitis may occur. The preauricular nodes usually can be palpated. Symptoms persist from 7 to 10 days. Conjunctival scrapings, as in other types of acute follicular conjunctivitis, contain many mononuclear cells and no inclusion bodies. Serologic studies usually indicate adenovirus type 3 to be the agent.

EPIDEMIC KERATOCONJUNCTIVITIS (EKC). The clinical findings associated with this disorder are a severe, acute follicular conjunctivitis (Plate 11*D*); swollen, tender, and sometimes grossly visible ipsilateral preauricular lymph nodes, which develop a few days after the conjunctivitis; and a keratitis characterized by small, round subepithelial infiltrates that usually appear about 7 to 10 days after the onset of the conjunctivitis and may persist causing severe discomfort for months (Plate 11*E*). Local steroids at this stage are helpful in alleviating symptoms. EKC is the most se-vere type of adenovirus conjunctivitis. A conjunctival pseudomembrane develops in about one third of affected patients, and scarring of the cornea may occur. Mild, influenza-like symptoms occur occasionally in children. Many minor epidemics have been traced to contaminated instruments and solutions in hospitals, clinics, and physicians' offices. Adenovirus type 8 is the principal etiologic agent. Antibiotics are not effective against this agent but help to sup-press secondary bacterial infection.

Other Viral Diseases. Ocular complica-tions of rubella, cytomegalic inclusion dis-ease, measles, and mumps are discussed in

TABLE 6-2   SUPPLEMENTARY LIST OF OCULAR COMPLICATIONS IN SELECTED SYSTEMIC VIRAL INFECTIONS

Viral Diseases	Possible Ocular Manifestations
Measles (rubeola)	Koplik's spots on the caruncle and semi-lunar fold; conjunctival injection and mucoid discharge; punctate staining of cornea with photophobia; (rare): metastatic uveitis, optic neuritis, esotropia.
Congenital rubella	Microphthalmos, glaucoma, corneal edema, aniridia and iris atrophy, cataract, retinopathy, optic atrophy, nystagmus.
Postnatal rubella	Mild catarrhal conjunctivitis.
Mumps	Dacryoadenitis, conjunctivitis, keratitis; (rare): episcleritis, uveitis, optic neuritis, retrobulbar neuritis, thrombosis of the central retinal artery, paresis of the internal and external ocular muscles.
Cytomegalic inclusion disease	Uveitis and retinitis; cararact.
Verrucae (warts)	Cutaneous lesions, conjunctivitis, keratitis (secondary to mechanical irritation from lesions at lid margin).
Newcastle disease	Follicular conjunctivitis, superficial punctate keratitis, preauricular lymphadenopathy.
Yellow fever	Hemorrhages of eyelids or conjunctiva, scleral jaundice.
Rift Valley fever	Chorioretinitis.
Dengue fever	Conjunctivitis, keratitis, iritis, paresis of ocular muscles.
Louping ill	Retrobulbar neuritis, diplopia.
Sandfly fever	Conjunctivitis, neuroretinitis.
Foot-and-mouth disease	Conjunctivitis, keratitis, preauricular lymph-adenopathy.

detail in the chapter on pediatric ophthalmology (p. 105). Table 6-2 summarizes these and other viral disorders in which ocular complications occur infrequently. Diplopia and ocular muscle paresis may occur in certain other viral diseases: poliomyelitis, lymphocytic choriomeningitis, Australian X disease, St. Louis encephalitis, rabies, equine encephalomyelitis, and, especially, encephalitis lethargica.

Systemic Rickettsial Diseases

The biological features of rickettsiae are intermediate between those of viruses and bacteria. They multiply only in certain cells of susceptible species, reproduce by binary fission, possess metabolic enzymes, and contain both ribose and deoxyribose nucleic acid. Rickettsiae are transmitted by arthropods and cause diseases characterized by fever and rash. The eight major diseases that they produce in man respond to vaccines and antibiotics, particularly the tetracyclines and chloramphenicol.

Typhus Fever (*Rickettsia prowazekii*). This acute infection, transmitted by lice, occurs in both epidemic and endemic forms. It results in sustained high fever, severe headache, generalized macular or maculopapular rash. It terminates by lysis in about two weeks. No specific eye lesion is associated with this disease, but in most fatal cases conjunctival exanthem, consisting of red spots on the conjunctiva, occurs. Corneal ulcers, iritis, endophthalmitis, and neuroretinitis have been reported occasionally.

Scrub Typhus or Tsutsugamushi Fever (*Rickettsia tsutsugamushi*). This disease, which clinically resembles epidemic typhus, is transmitted by mites. Conjunctival injection. engorgement of retinal veins, and retinal edema are seen in a significant number of patients. Ocular changes, including subconjunctival hemorrhages, retinal hemorrhages, retinal exudates, uveitis, and vitreous opacities, occur less frequently.

Rocky Mountain Spotted Fever (*Rickettsia rickettsii*). In this disorder a majority of patients have a mild catarrhal conjunctivitis often associated with photophobia. Swelling of the lids, associated with severe facial edema, also has been described.

Q Fever. Uveitis has been described in association with *Q fever*, a disease caused by *Rickettsia burneti*.

Systemic Mycotic Diseases

Fungi are a large group of plantlike microorganisms which grow in the form of filaments (hyphae) and produce spores. Approximately 50 of the thousands of known species of fungi produce disease in man. The eyes may be affected from generalized mycotic infections that extend from neighboring areas, through blood-borne metastases, or from hypersensitivity.

Histoplasmosis. The yeastlike fungus, *Histoplasma capsulatum*, which causes this disease, rarely has been identified in the human eye. A large number of patients hypersensitive to histoplasmin and with typical calcifications in the lung fields and anergy to tuberculin have been found to have similar ocular findings: scattered, small, discrete, atrophic chorioretinal scars in the midperiphery and far-periphery of the fundus (Plate 11*F*), and a lesion at or adjacent to the macula (Plate 11*G*). This often is cystic and surrounded by a zone of hemorrhage and edema. The central lesion eventually may appear as a green-gray, elevated subretinal mass, which may resemble a malignant melanoma and the disciform degeneration of Kuhnt-Junius (p. 284). The final picture usually is that of a pigmented scar or area of atrophy. An area of choroiditis surrounding the disc frequently is an additional finding.

As with tuberculosis, granulomatous uveitis is quite rare in patients with active pulmonary and disseminated histoplasmosis. Lesions of the retina and uveal tract, however, have been produced experimentally by the injection of *H. capsulatum* into the eyes of animals.

The clinical diagnosis depends on the ocular changes involved, a positive skin test with histoplasmin, the demonstration of complement fixation, the demonstration of other antibodies to histoplasmosis, and evidence of pulmonary calcification. Even in the presence of these criteria, however, the diagnosis is presumptive. Systemic corticosteroids are used widely in the treatment. Amphotericin B therapy is presently not advocated. Desensitization with histoplasmin has been employed.

Other Systemic Mycotic Infections. Involvement of the orbit has been described in actinomycosis secondary to infection of the jaw and sinuses. The lids, conjunctiva, cornea, and lacrimal glands also may be involved. The mycotic agent causing aspergillosis may infect the cornea, resulting in a necrotic ulcer, and also may infect the mucous membranes of the eye; obstruction of the canaliculus has been reported. In North American blastomycosis the most common site of ocular infection is the eyelids, but the orbit, conjunctiva, cornea, and uveal tract may be involved. The fungus causing coccidioidomycosis may cause a phlyctenular conjunctivitis or involve the optic nerve. The fungus of cryptococcosis has a predilection for the meninges; ocular complications include neuroretinitis, papilledema, optic atrophy, and strabismus.

Candida albicans (moniliasis) may infect the eyelids, cornea, and conjunctiva. The ocular complications of rhinosporidiosis are granulomatous lesions on the conjunctiva and infection of the lacrimal sac, with blockage of the lacrimal duct and epiphora. Associated eye findings in rare instances include nodules and ulcers of the eyelids and conjunctiva, which have occurred from sporotrichosis.

Systemic Protozoan and Metazoan Diseases

These diseases occur primarily in tropical countries. In endemic areas ocular complications including blindness are common. Service personnel and travelers returning from such regions may carry the diseases with them. Except for toxoplasmosis and toxocara, ocular protozoan and metazoan eye lesions are ophthalmologic curiosities in the United States.

Toxoplasmosis. *Toxoplasma gondii* is a protozoan having a worldwide distribution not only in humans but also in domestic and wild animals. In man the organism causes either congenital or acquired toxoplasmosis. Congenital toxoplasmosis is discussed in the chapter on pediatric ophthalmology (p. 142).

ACQUIRED TOXOPLASMOSIS. The method of transmitting toxoplasmosis has not been proved. Food ingestion, insect vectors, and direct contact have all been suggested. The disease may take any of the following forms: an atypical pneumonitis with a rash; a cerebrospinal form with fever, delirium, and convulsions; a febrile lymphadenitis; and a nonfebrile, subclinical lymphadenopathy. Ocular lesions are associated with only a few forms. Frequently, however, in patients between 10 and 40 years of age one sees focal retinochoroiditis that is similar to the lesions described for congenital toxoplasmosis. The affected areas usually are near the posterior pole, and during the acute stage are associated with severe vitreous opacities. Surrounding hemorrhages and satellite foci of inflammation may occur. These foci eventually develop into localized glial scars. It is impossible to distinguish with certainty between congenital toxoplasmosis retinochoroiditis and acquired lesions. Many instances of ocular toxoplasmosis diagnosed in older individuals probably represent reactivated congenital lesions that have been latent for a long period. The differential diagnosis and treatment of the two varieties is the same.

Malaria. This disease is caused by several species of Plasmodium, a protozoan transmitted by the Anopheles mosquito. Ocular complications include retinal hemorrhages, probably from secondary anemia, and dendritic ulcers of the cornea from concurrent infection with herpes simplex. True malarial involvement of the ocular tissue is rare; iritis, chorioretinitis, and optic neuritis have been described. These findings usually disappear with antimalarial therapy.

Worm Infestations of the Eye. Ocular disease results either from a mobile, adult worm or a larva that is often sessile and forms a cyst.

ONCHOCERCIASIS. Infection by microfilariae, the advanced stage embryo of the threadworm *Onchocerca volvulus*, causes this serious metazoan disease of the eyes. The disease is endemic in Central America and tropical Africa. The black fly transmits the infection, with man the definitive host. Microfilariae travel in the skin and tissue spaces and frequently enter the eyes. They may be seen swimming vigorously in the aqueous humor with the slit lamp biomicroscope and are present in conjunctival biopsies. Whereas living microfilariae are relatively harmless, substances released upon their death cause severe inflammation, which results in corneal opacities, iritis, complicated cataract, chorioretinitis, and optic atrophy. The onset is insidious and the inflammatory changes are chronic. Treatment consists of surgical removal of subcutaneous nodules inhabited by adult onchocerca and of chemotherapy (diethyl-carbamazine and suramin). Prevention depends upon the use of wells for drinking water (rather than running streams in which the black fly lives) and the use of D.D.T. and other insecticides. Hygienic living conditions and an adequate intake of vitamin A also are preventive measures.

TOXOCARA (VISCERAL LARVA MIGRANS). *Toxocara canis* and *Toxocara cati* are common parasites of puppies and cats. Infection in humans is acquired by ingestion of eggs from animal feces. This disease is limited almost exclusively to young children. After hatching in the stomach and intestines, the larvae migrate into the blood, lymph, and tissue spaces. Ultimately they may lodge in the choroid or

retina, and from here frequently wander into the vitreous. When the parasite dies, extensive granulomatous inflammation occurs. The resulting ophthalmologic picture may range from a translucent elevation of the retina to a massive retinal detachment and pseudoglioma closely resembling a retinoblastoma clinically.

A positive diagnosis can be made by a biopsy of tissue containing the larva. At the present time there is no reliable serum complement fixation test or skin test. A presumptive diagnosis may be made from the ocular findings and eosinophilia, together with a history of dirt-eating (geophagia) or intimate contact with infected animals. Other organs besides the eye may be infected. The presence of pneumonitis and hepatomegaly concurrently is particularly

TABLE 6-3 SUPPLEMENTARY LIST OF OCULAR FINDINGS IN SELECTED SYSTEMIC PROTOZOAN AND METAZOAN DISEASES

Diseases	Possible Ocular Complications
Amoebic dysentery (*Entamoeba histolytica*)	Iridocyclitis, central choroiditis.
Sleeping sickness (blood parasites of the genus Trypanosoma)	Lid edema, ptosis, conjunctivitis, keratitis, iridocyclitis, papilledema, ocular muscle palsies.
Schistosomiasis (flukes of the genus Schistosoma)	Edema of the lids; visual disturbances and blindness secondary to infection of meninges and brain.
Cysticercosis (*Taenia solium*, bladderworm stage)	Cysts found in the orbit, beneath the conjunctiva, and in the iris, anterior chamber, vitreous, and subretina; retinal detachment.
Hydatid disease (larvae of *Echinococcus granulosus*)	Orbital cysts and proptosis, intraocular cysts.
Bancroft's filariasis	Edema and inflammation of lids, microfilariae in the aqueous or posterior chamber.
Leishmaniasis (member of the genus Leishmania)	Lid lesions, nodules on cornea and sclera, iritis, retinal hemorrhages.
Hookworm (*Necator americanus*)	Intraocular granulomatous tissue reaction (resembling *Toxocara canis*).
Loiasis (*Loa loa*)	Conjunctivitis, keratitis, uveitis.
Thelaziasis (*Thelazia californiensis* and *T. callipaeda*)	Conjunctivitis, keratitis, inflammation of lacrimal passages.
Ophthalmomyiasis externa (*Oestrus ovis*)	Edema of lids, conjunctivitis and conjunctival hemorrhages, episcleritis.
Ophthalmomyiasis interna (*Hypoderma bovis* and *Wolfarthia magnifica*)	Uveitis, dislocation of lens, perforation of globe, exposure of lacrimal sac.

suggestive of toxocara. Since the larvae do not complete their life cycle within the human host, stool examinations are non-contributory. Corticosteroids suppress the allergic reactions, and chemotherapy may be indicated if there is generalized infection by the parasite.

TRICHINOSIS. This disease is caused by larvae of a nematode, *Trichinella spiralis*, which are encysted in striated muscle and other tissues. Marked edema of the lids and conjunctiva may be the initial sign of trichinosis. This is followed by pain and tenderness on movement of the eyes, and even by ophthalmoplegia. Diagnosis may be confirmed by a positive skin test and identification of the larvae in biopsy specimens. The treatment is supportive and symptomatic.

Other Protozoan and Metazoan Diseases. *Ocular myiasis* is infection of the eye and adnexa by insect larvae. This occurs in areas where hygienic conditions are poor and where flies abound. Ocular lesions associated with additional protozoan and metazoan diseases are listed in Table 6-3.

INFECTIONS LIMITED PRIMARILY TO THE EYE, ORBIT, AND ADNEXA

The Orbit

Bacterial, viral, and fungal infections seldom are primary in the orbit. Generally they reach the orbit from elsewhere, particularly by way of the paranasal sinuses or the bloodstream. Frequently the source of the infection evokes only a few mild clinical symptoms, whereas the resulting orbital inflammation gives rise to severe symptoms. Inflammation primarily may involve the periosteum (periostitis) and the loose areolar tissue of the orbit.

Acute Infection and Inflammation. Orbital cellulitis, especially prevalent in young children, generally results from infection in the paranasal sinuses (Fig. 6-3). It is characterized clinically by ocular pain, lid

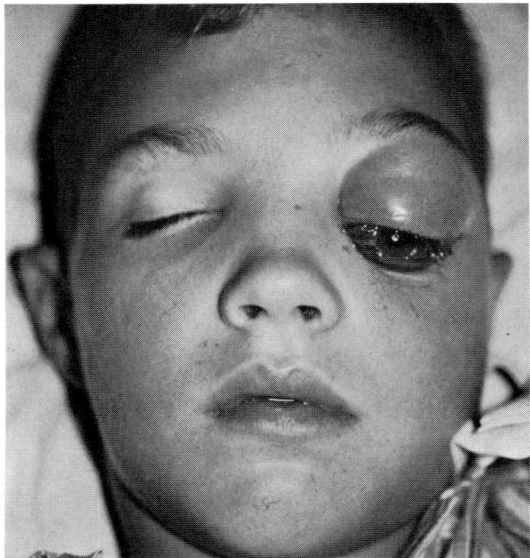

Figure 6-3   Orbital cellulitis.

edema, chemosis, proptosis, and limited ocular movements. The patient is acutely ill; fever and leukocytosis are present. This condition generally responds to parenteral antibiotics, but treatment must be sufficient to clear any sinusitis. Surgery on the sinus or the orbit may spread the infection, and it should be approached accordingly.

If orbital cellulitis becomes a suppurative process, it may be walled off and form an abscess, or it may result in destruction of the orbital septum and widespread extension. Additional complications of orbital cellulitis are cavernous sinus thrombosis, panophthalmitis, infarction of the retina, and optic neuritis. Mucormycosis is a frequent cause of acute, necrotizing, orbital

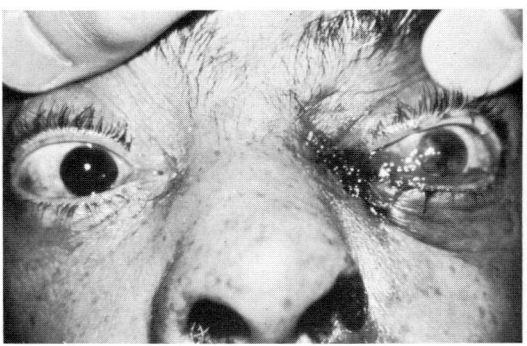

Figure 6-4   Mucormycosis infection of the orbit.

inflammation in debilitated patients (Fig. 6-4).

Cavernous Sinus Thrombosis. The cavernous sinuses are venous sinuses formed between the meningeal and periosteal layers of the dura. They lie on either side of the sphenoid bone and extend from the superior orbital fissure in the front backward to the apex of the petrous portion of the temporal bone. The cavernous sinus is unique in having nerves in its outer wall (oculomotor, trochlear, and the ophthalmic and maxillary divisions of the trigeminal nerve) and the internal carotid artery and abducens nerve passing through it.

Thrombosis of the cavernous sinus almost invariably occurs as a result of blood-borne infection, most often with streptococcus. The general signs vary within wide limits, but usually include headache, nausea, vomiting, somnolence and fever, and chills. A markedly elevated white count and frequently a positive blood culture may be obtained. Convulsions may occur. The ocular signs in the majority of patients include edema of the lids, exophthalmos and chemosis, and paralysis of the muscles of the eye. On ophthalmoscopic examination, engorgement of the retinal veins and low-grade papilledema may be observed. Until the advent of antibiotics this condition nearly always was fatal. Today, orbital sinus infections usually can be treated effectively with chemotherapy. Where thrombosis has developed, a number of cures have been reported following antibiotic therapy.

Chronic Infection and Inflammation. Chronic inflammation of the orbit occasionally occurs as the result of sarcoidosis, syphilis, certain fungi, and protozoan and metazoan parasites. The majority of chronic inflammatory lesions of the orbit are of unknown etiology. The lesions occur as a heterogeneous group that is poorly understood and that often presents a severe diagnostic problem to both the clinician and the pathologist. These lesions generally are labeled together under the terms orbital pseudotumor, inflammatory pseudotumor, chronic granuloma, or orbital granuloma.

The Lids

Infection may involve any of the layers and tissue components of the lids, resulting in a diversity of clinical pictures, such as

dermatitis, blepharitis, cellulitis, gangrene, granulomas, papillomas, and other elevated lesions. A wide spectrum of pathologic agents can involve the lid. The most important agents and the resulting lesions are listed in Table 6-4.

Blepharitis (Inflammation of the Eyelids). This condition often occurs in children, involves both upper and lower lids, and tends to become chronic. The most common cause is seborrhea. Blepharitis may become aggravated by secondary infection, usually from Staphylococcus. Always some degree of conjunctivitis is associated, and occasionally keratitis occurs. The lid margins have a red, irritated appearance, with scales clinging to the base of the lashes. Ulcers may appear on the lid margins and result in patchy loss of lashes or may cause misdirected lash growth (trichiasis). Cure is difficult, but the condition can be kept under control if treatment is instituted before serious ocular involvement can occur. Local antibiotics are used to control infection and local steroid therapy is helpful. Hyperopic refractive errors may play an important part. Autogenous vaccines and staphylococcal antitoxin have been used.

Hordeolum (Stye). This lesion is a localized staphylococcal infection of the lash follicles. *Internal hordeolum* is an acute infection involving a meibomian gland of the tarsal plate (Fig. 6-5). These internal infections are much more painful than the ordinary stye because the lesions are encased in fibrous tissue and are also deeper within the lid. They usually drain through the conjunctival surface of the lid, although they also may involve the glands of Zeis and Moll and drain externally (*external hordeolum*). Hot compresses and local antibiotics are used in the treatment of both types of hordeolum. Refractive errors should be excluded.

Chalazion. A chalazion is a benign, chronic, granulomatous mass resulting from chronic inflammation of a meibomian or Zeis gland (Figs. 6-6, 6-7, 6-8). It may follow an acute infection of an internal hordeolum. Clinically a chalazion is a localized, progressive, painless swelling of the lid. In rare instances it may press upon the cor-

TABLE 6-4 INFECTIONS OF THE EYELIDS

Agent	Types of Lid Lesions
Bacterial	
Staphylococci	Acute and chronic inflammation; lid margins red and inflamed; suppurative lesions; may result in ulcerative blepharitis.
Hemolytic streptococci (including erysipelas and impetigo)	Swelling and inflammation of lids, vesicles, pustules, superficial ulcers; rarely may cause gangrene.
Pseudomonas aeruginosa	Meibomitis.
Klebsiella pneumoniae	Meibomitis.
Corynebacterium diphtheriae	Red, swollen eyelids; diphtheritic membranes on inner surfaces.
Bacillus anthracis	Malignant pustule.
Moraxella lacunata	Inflammation at angles of lids; common in Southwestern United States.
Hemophilus ducreyi	Soft chancre of the eyelids.
Pasturella tularensis	Lids swollen and inflamed.
Neisseria gonorrhoeae	Lids swollen and indurated.
Mycobacterium tuberculosis	*Lupus vulgaris*: nodules, ulceration, and scar formation.
Mycobacterium leprae (Lepromatous leprosy)	Red, elevated nodules.
Spirochetal	
Treponema pallidum	Lids may be involved in primary, secondary, or tertiary stages; can cause chancre of the lids, syphilitic exanthema, or gumma.
Spirillum minus (rat bite fever)	Local hyperemia, edema, and tenderness.
Viral	
Trachoma	Tarsus almost always involved; in severe infections all the layers of the lid may be affected; tarsus acutely appears gray-red and edematous; softening, necrosis, and scarring are late complications.
Vaccinia	Vesicles and pustules.
Herpes simplex	Intraepidermal vesicles.
Herpes zoster	Vesicular rash.
Molluscum contagiosum	Nodules, with central depressions and caseous core located on or near lid margins.
Verrucae (warts)	Solid, elevated growths (verruca vulgaris); flat, smooth, occasionally pigmented lesions (verruca plana).
Fungal	
Actinomyces	Granulation tissue and large abscesses with "sulfur granules."
American blastomycosis	Fungating plaques and ulcerative granulomas.
Pityrosporon ovale	May be an etiologic agent of squamous blepharitis.

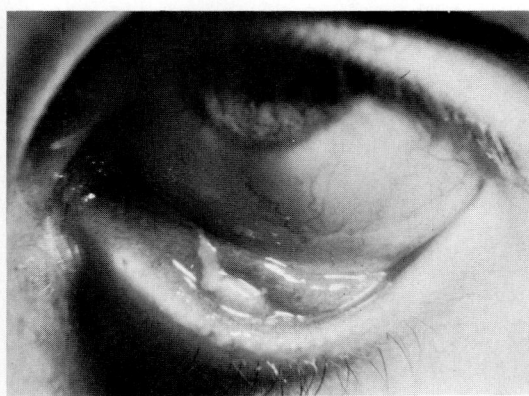

Figure 6-5   Internal hordeolum.

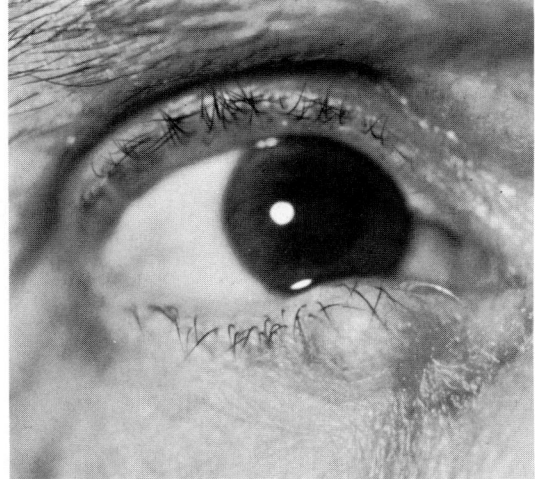

Figure 6-6   Chalazion of the lower lid.

Figure 6-7   Chalazion pointing on conjunctival surface of the upper lid.

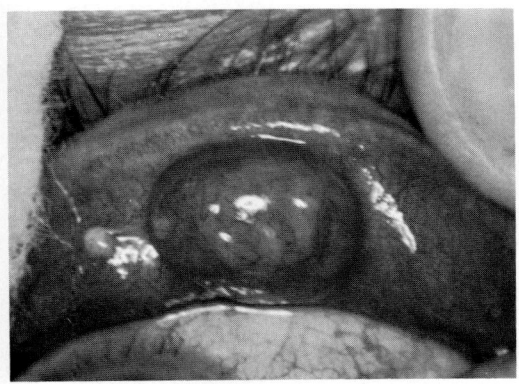

Figure 6-8 Conjunctival pyogenic granuloma secondary to a spontaneously draining internal hordeclum.

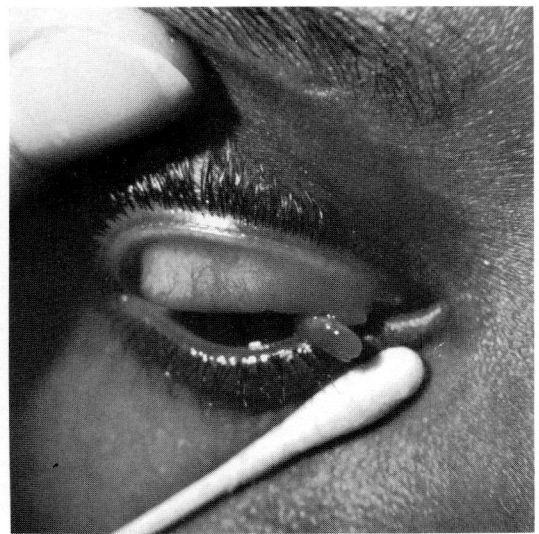

nea and distort vision. An incision through the conjunctival surface and thorough curettage usually is adequate. If a chalazion occurs repeatedly or has a solid appearance, a biopsy should be taken to exclude sebaceous gland carcinoma.

Molluscum Contagiosum. This is a mildly contagious viral disease that chiefly affects the skin of the lids (Fig. 6-9). The lesions are elevated above the surface and consist of one or more transparent nodules, usually about 2 to 3 mm. in diameter, with a central depression. When pressed upon, the lesions extrude a white, cheesy mass which contains microscopic molluscum bodies. If they are near the lid borders, molluscum lesions occasionally cause a chronic conjunctivitis. Other members of the family often show characteristic lesions also. Treatment consists of incising the nodule and expressing its contents.

Verruca Vulgaris and Verruca Plana. Verruca vulgaris is a solid papillomatous growth caused by a virus. This lesion frequently is located on the lid margin where it causes a conjunctivitis that cannot be cured without removing the verrucae. Verruca plana is a smoother, flatter growth, sometimes pigmented, which is caused by an identical or closely related strain of virus. Conjunctivitis and keratitis occur secondary to these lesions and resolve following excision of verruca.

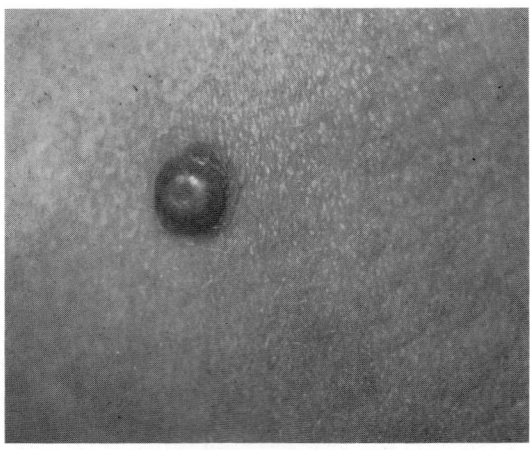

Figure 6-9 Molluscum contagiosum.

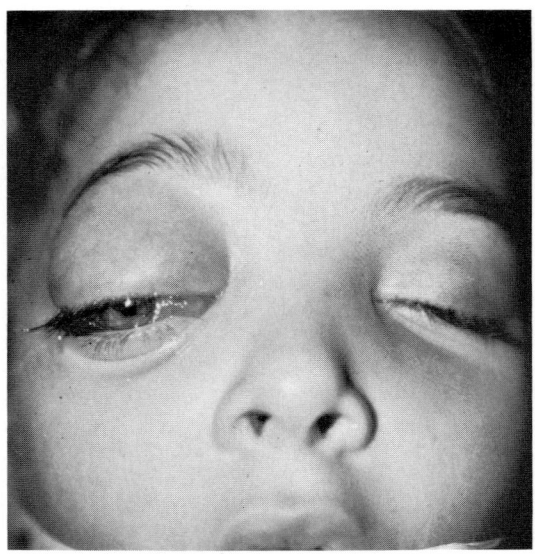

Figure 6-10 Lid abscess.

Abscesses. Lid abscesses may follow superficial infections of the lid, such as styes or blepharitis, or of the eyebrow (Fig. 6-10). They also may result from metastasis of infectious agents from other parts of the body. An acute frontal sinusitis rarely may break through to the lid and cause abscesses. A purulent infection of the root of a tooth may erode into the antrum and subsequently involve the lid. A lid abscess is treated like any other pyogenic infection of the body. Surgery should be done only after the pus has become well localized.

Gangrene. Gangrene of the lid is unusual because of the rich blood supply of that structure. It sometimes follows herpes zoster, erysipelas, and anthrax. Severe trauma, burns, and freezing can obstruct the local circulation so that dry gangrene occurs. Infrequently gangrene also develops after common exanthemata when there has been secondary infection of the skin with staphylococci and streptococci. Debilitated patients, particularly diabetics and alcoholics, are most susceptible to the development of gangrene.

The Lacrimal Gland and Lacrimal Drainage Apparatus

Acute inflammation of the lacrimal gland (dacryoadenitis) is manifest by swelling, pain, and redness over the upper temporal aspect of the eye (Fig. 6-11). This occurs as a complication of mumps, measles, and infectious mononucleosis and a number of other systemic diseases (Table 6-5). It also may occur following inflammation of the lids or conjunctiva or after a penetrating injury to the lacrimal gland. Chronic dacryoadenitis, in contrast, is painless and develops slowly. This form is usually due to chronic granulomatous diseases, including syphilis, tuberculosis, and sarcoid.

Dacryocystitis (inflammation of the lacrimal sac) almost always is associated with obstruction of the nasolacrimal duct (Fig. 6-12). Etiologic agents causing this infection

are found in Table 6-5. Acute dacryocystitis usually is bacterial in origin and presents as an acute, red, tender swelling below the lid margin on the side of the nose. Initial treatment is warm compresses and local and systemic antibiotics. If inflammation continues, the sac should be incised and drained. Chronic dacryocystitis is common in infants with congenital obstruction of the nasolacrimal duct and in adults following injury in the region of the lacrimal duct or due to nasal disease. Affected patients have

TABLE 6-5   INFECTIONS OF THE LACRIMAL APPARATUS: ETIOLOGIC AGENTS

Dacryoadenitis

Bacterial
   Klebsiella pneumoniae
   Coliform organisms
   Staphylococci
   Streptococci
   Diplococcus pneumoniae
   Neisseria gonorrhoeae
   Mycobacterium tuberculosis
Spirochetal
   Treponema pallidum
Viral
   Mumps
   Measles
   Infectious mononucleosis
   Influenza
Other
   Boeck's sarcoid
   Chronic swelling of the lacrimal glands also may occur as
      a result of leukemias, Hodgkin's disease, lympho-
      sarcoma, and reticuloendothelial disease.

Dacryocystitis*

Bacterial
   Staphylococci
   Diplococcus pneumoniae
   Streptococci
   Hemophilus influenzae
   Klebsiella pneumoniae
   Pseudomonas aeruginosa
   Mycobacterium tuberculosis
Spirochetal
   Treponema pallidum
Viral
   Trachoma (occurring with severe conjunctival infection)
Fungal
   Rhinosporidiosis
   Streptothrix (*Actinomyces israelii*)
   Candida albicans
   Aspergillus species

*Infection usually occurs secondary to blockage of the nasal lacrimal duct.

Panophthalmitis and Endophthalmitis. Infections of the globe may follow penetrating wounds, intraocular surgery, and corneal ulcers, or may result from metastatic spread from foci of infection elsewhere in the body. Practically all pathogenic bacteria, viruses, fungi, and protozoa may cause panophthalmitis or endophthalmitis. Pyogenic bacteria such as *Staphylococcus aureus, Pseudomonas aeruginosa, Streptococcus pyogenes, Diplococcus pneumoniae,* and the coliform organisms are the most common etiologic agents. *Proteus vulgaris, Clostridium perfringens,* and fungi such as actinomycosis, sporotrichosis, mucormycosis, and aspergillosis less commonly cause infection of the globe. Rarely, blastomycosis, tuberculosis, syphilis, mycrofilaria, and the larvae of various helminths are encountered.

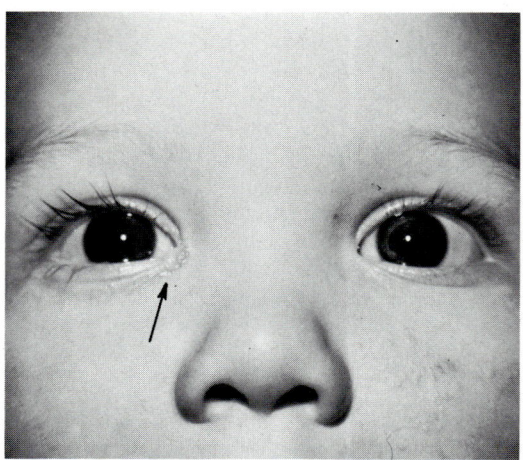

Figure 6-11 Obstruction of tear duct with epiphora and mucopurulent discharge.

epiphora, and, with pressure on the lacrimal sac, pus is pushed through the puncta. Local medications and probing may bring transient relief, but surgery usually is required. Acute infection of the sac may intervene at any time. The procedure of choice is to establish communication between the lacrimal sac and the nose (dacryocystorhinostomy). Inflammation of the canaliculi (canaliculitis) occurs because of infection, particularly with one of the Actinomyces *(Streptothrix).*

The Conjunctiva

Inflammation of the conjunctiva (conjunctivitis) is the commonest of all eye diseases. Classically it manifests itself by conjunctival hyperemia associated with a discharge that accumulates on the eyelids. Conjunctivitis, however, occurs in many different forms and its causes are legion.

Differential Diagnosis of the "Red Eye." Conjunctival hyperemia and discharge are not always due to simple infection of the conjunctiva. A number of other local and systemic conditions can result in a similar picture. In particular, care must be taken to differentiate simple conjunctivitis from iridocyclitis and the acute congestive phase of narrow angle glaucoma, which also cause a "red eye." If these are not recognized and treated promptly, serious sequelae may result. In conjunctivitis, pain is minimal, the cornea is clear, and the pupillary reactions are normal. Iridocyclitis causes greater discomfort and blurring of vision than does conjunctivitis. Also, in iridocyclitis there is a circumlimbal halo of dilated, deep, ciliary vessels; the anterior chamber may be hazy; and the pupil usually is miotic and responds poorly to light.

In narrow angle glaucoma the pupil is semidilated and fixed. The globe is hard to palpation and the cornea is steamy. Other serious causes of "red eye" are corneal

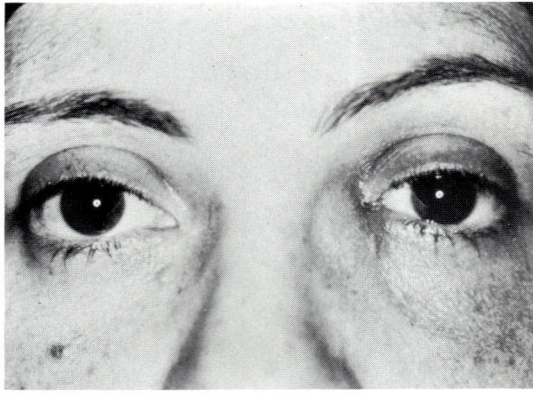

Figure 6-12 Infection of nasolacrimal sac.

foreign bodies, abrasion, and ulceration. Before a diagnosis of acute conjunctivitis is made the cornea should be carefully examined for these conditions. Whenever the general physician sees a patient with a red eye that has a pupil larger or smaller than the fellow eye, referral to an ophthalmologist is indicated.

Clinical Findings and Treatment. Bacterial infections of the conjunctiva vary in severity (Fig. 6-13). Usually they are accompanied by a mucopurulent or purulent discharge. Organisms provoke differing tissue responses, including follicle and papillae formation, membranes, ulcers, and granulomas. Most acute conjunctivitis of bacterial etiology clears in two or three days with appropriate antibacterial therapy. Topical application of either sulfonamide or broad spectrum antibiotic preparations usually is effective. Antibiotic ointment instilled at bedtime prevents the discharge from drying and the lashes and lid margins from adhering. Warm compresses may be used.

Viral conjunctivitis characteristically produces copious tearing, usually with minimal exudate, resists treatment, and lasts from 14 to 21 days (Fig. 6-14). Conjunctival discharge and conjunctival culture usually are examined in severe or resistant infections. The cytological picture can be helpful: a preponderance of polymorphonuclear cells is typical of an acute bacterial infection. (Two exceptions are *Neisseria catarrhalis* and *Moraxella lacunata*, which are not pyogenic in type.) In the later or subacute stage of bacterial conjunctivitis more mononuclear cells are evident, although polymorphonuclear cells still predominate.

Viral infections cause a mononuclear re-

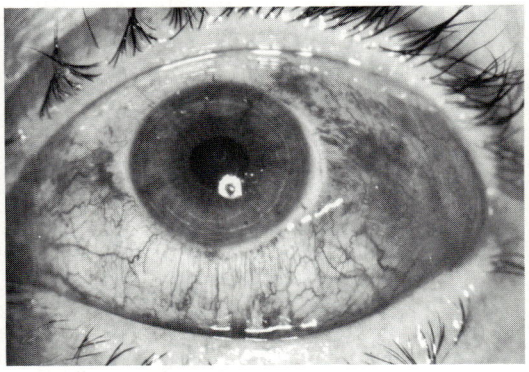

Figure 6-13 Bacterial conjunctivitis.

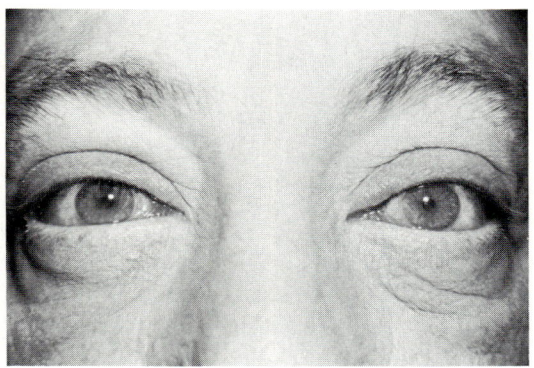

Figure 6-14 Viral conjunctivitis.

action, except for the large-sized viruses of trachoma, inclusion conjunctivitis, lymphogranuloma, and psittacosis (Chlamydiaceae) where polymorphonuclear cells predominate. Eosinophils and basophils indicate allergic inflammation.

Clinical features associated with individual infectious agents are discussed in Table 6-6. Pneumococcus and Staphylococcus are the bacteria that most commonly produce conjunctivitis, while trachoma and adenovirus types 3, 7, and 8 are the most frequent viral causes of conjunctivitis.

Trachoma. This disease is the chief cause of blindness in many areas of the world. Spread by direct contact, it is rampant in poor economic areas, particularly where the lack of water requires the use of common wash basins and communal towels. It is endemic in the countries along the Mediterranean Sea, in the Middle East, India, China, Mexico, Central America, Brazil, and Argentina. In the United States the disease occurs among the Indians, in the mountains of Tennessee and Kentucky and along the delta of the Ohio River, and among farmers of South Dakota, Nebraska, and Iowa, especially those living near Indian reservations. The disease does not affect tissues outside the eye, and the virus lives in the conjunctival and corneal epithelia. The clinical picture can be divided into four stages according to the classification of MacCallan:

1. Trachoma usually begins as a mild infection characterized by minute con-

TABLE 6-6 ETIOLOGY AND CLINICAL MANIFESTATIONS OF CONJUNCTIVITIS

Agent	Clinical Characteristics
Bacterial	
Diplococcus pneumoniae	Acute catarrhal conjunctivitis with subconjunctival hemorrhages; occurs most frequently during winter months; may cause epidemics; usually does not become chronic.
Staphylococcus aureus	Acute catarrhal conjunctivitis often associated with blepharitis and punctate keratitis (with staining most prominent over lower half of cornea); often occurs with chronic blepharoconjunctivitis; an important cause of angular conjunctivitis.
Neisseria meningitidis	Causes both purulent conjunctivitis (closely resembling that due to *N. gonorrhoeae*) and catarrhal conjunctivitis.
Neisseria gonorrhoeae	Hyperacute, purulent conjunctivitis.
Neisseria catarrhalis	Acute catarrhal conjunctivitis.
Hemophilus aegyptius (Koch-Weeks bacillus)	Causes acute, purulent conjunctivitis with subconjunctival hemorrhages; also acute catarrhal conjunctivitis; corneal complications occur; it is epidemic usually in the spring, and endemic in regions with a warm climate; incidence greatest in preschool children.
Hemophilus influenzae	Subacute conjunctivitis frequently with a mucopurulent exudate; often occurs in association with upper respiratory infections; may be associated with corneal ulceration; rarely becomes chronic.
Streptococcus viridans	May produce membranous, pseudomembranous, or acute catarrhal conjunctivitis.
Pseudomonas aeruginosa	Primarily produces corneal ulcers; occasionally causes conjunctivitis in absence of corneal involvement.
Corynebacterium diphtheriae	Causes membranous and pseudomembranous conjunctivitis.
Moraxella lacunata (Morax-Axenfeld bacillus)	Inflammation affecting the canthi and lid margins; marginal ulcers may occur; zinc as well as antibiotics are effective in treatment.
Pasturella tularensis	Single or multiple necrotic papules usually on lower cul-de-sac, followed by generalized conjunctivitis and ipsilateral preauricular lymph node enlargement (p. 196).

TABLE 6-6 ETIOLOGY AND CLINICAL MANIFESTATIONS OF CONJUNCTIVITIS (*Continued*)

Agent	Clinical Characteristics
Mycobacterium tuberculosis	Ulcers, nodules and phlyctenular kerato-conjunctivitis (p. 187).
Spirochetal *Treponema pallidum* (syphilis)	Primary syphilitic lesions; gumma of con-junctiva can occur in tertiary syphilis.
Viral Trachoma	Keratoconjunctivitis characterized by fol-licle formation, papillary hyperplasia, and pannus (p. 209).
Adenovirus Types 3 and 7	Pharyngoconjunctival fever (p. 196).
Type 8	Epidemic keratoconjunctivitis (p. 196).
Inclusion conjunctivitis	Acute follicular conjunctivitis in infants (important type of ophthalmia neona-torum; p. 146), children, and adults caused by a virus that is indistinguishable from that causing trachoma; response to sulfonamides or antibiotics.
Herpes simplex	Keratoconjunctivitis; corneal lesion is of paramount importance (p. 195).
Molluscum contagiosum and verrucosum	Follicular or papillary conjunctivitis may occur secondary to lesions on the lid mar-gins; rarely primary lesions may occur on conjunctiva.
Variola and vaccinia	Conjunctivitis may occur in association with cutaneous eruption on eye lids, hypopyon ulcers of cornea, uveitis, and vitreous opacities.
Others: infectious mono-nucleosis, lymphogranu-loma venereum, cat-scratch fever, rubeola, rubella, and Newcastle disease	Discussed in section on ocular manifesta-tions in systemic viral infections (p. 194).
Fungal (fungi are rare cause of conjunctivitis) *Candida albicans* *Actinomyces israelii* (Streptothrix) *Sporotrichum schenckii* Leptotrichiae (questionable cause of conjunctivitis)	

junctival follicles and subepithelial infiltrates. These changes give the conjunctiva a velvety appearance. Trachoma follicles involve primarily the conjunctiva of the upper tarsus, fornix, and limbus.

2. A month or six weeks after onset the follicles enlarge and become surrounded by inflammatory tissue so that they form hard, densely packed papillae. These lesions are arranged in rows or ridges; at first, they are beefy red, but later may appear gray or yellow. The upper part of the cornea usually is invaded by vessels from the limbus, marking the onset of trachomatous pannus.

3. Severe cicatrization and contraction ensue. Scarring is at first most marked in the palpebral conjunctiva of the upper lid, often taking the form of a heavy linear scar. The lids become deformed and shortened, and symblepharon occurs. Entropion of the upper lid and occasionally of the lower lid (Fig. 6-15), trichiasis, and corneal scarring result (Fig. 6-16).

4. Even without treatment the disease is self-limited, and complete arrest occurs. The serious sequelae are permanent.

Smears of conjunctival epithelial scrapings stained with Giemsa contain inclusion bodies in the epithelial cells, particularly

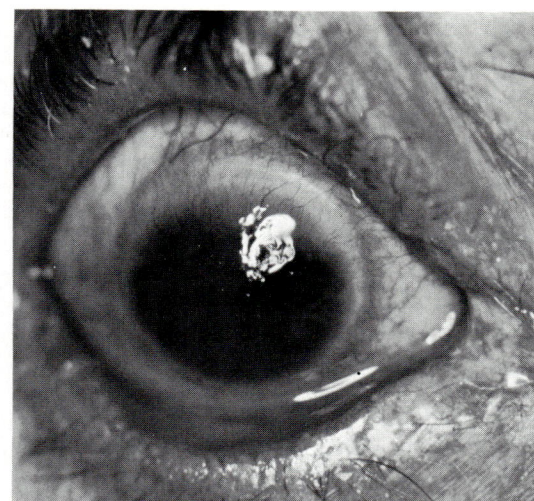

Figure 6-16   Corneal scarring from trachoma.

during the onset in stage 1. A polymorphonuclear exudate is present in the early stages. Large macrophages (Leber's cells) also occur. The trachoma virus is sensitive to sulfonamides, tetracycline, and streptomycin. Sulfonamides are most effective given systemically and the antibiotic drugs topically. The two methods may be combined for maximum effect.

The Cornea

The cornea is an avascular tissue vulnerable to trauma and contamination with microorganisms. Infections of the cornea are surprisingly uncommon, but when present are extremely serious, since they can lead to scarring, perforation, extensive intraocular infection, and loss of the eye.

Corneal Ulcers.   Corneal ulcers can be central or marginal. The principal causes are summarized in Table 6-7.

CENTRAL CORNEAL ULCERS.   These are due to primary infection of the cornea by bacteria, virus, or fungi (Plate 11*H*). The corneal epithelium forms an effective barrier against such invasion. The corneal stroma, in contrast, is very susceptible to infection even by organisms of low pathogenicity. The majority of infectious corneal ulcers follow trauma to the epithelium and are caused by bacteria. *Neisseria gonorrhoeae, Corynebacterium diphtheriae,* and some Koch-Weeks bacilli, however, are capable of infecting the cornea through an intact epi-

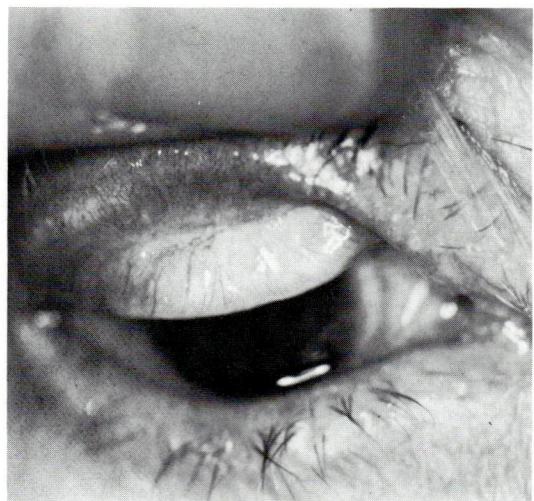

Figure 6-15   Scarring of the palpebral conjunctiva of the upper lid from trachoma.

thelium. Microscopic examination of scrapings often is sufficient for an etiologic diagnosis, which can be verified by culture of the ulcer. Rapid and effective treatment usually can prevent most of the disabling complications.

Diplococcus pneumoniae is the commonest bacterial cause of corneal ulcer. It produces a well circumscribed ulcer which frequently starts at the margins of the cornea and progresses to the center. The resulting snakelike appearance of the lesion commonly is referred to as a serpiginous ulcer. A hypopyon (Plate 12*A*) is a common finding and probably is due to the passage of toxins into the anterior chamber. Penicillin or any of the broad spectrum antibiotics may be used to treat pneumococcic corneal ulcers. Beta-hemolytic streptococcus occasionally causes corneal ulcers. These lesions have no creeping tendency but otherwise are similar to pneumococcal ulcers in their appearance, course, and response to treatment. *Pseudomonas aeruginosa*, a gram-negative, nonencapsulated rod, is the most virulent of all the agents causing central corneal ulcers. The lesion characteristically starts

in a small, usually central, area and spreads rapidly across the lower half of the cornea. Pseudomonas usually produce a green pigment which is pathognomonic for this type of infection. Perforation of the cornea and loss of the eye may occur within 24 to 48 hours after the initial infection. Treatment should, therefore, be instituted immediately. These ulcers usually respond to polymyxin B, colistin, and streptomycin. Some of the broad spectrum antibiotics also are effective. Pseudomonas thrive in fluorescein and other solutions and may be transmitted by the physician.

Moraxella liquefaciens (diplobacillus of Petit) is a gram-negative bacillus of low pathogenicity which causes corneal ulcers in debilitated or aged patients and particularly in alcoholics. Characteristically these are indolent ulcers located in the central cornea. Zinc preparations, broad spectrum antibiotics, and sulfonamide drugs are all effective in treatment. *Kleb-*

TABLE 6-7 ETIOLOGY OF CORNEAL ULCERS

Central Corneal Ulcers

Bacterial
    Diplococcus pneumoniae
    Beta hemolytic streptococcus
    Pseudomonas aeruginosa (Bacillus pyocyaneus)
    Klebsiella pneumoniae (Friedländer's bacillus)
    Moraxella liquefaciens (Diplobacillus of Petit)
    Escherichia coli
    Proteus vulgaris
    Others
Viral
    Herpes simplex virus
    Variola virus
    Vaccinia virus
Fungal
    Candida albicans (Monilia)
    Nocardia
    Aspergillus
    Mucor
    Cephalosporium
    Candida parapsilosis

Marginal Corneal Ulcers

Simple catarrhal ulcers
    Staphylococcus aureus
    Hemophilus influenzae
    Hemophilus aegyptius
    Moraxella lacunata (Morax-Axenfeld bacillus)
    Neisseria gonorrhoeae
Ring ulcers
    Unknown allergens or toxins

siella pneumoniae (Friedländer's bacillus), *Escherichia coli, Proteus vulgaris* and many other bacteria have been reported as causes of central corneal ulcer.

Herpes simplex is the major viral cause of corneal ulcers. Variola and vaccinia viruses in rare instances have been reported to cause this lesion. Fungal corneal ulcers develop after damage to the corneal epithelium by trauma or inflammation. They frequently follow prolonged treatment of an abrasion or bacterial and viral ulcers with antibiotics or corticosteroids. They appear initially as a white spot on the cornea which progresses into a gray, indolent, shallow ulcer with surrounding infiltrate and frequently hypopyon. Characteristically the inflammatory reaction in the early stages is mild. Local application of nystatin or amphotericin B may be effective. Some organisms respond to other antibiotics or sulfonamides.

MARGINAL CORNEAL ULCERS. These ulcers are more common and generally more benign than those in the central cornea (Plate 12*B*). They rarely are the result of primary infection of the peripheral cornea, but rather are the result of toxic, metabolic, and metastatic processes often associated with conjunctival infection. Topographically two major groups of marginal ulcers occur: simple, catarrhal ulcers and ring ulcers.

Simple, catarrhal ulcers are seen as ulcerations of the corneal periphery. Clinically they are superficial, gray, crescent-shaped ulcers. Usually these lesions occur as a complication of a chronic conjunctivitis, particularly that caused by *Staphylococcus aureus.* Scrapings from marginal ulcers, however, rarely contain any bacteria. Similar marginal ulcers may occur secondary to conjunctival or systemic allergy. Catarrhal ulcers are benign and do not spread centrally, but frequently recur. Treatment should be directed toward the conjunctivitis. Broad spectrum antibiotic or sulfonamide preparations are sometimes effective. Inclusion of a corticosteroid often is of value in clearing the corneal lesion. Desensitization may be of some benefit if recurrences are frequent.

Ring ulcers, as the name implies, extend around a portion or the whole of the corneal periphery. Unlike simple catarrhal ulcers, there is no association between the corneal lesion and conjunctivitis or blepharitis. The ring ulcer appears to be the result of a hypersensitivity reaction. Smears and cultures from the involved area are negative. Ring ulcers usually remain confined to the superficial stroma and rarely lead to perforation or extensive corneal damage. The lesions tend, however, to become heavily vascularized. The treatment is symptomatic, with local steroids often giving a good response. Mydriatics and warm compresses are sometimes helpful adjuncts.

A condition which bears some similarity to a ring ulcer but has a more severe prognosis is Mooren's ulcer (chronic, serpiginous ulcer). This is a superficial ulcer of unknown etiology that occurs in elderly persons. The corneal periphery is involved initially. In contrast to ring ulcer, Mooren's ulcer characteristically has an undermined border. The ulcer progresses gradually toward the center and eventually may involve the entire cornea.

Other conditions to be considered in the differential diagnosis of ring ulcers are as follows: ring abscesses, which are purulent lesions in the deep corneal stroma that are rapidly progressive and destructive; marginal dystrophy of the cornea, a degenerative condition in patients below the age of 40 that causes thinning of the stroma while leaving the epithelium intact; and necrotizing nodular scleritis, a disorder causing widespread necrosis of the sclera accompanied by severe pain and inflammation.

Other Corneal Infections. These include *superficial keratitis* (Table 6-8) and *deep keratitis* (p. 193).

The Uveal Tract, Retina, and Vitreous

The Uveal Tract. Infection may involve the uveal tract in (1) exogenous infection caused by the introduction of organisms through a perforating injury or operative site, or by the entry of parasites into the eye; (2) in the spread of infection to the uvea from adjacent structures outside the eye, (e.g., orbital abscesses or suppurative meningitis) or from other parts of the eye itself

TABLE 6-8 ETIOLOGY AND CLASSIFICATION OF SUPERFICIAL KERATITIS

Bacterial keratitis secondary to bacterial conjunctivitis.
    Staphylococcus aureus
    Hemophilus aegyptius (Koch-Weeks bacillus)
    Neisseriae gonorrhoeae (gonococcus)
    Neisseriae meningitidis (meningococcus)
    Other bacterial conjunctivitis
Viral keratitis, either primary or secondary to viral conjunctivitis, viral disease of the lids, viral and respiratory infection, and genitourinary and other infections.
    Herpes simplex
    Herpes zoster
    Trachoma
    Adenovirus (epidemic keratoconjunctivitis and pharyngoconjunctival fever)
    Lymphogranuloma venereum
    Vaccinia
    Varicella
    Measles
    Myxovirus infections (mumps, influenza, and Newcastle disease)
    Inclusion conjunctivitis
    Molluscum contagiosum
    Verruca vulgaris
Keratitis of suspected viral origin.
    Superficial punctate keratitis
    Reiter's disease
Allergic disorders with superficial keratitis.
    Complication of allergic blepharitis and conjunctivitis
    Vernal conjunctivitis
    Phlyctenular disease
Exposure keratitis (lower third of the cornea predominantly involved) and neurotrophic keratitis due to exposure and subsequent drying of the cornea.
    Paralysis of the seventh nerve
    Lagophthalmos
    Fifth nerve lesions
    Loss of corneal sensation
    Endocrine exophthalmos and other types of exophthalmos
    Injury or deformity of lids
Superficial keratitis associated with diseases of the skin.
    Rosacea
    Erythema multiforme
    Benign mucous membrane pemphigoid
    Psoriasis
    Ichthyosis
    Follicular hyperkeratosis of the palms and soles
    Leprosy
    Avitaminosis A: xerophthalmia, Bitot's spot, and keratomalacia
Superficial keratitis due to drug irritation (contact keratitis).
Superficial keratitis due to trauma.
    X-ray
    Ultraviolet light
    Trichiasis

(e.g., conjunctivitis, keratitis, scleritis, and retinitis); and (3) by endogenous infection occurring either in a generalized systemic infective disease or related to a focus of infection elsewhere in the body.

The relation of uveitis to focal infections is a controversial and unsettled topic. In the early part of the twentieth century it was believed that foci of infection in the teeth, tonsils, nasal sinuses, respiratory tract, gastrointestinal tract, prostate, and urinary tract caused uveal inflammation by bacterial metastasis. Now it seems more likely that if uveitis is at all related to focal infection, it is by a mechanism of allergic response or by the initiation of a process of auto-immunity in the uvea.

A summary of the organisms reported to cause infection of the uveal tract are listed in Table 6-9. It should be kept in mind, however, that proven infections of the uveal tract account for only a small portion of the incidence of uveitis. The vast majority of cases of uveitis are of unknown etiology.

TABLE 6-9 ETIOLOGY OF UVEITIS

Bacterial
  Mycobacterium tuberculosis (p. 190)
  Mycobacterium leprae
  Neisseria gonorrhoeae (p. 192)
  Rare:
  Beta hemolytic streptococcus
  Diplococcus pneumoniae
  Neisseria meningitidis (meningococcus)
  Salmonella typhosa
  Coliform bacilli
  Klebsiella pneumoniae
  Staphylococcus aureus
Spirochetal
  Treponema pallidum
Viral
  Herpes simplex virus
  Herpes zoster virus
  Cytomegalic inclusion virus
  Variola
  Vaccinia
  Infectious mononucleosis virus
  Lymphogranuloma venereum
  In addition, numerous other systemic viral infections (e.g., varicella, measles, mumps, influenza, and infective hepatitis) may cause a mild and transient uveitis.
Rickettsial
  Rickettsia prowazekii (typhus fever)
  Rickettsia tsutsugamushi (scrub typhus)
Fungal
  Histoplasma capsulatum (histoplasmosis): this is suspected to be a frequent cause of uveitis.
  Rare:
  Blastomyces dermatitidis
  Aspergillus
  Mucor
  Coccidioides immitis
  Candida albicans (Monilia)
Protozoan and Metazoan
  Toxoplasma gondii
  Entamoeba histolytica (amoebic dysentery)
  Plasmodium species (malaria)
  Parasites of the genus Trypanosoma (sleeping sickness)
  Members of the genus Leishmania
  Onchocerca volvulus (onchocerciasis)
  Toxocara canis
  Toxocara cati
  Taemia solium —bladder worm stage

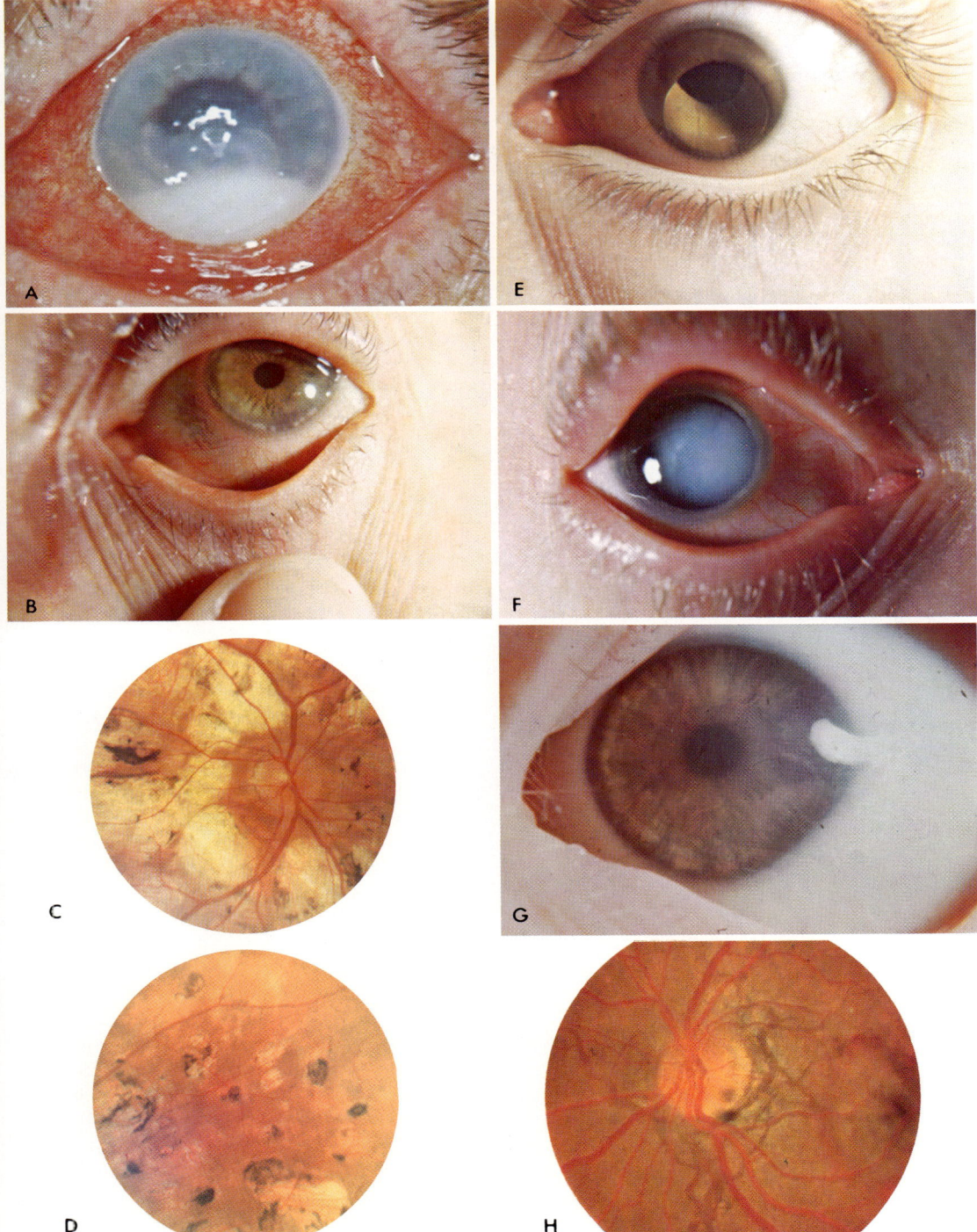

Plate 12 *(A)* Central corneal ulcer with hypopyon. *(B)* Marginal keratitis. *(C)* Embolic retinitis. *(D)* More peripheral view of same fundus as in 12C. *(E)* Homocystinuria. Anteriorly dislocated lens with secondary glaucoma *(F)* Homocystinuria. Subluxated lens and complete cataract. *(G)* Mucopolysaccharide disease, type 5 (after McKusick). Typically diffuse corneal haze. *(H)* Fundus of patient with pseudoxanthoma elasticum showing angioid streaks and macular degeneration.

217

The Retina. Septic emboli arrested in the retinal circulation cause foci of retinal edema and necrosis that are seen ophthalmoscopically as opaque, white areas often associated with hemorrhage (Plate 12C, D). Systemic infections caused by such agents as meningococci, gonococci, and streptococci may cause a purulent retinitis with widespread inflammation and necrosis. Infections affecting the choroid usually involve the retina as well. Tuberculosis, syphilis, and certain viral infections such as cytomegalic inclusion disease, toxoplasmosis, and nematode infections, are among the principal agents that may involve the retina primarily.

The Vitreous. The vitreous may be infected by bacteria found in suppurative conditions of the eye. Infection also may result from fungi such as Aspergillus and Cephalosporium, cysticercus, microfilaria, Echinococcus cysts, and the larvae of *Toxocara canis* and *Toxocara cati*.

HERITABLE DISEASES OF CONNECTIVE TISSUE AND OTHER INBORN ERRORS OF METABOLISM

Hereditary Disorders Affecting Amino Acid Metabolism

Alkaptonuria and Ochronosis. Alkaptonuria is characterized by a deficiency of homogentisic acid oxidase, an enzyme normally present in the liver and kidneys. This enzyme breaks down homogentisic acid, a normal intermediary in phenylalanine and tyrosine metabolism. In affected individuals homogentisic acid is both excreted in the urine in large amounts and stored in the tissues, especially in cartilage. The condition, usually present at birth, continues throughout life; it is asymptomatic until the second or third decade of life. Clinical features are blackness of the urine and pigmentation of cartilaginous and collagenous structures (ochronosis) due to the gradual accumulation of a black polymer of homogentisic acid. The pigmented tissue de-

generates, causing severe osteoarthritis, valvular heart disease, and atherosclerosis. Ocular complications are scleral pigmentation, which usually is most marked near the insertions of the recti muscles, and pigmentation of the cornea, conjunctiva, and tarsal plates. The lens, vitreous, and retina remain free of pigment. No effective treatment has been found.

Homocystinuria. The characteristic extraocular features of this inborn error of amino acid metabolism are a fair complexion, sparseness of hair, mental deficiency, pes cavus, genu valgum, and a predisposition for thromboembolism. Patients have high plasma levels of methionine and homocystine, and excrete increased amounts of homocystine. Congenital dislocation of the lenses is the principal ocular finding (Plate 12E, F). They may dislocate anteriorly to cause severe glaucoma. Homocystinuria in the past has been frequently misdiagnosed as Marfan's syndrome and less frequently as Marchesani's syndrome (p. 222).

Hereditary Disorders Affecting Carbohydrate Metabolism

Galactosemia. Congenital galactosemia is caused by the absence of one enzyme (P-galactose-uridyl-transferase), resulting in the inability to metabolize galactose. Affected infants appear normal at birth, but within a few days vomiting and diarrhea begin. Malnutrition, stunting, hepatomegaly, ascites, and edema subsequently develop. Those who are untreated and survive are stunted, become mentally retarded, and develop cataracts. The primary factor initiating galactose cataracts is the high concentration of galactose in the aqueous humor. The cataracts may be nuclear or zonular. If milk and other galactose-containing foods are excluded from the diet in the early stages of cataract formation, the lenses may clear.

Other Hereditary Disorders of Metabolism Affecting Multiple Organs

Gout. Resulting from a disturbance in purine metabolism, this disease is associated with recurrent attacks of acute arthritis, which may become chronic and deforming. Ocular complications probably are the result of deposition of uric acid in the ocular tissues. Crystals of uric acid can be seen in the cornea of some of these patients by slit lamp biomicroscopy. Increased incidences of chronic iridocyclitis, recurrent episcleritis, and scleritis have been reported.

Hemochromatosis (Bronze Diabetes). In this rare disease a metabolic defect presumably causes exaggerated absorption of iron from the intestinal tract. Cirrhosis of the liver, diabetes mellitus, and bronze skin form the classic triad of signs in about 75 per cent of affected patients. Diabetic changes may occur in the retina. A blue discoloration, involving the discs and posterior pole of the retina also has been described.

Cystinosis. An inherited metabolic disorder of childhood, cystinosis is characterized by deposits of cystines in various organs, renal tubular defects resulting in glycosuria, albuminuria and aminoaciduria, dwarfism, infantilism, and rickets. Cystinosis carries a poor prognosis because of renal failure. Homogeneously dispersed crystals, appearing as refractile opacities in the cornea and conjunctiva, are seen on examination by slit lamp biomicroscopy. A pigmentary disturbance in the peripheral fundus also has been observed in patients. Adult cystinosis is a rare disorder of a benign nature, in which crystalline opacities have been observed in the cornea and conjunctiva, and cystine crystals in bone marrow aspirates.

Hurler's Disease. The underlying defect here is a disturbance in the deposition and excretion of mucopolysaccharides of connective tissue. Many different organ systems are involved. In the fully developed disease, gargoylism, the cardinal features include dwarfism with skeletal deformity, limited joint motion, hernia, hepatosplenomegaly, deafness, cardiac abnormalities, mental retardation, and corneal haze (Fig. 6-17). This may be confused with congenital glaucoma, corneal dystrophy, and interstitial keratitis. The corneal haze is diffuse, and the cornea is edematous and increased in thickness. Recently several related types of this disease—the entire group being called mucopolysaccharidoses—have been

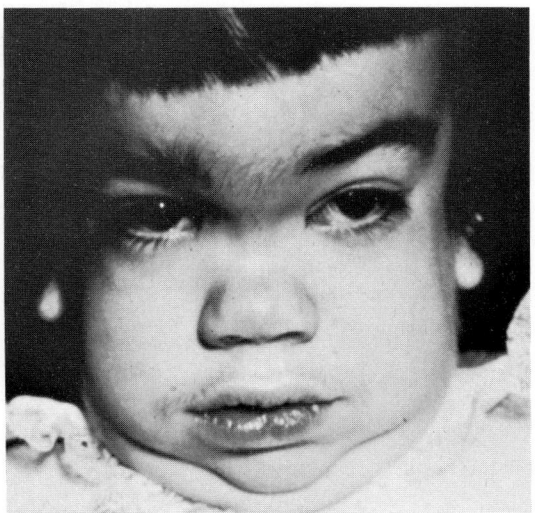

Figure 6-17 Hurler's syndrome. Typical facies.

described in which corneal haze may or may not be present, and involvement of other tissues is usually less severe (Figs. 6-18, 6-19; Plate 12G). These diseases are diagnosed by demonstrating mucopolysaccharides in the urine, by taking a biopsy of skin or conjunctiva, and by typical x-ray findings. The metabolic disturbance is rather characteristic for each type.

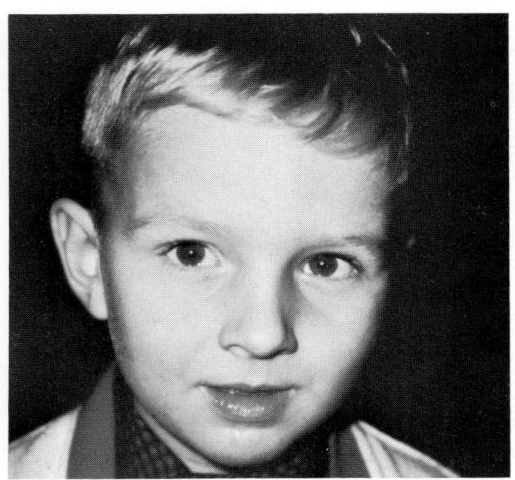

Figure 6-18 Mucopolysaccharide disease, type 5. (After McKusick.)

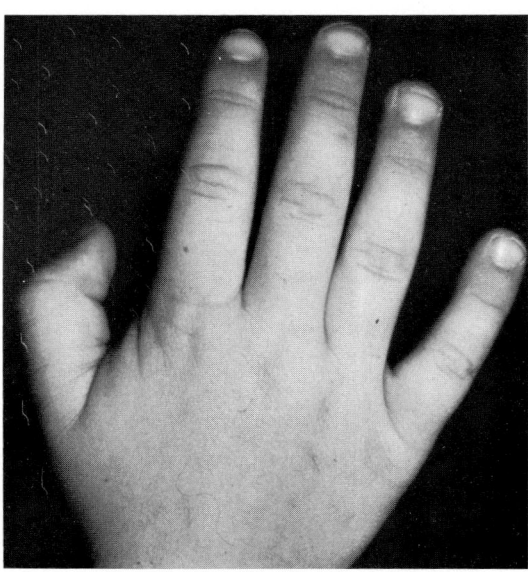

Figure 6-19 Same child as in Figure 6-18. Broad, spadelike hand.

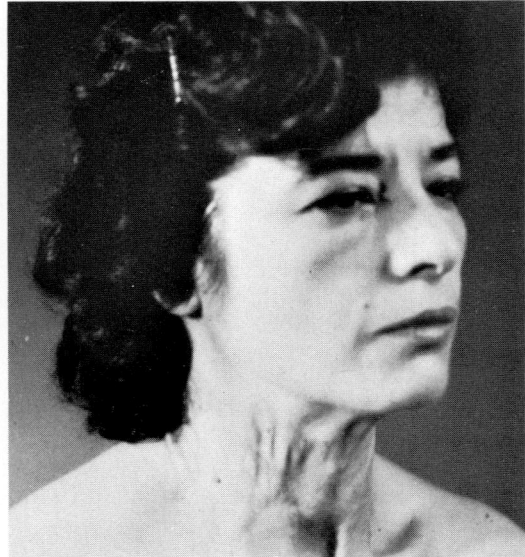

Figure 6-20 Pseudoxanthoma elasticum. Typical folds of skin due to loss of elasticity.

Pseudoxanthoma Elasticum. This is a familial disease affecting the elastic component of tissues, with resultant abnormalities in the skin, cardiovascular system, and eyes. The skin is inelastic, softened, and redundant, particularly in the face, neck,

axilla, periumbilical areas, and inguinal region (Figs. 6-20, 6-21). Defects in the arterial walls may result in hemorrhages in any organ system. Angioid streaks are a common finding in this condition (Grönblad-Strandberg syndrome) (Plate 12*H*). Pigmentary disturbances of the macula with loss of central vision may develop. There is no known treatment for this disease.

Ehlers-Danlos Syndrome. This is an uncommon connective tissue disorder with the basic defect probably an abnormal organization of collagen fibers. The skin is velvety, lax, and redundant (Figs. 6-22,

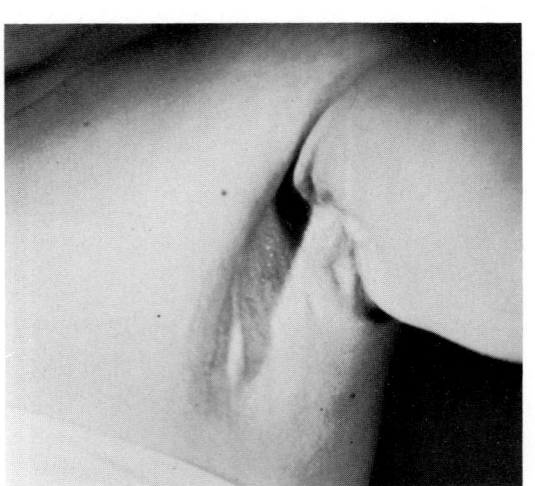

Figure 6-21 Same patient as in Figure 6-20. Skin folds in axilla.

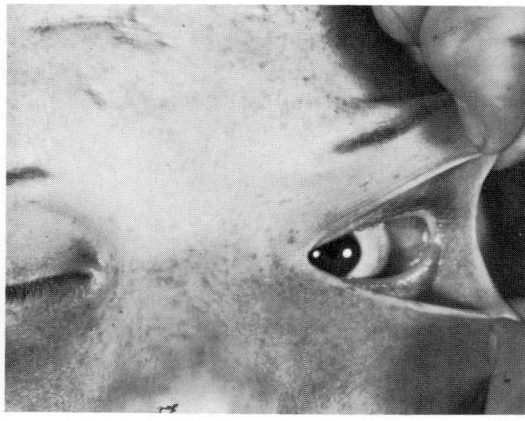

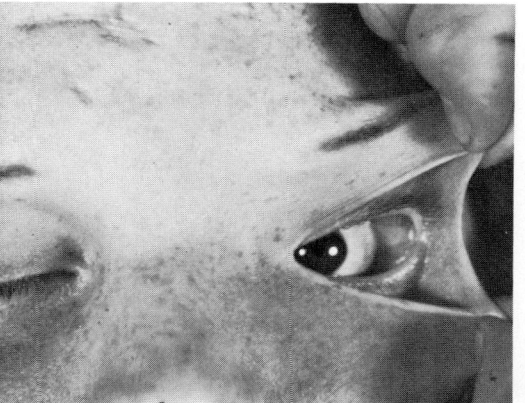

Figure 6-22 Ehlers-Danlos syndrome. Hyperelasticity of skin.

Figure 6-23 Ehlers-Danlos syndrome. Hyperelasticity of cervical skin.

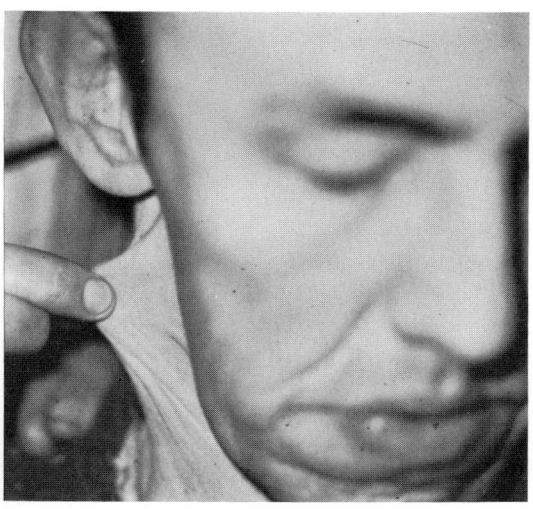

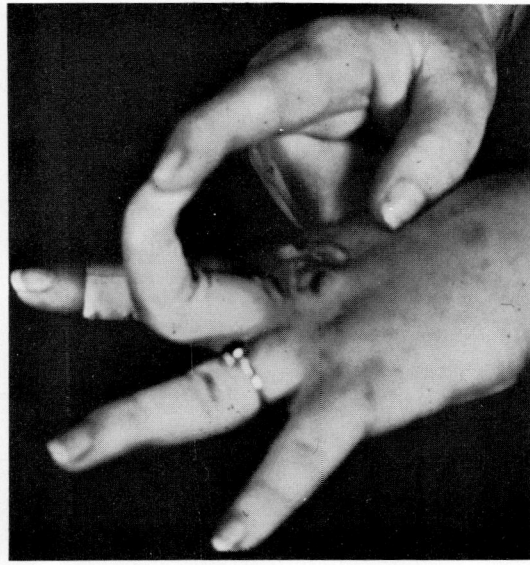

Figure 6-24 Same patient as in Figure 6-23. Hyperextensibility of fingers.

Figure 6-25 Same patient as in Figure 6-23. Hyperextensibility of toes.

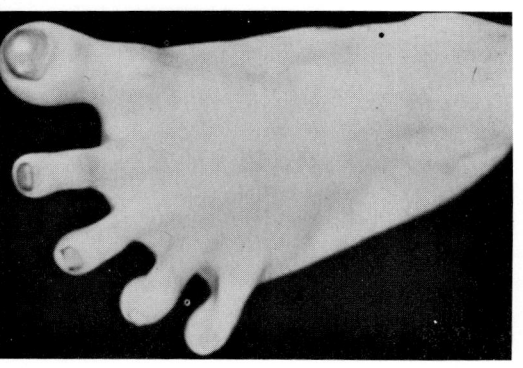

6-23). Musculoskeletal changes include hyperextensibility of joints (Figs. 6-24, 6-25), flat feet, kyphoscoliosis, and hernias. Diaphragmatic hernia, spontaneous lung rupture, and dissecting aortic aneurysm have been reported. Frequent ocular manifestations are blue scleras, epicanthal folds, and strabismus. Less common findings are microcornea, myopia, and keratoconus.

Osteogenesis Imperfecta. This is a generalized connective tissue disorder involving the bones, skin, ligaments, tendons, fascia, sclera, and inner ear. Common findings are multiple fractures and deformities, deafness (due to otosclerosis), thin skin, loose jointedness, and hernias. Bone abnormalities result from a defect of the bone matrix with a disorder of osteoblastic activity. In other tissues collagen fails to mature beyond the reticular fiber stage. Blue scleras are the hallmark of the disease (Plate 13A). Embryotoxon, a congenital opacity deep in the periphery of the cornea, is common. Thin corneas, hypermetropia, keratoconus, megalocornea, and glaucoma can occur.

Marfan's Syndrome. This is an inherited disease of connective tissue. It has been suggested that the element of connective tissue primarily affected is either the elastic fibers or collagen fibers; the precise defect, however, has not been identified. The disorder is passed as a simple mendelian dominant which affects the sexes equally. The characteristic skeletal abnormalities are arachnodactyly, long and slender extremities, kyphoscoliosis, pectus excavatum, laxity of bones and ligaments, high arched palate, and a dolichocephalic skull (Plate 13B). The principal cardiovascular complications are dilatation of the aortic ring with aortic regurgitation, dissecting aortic aneurysm, coarctation of the aorta, patent ductus arteriosus, and pulmonary artery defects.

The most characteristic ocular change is dislocation of the lens (ectopia lentis), which nearly always is bilateral (Plate 13C). Because of lack of support of the lens, the iris is tremulous. Occasionally heterochromia iridis and blue sclera are present. Myopia and retinal detachment also can occur. Visual impairment ranges from blurred vision to uniocular diplopia. The poorer eye often deviates, developing into a divergent or convergent strabismus with amblyopia. Nystagmus may be present. Other ocular anomalies include notching of the lens, eccentric or multiple pupils, and persistent pupillary membranes.

The visual defects should be recognized and treated as early as possible. Corrective glasses are helpful, but surgical removal of the subluxed lens may be required for adequate vision.

Marchesani's Syndrome. Persons affected by this rare hereditary syndrome are short in stature with short limbs, have spade-like hands with stubby fingers, and are brachycephalic. The lens is an abnormally small sphere, and a deficiency of the lens zonules results in partial or complete luxation. Secondary glaucoma, from pupillary block by the spherical lens is a common complication.

Wilson's Disease (Hepatolenticular Degeneration). The primary disturbance in this autosomal recessive, inherited disease is an increase in the net absorption of copper. The concentration of serum ceruloplasmin and total serum copper is decreased; the concentration of nonceruloplasmin copper is increased. These changes result in an accumulation of copper in the eye and other tissues. The characteristic ocular lesion is a brown or brown-green ring of copper deposits at the periphery of the cornea (Plate 13D). In many patients this ring is grossly visible when the cornea is illuminated laterally. On examination with the slit lamp biomicroscope, the ring is seen to be composed of small granules located deep in the cornea close to Descemet's membrane. If untreated, affected patients develop increasingly severe extrapyramidal disease and cirrhosis of the liver in addition to the ocular findings. Good results have been reported following treatment with the copper-complexing agent, D-penicillamine, and dimercaprol (British Anti-Lewisite) used in conjunction with a low copper diet. Fading or complete disappearance of the Kayser-Fleischer ring has been reported following treatment.

Albinism. This is a genetically determined, metabolic defect in which melanin is either scarce or absent because tyrosine is not converted to DOPA (3,4 dihydroxyphenylalanine), a precursor of melanin. Albinism occurs in a variety of forms and

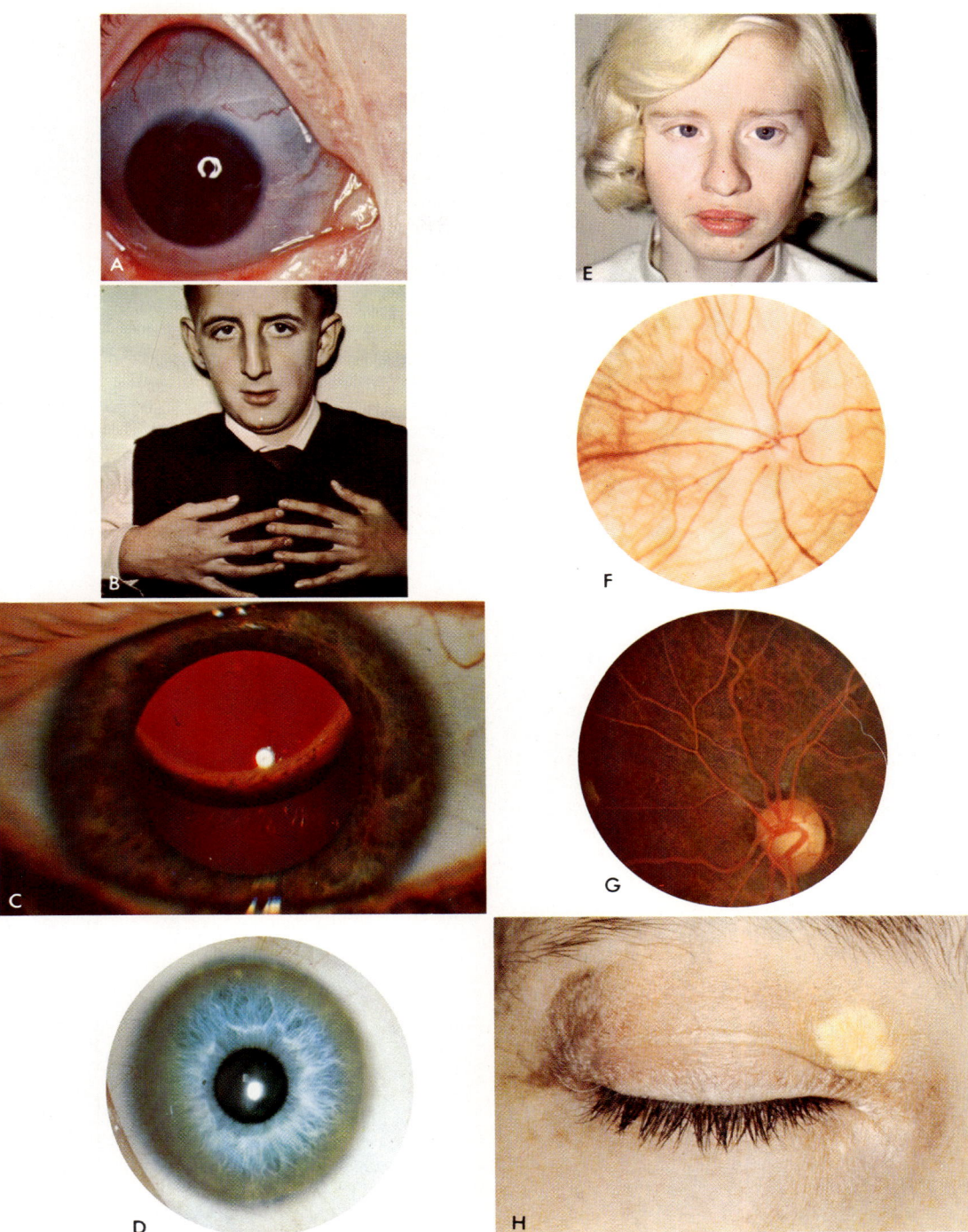

Plate 13 *(A)* Osteogenesis imperfecta. Blue sclera. *(B)* Marfan's syndrome. Characteristic physical appearance. *(C)* Same patient as in 13*B*. Subluxated lens. *(D)* Wilson's disease. Kayser-Fleischer ring. *(E)* Albinism showing characteristic skin and hair color. *(F)* Same patient as in 13*E*. Albinotic fundus. *(G)* Lipemia retinalis occurring in primary hypercholesterolemia. *(H)* Xanthelasma palpebrarum.

may affect the eyes alone or the skin, hair, and eyes (Plate 13E, F) (p. 6).

Chediak-Higashi Syndrome. This rare autosomal recessive disease usually is fatal in childhood. The principal features are generalized, decreased pigmentation with localized hyperpigmentation, peculiar cytoplasmic inclusions of the leukocytes, hepatosplenomegaly, and a predisposition to malignant lymphomas. The ocular manifestations are albinism of the eye, photophobia, increased lacrimation, and nystagmus.

Amyloidosis. This is characterized by the widespread deposition of an abnormal protein complex, amyloid. Two forms of the disease are described, primary and secondary. Primary amyloidosis has been observed both as a familial disease and a sporadic form. The primary form has been considered by some to be a storage disease similar to the lipoidoses, and by others to have an immunologic or autosensitive etiology. Secondary amyloidosis usually is associated with diseases, such as tuberculosis, syphilis, and lung abscesses, in which chronic suppuration and tissue necrosis are outstanding features. The secondary type also occurs in some nonsuppurative diseases, such as multiple myeloma and rheumatoid arthritis.

Ocular involvement has been reported in a number of patients with amyloidosis. Findings include amyloid nodules in the conjunctiva and in the eyelids; ptosis; proptosis; and hemorrhage into the lids, conjunctiva, sclera, and retina. Vitreous opacities having a glass-wool appearance are common. These have been described as part of the syndrome of primary familial amyloidosis. Additional findings are ocular muscle palsies, pupillary abnormalities, iritis, glaucoma, and involvement of the optic nerve.

The diagnosis of amyloidosis is best confirmed by biopsy. An elevated alpha-2 gamma globulin, seen on paper electrophoresis, may be diagnostically helpful, although this probably is not specific for amyloidosis. The Congo red test frequently is positive in secondary amyloidosis, less frequently in primary amyloidosis. Therapy for the primary type is symptomatic. In rare instances vitreous transplantation has been carried out. Treatment of secondary amyloidosis should be directed to the underlying cause.

LIPOIDOSES

The lipoidoses are a group of diseases characterized by lesions which contain lipid substances. They may be local or generalized disturbances of the lipid metabolism. A classification of these disorders, suggested by Thannhauser and Lever, is given in Table 6-10. Only the most common conditions are discussed in this chapter.

Systemic Lipoidoses with Increased Serum Lipids. This group of abnormalities may be sporadic or familial. Fat metabolism may be disturbed primarily or fatty substances may accumulate from other disorders. In the bloodstream fat is transported almost entirely in bound form as lipoprotein complexes. It is stored in depots and later is metabolized by the liver and other organs. The lipoprotein complexes are composed of phospholipids, cholesterol, and triglycerides. In addition, a small portion of the lipid component of the plasma is present as free fatty acid. Pure, primary hypercholesterolemia is marked by an increase in cholesterol and phospholipid alone, with no increase in triglyceride. A mixed form also occurs in which all three increase. In idiopathic hyperlipema (essential, familial hypertriglyceridemia), primarily the triglyceride increases, although the phospholipids and cholesterol concentrations may be elevated as well.

PRIMARY HYPERCHOLESTEROLEMIA. This is a dominantly inherited group of diseases characterized clinically by xanthoma, particularly on the eyelids (xanthelasma palpebrarum), elbows, and knees (Plate 13G). In addition, atherosclerotic disease, a frequent occurrence, may lead to coronary occlusion in early life. Ocular findings include arcus juvenilis or arcus senilis (gerontoxon). Rarely lipid keratopathy, which is characterized by the appearance of a fatty plaque in the cornea, and yellow deposits on the irides are found. When serum triglyceride levels are normal, the serum appears clear, and lipemia retinalis is not present. Diet or drugs can lower serum phospholipid and cholesterol.

IDIOPATHIC HYPERLIPEMIA. Although this condition may be recessively inherited, it usually is not a familial disease. Xanthoma may occur in various parts of the body, but xanthelasma of the eyelids usually is absent, as are arcus juvenilis and arcus senilis. Lipemia retinalis is a visible indication of a high increase in triglyceride (Plate 13H). The retinal vessels typically appear as broad, cream- or salmon-colored ribbons, often upon a milky background due to lipemic choroidal vessels. Lipemia retinalis develops first in the peripheral vessels and, as the triglyceride levels increase, the larger vessels and the disc become involved. Conversely, as the triglyceride level diminishes, the lipemia retinalis recedes from the central fundus and is last detectable in the periphery. Lipemia retinalis is produced when fat emulsifies as chylomicra of greater than 0.1 micron in diameter. Idiopathic hyperlipemia is treated by dietary control and reduced fat intake.

SECONDARY HYPERLIPEMIA. Certain systemic disorders give rise to hyperlipemia (Table 6-10). The most common cause of lipemia retinalis is diabetic acidosis.

Systemic Lipoidoses with Normal Serum Lipids. Histiocytosis (reticuloendotheliosis) is a group of three rare and closely related diseases of unknown etiology: Hand-Schüller-Christian disease, Letterer-Siwe disease and eosinophilic granuloma. Hand-Schüller-Christian disease usually is characterized by the triad of diabetes insipidus, exophthalmos, and multiple defects of the bones, involving particularly the cranium. Enlargement of the liver, spleen, and lymph nodes is common. The disease begins in childhood or young adulthood and takes a chronic course; the mortality is about 50 per cent. Exophthalmos develops when the lesions that are composed of lipid-laden histiocytes extend into the soft tissues of the orbit.

Letterer-Siwe disease affects infants and very young children and almost always is fatal within a few months. The principal clinical manifestations are fever, anemia, enlargement of the liver and spleen, pulmonary infiltrations, and lymphadenopathy. Microscopically the lesions are composed of large, mononuclear cells with little or no lipid.

Eosinophilic granuloma, the least severe disorder in this group, usually takes the form of one or several infiltrative lesions of the bone. Occasionally the orbital bones may be involved. The lesions are composed of eosinophils, reticulum cells, and frequently include lipid-laden histiocytes.

These three disorders probably represent variations of the same basic disease process. Localized lesions sometimes respond to x-ray therapy. Corticosteroids, ACTH, and folic acid antagonists also have been em-

TABLE 6-10 LIPOIDOSES

Systemic Lipoidoses with Increased Serum Lipids
    Primary hypercholesterolemia
    Secondary hypercholesterolemia (myxedema, biliary cirrhosis, diabetes
      mellitus, and nephrotic syndrome)
    Idiopathic hyperlipemia
    Secondary hyperlipemia (diabetes mellitus, nephrotic syndrome, glycogen
      storage disease (von Gierke's disease), pancreatitis, and acute, fatty
      liver
Systemic Lipoidoses with Normal Serum Lipids
    Histiocytosis (Hand-Schüller-Christian disease)
      Fulminating type: Letterer-Siwe disease
      Regular type: Hand-Schüller-Christian disease
      Abortive type: eosinophilic granuloma
    Niemann-Pick disease (sphingomyelin lipoidosis)
    Gaucher's disease (kerasin lipoidosis)
    Lipoid proteinosis
Cutaneous Lipoidoses with Normal Serum Lipids
    Extracellular cholesterosis
    Necrobiosis lipoidica
    Xanthelasma palpebrarum
    Juvenile xanthogranuloma (nevoxanthoendothelioma)

ployed in treatment. Niemann-Pick disease and Gaucher's disease are discussed in the chapter on pediatric ophthalmology (pp. 134 and 135).

Cutaneous Lipoidoses with Normal Serum Lipids. The ophthalmologist encounters abnormalities of this category most frequently as xanthelasma palpebrarum. This is a soft, yellow plaque present on the eyelids. In rare cases, similar lesions may occur on the conjunctiva, cornea, or sclera. It is stated that 50 per cent of all patients with localized xanthelasma palpebrarum have normal serum lipids. Since similar lesions can also occur as part of the picture in the systemic lipoidoses, with essential hyperlipemia and hypercholesterolemia, diagnostic laboratory studies are indicated. Juvenile xanthogranuloma has been discussed in a previous chapter (p. 156).

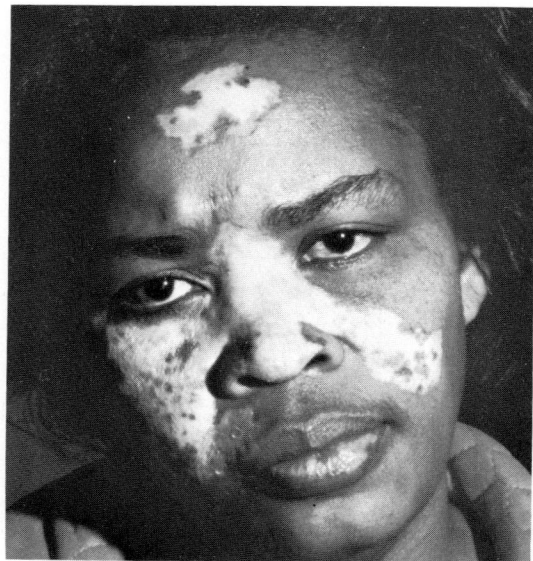

Figure 6-26 Lupus erythematosus. Typical butterfly distribution of erythematoid scar.

THE COLLAGEN DISEASES

Systemic Lupus Erythematosus. Many organ systems are affected by this disease, which most commonly occurs in women in their twenties and thirties. The clinical forms and degrees of severity of systemic lupus erythematosus vary greatly. In a severe case there is commonly fever, skin rash (Fig. 6-26; Plate 14*A*), plural and pericardial effusions, polyarthritis, and central nervous system abnormalities. Typically the clinical course is prolonged, with exacerbations and remissions occurring over a period of years. As with the other collagen diseases, the cause is unknown, but considerable evidence suggests an autoimmune origin.

The most characteristic ocular change, cotton-wool exudates (cytoid bodies) (Plate 14*B*), usually appears suddenly in the posterior pole and then gradually disappears over a four to six week period. Additional fundal changes include superficial hemorrhages, retinal edema, and papilledema. The skin of the eyelid may show either discoid or disseminated lesions similar to those found elsewhere on the skin. The pale blue discoid lesions may contain well circumscribed patches of erythema and infiltration. Scaling, atrophy of the skin, and scarring frequently occur. With the disseminated lesions a more pronounced edema and erythema may give the affected part of the lids a purple color. Conjunctival involvement frequently begins with an area of intense hyperemia, which becomes atrophic and eventually appears as a white, depressed scar. Other ocular findings include inflammation of the cornea, which may vary from superficial staining to ingrowth of deep vessels and scarring, episcleritis, and iridocyclitis. Central nervous system involvement may result in ocular muscle palsies or nystagmus.

Systemic lupus erythematosus is diagnosed from clinical and laboratory findings. The most important of these is a positive LE preparation; others are an increased sedimentation rate, leukopenia, thrombocytopenia, anemia, hematuria, and elevated gamma globulin. The use of corticosteroid therapy, and to a lesser extent, antimalarial treatment, has improved the life expectancy of patients with this disease. Local corticosteroid preparations and mydriatics are used to treat the ocular inflammation.

Rheumatoid Arthritis. In this disease inflammatory changes in articular and periarticular structures predominate. These lesions may progress to ankylosis of the

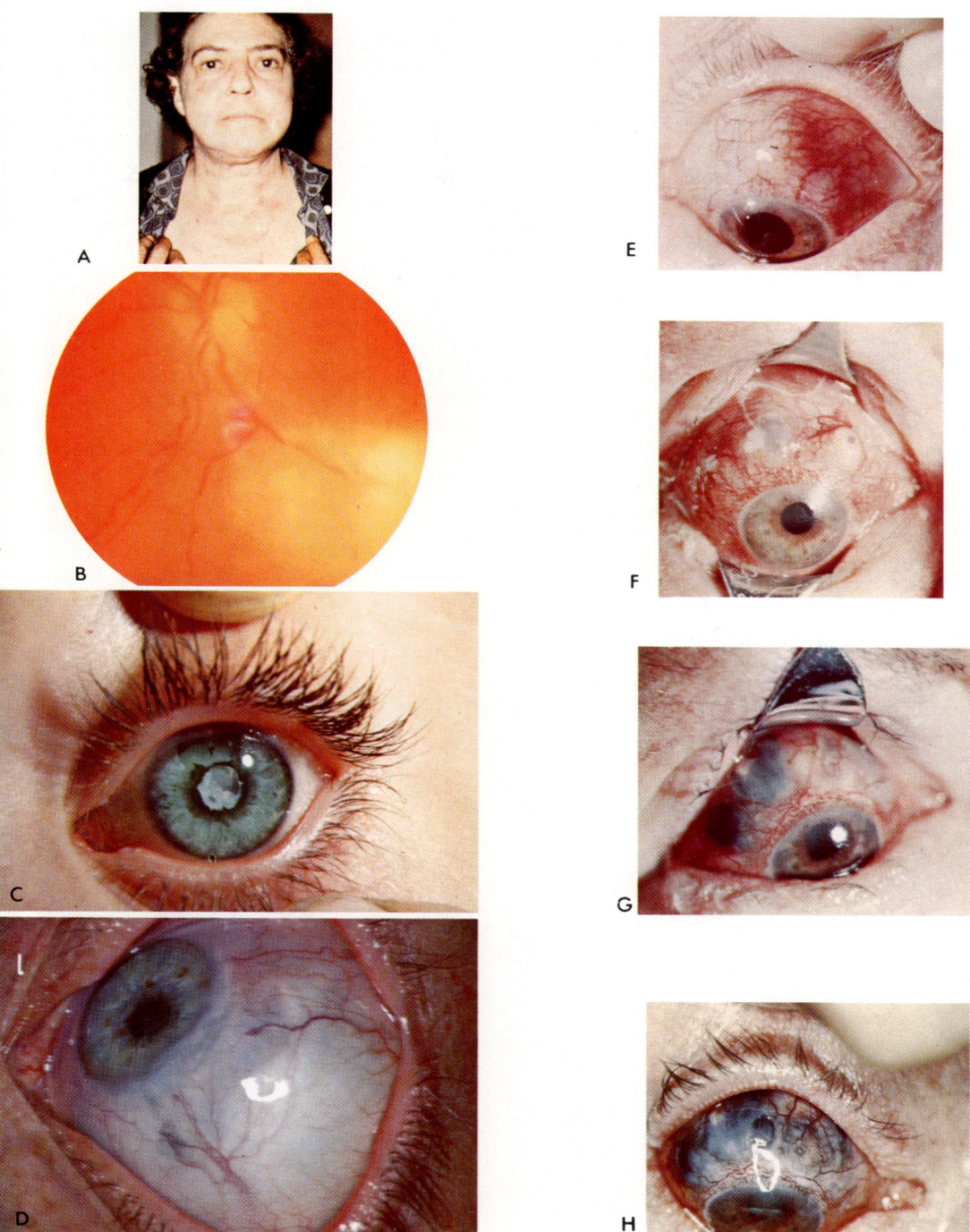

Plate 14 *(A)* Skin changes in systemic lupus erythematosus. *(B)* Cotton-wool exudate in systemic lupus erythematosus. *(C)* Secondary cataract and posterior synechiae in childhood rheumatoid arthritis. *(D)* Scleral thinning due to repeated attacks of nodular scleritis. *(E)* Rheumatoid scleritis progressing to scleromalacia perforans over a two-month period (14E to 14H). *(F)* Progressive stage of 14E. *(G)* Further progression of scleromalacia perforans. *(H)* Later stage of scleromalacia perforans.

joints and deformities. The clinical course usually is chronic, with spontaneous remissions and exacerbations.

JUVENILE RHEUMATOID ARTHRITIS. Sometimes one of the most significant complications in children with rheumatoid arthritis and Still's disease (Fig. 6-27) is chronic, bilateral, nongranulomatous iridocyclitis. The incidence of this disorder in the juvenile rheumatoid population is approximately 20 per cent. Band keratopathy occurs in most affected eyes. Grossly this appears as a horizontal band of corneal opacification, extending from the limbus across the palpebral aperture toward the central portion of the pupil. Secondary cataracts occur in many patients as a result of the chronic inflammation (Plate 14C). Additional sequelae of this type of uveitis are iris-lens adhesions (posterior synechiae), secondary glaucoma, and often phthisis bulbi. The inflammation should be promptly identified and treated to prevent, or at least delay, severe visual impairment.

ADULT RHEUMATOID ARTHRITIS. The significant ocular complications in adults with rheumatoid arthritis are episcleritis, scleritis, and keratitis sicca. Episcleritis usually is relatively mild and transient and responds to instilled corticosteroids.

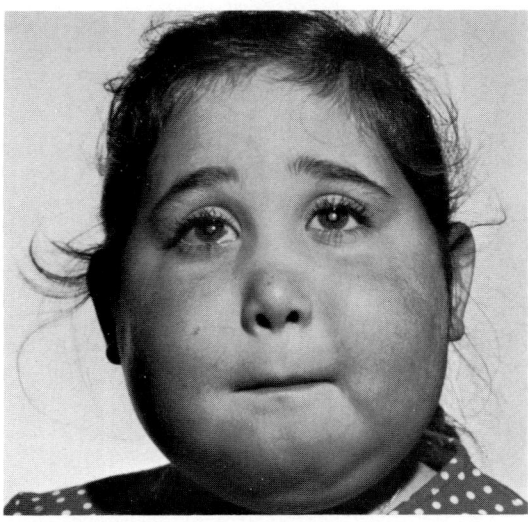

Figure 6-27 Juvenile rheumatoid arthritis. Typical moon facies after corticosteroid therapy.

RHEUMATOID SCLERITIS. Occasionally patients with long-standing rheumatoid arthritis, particularly women over the age of 50, may develop inflammation of the sclera. Clinically this may range from circumscribed changes to diffuse involvement. Discrete lesions usually begin as a yellow, necrotic nodule (rheumatoid nodule) (Plate 15A, B) that gradually absorbs to leave the sclera thinned (Plate 14D), or even results in a punched-out defect into which uveal tissue may herniate (focal scleromalacia perforans). In diffuse involvement the sclera either may become massively thickened (brawny scleritis) or so severely thinned that the uvea bulges through (scleromalacia perforans) (Plate 14E, F, G, H). Transplantation with fascia lata and cadaver sclera may correct the tissue deficiency in the latter.

Sjögren's Syndrome. This is characterized by deficient lacrimal secretion, a dry mouth, and polyarthritis (Plate 15C, D, E). It is especially common in women past middle age. The diminished lacrimation can be demonstrated by a filter paper (Schirmer) test. The conjunctival secretion often is foamy. Chronic conjunctivitis and punctate corneal erosions are common. Epithelial filaments may be attached to the erosions. Ocular symptoms are often exaggerated in a warm, dry environment (for example, while the person is riding in an automobile with the heater on) due to evaporation of the scant lacrimal secretion. When corneal erosions are present, these patients are extremely uncomfortable and may have great difficulty using their eyes or even holding them open. Treatment includes frequent instillation of "artificial tears" containing methyl cellulose or polyvinyl alcohol. Stensen's duct is sometimes transplanted into the conjunctival sac if the secretion from the parotid gland is adequate.

Periarteritis Nodosa (Polyarthritis). This is a diffuse, systemic disease in which necrosis and fibrinoid changes occur in the walls of of the medium-sized arterioles. It occurs most often in young men. The course may be subacute or chronic, and the outcome frequently is fatal. The clinical picture depends upon the systemic distribution of the lesions, which is variable and often patchy. The patient usually is febrile. Many show kidney involvement with hypertension. Gastrointestinal or cardiac problems,

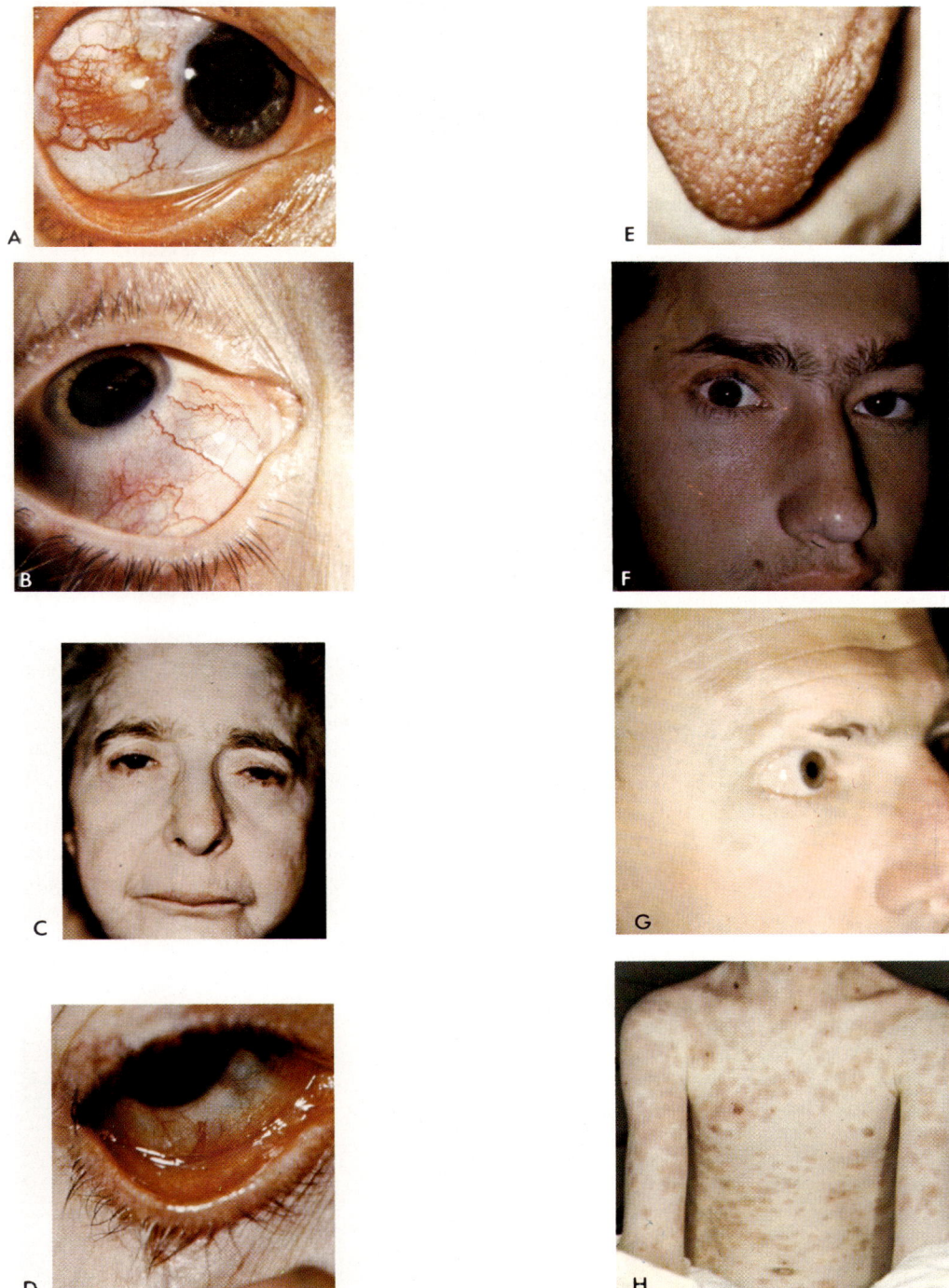

Plate 15 *(A)* Nodular scleritis. *(B)* Another example of nodular scleritis. *(C)* Sjögren's syndrome. *(D)* Same patient as 15*C*. Conjunctivitis and blepharitis due to lack of tears. *(E)* Same patient as 15*C*. Dry appearance of tongue and mouth. *(F)* Circumscribed scleroderma plaque adjacent to brow. *(G)* Scleroderma with partial loss of right upper lid. *(H)* Erythema multiforme. Acute skin lesions.

peripheral neuritis, myositis, arthralgia, and cutaneous disturbances may occur.

Ocular manifestations are as varied as the systemic signs. Mild to severe episcleritis and nodular scleritis may occur, even to the point of perforation of the globe. Marginal corneal ulcers, iritis, and uveitis have been reported. Nystagmus, ptosis, ocular palsy, pupillary disturbances, and hemianopia or blindness may develop, depending on the area of the central nervous system involved. Retinal changes constitute the most striking part of the eye picture. Cotton-wool exudates, flame-shaped hemorrhages, exudative retinal detachment, and papilledema may be seen. As hypertension develops, the picture of hypertensive retinopathy, usually of the malignant type, ensues. The central artery may occlude and optic atrophy follow. The ciliary vessels also can be involved, resulting in areas of choroiditis. Systemic findings and muscle biopsy may confirm the diagnosis. Temporal arteritis, a condition closely related to periarteritis nodosa, is discussed in the chapter on neuro-ophthalmology (p. 315).

Scleroderma. A disease of unknown etiology, scleroderma is characterized by hardening, thickening, and finally atrophy of the affected skin and subcutaneous tissues. Two types of scleroderma occur, circumscribed (morphea) (Plate 15F) and systemic. In the circumscribed type the eyelids or eyebrows may be involved. This form begins with brown or violaceous spots in the skin followed by a sclerosing process in the center of the lesions. The result is a white area surrounded by a violet edge. In the systemic form the skin of the face and lids may become reddened and edematous, and subsequently whitened and smooth. Considerable loss of the lid margin may occur (Plate 15G). Additional ocular complications include cataract formation and keratitis with marginal ulceration.

Dermatomyositis. This rare, subacute or chronic, inflammatory disease involving primarily the skin and muscles is characterized by edema, dermatitis, and progressive multiple myositis. The skin lesion resembles that seen in systemic lupus erythematosus. The eyelids not uncommonly become edematous, reddened, and tender. The ocular muscles may be involved, with resultant diplopia. Retinal hemorrhages and exudates also have been reported. Before the introduction of corticosteroids, dermatomyositis frequently was fatal. Even with their use, permanent atrophy and fibrosis of muscles may result.

Other Connective Tissue Diseases

Erythema Multiforme. An acute, self-limited dermatosis, erythema multiforme is characterized by macules, papules, vesicles, and bullae of the skin and mucous membranes (Plate 15H). In children it may be associated with a severe, purulent conjunctivitis (Stevens-Johnson syndrome). Blindness can result from conjunctival ulceration with necrosis of tissue, secondary infection, and scarring (Plate 16A). The conjunctival cul-de-sac may be completely obliterated and the eyelids bound to the cornea as a result of infection and ulceration (Plate 16B). Entropion, resulting in the lashes rubbing against the cornea, is a frequent complication and may cause severe photophobia and corneal damage (Fig. 6-28). Drug sensitivity, particularly to sulfonamides, seems to be an etiologic factor. Treatment consists of intensive local and systemic steroid therapy, local antibiotics if secondary infection is present, removal of lashes that rub against the cornea, and instillation of artificial tears or transplantation of the parotid duct.

Pemphigus. The conjunctiva may be involved in acute pemphigus. Bullae form,

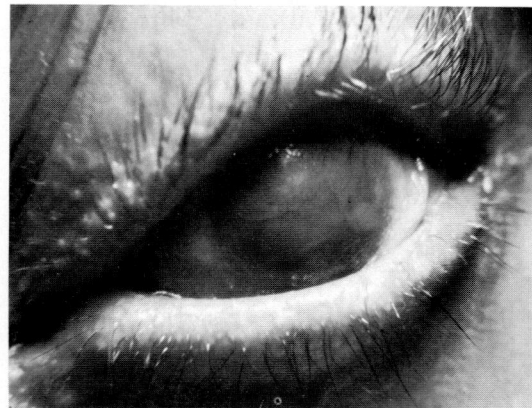

Figure 6-28 Stevens-Johnson disease with entropion, trichiasis, and corneal scarring.

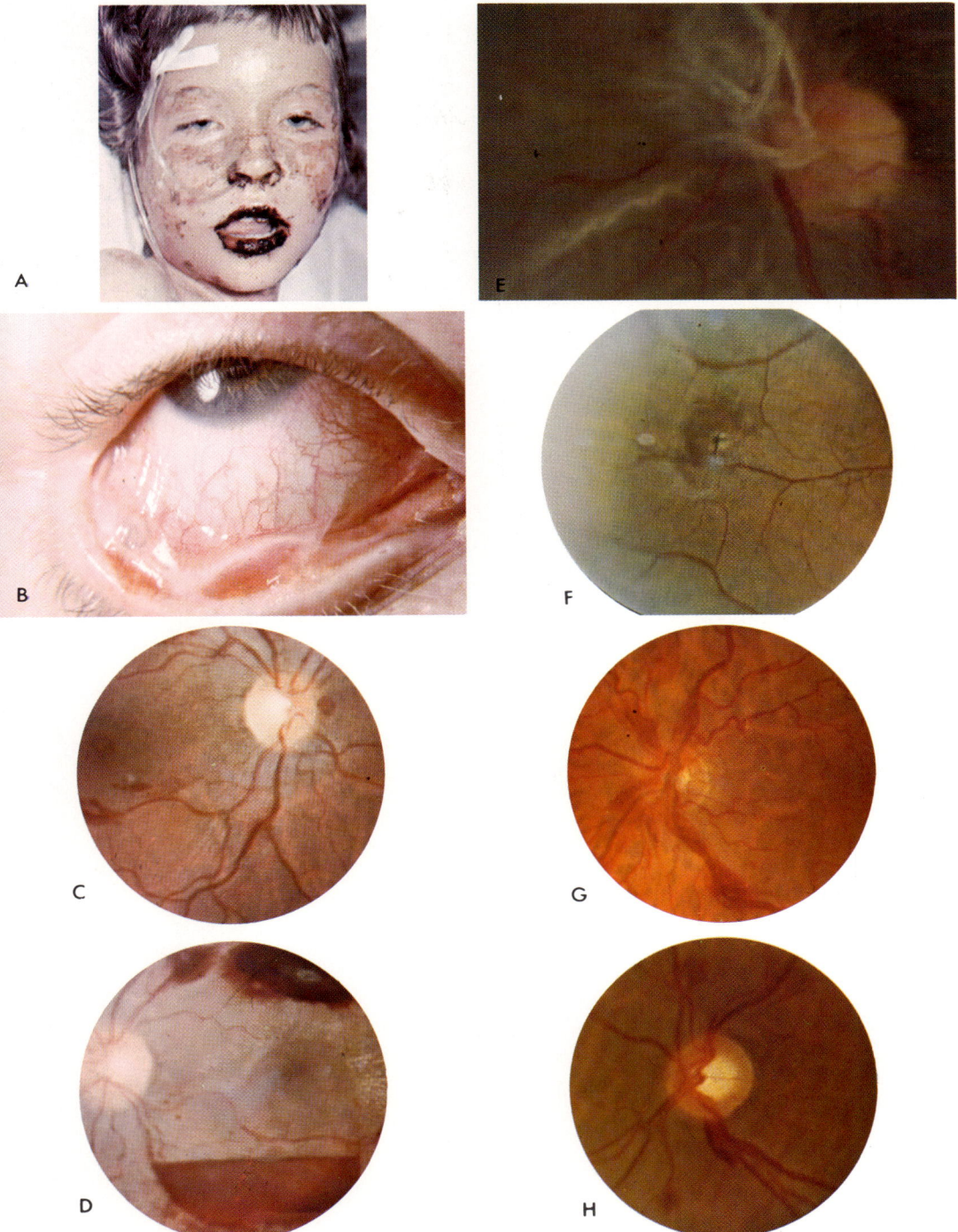

Plate 16 (A) Skin and mucous membrane lesions, including eye involvement in Stevens-Johnson syndrome. (B) Stevens-Johnson syndrome with symblepharon. (C) Aplastic anemia. View of fundus. (D) Aplastic anemia with preretinal hemorrhage. (E) Sickle cell disease showing retinitis proliferans. (F) A more peripheral view of fundus in patient with sickle cell disease. (G) Fundus appearance in polycythemia. (H) Fundus appearance in leukemia.

231

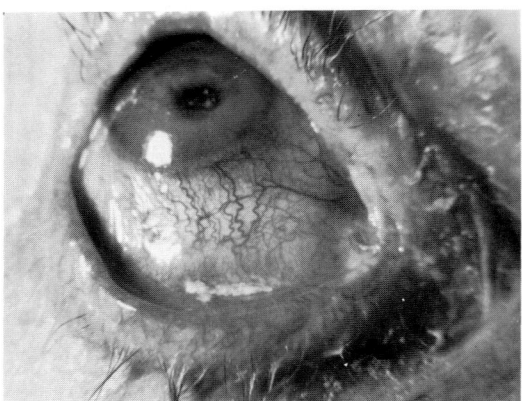

Figure 6-29 Ocular pemphigoid with shrinkage of the conjunctiva and symblepharon.

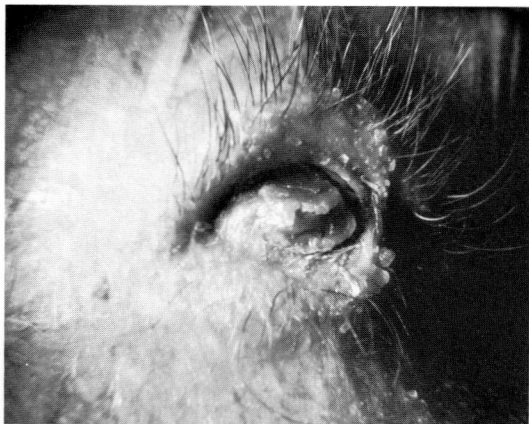

Figure 6-31 Fellow eye of same patient as in Figure 6-29. Terminal stage with complete symblepharon and an opaque cornea.

which rupture rather quickly, leaving ulcerated areas. A generalized skin eruption, with mouth and throat lesions, dominates the picture. The conjunctival lesions usually are of little diagnostic value. Corticosteroids have improved the prognosis of this disease.

Ocular Pemphigoid. This condition may occur without skin eruptions, and with or without lesions in the nose and throat. Often the bullous lesions are not seen, but cicatrization of the conjunctiva, most marked in the lower fornices, is characteristic (Figs. 6-29, 6-30). It occasionally is referred to as "progressive, essential shrink-

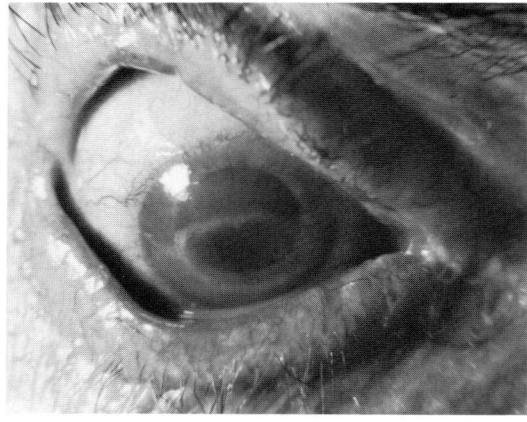

Figure 6-30 Same patient as in Figure 6-29. Subsequent corneal erosion.

age of the conjunctiva." The atrophy of the conjunctiva cuts off lacrimal and conjunctival secretion with a resultant dry eye (xerosis). Entropion, adhesions of the lids to the globe, and an opaque cornea are additional late complications (Fig. 6-31). Instillation of topical corticosteroids appears to be beneficial.

Granulomatous Diseases of Unknown Etiology

Sarcoid. This is a systemic disease, or group of diseases, of unknown etiology characterized histologically by the presence of epithelioid cell tubercles showing little or no necrosis. The disease may affect many organs including almost any part of the eye or ocular adnexa. Among the most frequently seen systemic changes are diffuse fibrosis of the hili of the lungs, and lymph node and cutaneous involvement with soft, brown or red papules, nodules, and plaques.

Iritis is the most frequent and important of the ocular complications of sarcoidosis. The characteristic picture is a nodular iritis which may be painless. The iris nodules are seen as multiple, small, white, superficial lesions in the crypts and on the margin of the iris. These gradually increase in size. The choroid is less frequently affected than the iris, but occasionally yellow nodules or discrete, localized areas of chorioretinitis are observed. Mutton fat deposits form on the posterior surface of the cornea. They may damage the endothelium and cause corneal edema. Additional ocular manifestations of this disease are numerous: nodules may appear in the episclera, particularly over the insertion of the recti muscles; nodules, large follicles, and calcareous deposits often occur in the conjunctiva; band keratopathy of the cornea is sometimes seen. Retinal involvement usually consists of periphlebitis (Figs. 6-32, 6-33); nodules, however, have been reported in the retina and optic nerve. Bead-like vitreous opacities have been described. Sarcoid nodules in the lids and painless swelling of the lacrimal gland occasionally are also encountered.

The condition is seen more frequently in Negroes than in the white race. The diagnosis of sarcoidosis is difficult to prove in many cases. Tuberculosis, lymphogranulomatosis, syphilis, neoplasm, leukemia, and leprosy must be ruled out. The important features to be considered in making a diagnosis are as follows: the history and clinical picture; anergy to tuberculoprotein; suggestive pulmonary or bone lesions seen by x-ray; characteristic skin lesions; a change in the albumin-globulin ratio with an elevated serum globulin. The Kveim test, consisting of the intracutaneous injection of a sterile antigen prepared from human sarcoid material, may be helpful. A histopathologic diagnosis can sometimes be made from a lymph node biopsy. Improvement may follow after corticosteroid or ACTH therapy. Local treatment of the

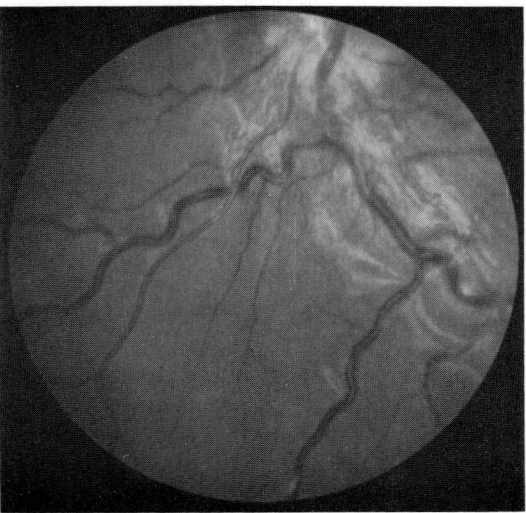

Figure 6-33 Another area of the fundus in same patient as in Figure 6-32.

iritis and other ocular complications is indicated.

Wegener's Granulomatosis. This condition, possibly a variant of periarteritis nodosa, is characterized by the following triad: necrotizing granulomatous lesions, primarily in the upper and lower respiratory tract; generalized, focal necrotizing vasculitis; and a necrotizing glomerulitis, which usually is the cause of death. The orbit often is involved by direct extension from the nose, nasal sinuses, and nasopharynx.

Lethal Midline Granuloma. In this disease there is insidious destruction of the center of the face beginning with edema of the nose and congestion of the nasal passages, subsequently followed by ulcerations around the nostrils and perforation of the nasal septum and palate. Frequently the orbit is involved in the extensive, mutilating progress.

BLOOD DISEASES

The physician viewing the fundus of the eye through the ophthalmoscope can directly examine the columns of arterial and venous blood. He may see evidence of ex-

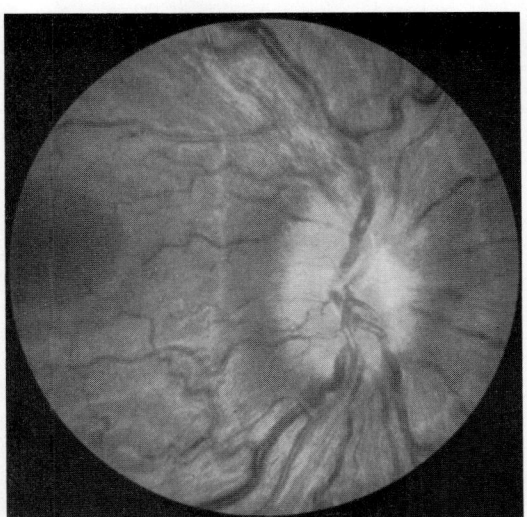

Figure 6-32 Sarcoidosis with periphlebitis and secondary edema of the disc.

cesses, deficiencies, or alterations in the various components of the blood, not uncommonly before signs of these disorders are manifest elsewhere in the body.

Anemias

Retinal changes occur in any of the anemias, whether macrocytic, microcytic, or normocytic in type, when the red corpuscles fall below 50 per cent of their normal concentration. The extent of the retinopathy increases in proportion to the anemia. The characteristic ophthalmoscopic signs are dilation of retinal veins (Plate 16*C*); retinal hemorrhages and, less frequently, extraretinal hemorrhages (Plate 16*D*); generalized pallor of the fundus and optic disc; retinal edema; retinal exudates; and subconjunctival hemorrhages. Sometime the venules and arterioles appear alike.

Blood Loss. Ocular changes may occur following sudden and massive blood loss. The fundus becomes pale, the arteries constricted, and the veins dilated. Hemorrhages generally do not appear unless the anemia becomes chronic. In rare instances vision may suddenly be lost. This usually follows recurrent hemorrhages associated with a marked drop in blood pressure, a situation occurring with gastric ulcers or uterine bleeding. The loss of vision is bilateral in 85 per cent of these patients. It may come on during the period of shock, but more often is delayed for as long as several weeks. The fundus picture may resemble that of central retinal artery obstruction, with the presence of a cherry red spot in the macula. About half the patients suffering such visual loss remain permanently blinded.

Pernicious Anemia. This is a macrocytic, hyperchromic anemia which results from a failure to absorb vitamin B_{12} due to a deficiency of "intrinsic factor" in the stomach wall. The fundus appears pale and slightly yellow; the disc usually shows some degree of pallor, and its margins may be blurred and edematous. The retinal veins are seen to be distended after leaving the disc. Superficial, flame-shaped hemorrhages appear in the posterior pole if the anemia is severe. Associated findings include glossitis, gastrointestinal ulceration, leucopenia, and thrombocytopenia. Neural degeneration, with retrobulbar neuritis, or primary optic atrophy sometimes occurs. Treatment consists of the injection of vitamin B_{12}.

HEMOGLOBINOPATHIES AND THALASSEMIA

Sickle Cell Anemia. This is a hereditary, chronic, hemolytic anemia which occurs in Negroes. Affected individuals are homozygous and carry two abnormal genes (SS or SC genotypes). Signs and symptoms typically include anemia, arthritis manifestations, leg ulcers, hematuria, hemoptysis, petechiae, and acute attacks of abdominal pain due to splenic or intestinal infarction. Ocular symptoms are many and varied: dilatation and tortuosity of retinal veins; stasis, sheathing, and occlusion of retinal arterioles, with localized edema and atrophy; chorioretinal scars related to ischemia; retinal hemorrhages and exudates; microaneurysms, neovascularization, and vitreous hemorrhage; and conjunctival capillary stasis (Plate 16*E, F*). The vasoproliferative response and incidence of vitreous hemorrhage are higher with SC than with SS disease. Less frequent ocular findings in sickle cell anemia include central retinal vein or artery occlusion, papilledema, and angioid streaks. Occasionally, occluded retinal vessels, stasis, and sheathing are found in patients with sickle cell trait (SA genotype). Stasis and obstruction of the small vessels causes the ocular changes. Diagnosis is made from clinical findings; blood smears; morphologic changes in red corpuscles in sealed, moist preparations (the sickle cell phenomenon); and hemoglobin electrophoresis.

Thalassemia. This is a severe childhood disorder occurring most frequently among peoples originating in the Mediterranean area. The fetal type of hemoglobin (hemoglobin F) persists beyond infancy in these patients. Homozygotes (Cooley's anemia; Thalassemia major) are severely affected and have a characteristic appearance that includes mongoloid facies with marked epicanthal folds, prominent frontal bossing, and enlargement of the spleen, liver, and heart. Additional ocular changes are rare.

Polycythemia. Polycythemia occurs with

congenital heart disease, severe emphysema, pulmonary arteriosclerosis, and polycythemia vera. Fundus changes develop when the red cell count is over 6 million and the hemoglobin level is 110 per cent or more (Plate 16G). Ophthalmoscopically, the fundus is dusky, and the veins are tortuous, markedly dilated, and dark violet. The arterioles are slightly dilated and have the color of normal veins. The optic disc is hyperemic and edematous, and its margins are blurred. Visual disturbances occur with considerable frequency in polycythemia vera, but are relatively uncommon in secondary polycythemia.

Thrombocytopenia. Platelet deficiencies result from an insufficient formation of these cells, from increased destruction of platelets, or from abnormalities in the platelets themselves. The occurrence of retinal hemorrhages in thrombocytopenia is inconstant. They are more likely to occur when thrombocytopenia is accompanied by severe anemia. When present, the hemorrhages usually are small, superficial, and appear in the region of the disc. Retinal edema and exudates may also be present.

Malignancies of the Blood and Reticuloendothelial System

Leukemia. A variety of ophthalmoscopic changes may occur with leukemia. Retinal vessels often are tortuous, dilated, and irregular in caliber, resembling a chain of sausages; venous sheathing may also be seen. Hemorrhages are extremely common and frequently have a white center (Plate 16H). Occasionally a white spot with a red center or a random distribution of red and white components is seen. The hemorrhages may be very small or may involve a large portion of the fundus and even rupture into the vitreous or subretinal space, with marked loss of vision. The optic disc may become edematous and blurred and show several diopters of papilledema. Exophthalmos sometimes occurs due to retrobulbar hemorrhage and leukemic infiltration of the orbits and lids. Severe involvement may cause optic atrophy. Hemorrhages of the lids, conjunctival petechiae, or ecchymoses are frequent. Bleeding into the orbit may result in proptosis (Plate 17A). Leukemic infiltration of the lids, conjunctiva, lacrimal sac, and lacrimal gland occurs as well.

Reticuloendothelial System. Malignant lymphoma and lymphosarcoma more commonly are observed in adults than in children. These tumors can involve almost any ocular tissue. In the orbit they often give rise to a firm and somewhat elastic mass. Malignant lymphomas and lymphosarcomas may cause painless swelling of the lids, followed by exophthalmos. When the lacrimal gland is involved, the globe is dislocated downward and medially. Invasion of the extrinsic eye muscle results in various forms of ocular palsy. Other symptomatology depends upon the portion of the eye or adnexa that is infiltrated. Most lymphomatous tumors respond to roentgen therapy, although they later recur or appear elsewhere.

Multiple Myeloma. This is a neoplasm of plasma cells that causes widespread skeletal destruction, anemia, hypercalcemia, renal impairment, and increased susceptibility to infections. The neoplastic plasma cells produce abnormal globulins. An unusual ocular finding occurring in this disease is the development of many cysts in the ciliary body and pars plana. On histopathologic examination an exudative material composed of PAS-positive, carbohydrate-bound protein is found between the pigmented and nonpigmented epithelial layers. Dilated veins and flame-shaped hemorrhages are seen in the retina. In rare instances myeloma cells may infiltrate the tissues of the eye. The neoplastic plasma cells produce abnormal globulins, which may be detected in the blood or urine.

Dysproteinemias and Paraproteinemias. These are a group of disorders in which abnormal globulins are present in the circulating plasma. The ocular findings in two of these disorders are particularly well documented: macroglobulinemia and cryoglobulinemia.

MACROGLOBULINEMIA. In this abnormality there is a disturbance in the cell populations normally responsible for the synthesis of gamma-M macroglobulins (IgM). This substance, which is present in low concentrations in normal serum, is found at markedly elevated levels. Primary or idiopathic macroglobulinemia was first described by Waldenström in 1944.

Elevated IgM also may occur with malignant lymphoma, chronic lymphocytic leukemia, lymphosarcoma, and related conditions. The clinical picture in macroglobulinemia includes anemia, bleeding and thrombotic tendencies, lymphadenopathy, hepatosplenomegaly, and ophthalmoscopic changes (Plate 17*B*). In the fundus hemorrhages often are accompanied by cotton-wool exudates. The retinal veins are tortuous and dilated, sometimes to extreme degrees, and edema of the optic nerve is commonly noted. Bilateral occlusion of the central retinal vein has occurred. Diagnosis depends upon demonstration of elevated IgM by ultracentrifugation or immunoelectrophoresis. Plasmapheresis may be used in treatment as a temporary measure. Chemotherapy with chlorambucil or melphalan may result in long remissions, and corticosteroids may be helpful in the control of capillary bleeding.

CRYOGLOBULINEMIA. In this condition abnormally high-molecular-weight plasma proteins, which precipitate on exposure to cold, are present in the serum. Large quantities of cryoglobulins are encountered in disorders of the reticuloendothelial system such as multiple myeloma, chronic lymphocytic leukemia, lymphosarcoma, rheumatoid arthritis, lupus erythematosus, polyarteritis nodosa, Sjögren's syndrome, and subacute bacterial endocarditis. Idiopathic, or essential, cryoglobulinemia, which accompanies no apparent underlying disease of the reticuloendothelial system, has been described. Eye findings consist of dilated veins, hemorrhages, exudates, vascular thrombosis, and sheathing of the terminal arterioles. In addition, there may be arterial narrowing and tortuosity, neovascularization, and retinitis proliferans. Thrombosis of the central retinal artery and vein has been reported, possibly due to stasis and sludging of blood.

This disease should be suspected in patients who show peripheral vascular disturbances, particularly on exposure to cold. Diagnosis is made by incubating centrifuged plasma at 4° C. for 48 hours. This causes precipitation of cryoglobulins and cloudiness or gel formation, which clears when the plasma is warmed to 37° C. The prognosis usually parallels the underlying disease process, and therapy should be directed toward the basic disturbance. Corticosteroids have been of some benefit.

CARDIOVASCULAR DISORDERS

Hypertension and Arteriosclerosis

Ophthalmoscopic examination is an important part of the evaluation of the hypertensive patient. The literature contains exhaustive descriptions of the fundus changes of hypertension and arteriosclerosis, which often are interpreted inaccurately. Confusion arises from the following: failure to emphasize that most of the retinal arterial tree is arteriolar in nature (Wagener, Friedenwald); failure to utilize the knowledge of known changes taking place in similar sized vessels elsewhere in the body; and inaccurate use of the word "arteriosclerosis," a generalized term including several types of arterial disease. The retinal arterial tree is arteriolar in nature except for the central retinal artery and its large branches (papillary arteries) near the disc. A true artery possesses an internal elastic lamina and a well developed muscular coat, whereas an arteriole has no elastic lamina and the muscular coat is not continuous.

Arteriosclerosis — General. Arteriosclerosis is a generalized term that includes several different types of degenerative disease involving the arterial tree. Some types of arteriosclerosis occur only in large arteries, some only in arterioles, and some throughout the arterial system. Obviously only those types producing changes in arterioles or very small arteries could produce alterations visible ophthalmoscopically. This should always be kept in mind in evaluating the fundus for evidence of arterial disease.

Arteriosclerosis may be separated into six types:

1. Regenerative intimal thickening that occurs in arteries of any size in atrophic organs where, owing to atrophy, the demand for blood has diminished (Fig. 6-34).

2. Elastic intimal thickening in medium and small arteries, consisting of reduplica-

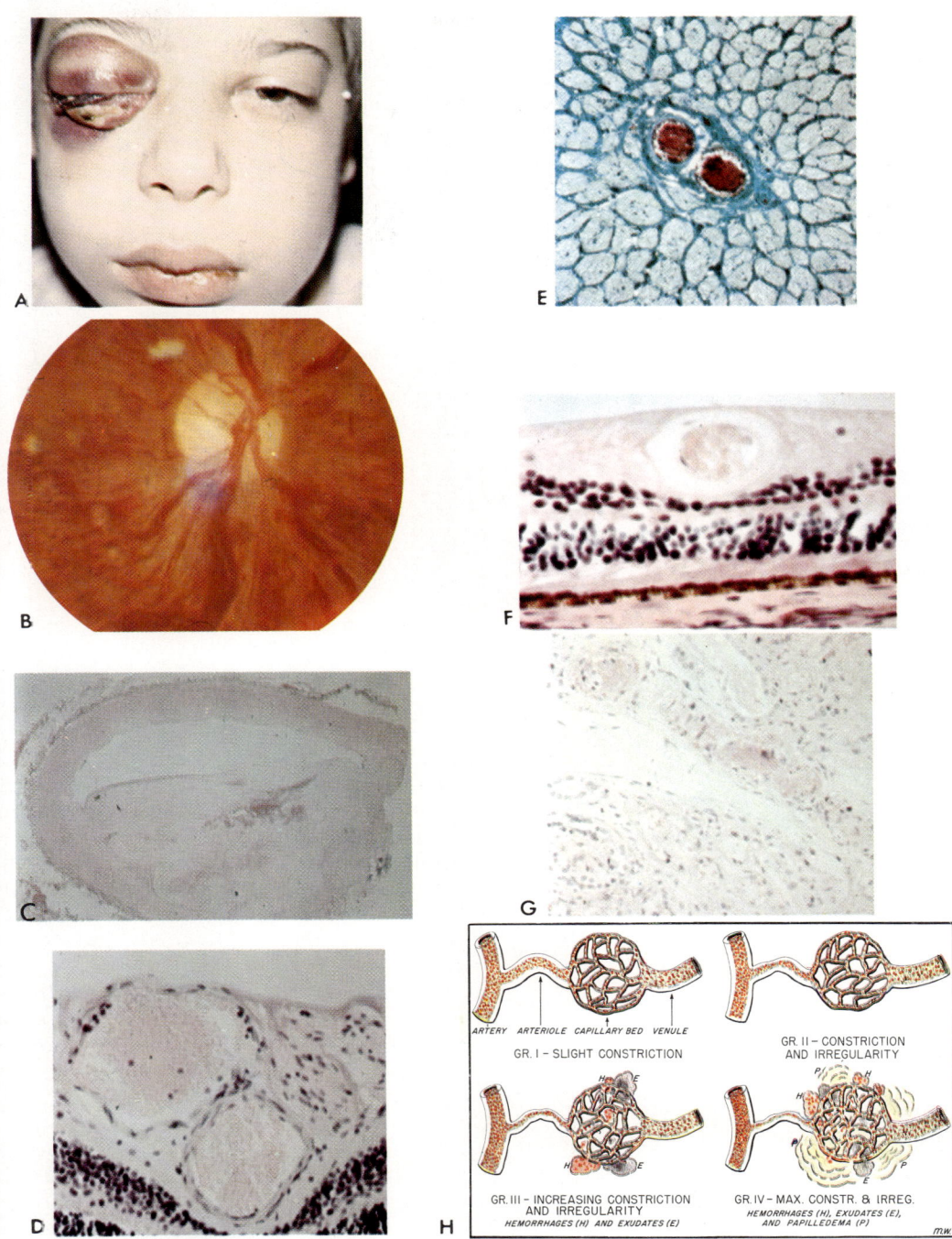

Plate 17 *(A)* Leukemia. Orbital hemorrhage. *(B)* Fundus changes in macroglobulinemia. *(C)* Cross section of aorta showing large atheroma. *(D)* Section showing retinal artery and vein at arteriovenous crossing. Endothelial wall of vein rests on media of artery. *(E)* Section showing common adventitial coat of central artery and vein within optic nerve. *(F)* Arteriolar sclerosis involving retinal arteriole. *(G)* Arteriolar sclerosis involving renal arterioles. *(H)* Schema for ophthalmoscopic classification of hypertension.

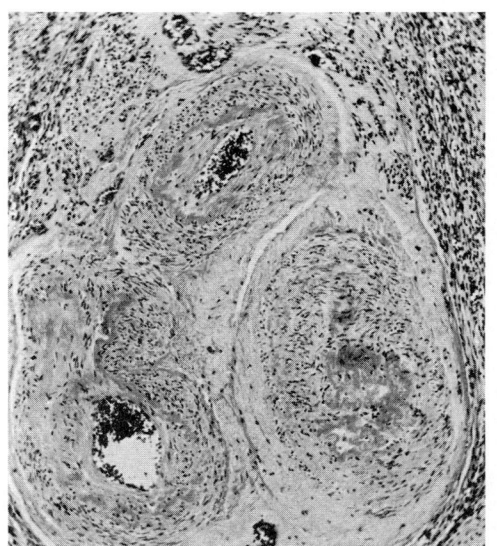

Figure 6-34 Cross section of uterine arteries showing regenerative thickening of the intima.

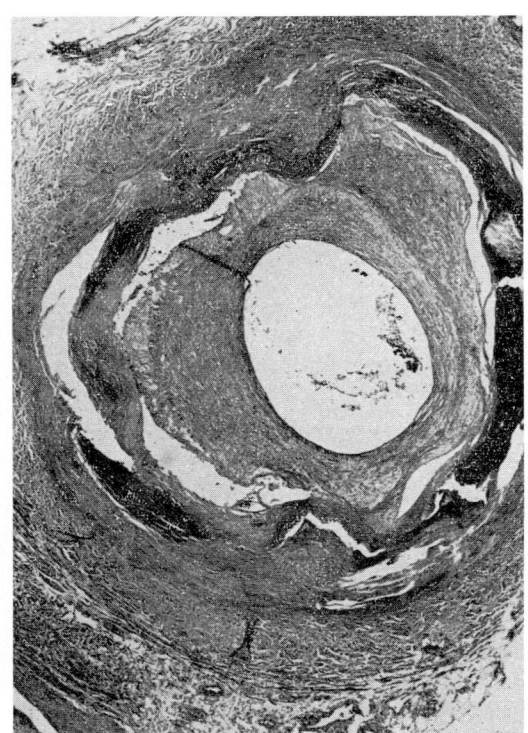

Figure 6-36 Cross section of artery of the lower extremity showing calcification of media.

tion of the internal elastic lamina (Fig. 6-35). This occurs throughout life but is accentuated by hypertension.

3. Senile ectasia, a disease of the aorta and large arteries.

4. Mönckeberg's sclerosis, or medial calcification, in large arteries (Fig. 6-36).

5. Intimal atherosclerosis, a plaquelike disease of the intima occurring in true arteries (Fig. 6-37).

6. Arteriolar sclerosis affecting arterioles. This is associated with, and is believed to be a consequence of, hypertension.

Of these six types, intimal atherosclerosis

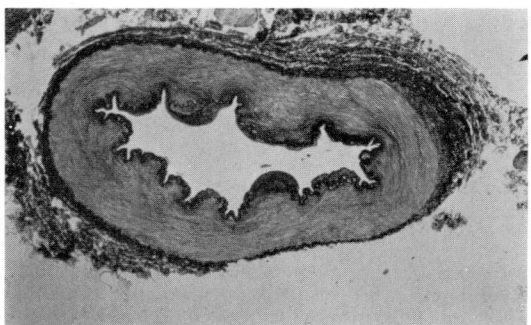

Figure 6-35 Cross section of artery showing reduplication of the elastic lamina.

and arteriolar sclerosis are the two most common types of arterial diseases occurring in retinal vessels. Although each is a distinct entity, they are frequently confused in the ophthalmologic literature, the two terms erroneously being used interchangeably. They should be carefully differentiated because of their individual natures and significance.

INTIMAL ATHEROSCLEROSIS. This disease of the intima is seen commonly in males over the age of 30. The primary lesion, or atheroma, is a small, round, yellow, elevated area of intimal thickening (Plate 17C, Figs. 6-38, 6-39). It consists of proliferation of connective tissue, edema with cholesterol crystals, and lipid deposits. Such lesions coalesce to form larger ones. As they enlarge, they may ulcerate and predispose to thrombosis formation with vascular obstruction, or, on the other hand, weaken the arterial wall and result in an aneurysm formation or calamitous rupture.

The course is characterized by sudden vascular accidents, exemplified by coronary occlusion, cerebral thrombosis, and cere-

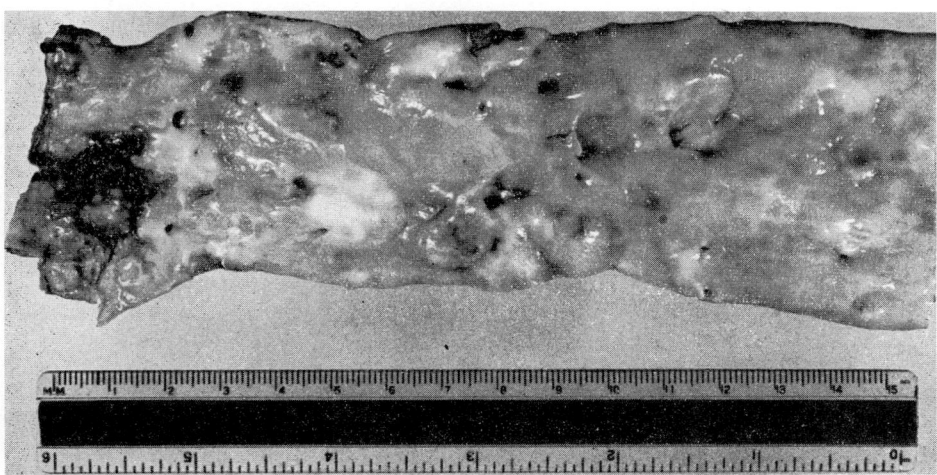

Figure 6-37 Photograph of aorta showing extensive lesions of intimal atherosclerosis.

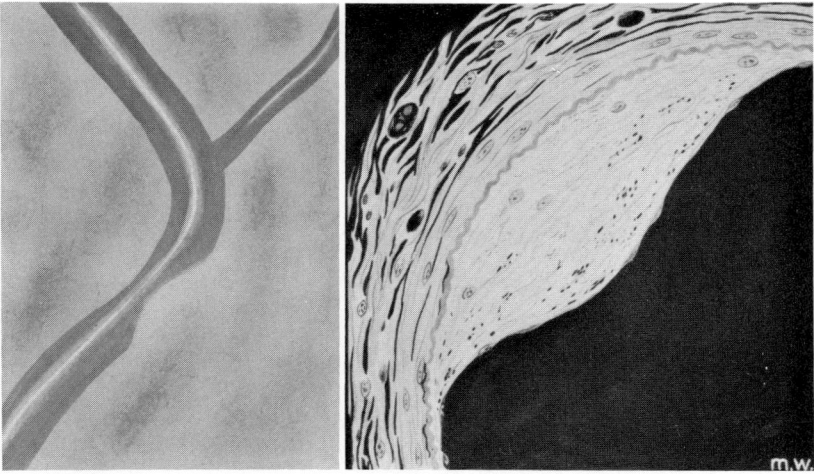

Fig. 6-38   Fig. 6-39

Figure 6-38 An atheromatous plaque in the retinal artery near the disc causing an indentation of the arterial wall.
Figure 6-39 Schematic cross section of an atheroma.

bral hemorrhage. In the eye atherosclerosis may manifest itself by thrombosis of the central retinal artery or one of its branches. The eye is one organ in the body where thrombosis of a vein results from intimal atherosclerosis. This occurs because the central retinal vein and artery and their branches are surrounded by a common adventitial sheath at their arteriovenous crossings (Plate 17D) as well as within the optic nerve (Plate 17E). The atheromatous process readily invades the vein, causing a similar atheromatous plaque on which a thrombosis may form. Atherosclerosis occurs in a spotty fashion throughout the body so that the arteries of either the brain, the heart, or the eyes may be extensively involved (Fig. 6-40A, B), with little or no change occurring in the other organs. Because of this inconstant distribution, ophthalmoscopic examination is not of great help in evaluating this disease.

ARTERIOLAR SCLEROSIS. This disease is caused by hypertension, and its changes represent damage of the arterioles from the stress and strain of elevated blood pressure. The vessel wall shows diffuse involvement rather than the spotty plaque-like lesions of intimal atherosclerosis. Hyaline material, containing lipid, deposits initially just beneath the endothelium. As the disease progresses, the muscularis becomes involved, and finally the entire vessel wall.

Arteriolar sclerosis involves arterioles throughout the body fairly uniformly (Plate 17F, G). This is an important point, because the characteristic changes in the fundus are a fairly accurate reflection of the changes occurring elsewhere in the body; for example, in the kidneys.

Ocular Changes in Arteriolar Sclerosis and Hypertension. The rapidity of onset and the degree of arteriolar sclerosis depend upon both the duration and the severity of the hypertensive process. Arteriolar sclerosis appears more rapidly in severe than in mild hypertensive states. However, if a mild hypertension is of sufficient duration, arteriolar sclerosis may be pronounced. Normally the retinal arterioles appear a clear pink with a small central light reflex from the wall. This light streak is formed by the reflection of light from the convex surface of the blood column and the blood vessel wall, which normally is almost transparent. The light streak in the arteries is always wider and brighter than that in veins of similar caliber.

The ophthalmoscopic changes of hypertension usually precede those of arteriolar sclerosis. The exact cause of hypertension is still obscure, but there is considerable agreement that an increase in resistance to blood flow results from constriction of the arterial bed throughout the body. The cause of the constriction is not definitely established. Early in the hypertensive state the peripheral arterioles show normal physiological responses to physical and chemical stimuli, evidence that the disturbance is functional. The ophthalmoscopic

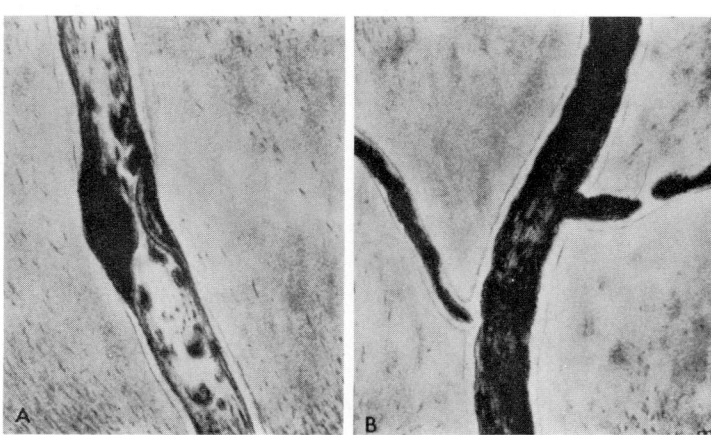

Figure 6-40 (A) Flat preparation (fat stain) showing intimal atherosclerosis in retinal arterial system. (B) Similar preparation showing arteriosclerosis in retinal arterial system. (After Friedenwald.)

changes seen in the retinal arterioles in hypertension support these findings. Because the retinal changes of hypertension stem from narrowing of the retinal arterioles, ophthalmoscopic examination is of little aid in determining the underlying cause. The ophthalmoscopic signs of hypertension associated with chronic glomerulonephritis may differ in no way from those of severe essential hypertension.

The ophthalmoscopic changes of hypertension all relate to constriction of arterioles. The earliest recognizable change is generalized attenuation of the retinal arterial tree, especially the smaller branches. When more severe, the irregularities in caliber (probably caused by local spasm) are superimposed upon generalized narrowing. In severe hypertension the capillary blood flow may be so impaired that nutritional damage to the vessel wall occurs. This results in hemorrhages, exudates, and edema.

The ophthalmoscopic signs of arteriolar sclerosis are secondary to hypertension and stem from thickening of the wall of the arteriole. First, reflection of light from the wall of the arteriole increases, causing widening of the light streak. As the light streak widens it eventually becomes so broad that it occupies most of the vessel, and the vessel assumes the appearance of burnished copper; hence the term "copperwire." A silver-wire appearance, or opaque vessel wall, is the advanced stage of the sclerotic process.

GRADING OF HYPERTENSION

The retinal changes of hypertension and arteriolar sclerosis should be graded separately because of their individual significance. Several systems have been suggested. The Keith-Wagener-Barker classification of retinal changes associated with hypertension has been used longer than any other system. It is described in Table 6-11. A simplified system for the separate grading of the retinal changes of hypertension and of arteriolar sclerosis also has been proposed (Scheie) (Plates 17H, 18A). Hypertension is evaluated from the narrowing of arterioles and focal spasm, hemorrhages, exudates, and edema of the disc. Criteria are utilized that can be duplicated with considerable uniformity by successive observers on the same patient. The changes are graded from normal to Grade IV. Patients with mild hypertension may have such minimal narrowing of retinal arterioles that it cannot be detected ophthalmoscopically.

When the hypertension is more severe, narrowing may be recognizable, particularly in the smaller secondary branches, and the changes are termed Grade I. These are well seen in early toxemia of pregnancy, and in hypertension of rapid onset

TABLE 6-11. KEITH-WAGENER-BARKER CLASSIFICATION OF DIFFUSE ARTERIOLAR DISEASE WITH HYPERTENSION

Group 1
Essential benign hypertension with adequate cardiac and renal function. Moderate arteriolar attenuation, often combined with focal constriction, and brightened arteriolar light reflex (with burnished copper wire or polished silver wire appearance).

Group 2
Patients have a continuously higher blood pressure but are still in good health. Arteriovenous changes may be present. Arterioles are quite attenuated with localized arteriolar constriction. Hard, shiny deposits and tiny hemorrhages may develop.

Group 3
Diffuse arterial changes with evidence of functional insufficiency of retina, brain, kidneys, and other organs. Marked attenuation of arterioles, retina appears wet and edematous, cotton-wool exudates, and hemorrhages.

Group 4
Patients in very serious condition with severe nervous system, visual, and other organ disturbances. Patients have ophthalmoscopic signs of Group 3, with papilledema.

in young persons where the duration has been insufficient for arteriolar sclerosis to have developed. Minimal changes such as these could easily be overlooked if the patient had not been referred with the diagnosis of hypertension.

Grade II hypertensive changes exist when the narrowing is still more pronounced and localized irregularity or focal constrictions are present. These are thought to be local spasm and contraction of the wall of the arteriole. When severe, especially in young persons, the prognosis is poor.

Grade III hypertensive changes include narrowing and irregularity, usually severe, accompanied by exudates and usually retinal hemorrhages.

Grade IV changes include those of Grade III plus papilledema, often with visible edema of the retina.

Two types of exudates may occur during severe hypertensive states. They in all likelihood result from nutritional disturbances secondary to severe arteriolar spasm. Cotton-wool exudates probably represent localized ischemic infarction of the nerve fiber layer of the retina, although some pathologists say that they are accumulations of fibrin. These are seen typically during acute phases of severe hypertensive state, but also may occur in other disorders such as lupus erythematosus and polyarteritis nodosa. Hard, shiny exudates indicate a protracted, severe hypertensive state and are due to lipid degeneration and infiltration of the deep layers of the retina. They have a predilection for the macular region, often in the form of a so-called macular star.

GRADING OF ARTERIOLAR SCLEROSIS

Arteriolar sclerosis results from hypertension and develops more rapidly if the hypertension is severe. However, marked sclerosis can result from relatively mild hypertension of many years duration. In arteriolar sclerosis the wall of the arteriole thickens and reflects more light to produce the following: widening of the light streak, the earliest change of arteriolar sclerosis; copper-wire arteries, the term indicating the appearance of the arteries as the light streak further widens to occupy most of the surface of the vessel; silver-wire arteries, indicating the extreme form of arteriolar sclerosis, in which the vessel wall is so thickened by hyalinization and lipid infiltration that it becomes opaque and obscures the blood column. The artery appears as a white cord even though a lumen may still be present. As the thickness of the arteriole wall increases, arteriovenous crossing defects appear. These are produced by compression of the vein by the arteriole where they cross and are bound in a common adventitial sheath. Because of this sheath, the thickened arteriole wall impinges on the lumen of the vein.

Ophthalmoscopically several different phenomena result that indicate the presence of arteriolar sclerosis. The commonest appearance is that of compression of the vein by the artery. This may vary in severity from a slight indentation to nearly complete interruption of the vein. Tapering of the vein at the arteriovenous crossing is seen occasionally if the sclerotic process extends into the adventitia of the vein. Owing to constriction or compression of the vein by the arteriole, blood return may be impeded, and the vein becomes distended for some distance peripheral to the crossing. This has been referred to as "banking." Deflection of a vein from its normal course is another common event at the point where the arteriole crosses (Plate 18B).

Scheie's grading system for arteriolar sclerosis is based upon alterations of the light reflex from the arterioles and the arteriovenous compression phenomena. This ranges from 0 to IV. Many patients with hypertension show no evidence of sclerosis and are termed Grade 0. The earliest recognizable increase in light reflex or in broadening of the reflex stripe associated with minimal arteriovenous compression is classified Grade I. When more marked these are termed Grade II. Presence of copper-wire arteries and more marked arteriovenous compression are indicated by Grade III. Silver-wire arteries indicate the severest degree of sclerosis, or Grade IV.

As already mentioned, the ophthalmic consultant should grade the fundus changes of hypertension separately from those of arteriolar sclerosis because of their different significance (Plates 18C to 21D). The ophthalmoscopic changes of hypertension stem from vasospasm and

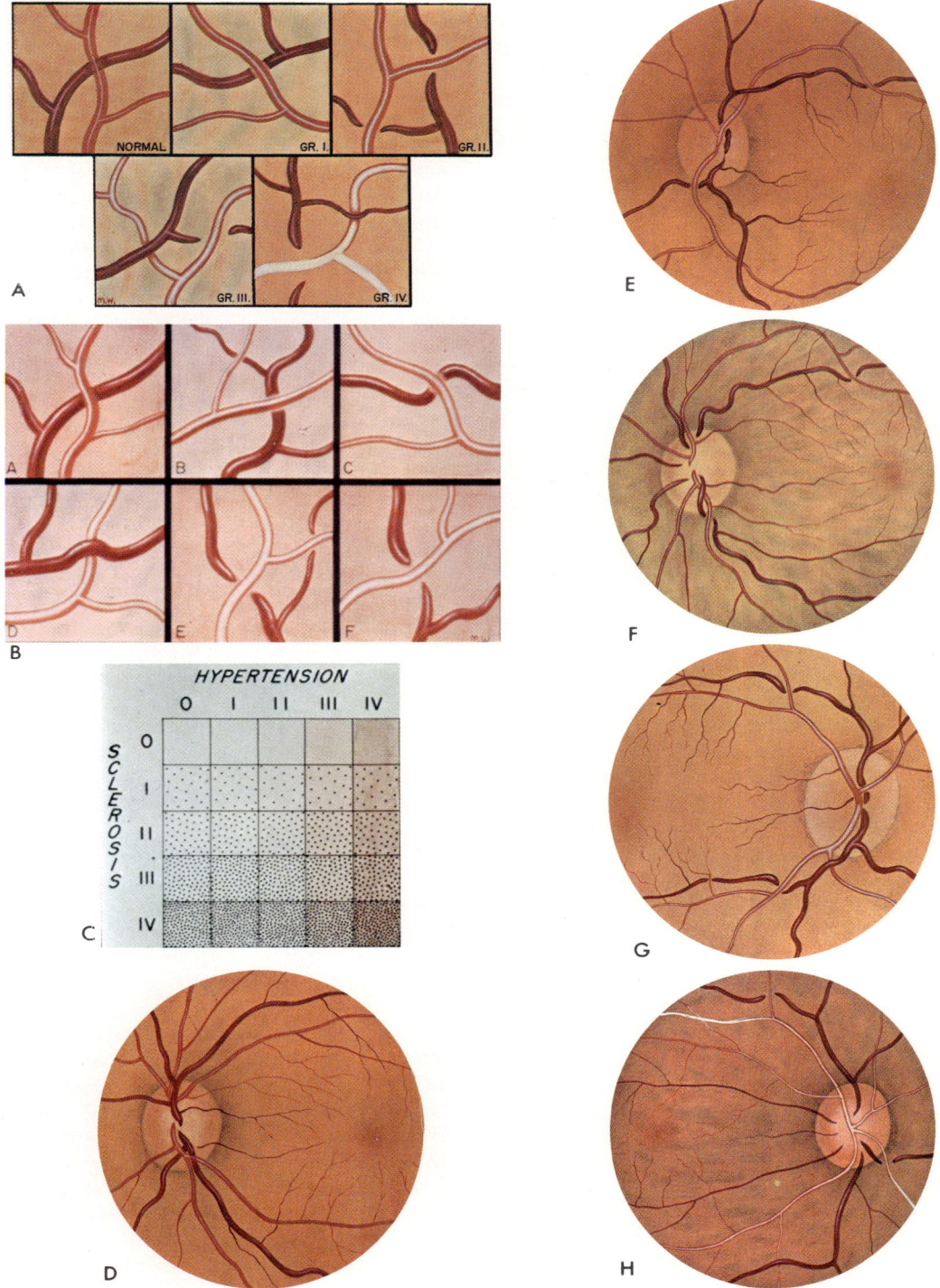

Plate 18 *(A)* Schema for ophthalmoscopic classification of arteriolar sclerosis. *(B)* Changes in arteriovenous crossing in arteriolar sclerosis: A, normal crossing; B, early arteriovenous compression; C, deviation of vein; D, humping of vein; E, tapering of vein; F, banking of vein. *(C)* Correlation of degree of retinal changes of hypertension and degree of retinal arteriolar sclerosis. *(D)* Grade 0 hypertension; grade 0 arteriolar sclerosis. *(E)* Grade 0 hypertension; grade I arteriolar sclerosis. *(F)* Grade 0 hypertension; grade II arteriolar sclerosis. *(G)* Grade 0 hypertension; grade III arteriolar sclerosis. *(H)* Grade 0 hypertension; grade IV arteriolar sclerosis.

243

rather accurately parallel the severity of the hypertensive process. The changes of arteriolar sclerosis, on the other hand, furnish an estimate of the damage to the arterioles due to the wear and tear of elevated intraarterial pressure.

Evaluating the severity of the sclerosis of the retinal arterioles is probably of greater value to the internist than estimating the hypertensive state. The severity of hypertension can readily be assessed by blood pressure measurements and other means, but the degree of sclerosis may be very difficult to determine. Furthermore, the amount of sclerosis serves as some indication of the duration of the hypertension. Little or none suggests recent origin, particularly if the hypertension is severe. Marked sclerosis indicates longer duration, even though sclerosis may develop more rapidly with severe hypertension. This can be helpful because even though the diagnosis and severity of hypertension can be determined with great accuracy, the duration often is difficult to ascertain. The history is notoriously unreliable.

Any degree of arteriolar sclerosis may occur with any degree of hypertensive change. Mild hypertension over a period of years may produce marked arteriolar sclerosis, whereas an acute, fulminating, malignant hypertension may cause death before sclerosis can develop. On the other hand, if superimposed on long-standing benign hypertension, it may be accompanied by severe arteriolar sclerosis.

Quantitative evaluation of the degree of sclerosis is of increasing value with the development of more effective means of lowering blood pressure. It is advantageous to know about the severity of the arteriolar sclerosis, because if none were present the hypertension would have caused little organic vascular damage; if the arteriolar sclerotic changes were severe, the damage would be marked and the prognosis more guarded.

OCCLUSION OF THE RETINAL ARTERIES

Causes of retinal artery occlusion are intimal atherosclerosis; emboli; inadequate blood supply to the retinal vessels from carotid occlusion, massive hemorrhage, and heart failure; and temporal arteritis (p. 315). Other cited causes include syphilis, rheumatic fever, hepatitis, lupus erythematosus, cryoglobulinemia, sickle cell disease, mucormycosis, and prolonged pressure on the globe. In many instances the cause cannot be determined.

Most occlusions of the central retinal artery and arterioles occurring among older persons result from spasms or thrombosis, usually secondary to intimal atherosclerosis. Transient loss of vision (*amaurosis fugax*), resulting from retinal ischemia, may precede occlusion of the central retinal artery. Such prodromal attacks are thought to be due to vasospasm. They are characteristically unilateral and persist for only a few seconds or minutes. On ophthalmoscopic examination during such an episode, one may note emptying of the retinal arterioles. The retinal arterial pressures should be measured with an ophthalmodynamometer in all patients with such attacks to detect the possible obstruction of the internal carotid artery.

Emboli may lodge in the central retinal artery or in its branches. Cholesterol and calcific emboli, common in older patients, probably arise from the walls of diseased carotid or vertebral vessels. When arrested in branch arterioles, these emboli often appear larger than the apparent lumen of the vessel. In younger patients emboli most commonly originate from post-rheumatic cardiac vegetations, particularly following cardiac catheterization or mitral valvotomies. Fat emboli may form after fracture of the long bones.

If occlusion of the central retinal artery persists for more than a few minutes, ischemic infarction results. The retina becomes milky-white for some distance around the disc due to swelling and necrosis of the ganglion cells. A cherry red spot is present in the very thin macular area (Plate 21*E*). The arterioles are severely constricted, the veins full. Venous pulsations are neither visible nor can be elicited with digital pressure on the globe. There may be fragmentation of the blood column in the arterioles and venules, particularly near the disc. After several weeks edema gradually subsides and the cherry red spot disappears. The arterioles may redilate to some extent or eventually become white, threadlike structures, and the optic nerve

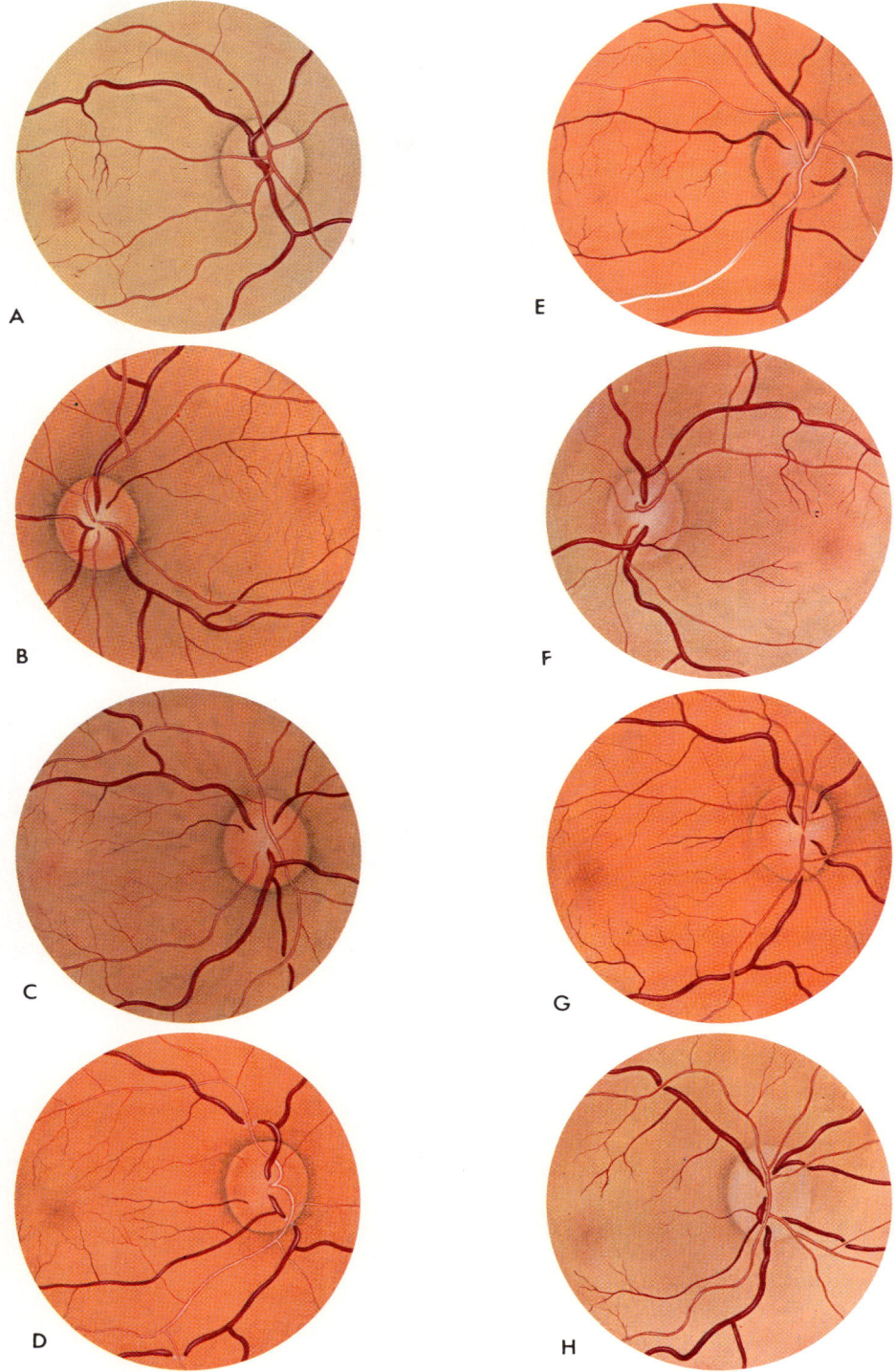

Plate 19 *(A)* Grade I hypertension; grade 0 arteriolar sclerosis. *(B)* Grade I hypertension; grade I arteriolar sclerosis. *(C)* Grade I hypertension; grade II arteriolar sclerosis. *(D)* Grade I hypertension; grade III arteriolar sclerosis. *(E)* Grade I hypertension; grade IV arteriolar sclerosis. *(F)* Grade II hypertension; grade 0 arteriolar sclerosis. *(G)* Grade II hypertension; grade I arteriolar sclerosis. *(H)* Grade II hypertension; grade II arteriolar sclerosis.

245

head may become more markedly white as atrophy develops.

Occlusion of the central retinal artery causes sudden, painless, total, or nearly total, loss of vision in the affected eye. If a branch arteriole occludes (Plate 21*F*), ischemic infarction is limited to the area of the retina supplied by that arteriole. The affected portion has a milky-white appearance; fragmentation and constriction of the blood column are seen in the involved arteriole (Plate 21*G*). Pallor of the sector of the disc may occur later, and a field defect, corresponding to the affected segment of the retina, will be present.

Retinal artery occlusion may be treated by anticoagulation, inhalation of oxygen or carbon dioxide, and vasodilatation with retrobulbar Priscoline, or by stellate ganglion block. The globe may be massaged to force the embolus through the occluded vessel. The intraocular pressure may be lowered by means of paracentesis of the anterior chamber or with pilocarpine drops. If treatment is not initiated promptly, permanent loss of vision can be expected. Patients should receive a careful systemic examination to determine the cause and to prevent occlusion in the other eye.

OCCLUSION OF THE RETINAL VEINS

Causes of occlusion of the retinal veins are external compression of the vein, particularly constriction against a rigid arterial wall; diabetes; degenerative venous disease (phlebosclerosis, with intimal proliferation or phlebitis); and thrombosis associated with abnormal states of the blood or with slowing of the bloodstream. Less common causes are granulomatous diseases, generalized infections, contiguous inflammation from the orbit or sinuses, gastrointestinal bleeding, and trauma. Occlusion often occurs in patients with atherosclerosis of the central artery or its branches and in patients with preexisting glaucoma. The retinal veins most commonly occlude in older persons.

In occlusion of the central vein, vision is reduced, but in contrast to central retinal artery occlusion, the patient usually can perceive light or hand movements. The fundus is "splashed with blood" from widespread retinal hemorrhage (Plate 21*H*). The retinal veins are greatly engorged, patches of white exudate may be seen among the hemorrhages, and some edema of the disc is present. Vision usually remains poor, even after subsequent recanaliculization of the occluded vein or the development of collateral circulation.

Secondary changes and complications following central vein occlusion are residual hemorrhages and microaneurysms, which may persist for long periods after the occlusion; venous sheathing; and new vessel formation. The new vessels may be numerous on the optic disc, forming a *rete mirabile*.

Secondary glaucoma ("hemorrhagic glaucoma") develops in 5 to 20 per cent of patients with central retinal vein occlusion, usually within three to four months of the occlusion. It generally is preceded by the appearance of new vessels on the iris (rubeosis iridis). Glaucoma of this type is difficult to control, and in a blind, painful eye retrobulbar alcohol injection or enucleation may be required.

Incipient occlusion of the central retinal vein presents a picture of generalized engorgement of the veins accompanied by a small to moderate number of retinal hemorrhages. These changes, present before the patient reports subjective symptoms, are an important sign of impending occlusion. Anticoagulant therapy may be beneficial in this as well as in fresh or incomplete occlusions. Anticoagulants also have been used prophylactically to attempt to prevent thrombosis in the other eye.

Occlusion of a branch vein frequently occurs at a point adjacent to a sclerosed arteriole. The venule distal to the obstruction is dilated; the surrounding retina is covered with flame- or spindle-shaped hemorrhages of varying sizes. Later the proximal portion of the venule, difficult to see following occlusion, may refill. Patients with occlusion of the central retinal vein or its branches should have a thorough systemic examination.

Vascular Disorders of the Choroid

Choroidal Hemorrhage. Localized choroidal hemorrhages usually are circular, and dark red to slate gray. They may occur in vascular sclerosis of the choroid. A choroidal hemorrhage in the macular area may extravasate between Bruch's mem-

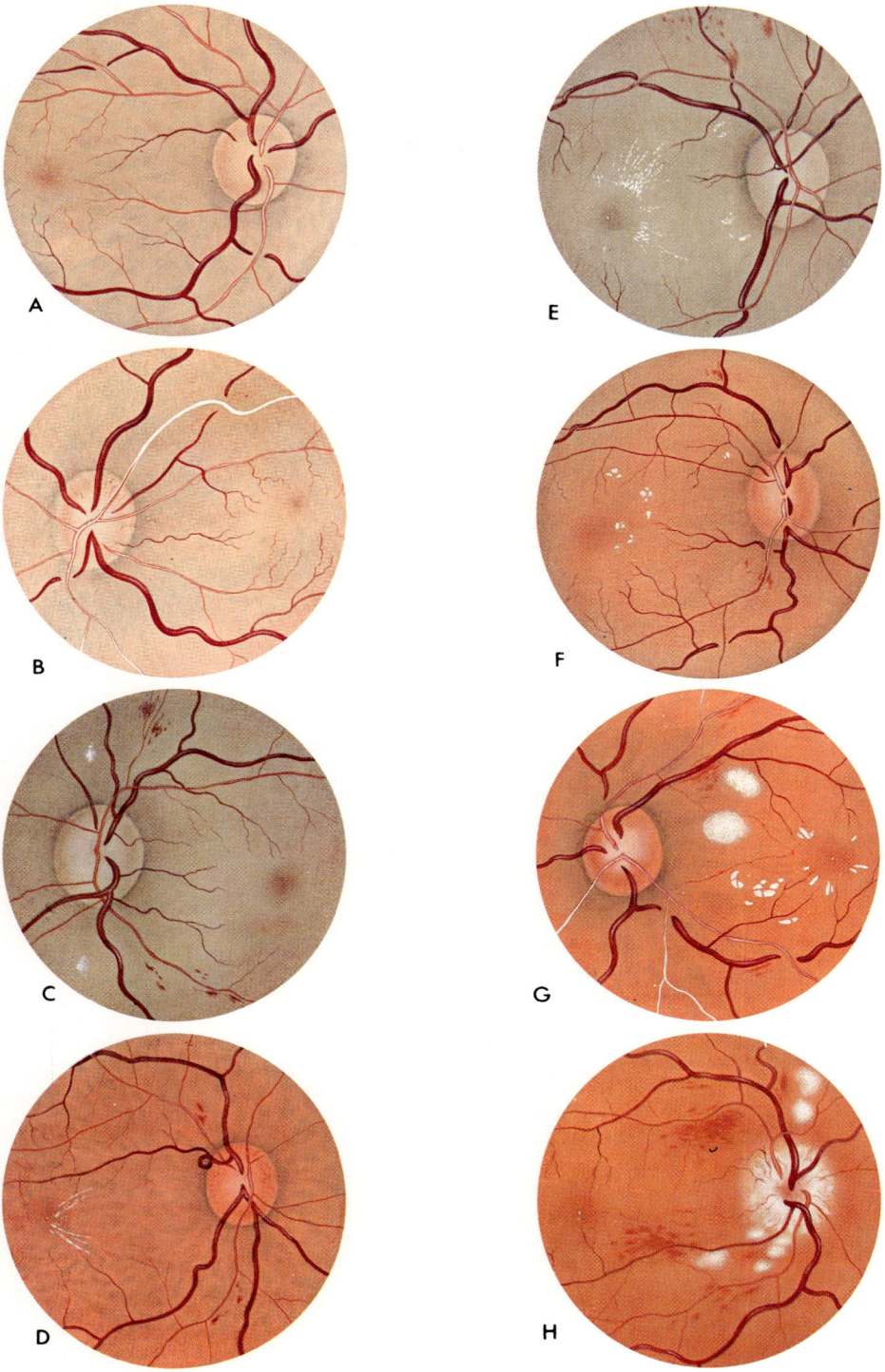

Plate 20 *(A)* Grade II hypertension; grade III arteriolar sclerosis. *(B)* Grade II hypertension; grade IV arteriolar sclerosis. *(C)* Grade III hypertension; grade 0 arteriolar sclerosis. *(D)* Grade III hypertension; grade I arteriolar sclerosis. *(E)* Grade III hypertension; grade II arteriolar sclerosis. *(F)* Grade III hypertension; grade III arteriolar sclerosis. *(G)* Grade III hypertension; grade IV arteriolar sclerosis. *(H)* Grade IV hypertension; grade 0 arteriolar sclerosis.

247

brane and the pigment epithelium, resulting in a disciform degeneration of the macula. Choroidal hemorrhages also may occur with choroiditis, in myopia, trauma, and occasionally in systemic diseases such as blood dyscrasia, diabetes, and Paget's diseases. Choroidal hemorrhage should be differentiated from malignant melanoma of the choroid.

Massive hemorrhage from the choroid is a rare but devastating complication of intraocular surgery. This occurs after the eye is opened, and is related to the sudden drop in intraocular pressure. The choroid may rupture and the contents of the globe flow out. In other instances, the blood may remain within the choroid. Massive hemorrhages of the choroid also have occurred spontaneously in the eyes of old, grossly arteriosclerotic patients, particularly in the presence of glaucoma.

Sclerosis Due to Aging. The outlines of choroidal vessels in most normal eyes are indiscernible with the ophthalmoscope. In some persons, however, the choroidal vessels may be seen clearly. They show a degree of sheathing that varies from two parallel white borders adjacent to the blood column to complete "pipe stem" sheathing without a visible blood column. This latter picture is referred to as sclerosis of the choroidal vessels. In spite of the ophthalmoscopic appearance, histopathologic examination of some of these eyes sometimes does not reveal the expected degree of sclerotic changes. Conversely, sclerosis of the choroidal vessels is found histopathologically in most patients above the age of 60, but these changes may not be recognized with the ophthalmoscope. Such sclerosis results in little functional disturbance of the choroid and retina. Microscopic examination of the choroid frequently reveals atheromatous plaques, but because of the extensive collateral system, occlusion of vessels is rare.

Renal Disease

Azotemic Type (Albuminuric Retinitis; Renal Retinopathy). These terms refer to retinal changes occurring in azotemic types and phases of renal disease (including chronic pyelonephritis; acute pyelonephritis associated with high blood pressure and nitrogen retention; urinary obstruction; and glomerulonephritis). It generally is recognized that high blood pressure is an essential factor in the production of retinopathy in renal disease. Considerable disagreement exists as to whether or not it is possible to distinguish the renal from other types of retinopathy by ophthalmoscopic findings. Some authorities state that certain features of the fundus picture in renal retinopathy differ qualitatively from those in other hypertensive states. These include marked edema of the disc and a retina with fundus details obscured by the opaque quality of the edema, extremely numerous cotton-wool exudates located in the posterior pole, and changes in the arterioles suggesting fibrosis. The presence of only moderate elevation of the diastolic pressure in association with these findings is stated to be further evidence for renal retinopathy.

Nephrotic Type. Retinal changes of this type are described as occurring in patients with renal disease characterized by edema, proteinuria, depletion of serum albumin, and often an increased serum cholesterol. Such disease may occur without antecedent infection, as a phase of acute, progressive glomerulonephritis, in diabetes mellitus, in systemic lupus erythematosus, and in other disorders. On ophthalmoscopic examination there is mild edema of the disc and retina, and the vessels are distinct with the veins dilated, tortuous, and dark in color. The arterioles are full and of normal color with absence of any changes of hypertensive retinopathy. A heightened reflex, apparently emanating from the internal limiting membrane of the retina, is seen. Anemia sometimes occurs in renal disease and produces the fundus changes previously described.

Toxemia of Pregnancy

The outstanding feature of this common and serious complication of pregnancy is a secondary type of diastolic hypertension, which usually occurs after the sixth month. Other principal findings include proteinuria, edema, hematuria, and other signs of acute nephritis. This disorder is known

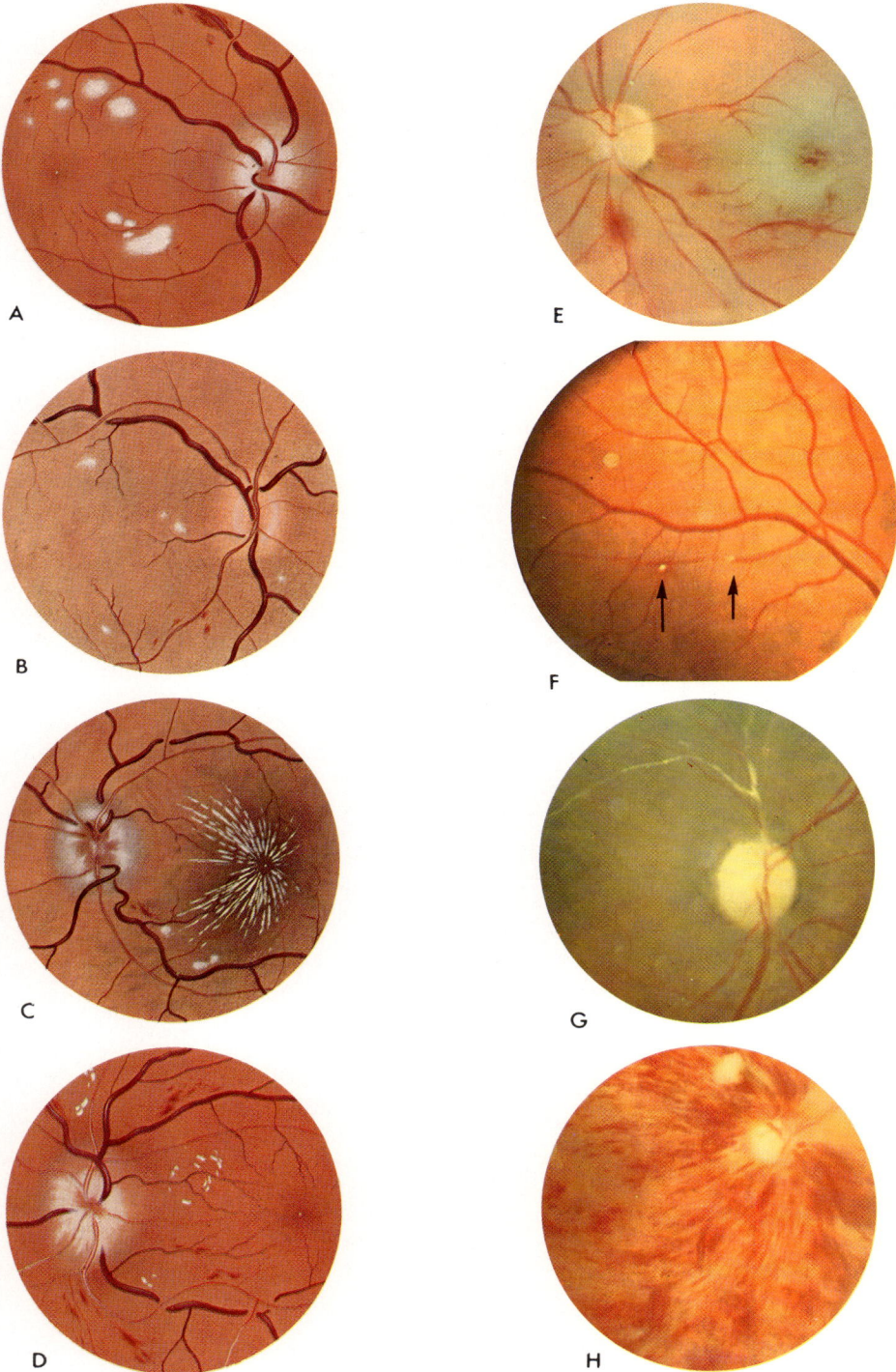

Plate 21 *(A)* Grade IV hypertension; grade I arteriolar sclerosis. *(B)* Grade IV hypertension; grade II arteriolar sclerosis. *(C)* Grade IV hypertension; grade III arteriolar sclerosis. *(D)* Grade IV hypertension; grade IV arteriolar sclerosis. *(E)* Central retinal artery occlusion with cherry-red spot of macula. *(F)* Embolus lodged in arteriole following carotid arteriogram. *(G)* Occlusion of superior temporal papillary artery. *(H)* Central retinal vein occlusion.

249

in its early stages as preeclampsia. It is termed eclampsia when headaches, vomiting, and convulsions or coma develop. The ophthalmoscopic findings are the same as those described for hypertensive retinopathy, with marked spasm of the arterioles, edema, exudates, and hemorrhages developing in severe cases. The edema and exudation may assume a star configuration in the macular area. A flat macular detachment or large retinal detachment is not uncommon. If the retinopathy is limited to narrowing of the arterioles, conservative treatment with rest, sedation, and controlled diet and fluid balance may suffice. Some of the hypotensive drugs may be helpful. If the toxemia is severe, and retinopathy advanced, termination of the pregnancy may be necessary to avoid permanent visual damage and possible death.

Occlusion of the Carotid Arteries

Carotid occlusion may result in a wide variation in symptoms, often including optic atrophy and blindness. The most common cause of carotid occlusion is atherosclerosis. Disorders of carotid occlusion are discussed in detail in the chapter on neuro-ophthalmology (p. 313). *Pulseless disease* is a term used to describe occlusion of the main branches of the aortic arch near their origin. It results in the absence of radial pulses, hypersensitivity of the carotid body, and ocular changes, including development of arteriovenous anastomoses and cataract. One form of pulseless disease (Takayasu's disease) is due to widespread arteritis and has been reported most commonly in young Japanese women.

Cyanosis of the Retina

In long-standing congenital or acquired cardiac insufficiency, the fundus may appear to have a dusky hue. The conjunctiva in such patients also may appear congested and cyanotic. Dark, tortuous, dilated, retinal veins, edema of the retina, and scattered hemorrhages also may occur as a result of an associated, compensatory polycythemia.

ENDOCRINE DISEASES

Endocrine Ophthalmopathy

Clinical Types and Findings. Since Parry first described exophthalmic goiter in 1786, the cause and classification of this disorder has aroused much interest and disagreement. A wide variety of ocular signs accompany thyroid dysfunction. In 1944 Mulvaney suggested that they could be resolved into two types: *thyrotoxic* and *thyrotropic* exophthalmos. The mild, thyrotoxic type, he proposed, results entirely from the effect of thyrotoxicosis on the smooth muscles of Müller in the lids, and on the vestigial muscle bundles in the connective tissue of the orbit. This effect, together with the accompanying sympatheticotonia, results in proptosis, lid retraction, stare, and minor degrees of extraocular weakness, but never in congestive or infiltrative phenomena.

In severe thyrotropic exophthalmos, by contrast, Mulvaney postulated that thyrotropin, acting directly upon the orbital tissues and extraocular muscles, produces edema and infiltrative changes. Although his theory continues to exert considerable influence, more recent interpretations suggest that these two types of ocular involvement are extremes of a spectrum rather than separate entities.

Mild endocrine ophthalmopathy occurs in females much more frequently than in males (Plate 22A). In common with more severe endocrine ophthalmopathy, it usually occurs after the age of 40 in 80 per cent of patients, and the onset in relation to the thyroid disease is variable. The milder changes cause few symptoms. These include a number of physical findings to which proper names have been attached. The most important are wide and palpebral fissure due to retraction of upper lid (Dalrymple's sign); infrequent blinking (Stellwag's sign), resulting in staring; lid lag on downward gaze (von Graefe's sign); and weakness of convergence (Möbius' sign). Exophthalmos is more apparent than real and probably is due to retraction of the lids, with widened fissure. The globe is freely moveable and can easily be pushed backward into the orbit without undue resistance.

The ocular disorder usually disappears or improves with control of the hyperthyroidism. However, in a small number of patients, the ocular signs may rapidly become severe, especially if the basal metabolic rate is lowered suddenly by certain types of medical or surgical therapy. In these patients exophthalmos may be extremely pronounced, and the globe resists being pushed backward into the orbit because of the increased volume of the orbital contents.

Severe endocrine ophthalmopathy may be accompanied by annoying symptoms, which include marked exophthalmos, tearing, foreign body sensation due to conjunctival and corneal irritation, and discomfort in the orbital area. The severe form of endocrine ophthalmopathy has no sexual predilection. When accompanied by a low basal metabolic rate, the initial symptoms of puffiness and itching of the eyelids with mild conjunctival injection may suggest allergy and lead to mistaken diagnoses. With increasing congestion and infiltration of the orbital contents, conjunctival hyperemia and edema increase, and the conjunctiva may push forward through the palpebral fissure (Plate 22B).

When the extraocular muscles are involved, diplopia may result and ocular rotations may be impaired (Plate 23A, B, C; Fig. 6-41A, B). Weakness of upward gaze usually is first and may be due to the superior rectus having to pull against an edematous or fibrotic inferior rectus muscle. The patient loses the protective mechanism of upward rotation of the eyes during sleep. Also, exophthalmos may prevent the lids from closing, and the corneas remain exposed (Plate 22C). The central zone shows erosions earliest, and indicates danger to the eye. Such lesions will stain with fluorescein. Continued erosion can lead to corneal ulceration or even perforation if complicated by infection.

Visual loss can result from papilledema, papillitis, or retrobulbar neuritis. These usually occur in patients with the most severe ophthalmopathy and are thought to be associated with increased orbital pressure. Visual loss from this cause usually is reversible, but occasionally blindness may result. Patients with severe exophthalmos, therefore, should be carefully observed to detect possible involvement of the optic nerve. Visual fields and visual acuity should be tested periodically. Careful ophthalmoscopic examinations also should be made for papilledema, papillitis, or retinal folds

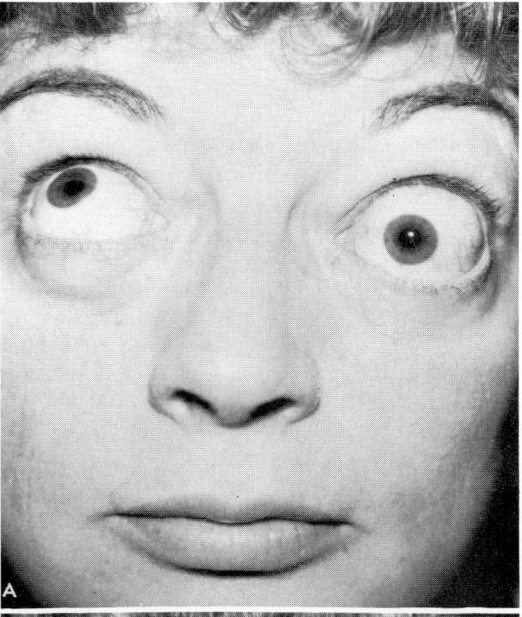

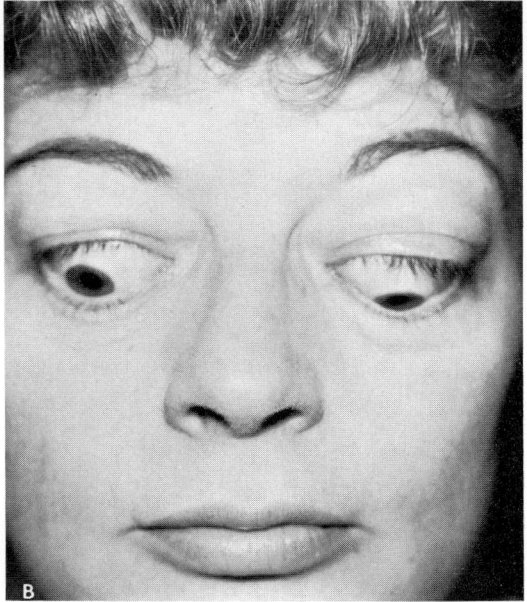

Figure 6-41 (*A*), (*B*) Endocrine ophthalmopathy with exophthalmos and limitation of motion.

from the increased orbital pressure. The severe type of exophthalmos usually runs a self-limited course of one or two years. Resolution almost never is complete, and some degree of exophthalmos persists.

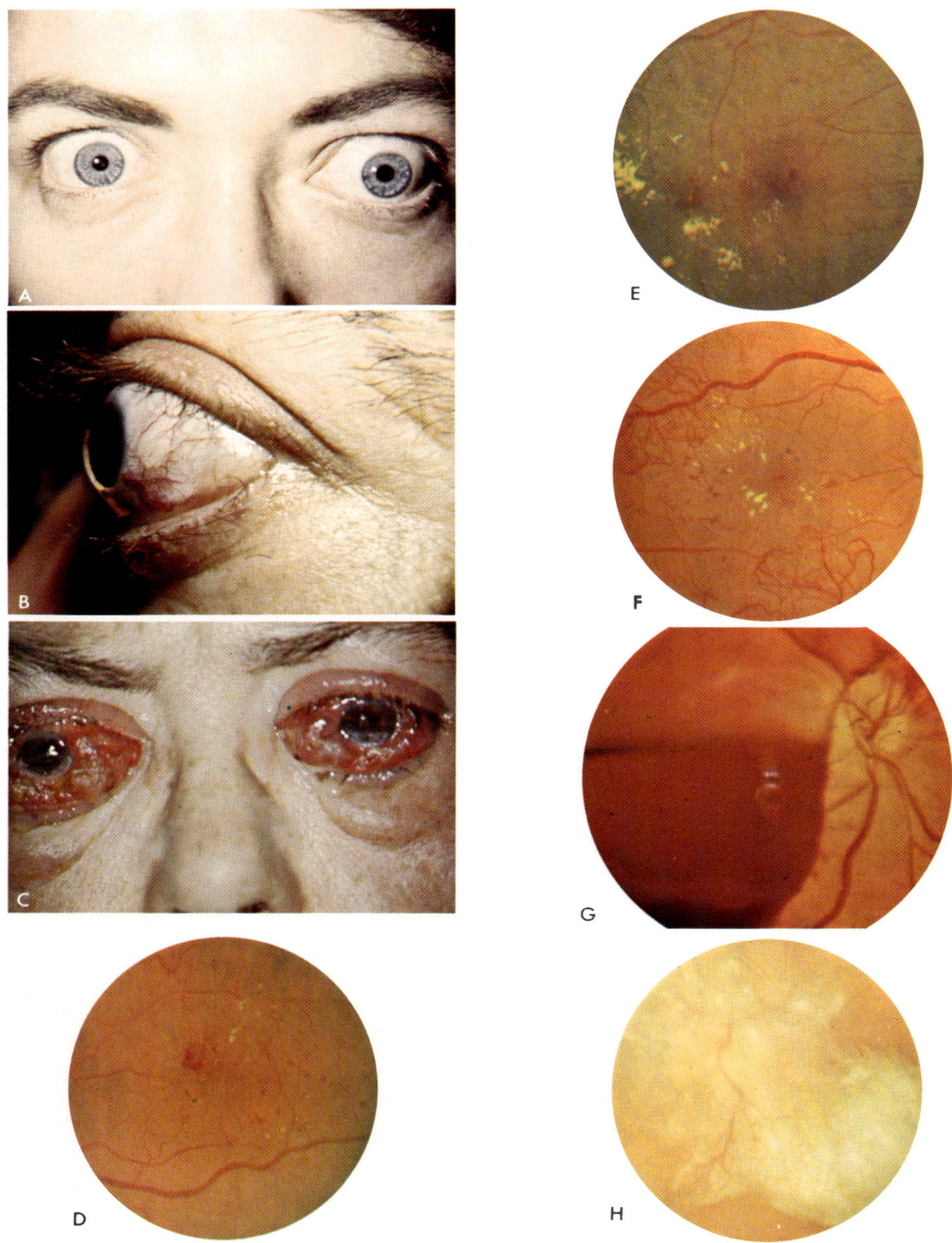

Plate 22 *(A)* Endocrine ophthalmopathy with exophthalmos and lid retraction. *(B)* Endocrine ophthalmopathy with exophthalmos and congestion. *(C)* Endocrine ophthalmopathy with exophthalmos, chemosis, and exposure keratitis. *(D)* Progressive stages in diabetic retinopathy (22D to 22H). Characteristic microaneurysms, yellowish exudates, and hemorrhagic phenomenon. *(E)* Progressive stage of 22D. *(F)* Progressive stage of 22E. *(G)* Diabetic retinopathy with preretinal hemorrhage. *(H)* Diabetic retinopathy with retinitis proliferans.

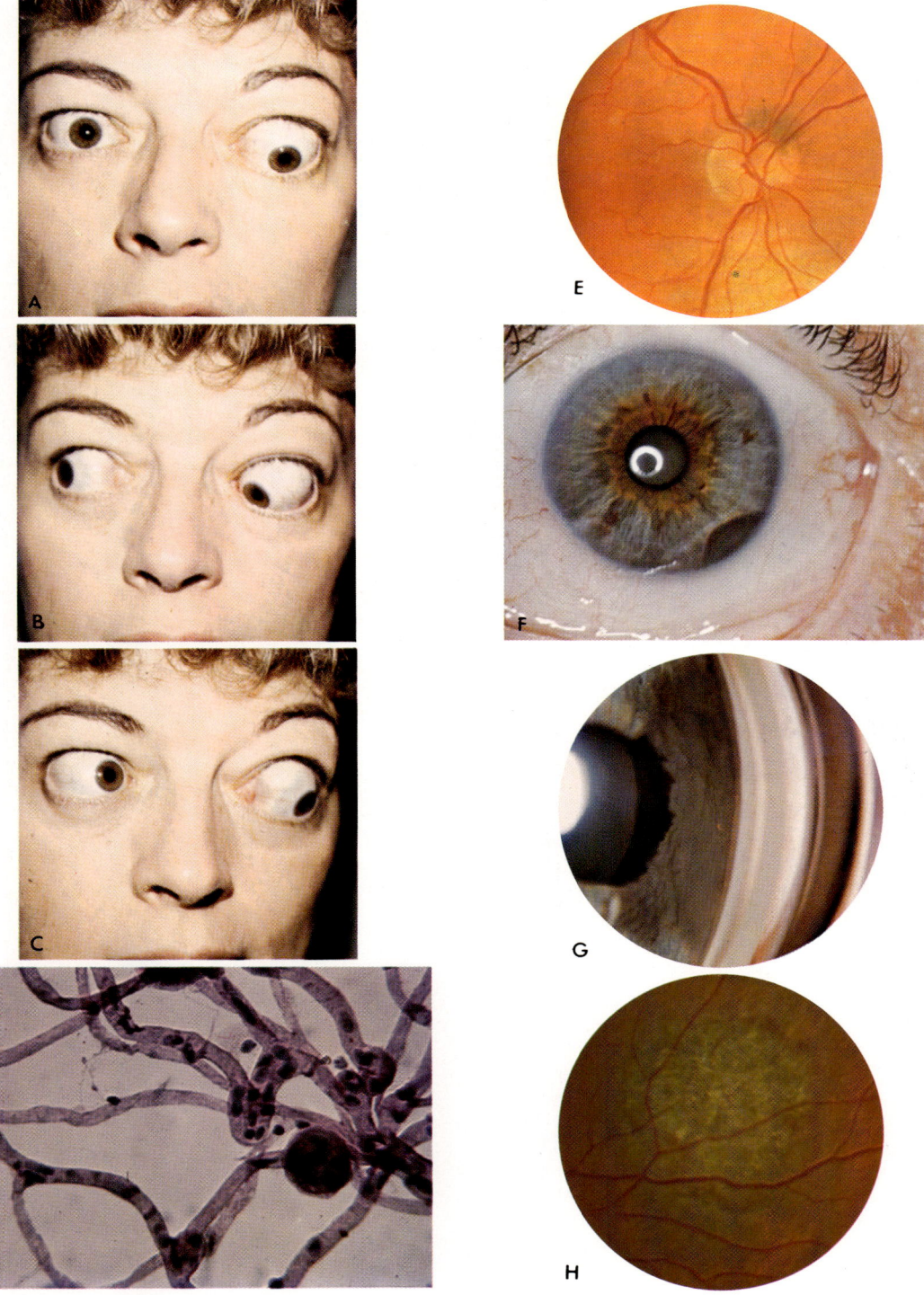

Plate 23 *(A)* Endocrine ophthalmopathy with exophthalmos and limitation of motion. Looking straight ahead. *(B)* Same as 23*A.* Looking to the right. *(C)* Same as 23*A.* Looking to the left. *(D)* Flat-mount preparation of trypsin digested retina (after Cogan and Kuwabara) demonstrating loss of mural cells and microaneurysms. *(E)* Choroidal nevus above disc. *(F)* Malignant melanoma of iris. *(G)* Iris melanoma. Gonioscopic view. *(H)* Choroidal malignant melanoma.

Secondary fibrotic changes may occur in the extraocular muscles, with permanent diplopia.

Etiology of Endocrine Ophthalmopathy. The precise cause of this disorder is largely conjectural. Pituitary and thyroid function and exophthalmos are related. Mulvaney's theory of *thyrotoxic* exophthalmos probably is not valid. It is doubtful that in many patients the contraction of the muscles of Müller and other smooth muscle fibers can exert sufficient traction on the globe to cause proptosis. Spasm of the smooth musculature of the lids, resulting from thyrotoxic sympatheticotonia, however, may be responsible for lid retraction and stare, phenomena that tend to resolve after thyrotoxicosis regresses.

Exophthalmos can be produced in experimental animals by the injection of thyroid stimulating hormone (TSH). Experimental exophthalmos produced in the guinea pig by TSH tends to be inhibited by thyroid hormone and is intensified by removal of the thyroid gland. In man, however, administration of TSH does not necessarily produce exophthalmos. Bio-assay results for TSH in patients with severe exophthalmos vary widely. In addition, patients with either hypothyroidism or hyperthyroidism may have high levels of TSH. Exophthalmos can occur with both. Thus it is generally concluded that in man TSH is not solely responsible for the exophthalmos associated with thyroid disease. The possibility of a separate ophthalmotropic or exophthalmos-producing substance has been postulated for many years.

In 1958, Adams demonstrated a thyrotropic substance found in the serum of patients with Graves' disease that has become known as the long-acting thyroid stimulator (LATS). Although its chemical structure and immunologic characteristics have not been determined definitely, LATS may represent a rearrangement of the amino acid sequence in the peptide molecule of thyrotropin. Alternatively, LATS might be thyrotropin that is abnormally bound to a serum protein carrier and has prolonged survival in the plasma.

Autoimmunity may influence the pathogenesis of endocrine ophthalmology. The possibility that local factors are important in the development of this disorder is suggested by the occasional unilateralism, asymmetry, and asynchronism that is seen. It may be that several etiologic factors combine to cause an increase in orbital connective tissue and hyaluronic acid, a substance with strong water-binding capacity. These may result in the clinical findings of endocrine ophthalmopathy. Fibrosis, particularly of the extraocular muscles, may occur subsequent to this.

Treatment of Thyroid Ophthalmopathy. Therapy of the milder form of ophthalmopathy involves proper management of the thyrotoxicosis. Ocular signs should be observed carefully throughout therapy. Abrupt lowering of the basal metabolic rate by medical or surgical means should be avoided, particularly in the presence of eye involvement. Failure to observe this precaution may aggravate or precipitate a severe ophthalmopathy.

Management of the severe type of ophthalmopathy may be very demanding and should involve cooperation of both the ophthalmologist and the general physician or endocrinologist. Attempts should be made to inhibit pituitary function. Corticotropin or cortisone, desiccated thyroid, and iodine therapy are helpful. Roentgen therapy of the pituitary and orbit has been suggested.

When exophthalmos is present, antibiotic or bland ointments, methylcellulose solution, and airtight goggles help protect the cornea, particularly during sleep. If exposure becomes a serious threat and the corneas stain with fluorescein, lid adhesions should be created (tarsorrhaphy). In addition to protecting the cornea, this often improves the cosmetic appearance as well. The lid adhesions are removed when the ophthalmopathy has run its course.

If papilledema or retrobulbar neuritis develops and vision is failing, orbital decompression is indicated. Removal of the lateral or inferior orbital wall permits the orbital contents to herniate and lowers the orbital pressure. Late fibrosis and contracture of the extraocular muscle may cause an annoying diplopia. This may be severe enough to require surgical correction of the ocular deviation. Extraocular muscle surgery, however, should be withheld until the disorder has stabilized. If surgery is done while the process is acute, marked orbital edema may result.

Hypothyroidism. Hypothyroidism may occur spontaneously in middle age, may develop after thyroidectomy, or may be a congenital defect giving rise to cretinism in childhood. The principal ocular manifestations are part of the general picture of myxedema. The lids and surrounding skin are baggy and swollen, resulting in slitlike palpebral fissures. Loss of the outer half of the eyebrows is common. Less common findings are discrete, superficial, gray areas in the central part of the cornea, superficial cortical lens opacities, bilateral retrobulbar neuritis, and optic atrophy. Administration of thyroid produces a dramatic response.

Disorders of the Parathyroid Glands and Calcium-Phosphorus Metabolism

Hypoparathyroidism. This disorder usually occurs after removal of, or damage to, the parathyroid glands during thyroidectomy. Spontaneous hypoparathyroidism also has been reported. Inadequate parathyroid function results in a decreased concentration of ionized calcium in the blood and diminished calcium excretion. Hyperirritability of nervous tissue and tetany result. The occurrence of cataract in association with tetany is a well known finding. The lenticular opacities occur months or years after the onset of hypoparathyroidism, and characteristically appear by slit lamp biomicroscopy as small, discrete, punctate opacities in the cortex, often associated with crystal-like structures of different colors. These opacities are bilateral, develop slowly, and seldom interfere with vision. Optic neuritis and papilledema associated with increased intracranial pressure may develop. Diagnosis is made on the basis of the clinical findings and laboratory studies, which reveal low serum calcium, elevated serum inorganic phosphorus, and decreased urine phosphorus with normal alkaline phosphatase. The Ellsworth-Howard test (intravenous injection of active parathyroid extract with subsequent measurement of urinary phosphate content) results in a tenfold or greater increase in urinary phosphorus. After parathyroid extract is given, serum calcium and phosphorus levels revert to normal. This

disorder is managed with vitamin D or dihydrotachysterol, calcium salts, and a low phosphorus diet.

Pseudohypoparathyroidism. Less common than hypoparathyroidism, pseudohypoparathyroidism is characterized by an absence of response to normally produced parathyroid hormone, presumably because of a renal end-organ defect. The parathyroid glands may be normal or hypertrophied. The average age of onset is about 8 years, and the disease usually becomes manifest by age 20. It is twice as frequent in women than in men. Patients usually have a round face, short stature, and stocky build. Shortening of the metacarpals and, less often, of the metatarsals and phalanges is common. The disease shares with hypoparathyroidism the metabolic abnormalities of hypocalcemia, hyperphosphatemia, and decreased urinary phosphate excretion, with the attendant signs of tetany or convulsions. In addition to the metabolic defect, two other components are present: extraskeletal ossification and calcification, and bony dysplasia. Cerebral calcification, identical with that seen in hypoparathyroidism, occurs. Mental retardation is common. Cataracts, of the type found in hypoparathyroidism, and blurring of disc margins have been reported. The Ellsworth-Howard test is negative. Characteristically, less than a twofold increase in urinary phosphorus excretion occurs. Patients respond to vitamin D and dihydrotachysterol, but not to parathyroid extract.

Pseudo-Pseudohypoparathyroidism. In this rare disorder the metabolic abnormalities of hypocalcemia and hyperphosphatemia are lacking, but the dyschondroplastic changes and ectopic calcification and ossification of pseudohypoparathyroidism are typically present. Mental retardation is common. Blue sclerae, cataract, and esotropia have been described.

Diabetes Mellitus

The belief that diabetes mellitus is a simple insulin deficiency has long since given way to the understanding that this disease is a complex entity with many underlying factors. The pathogenesis of the diabetic state probably involves abnormal binding of certain chains in the insulin molecule, insulin antibodies, local changes affecting insulin action on fat cells, alteration of the effect of adrenal steroids upon glycogenolysis, and aberrations of certain enzymes inhibitory to insulin. Certain adenohypophyseal hormones appear to play an important role in the development of diabetic vascular disease. Diabetic retinopathy affects to some extent about 80 per cent of all diabetic patients. The incidence of retinopathy increases with the duration of the diabetes. The age of the patient, the severity of the diabetes, and the adequacy of its control, however, are not the only factors influencing the development and severity of retinopathy. Diabetes may affect any of the structures of the eye, but retinopathy is the most severe complication, being progressively difficult to treat and frequently leading to blindness.

Diabetic Retinopathy. The retinopathy of diabetes is characterized by microaneurysms, punctate hemorrhages, and numerous white and yellow spots referred to as exudates. These changes first appear in the macular area. Diabetic retinopathy usually is progressive (Plate 22D, E, F, G, H). Superficial, flame-shaped hemorrhages develop in addition to the round, deep ones, and retinal hemorrhages eventually may break into the vitreous. The hemorrhage organizes, connective tissue bands form, and the retina may detach. This latter complication is much more likely to occur in juvenile than adult diabetics. Retinopathy with Kimmelstiel-Wilson disease is the most severe type.

On electron microscopic study the principal change is a diffuse and irregular thickening and reduplication of the basement membrane in the capillaries. This may precede the development of microaneurysms, or even of clinical diabetes. Cogan and Kuwabara have shown in light microscopic studies of flat mount preparations of the retina that "ghosting" and disappearance of the mural cells (pericytes) is one of the earliest histologic changes (Plate 23D). They suggested that these cells may control the tonus of the capillaries, and when they are lost the capillary dilates and fills with blood. Microaneurysms then develop as saccular, thin-walled out-pouchings. Other capillaries in the area degenerate and infarct. The microaneurysms themselves undergo a series of changes resulting in occlusion. In the absence of coincidental arteriolar sclerosis and hypertension, the retinal arterioles are morphologically normal. The retinal veins, however, frequently are distended, probably as a result of increased blood viscosity.

The treatment of diabetic retinopathy is presently unsatisfactory. Proper diet and insulin therapy is important to the general health of the patient, and it is felt by many authorities that the complication of retinopathy is less frequent and severe in the well managed diabetic. Surgical hypophysectomy and various other methods to ablate or suppress the adenohypophysis have been tried with varying success. Treating neovascularization by light or laser coagulation may retard the retinopathy. Among the therapies tried and found wanting have been administration of anticapillary fragility factors; anticoagulants; lipotropic substances; low-salt, low-fat, and high-unsaturated-fat diets; massive vitamin B_{12} and B-complex administration; ocular x-ray irradiation; and adrenalectomy.

Other Ocular Changes in Diabetes

LENS CHANGES. Sudden shifts in the blood sugar concentration cause marked changes in the refractive power of the eye. A severe drop in the serum glucose results in an increase in the amount of hyperopia or a decrease in the amount of myopia. Diabetes should be suspected, therefore, when there are large and otherwise unexplained fluctuations in the refractive error. These changes probably are due to alterations in the water balance of the lens, with resulting swelling and thinning.

Senile cataract occurs earlier in diabetics, and the progress is more rapid than in normal persons of the same age. In addition, a type of cataract characteristic of diabetes has been described. It consists of multiple, white, snow-flake dots located over a network of vacuoles; the opacities are directly under both the anterior and the posterior lens capsules. Young diabetics are particularly prone to the development of this type of cataract.

OCULAR MUSCLES. Accommodation usually fails earlier in diabetics than in normal persons, possibly as a result of early lens sclerosis. Extraocular muscle paralysis is not uncommon in diabetics. Paralysis of the third nerve typically occurs in middle aged individuals who have had mild diabetes for many years. The onset is acute and frequently accompanied by homolateral headache. The external third nerve paralysis may be partial or complete, but the pupillary responses characteristically are spared. This is in contradistinction to third nerve paralysis caused by tumor or aneurysm, in which the pupil nearly always is involved.

THE IRIS. The pigment epithelium in diabetics becomes vacuolated, thickened, and appears to contain an excess of glycogen. Blood vessels sometimes form on the anterior surface of the iris (rubeosis iridis) and result in glaucoma. A characteristic type of iritis has been described in diabetics. This is marked by vascularity of the tissues around the cornea, edema of the conjunctiva, thick anterior chamber exudate and numerous vessels on the iris similar to those seen in rubeosis iridis, but with a normal or diminished intraocular pressure.

INTRAOCULAR PRESSURE. The intraocular pressure in comatose patients with diabetic acidosis is extremely low, probably due in part to dehydration.

DISEASES OF THE SKIN

Disorders Limited to the Lids

The skin of the lids may be affected by a large variety of localized inflammatory, infectious, and degenerative diseases, as well as by a number of systemic diseases.

Hyperemia. Active or passive hyperemia may involve the lids. *Active hyperemia* is seen in many local inflammatory and allergic conditions and accompanies fever and certain forms of intoxication, such as atropine poisoning. It also may occur in onchocerciasis and trichinosis. Hyperemia of the nasal part of the skin of the upper lid may come from acute empyema of the frontal sinus, whereas hyperemia that is limited to the region overlying the lacrimal

sac should suggest disease of this structure. *Passive hyperemia* usually appears bluer than active hyperemia owing to dilatation of the veins. In patients with general circulatory disturbances, both lids may appear cyanotic. Unilateral, passive hyperemia follows compression of the veins in the region of the orbit with blood backing up into the lids. This can be caused by thrombosis of the orbital veins, arteriovenous aneurysm, and tumors of the orbit.

Hemorrhages in the Lids. These vary from small petechiae to massive ecchymoses. The most frequent cause of lid hemorrhage ("black eye") is a direct blow from a fist. The eye should be examined carefully in these cases. Frequently the lids contain hemorrhage immediately after trauma that breaks the nose. In large hemorrhages the blood may spread onto the adjacent skin of the face, especially across the bridge of the nose and into the opposite lids. Hemorrhage also may diffuse back into the orbit and cause exophthalmos. Hemorrhages occurring in the lids 24 hours after a severe fall suggest fracture of the base of the skull. Lid petechiae sometimes occur spontaneously.

Edema of the Lids. This condition may result from any inflammatory disease of the globe or other tissues in the orbit. Among the generalized disorders that lead to noninflammatory edema are allergic reactions and chronic heart and kidney diseases. Edema of the lids is an early sign in endocrine ophthalmopathy and an initial finding in patients with Trichinella infestation. Skull fracture with leakage of cerebrospinal fluid may cause swelling of the lids.

Inflammation of the Lids. A broad spectrum of diseases may result in inflammatory changes in the skin of the lids. The inflammation may arise in the lids or spread there from neighboring parts.

Blepharitis occurs in three forms: *squamous, ulcerative,* and *angular.* In the squamous type the skin of the lid margin is covered with small, white or gray scales, resembling dandruff. When the scales are removed, the skin is seen to be hyperemic but not ulcerated. Squamous blepharitis almost always is associated with seborrheic dermatitis of the scalp. Ulcerative blepharitis is characterized by small ulcerated areas along the lid margin, multiple suppurative lesions, and loss of lashes. Staphylococcal infection of the eyelid is the most common cause of ulcerative blepharitis. Angular blepharitis, an inflammation of the angles of the lids, usually is associated with an angular conjunctivitis. The most frequent causes are *Moraxella lacunata* and *Staphylococcus aureus*. The principal symptoms in all three types of blepharitis are irritation, itching, and burning of the lid margins.

Degenerative Processes. The skin of the lids atrophies in old age and also from any chronic inflammatory process involving the skin. *Blepharochalasis* is caused by hypertrophy and loss of elasticity of the skin of the upper lids. The skin sometimes overhangs the cilia and obscures vision. In younger persons it may follow inflammatory swelling of the lids. Blepharochalasis also may be congenital or may occur without inflammation in older persons. Cosmetic surgery may be desired by the patient.

Pigment Abnormalities. A congenital lack of pigment in the lids occurs in albinos. Decreased pigmentation occurs after severe, generalized infections. In one form, termed *vitiligo*, oval, usually symmetrical, depigmented areas develop on the skin of the lids and affect the associated cilia. Whitening of the hairs, called *poliosis*, occurs with uveitis in the Vogt-Koyanagi syndrome.

Hyperpigmentation and Abnormal Pigmentation of the Skin. Large, brown, irregular spots *(chloasma)* may occur on the lids and the brow during pregnancy. They seem to be comparable to the pigmentation of the linea alba. Chloasma also may occur in cachectic states, especially in pulmonary tuberculosis. Graves' disease, Addison's disease, ochronosis, and "bronzed diabetes" also may cause pigmentation, as may injection or ingestion of silver nitrate and arsenic. Exposure to sunlight or to ultraviolet radiation from arc lamps also increases melanin production.

Diseases of the Glands of the Lids. Anhidrosis of the lids, or absence of sweating, occurs from many inflammatory skin diseases such as ichthyosis and psoriasis. It also occurs as the result of scar formation in the skin of the lids. *Unilateral anhidrosis* of the lid follows damage to the sympathetic nerve on the same side (Horner's syndrome). It is also a sequela of progressive facial hemiatrophy. *Unilateral hyperhidrosis* results from peripheral, irritative lesions of the sympathetic nerve. Small, clear cysts of the sweat glands, about the size of a pinhead, often are found at the edge of the lid. When symptomatic, they may be opened with the tip of a blade.

The sebaceous glands in the lids sometimes produce excessive secretion. This mixes with tears to form a white, soapy emulsion in the cul-de-sacs. Bacteria split the emulsion into irritating, fatty acids, resulting in conjunctivitis. If the sebaceous glands become infected, a bilateral, chronic inflammation (meibomianitis) develops. This generally is associated with blepharitis.

Retention cysts of the sebaceous glands occur in the form of *comedones, milia,* and *atheromas.* A comedo appears as a black pinpoint in the dilated mouth of a sebaceous gland. They frequently arise in adolescence and may be related to excessive secretion. If the associated follicle is secondarily infected, acne pustules develop. Comedones in the skin of the lid usually are associated with similar lesions of the face.

Another form of retention cyst, the milium, affects only the skin of the lids. Milia are small, white bodies (whiteheads) consisting of encysted, horny cells in the epidermis. Atheromas are similar to milia but occur in a follicle deeper in the skin. They frequently are seen around the eyebrows and can form large, rather flat, yellow-white nodules whose contents may calcify. Atheromas should be removed by incision through the skin and curettement.

Ocular Complications of Generalized Skin Disorders

The lids may be involved in many generalized dermatologic disorders. In addition, the lens, corneal epithelium, and lacrimal gland are formed from surface ectoderm. Consequently, pathologic changes of these structures occurring in association with skin lesions should lead the physician to suspect a diffuse disorder of tissues derived from surface ectoderm.

An outline of the major oculodermal processes is given in Table 6-12.

Eczema. This is a general term for that form of dermatitis in which the inflammatory changes of the skin do not follow a clear-cut course or pattern of distribution. The lids commonly are involved, and all clinical phases of dermatitis may be seen, from acute inflammation with reddened, swollen, weeping skin to chronic conditions with indurated, brawny-appearing skin. Included in the general category of eczematoses are infectious eczematoid dermatitis, dermatomycosis, localized neurodermatitis, and the "id" eruptions caused by yeast, fungi, bacteria, and metabolic products. Atopic eczema is a special form influenced by inheritance and distinguished by specific, circulating antibodies in the blood. The eyelids frequently are involved. Progressive cataracts may be associated, even in the young, and usually require surgery (Fig. 6-42).

Rosacea. Primarily an accentuation of the normal flush reaction of the face, this disorder may be associated with seborrheic dermatitis, pustules (acne rosacea), and eventually with dilated veins and telangiectasis (Fig. 6-43). The onset is in childhood or early adult life and initially the flush is usually episodic. The development of rosacea is influenced by heredity, and individuals of certain origins, particularly English and Irish, are most frequently affected. Chronic blepharitis and conjunc-

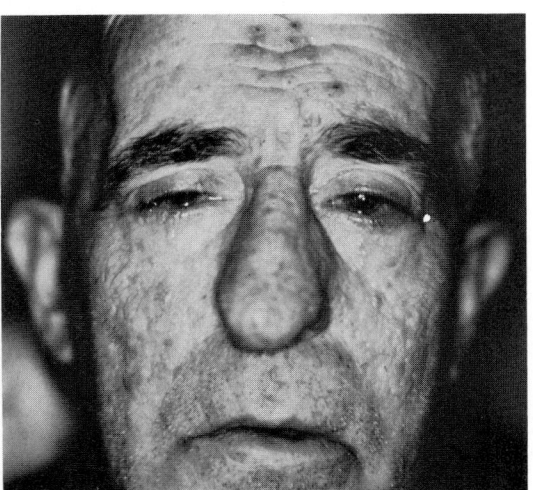

Figure 6-43 Rosacea keratitis.

tivitis occur in more than half the affected patients. Less frequent but more severe ocular complications are keratitis (Fig. 6-44), iritis, and episcleritis. Rosacea keratitis consists of phlyctenule-like lesions at the limbus and superficial and deep corneal infiltrates. It may be followed by pannus. Therapy includes dietary control, avoiding extremes of heat and cold, and reducing emotional tension. Ocular complications

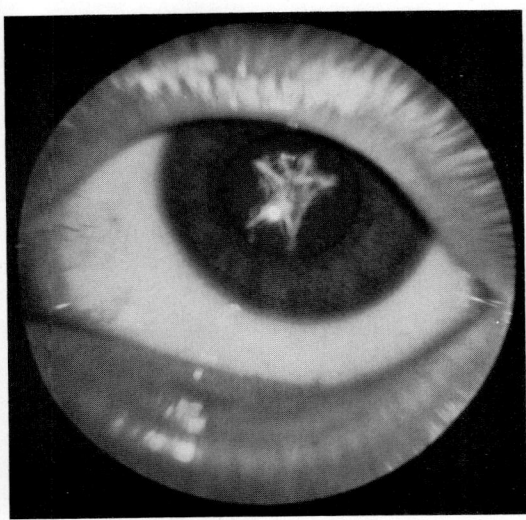

Figure 6-42 Atopic eczema with a secondary cataract.

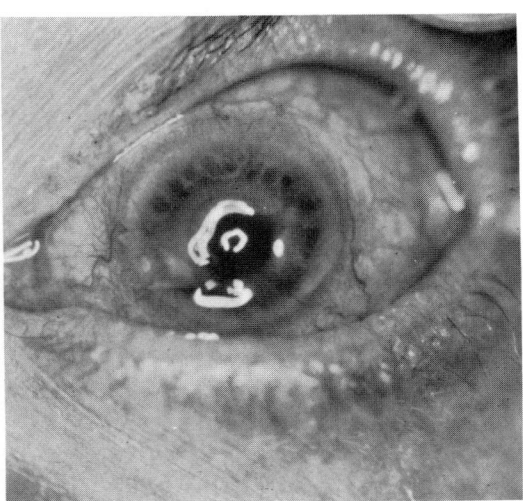

Figure 6-44 Close-up view of cornea of same patient as in Figure 6-43 showing scarring from repeated ulceration.

TABLE 6-12   SOME DISEASES INVOLVING THE SKIN AND EYES*

I. Heredocongenital and developmental anomalies
   A. Phakomatoses
      1. Tuberous sclerosis (Bourneville)
      2. Neurofibromatosis (von Recklinghausen)
      3. Nevus flammeus with glaucoma (Sturge-Weber)
      4. Angiomatosis retinae et cerebelli (von Hippel-Lindau)
   B. Pseudoxanthoma elasticum and angioid streaks of the retina (Grönblad-Strandberg)
   C. Rothmund's syndrome
   D. Werner's syndrome
   E. Nevoxanthoendothelioma (Juvenile xanthogranuloma)
   F. Porphyria congenita
   G. Ocular manifestations of sickle cell disease
   H. Pityriasis rubra pilaris
   I. Keratosis follicularis spinulosa decalvans (Siemens)
   J. Dermochondrocorneal dystrophy
   K. Ataxia-telangiectasia (cerebellar ataxia, oculocutaneous telangiectasia)
   L. Retrolental fibroplasia and hemangioma of the skin
   M. Ophthalmoplegia, steatorrhea, phlebectasis, and vascular lipoma
   N. Symmetric lower lid defects associated with abnormalities of the zygomatic processes
   O. Xeroderma pigmentosum
   P. Epidermolysis bullosa
   Q. Albinoidism, piebalding, and poliosis
   R. Dermoids and teratomas
   S. Various deformities of eyelashes
   T. Onycholysis partialis semilunaris recidivans and zonular cataract
   U. Pachyonychia congenita with dyskeratosis of cornea (cataracts, opacities, and partial blindness)
   V. Blepharochalasis, palpebral dermatolysis
   W. Others, including ichthyosis and colobomata
II. Infective processes
   A. Bacterial infections: staphylococci (impetigo, folliculitis, furunculosis, and carbuncles); streptococci [erysipelas (beta-hemolytic streptococci)]; granuloma pyogenicum; Morax-Axenfeld diplobacillus; diphtheria; anthrax; glanders; chancroid; tuberculosis; leprosy; rhinoscleroma; granuloma inguinale; and spirochetal
   B. Viral infections: vaccinia, varicella, herpes simplex, herpes zoster, Kaposi's varicelliform eruption, verrucae, molluscum contagiosum, cat-scratch disease, and lymphogranuloma venereum
   C. Rickettsial infections: scrub typhus, Rocky Mountain spotted fever, and others
   D. Fungal infections: actinomycosis, blastomycosis, coccidioidomycosis, moniliasis, rhinosporidiosis, tinea, favus, and torulosis (cryptococcosis)
   E. Parasitic infections:
      1. Protozoan: leishmaniasis (Oriental sore), trypanosomiasis, and toxoplasmosis.
      2. Metazoan infestations of Ascaris, Oxyuris, Ancylostoma, Necator, Trichina, Filaria, *Loa loa*, Dracunculus, Schistosoma, Wuchereria, Onchocerca, and leeches
      3. Arthropoda: lice (pediculosis capitis and corporis)
      4. Scabies: *Demodex folliculorum*, and myiasis
      5. Bites and stings: ticks, spiders, chiggers, centipedes, and caterpillar (hairs)

*Adapted from Beerman, H., Kirschbaum, B., and Cowan, L.: Oculocutaneous diseases and internal medicine; a review of the literature. Am. J. Med. Sci. *238*: (Oct.) 1959.

TABLE 6-12 SOME DISEASES INVOLVING THE SKIN AND EYES *(Continued)*

III. Other Inflammatory Processes
    A. Syndromes and disease entities
        1. Vogt-Koyanagi and Harada's syndromes
        2. Behçet's syndrome
        3. Erythema multiforme and Stevens-Johnson syndrome
        4. Pemphigoid
        5. Reiter's disease
        6. Sjögren's syndrome
        7. Mikulicz's disease
        8. Erythema nodosum
        9. Lichen planus
        10. Psoriasis
        11. Dermatitis herpetiformis
        12. Xeroderma pigmentosa
        13. Rosacea
        14. Sarcoidosis
    B. Allergic
        1. Drugs
        2. Pollens
        3. Bacterial products
        4. Animal and vegetable proteins
        5. Atopic dermatitis
        6. Other contactants and sensitizers
IV. Traumatic and Toxic
    A. Physical (thermal; cold; radiation, including ultraviolet, x-ray, and radium)
    B. Chemical: acids, alkalies, others
    C. Mechanical: traumatic deformities
V. Metabolic and Pigmentary
    A. Intrinsic and hereditary: ochronosis, bile pigments, diabetes mellitus, xanthomatoses, lipoidoses, and porphyrias
    B. Extrinsic: silver, gold, iron, and copper
VI. Neoplastic and Related Lesions
    A. Nevi
    B. Precancerous conditions
    C. Pseudocancerous lesions
    D. Malignancies
VII. Degenerative
    A. Senile elastoses
    B. Xerosis
    C. Cornification
    D. Hyalin degeneration
    E. Amyloid degeneration
    F. Collagen degeneration
    G. Fatty and calcareous degeneration
    H. Aging and exposure
VIII. Collagen Diseases
    A. Lupus erythematosus
    B. Scleroderma
    C. Dermatomyositis
    D. Polyarteritis nodosa
    E. Rheumatoid nodules
IX. Vitamin Deficiencies
    A. Vitamin A
    B. Vitamin B–group
    C. Vitamin C
    D. Vitamin D
X. Psychogenic
    A. Neurodermatitis
    B. Facitial

may require applying topical corticosteroids and eliminating secondary bacterial infection with antibiotic or sulfonamide medications.

Dermatitis Herpetiformis. This chronic, recurrent, pruritic disease is characterized by symmetrically distributed groups of papules and vesicles surrounded by erythema. Bullae may be present in rare instances. The extensor surfaces of the extremities, the shoulders, and the buttocks are principally affected. Lesions of the mucous membranes are uncommon. When conjunctival and corneal complications occur, they are similar to those of ocular pemphigus and consist of recurrent bullae, ulceration, and cicatrization. Remissions may follow treatment with sulfapyridine and the sulfones.

Epidermolysis Bullosa. The major characteristic of this uncommon disease is a poor adherence of the epidermis to the dermis, with the appearance of bullae after minimal trauma (Fig. 6-45). The two major forms are *simple*, a relatively benign process, and *dystrophic*, a destructive mutilating disorder. Ocular complications, when they occur, take the form of cicatrizing conjunctivitis and keratitis. Treatment is entirely symptomatic.

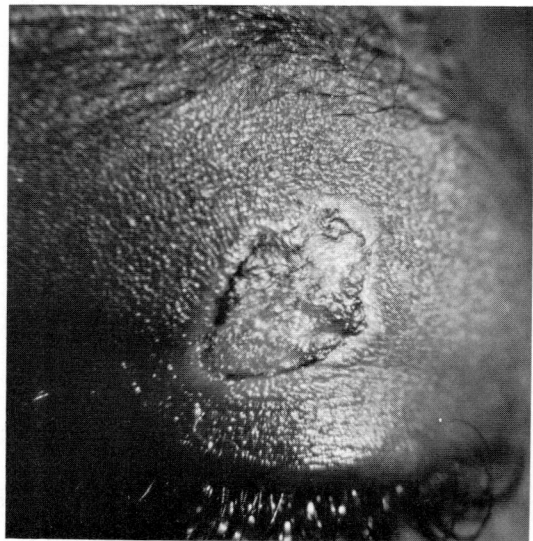

Figure 6-45 Lesion above lid in epidermolysis bullosa.

Hydroa Vacciniforme. In this rare recurrent disease of children, vesicles and bullae may erupt on the face and other exposed parts of the body; the lids commonly are affected. The eruption results from a congenital, abnormal sensitivity to ultraviolet radiation and sunlight. The onset usually is in infancy or early childhood and generally disappears after puberty.

Other dermatoses resulting from photosensitivity, in which the eye or adnexa may be involved, include *acute solar dermatitis*, a disorder in which an erythematous vesicular or bullous skin eruption occurs together with conjunctivitis and keratitis, and *xeroderma pigmentosum*, a rare, congenital, precancerous condition.

Erythema Nodosum. This is a distinctive reaction pattern in the skin and subcutaneous tissues to a variety of etiologic factors, including drugs and bacterial, viral, and fungal infections. The lesions consist of multiple, red, tender, slightly raised nodules usually on the anterior surface of the legs, extensor surface of the arms, and buttocks. These nodules occasionally occur on the lids and conjunctiva, and uveitis may occur. Determining and treating the underlying cause is important. Bedrest, local heat, salicylates, and corticosteroid therapy (if not contraindicated by an underlying systemic infection) are sometimes effective.

OTHER OCULAR COMPLICATIONS OF SKIN DISORDERS

Psoriasis, a chronic skin disorder whose principal features include a scaling eruption, may be associated with conjunctivitis and keratitis. *Ichthyosis* is a congenital abnormality of keratinization that may involve a hyperkeratosis of the skin of the lids as well as of the face. Corneal and conjunctival changes also have been described. *Lichen planus*, a papulosquamous eruption of unknown cause, may affect the eyelids and conjunctiva. *Elephantiasis* is caused by stases in the flow of lymph. This leads to a chronic edema and inflammation in the lids. Elephantiasis of the lids can result from erysipelas, chronic lid eczema, and occasionally filiariasis. *Alopecia areata* is characterized by a sudden, complete loss of hair and sharply defined, round or oval patches with no evidence of inflammation or atrophy. The eyebrows and eyelashes may be involved.

TUMORS

Ocular tumors have a special significance among eye diseases: they are the only life-threatening condition arising in the eye or adnexa with which the ophthalmologist must deal. In addition, they result in visual loss and cosmetic problems. Ocular tumors may be intraocular; external, involving the lids and conjunctiva; and orbital.

Intraocular Tumors

Nevi of the Uveal Tract (Benign Melanomas). These benign lesions may occur in any part of the uveal tract. Iris nevi appear as dark areas ranging in size from a pinpoint to a large segment of the iris. Choroidal nevi are less common and generally vary in size from one to several disc diameters and in color from brown to slate gray (Plate 23E). Nevi of the ciliary body are unusual and invisible clinically unless quite large. Nevi of the uveal tract appear histopathologically as masses of plump, pigmented cells. Although these lesions do not affect vision, there is considerable evidence that most malignant melanomas arise from preexisting nevi. They should be watched, therefore, for any growth or change in appearance.

Malignant Melanomas. This group of neoplasms constitute the most common, malignant, intraocular tumors. They may arise anywhere in the uveal tract and exhibit a spectrum of cell types and degrees of pigmentation and biological activity. Malignant melanomas occur most commonly in the fifth and sixth decades of life and usually are solitary lesions involving one eye. These lesions are rare in children and also in non-Caucasians of all ages.

MALIGNANT MELANOMAS OF THE IRIS. These comprise 6 to 8 per cent of melanomas of the uveal tract (Plate 23F, G). The tumor may appear grossly as a discrete, pigmented or fleshy mass in the iris, or as a diffuse discoloration and thickening. Some affected patients have a history of a pre-existing pigmented lesion that eventually began to change in size and color. Other patients are unaware of the preexisting tumor. Malignant melanomas of the iris, usually symptomless, are discovered incidentally. When symptoms occur, they usually are due to necrosis or inflammation of the iris stroma, resulting in iridocyclitis or glaucoma. Rarely the patient may notice a distortion of the pupil. The presenting signs also may be hemorrhage into the anterior chamber or alteration of the refractive error as a result of invasion of the ciliary body. Clinical features indicating that an iris lesion is a malignant melanoma, rather than a nevus, include observing an increase in size on repeated examination; the presence of nutrient vessels; the presence of satellite lesions on the iris; extension of the lesion into the filtration angle, as seen by gonioscopic examination; and the onset of glaucoma or iridocyclitis.

MALIGNANT MELANOMAS OF THE CILIARY BODY. These are slightly more common than those of the iris (about 9 per cent of uveal malignant melanomas). Early lesions may be detected by gonioscopic observations of angle changes produced by the tumor. Frequently they are not diagnosed until after they invade the iris, angle, or choroid, and they are visible grossly or by ophthalmoscopy.

After the tumor has penetrated the sclera, the patient may present with a black, subconjunctival mass. The presenting symptoms of ciliary body melanomas are blurred vision, field loss, and pain resulting from glaucoma or inflammation.

MALIGNANT MELANOMAS OF THE CHOROID. These comprise about 85 per cent of melanomas of the uveal tract (Plate 23H, Figs. 6-46, 6-47, 6-48). The most common symptom is a change in visual acuity, arising from detachment of the retina. Less commonly, there may be metamorphopsia when the macular region is involved, or photopsia, particularly with lesions involving the peripheral retina. Large, necrotic melanomas or melanomas of the anterior choroid may be associated with the symptoms of uveitis and secondary glaucoma.

When observed early, the malignant melanoma of the choroid characteristically

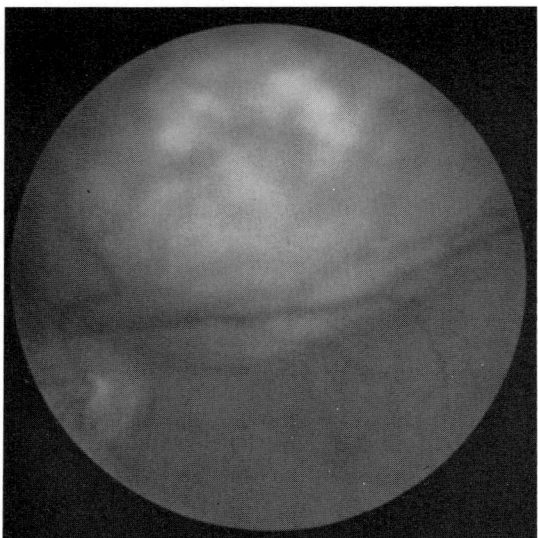

Figure 6-46 Ophthalmoscopic appearance of lightly pigmented choroidal malignant melanoma.

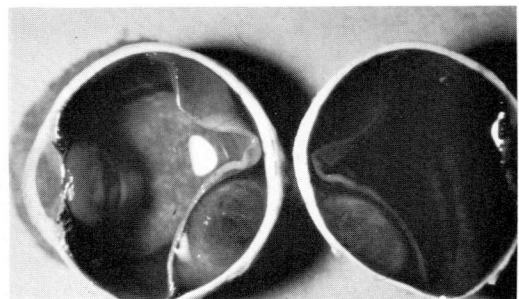

Figure 6-48 Sectioned globe containing choroidal malignant melanoma.

appears as a somewhat elevated brown or gray lesion. As the melanoma grows and breaks through Bruch's membrane, it frequently assumes a mushroom shape. A constriction is present at the site of penetration through Bruch's membrane. The mass protruding toward the vitreous cavity

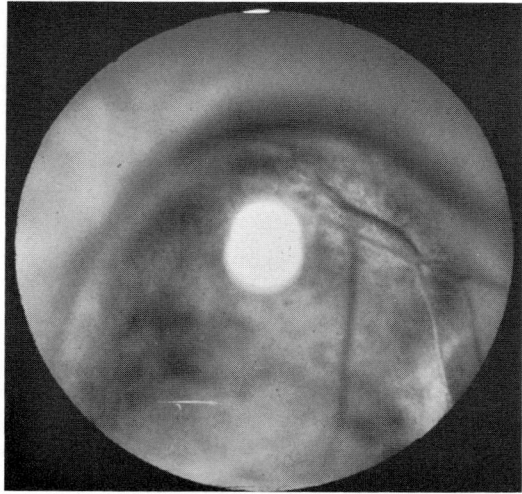

Figure 6-47 Ophthalmoscopic appearance of large choroidal malignant melanoma.

is relatively large and round. With further enlargement, the lesion appears as a solid, retinal detachment commonly associated with a serous detachment in the dependent portion of the fundus. Additional findings suggestive of malignant melanoma are an abnormal vascular pattern over the surface of the lesion, dilated episcleral and iris vessels corresponding to the sector in which the tumor lies, retinal striae, and drusen and clumps of pigment overlying the neoplasm. Hemorrhages are seen infrequently.

A number of clinical tests are useful in diagnosing these lesions, the most important of which are transillumination and retroillumination. With transillumination a bright focal light is passed across the sclera in the area of the lesion; a solid mass, such as a melanoma, will not transmit light. On retroillumination a bright ophthalmoscope light is focused beneath the lower border of the lesion. Reflected rays will not penetrate the melanoma and the margin of the lesion will appear as a dark zone, and the vessels coursing over the tumor will appear to fluoresce. Additional diagnostic studies include the use of radioisotopes, particularly P^{32}; fluorescein angiography; and the use of ultrasonic reflection. Other lesions may simulate malignant melanomas and must be considered in the differential diagnosis: inflammation, macular degeneration, benign melanoma of the choroid, metastatic carcinoma, serous detachment of the retina, hyperplasia of the pigment epithelium, hemorrhage, hemangioma of the choroid, Coats' disease, congenital crater of the optic disc, and angioid streaks (from Reese).

The prognosis of malignant melanomas of the uveal tract depends on many factors, among the most important of which are the location and cytology. Iris tumors clearly have a more favorable prognosis than those of the posterior uvea. Callender's cytologic classification of the uveal melanomas has proved useful in estimating the prognosis. The most benign tumors in this grouping are those composed almost entirely of spindle cells (less than 20 per cent proved fatal within 15 years after enucleation), whereas at the other extreme are the pure epithelioid cell tumors (more than half of these patients are dead within five years after enucleation). Small size and heavy reticulin fiber content generally are favorable features.

Treatment depends on the site of the lesion. Iridectomy is the treatment of choice for localized iris tumors. In recent years iridocyclectomy has been employed for resectable tumors of the ciliary body. Eyes containing choroidal melanomas should be enucleated. Possibly excepted are small lesions (1 to 4 disc diameters in size) occurring in eyes with good vision and not associated with any significant complications. Some authorities recommend careful observation until it is determined that these lesions are progressive. Additional methods of treatment include diathermy, photocoagulation or laser treatment, and the use of cobalt-60 applicators, radon seed implantation, and cryosurgery.

Melanocytomas. These locally invasive, nonmalignant, primary melanotic tumors usually arise from the optic disc (Fig. 6-49). The characteristic clinical features are small size, deep pigmentation, slow growth, and rare interference with visual acuity. Generally they are situated eccentrically on the nerve head and extend into the adjacent

retina. In contrast to melanomas, melanocytomas are frequent in non-Caucasians. Histopathologically the lesion is composed of remarkably uniform, plump, ovoid to polyhedral cells, heavily laden with pigment granules.

Tumor Metastasis to the Eye. Until recently, metastatic tumors involving the eye were considered unusual. Patients with metastatic disease rarely were examined by ophthalmologists, and ocular tissue from such patients seldom was submitted to an ocular pathology laboratory. Subsequently it has been found that ocular and orbital metastases are relatively common. Moreover, the eye and orbit may be the first site of malignant spread, and eye symptoms can precede diagnosis of the primary tumor.

Leukemic infiltration of the uvea and retina frequently occurs in the terminal stages of this disease (p. 235). Reports of intraocular metastasis from a solid tumor in the infant or child are extremely rare. In adults, metastatic carcinoma in the eye most commonly results from primary breast carcinoma in women and primary bronchogenic carcinoma in men. Other sources of ocular metastasis are malignancies in the alimentary tract, ovary, thyroid gland, prostate, and testicle.

Metastatic carcinomas are found mainly in the posterior choroid, with blurred vision and pain usually the principal symptoms (Plate 24A). Bilateral involvement occurs in about 25 per cent of affected patients. Ophthalmoscopically the lesions appear as yellow to gray, mottled, slightly elevated areas. Metastases characteristically are flatter and lighter in color and grow more rapidly than malignant melanomas of the choroid. Unlike ocular melanomas, multiple tumor foci often are seen with metastatic tumors. A more or less solid appearing detachment of the retina may be present, particularly in the posterior pole. Metastatic carcinomas of the choroid usually permit normal transillumination because of their thinness.

Only about 12 per cent of metastases to the uveal tract involve the iris or ciliary body. Lesions in these areas may be discrete or diffusely infiltrating, and fre-

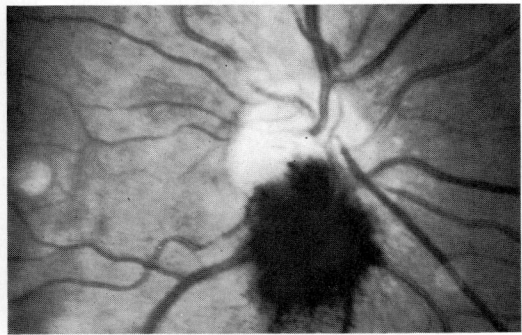

Figure 6-49 Melanocytoma.

quently give rise to a clinical picture of a peculiar uveitis that sometimes is accompanied by secondary glaucoma. Metastases to the retina and optic nerve are extremely rare.

The prognosis for life in a patient with metastatic malignancy is very poor. No report can be found in which a cure of the malignant disease was effected by enucleation and removal of the primary tumor. Other metastases, if not present when the ocular lesion is discovered, rapidly appear. The goals in treatment are maintenance of vision and comfort. Irradiation may be beneficial. Metastases from breast carcinomas, when treated by hormone therapy, castration, or adrenalectomy, frequently are followed by regression of the ocular lesions. If pain from uveitis or secondary glaucoma becomes intractable, enucleation may be necessary.

Hemangiomas. These are tumors arising from the endothelial cells. Reese considers them neoplasms, although they do not have the features of unlimited growth, infiltration, or metastasis. Frequently hemangiomas are components of von Hippel-Lindau disease (angiomatosis retina) and Sturge-Weber disease. Most frequently they are located in the choroid. The lesion is lighter in color than the surrounding fundus and may appear honeycombed. Hemangiomas are one of the disorders to be considered in the differential diagnosis of malignant melanomas. Unlike melanomas, hemangiomas do not have clumps of pigment on the surface, and they transmit light fully on transillumination. Choroidal hemangiomas may be associated with retinal detachment. Hemangiomas rarely may occur on the iris. If the anterior chamber angle is involved, glaucoma may be present.

Epithelial Tumors of the Uveal Tract. The following are uncommon tumors arising primarily from the ciliary body:

1. *Pseudoadenomatous hyperplasia of the ciliary epithelium,* a benign tumor, occurs following injuries or inflammatory processes and as an aging phenomenon. The lesion consists of nodules or masses that grow from the epithelium of the ciliary processes and pars plana into the vitreous cavity.

2. *Benign epitheliomas,* adenoma-like structures, arise from the nonpigmented epithelium of the ciliary processes.

3. *Diktyoma* is a tumor which may be benign or malignant and which arises from the epithelial layers of the ciliary body. In many respects it resembles embryonic retina. It occurs principally in children and is a cause of the white pupil. The tumor may contain poorly differentiated neural tissue or cartilage.

4. *Carcinoma or adult type of medullo-epithelioma,* usually appears as white, fluffy masses on the inner surface of the ciliary body. This tumor consists of cuboidal or columnar epithelial cells having a tubular structure.

OTHER INTRAOCULAR TUMORS

Retinoblastoma is the principal tumor of the retina and is the most frequent, malignant, ocular neoplasm of childhood. This tumor is discussed in the chapter on pediatric ophthalmology (p. 152). *Leiomyoma* is a benign tumor arising from the dilator and sphincter muscles of the iris. Clinically appearing as pink-to-brown nodules, the tumor usually involves the pupillary area of the iris and is clinically indistinguishable from nevi and lightly pigmented malignant melanomas. *Neurilemomas* are benign, localized, encapsulated tumors arising from the Schwann's cells of peripheral, cranial, and sympathetic nerves. They usually involve the ciliary nerves, but also occur in the orbit, lid and conjunctiva. *Astrocytomas* usually occur in patients with tuberous sclerosis, which is discussed with phakomatoses in the chapter on pediatric ophthalmology (p. 172). *Juvenile xanthogranuloma* (nevoxanthoendothelioma) is a rare disease in which small, yellow nodules composed of large, pale-staining, multinucleated, Touton giant cells and eosinophils are present on the skin, conjunctiva, orbit, and iris (p. 156).

External Tumors: The Lids

Basal Cell Carcinoma. The most common malignancy involving the eyes and adnexa, basal cell carcinoma comprises

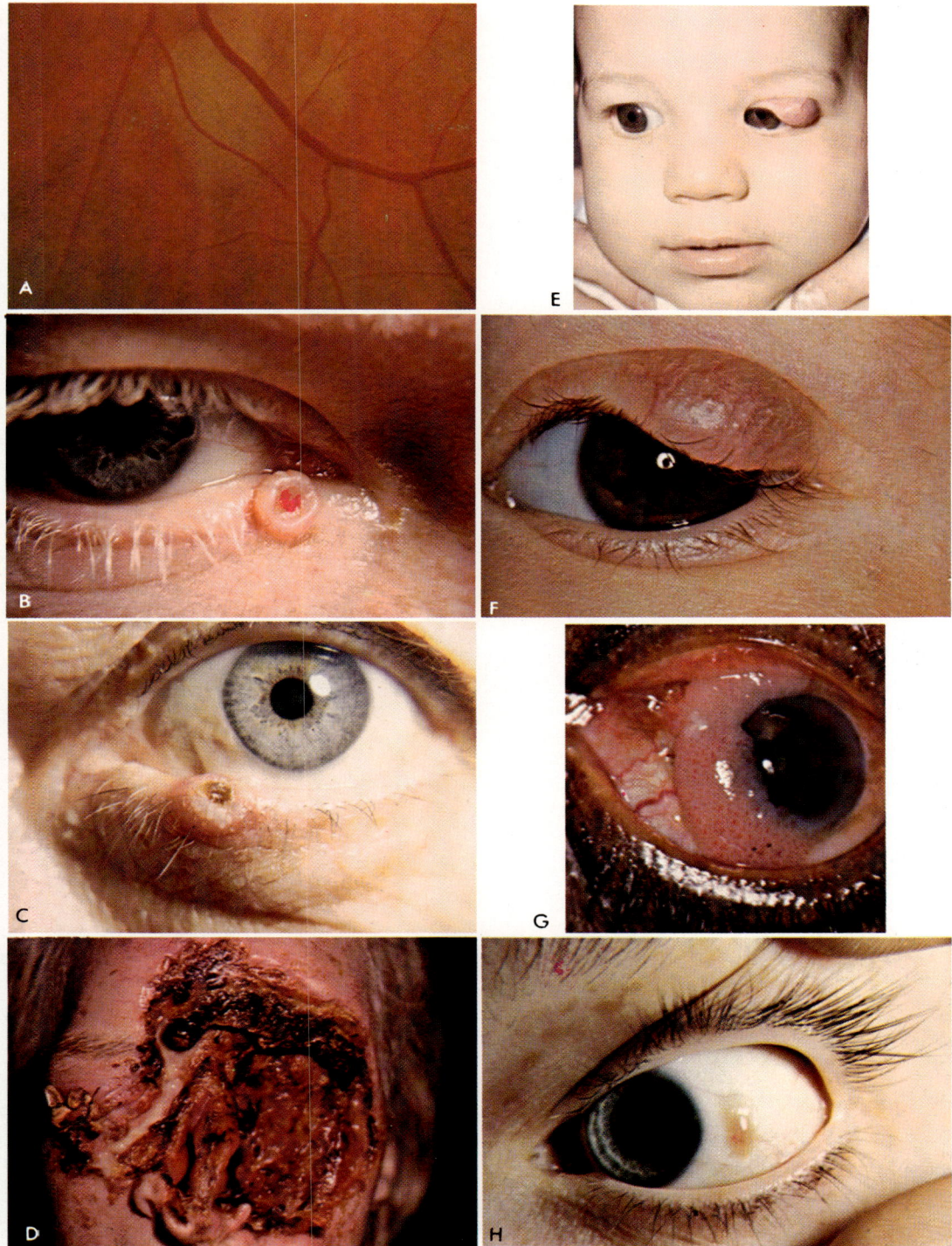

Plate 24 *(A)* Choroidal metastasis from breast carcinoma. *(B)* Basal cell carcinoma. *(C)* Basal cell carcinoma with local infiltration. *(D)* Massive invasion and destruction from untreated basal cell carcinoma. *(E)* Hemangioma of lid. *(F)* Close-up view of same lesion as shown in 24E. *(G)* Extensive papilloma of the conjunctiva. *(H)* Lightly pigmented malignant melanoma of the conjunctiva.

267

more than 90 per cent of all malignant tumors on the lids. This tumor occurs with increasing frequency with age and affects men more commonly than women. It occurs most frequently on the lower lid and at the inner canthus. The lesion begins as a small, slightly elevated nodule (Plate 24B). A central dimple with a slightly irregular, pearly border is characteristic. When atypical, it may be mistaken for a verruca, papilloma, or nevus. Ulceration may occur. Basal cell carcinomas spread by direct extension (Plate 24C) and may be highly invasive (Plate 24D), but they do not metastasize. Histopathologically the cells composing the tumor resemble those of the basal cell layer of the epithelium. Basal cell carcinomas can be treated by surgical removal or radiation therapy. Most early lesions can be removed by simple excision. Radiation therapy requires careful protection of the eye, or it may be followed by such complications as keratinization of the cornea, keratitis, corneal ulcers, cataract, and skin necrosis.

Squamous Cell Carcinoma. This malignancy accounts for less than 5 per cent of malignant tumors of the lids. Squamous cell carcinoma occurs predominantly in older males and is found most commonly on the upper lid. It begins as a wartlike, keratotic lesion which may grossly resemble the basal cell carcinoma. Later it becomes ulcerated and fissured. As the lesion further enlarges, it appears as a shallow, crusted ulcer with a granular, red base. Metastases occur along the channels of lymphatic drainage. The lesion is more difficult to manage than basal cell carcinoma and carries a more serious prognosis. Early recognition and excision are essential.

Miscellaneous Malignant Tumors. *Sebaceous gland carcinomas* are insidious, yellow-white tumors on the tarsal portion of the lids. They often are mistaken for, or associated with, chalazia. For this reason, recurrent chalazia should be biopsied and the diagnosis established histopathologically. Sebaceous gland carcinomas are treated by wide local excision. *Malignant melanomas of the skin* are highly malignant neoplasms which carry a worse prognosis than intra-ocular melanomas. Metastases to the lids, usually rare lesions, also have been reported to appear clinically similar to chalazia.

Precancerous Lesions. *Senile keratoses* usually develop as multiple lesions, less than 1 cm. in size. They occur in persons past middle age, particularly those with a history of prolonged exposure to sunlight. The appearance of the lesions is variable; most are flat and brown at the onset, and usually progress to well demarcated keratotic papules. *Bowen's disease* is seen as a single, scaly, dull red patch of irregular outline that gradually increases in size. It is clinically indistinguishable from basal cell carcinoma. *Xeroderma pigmentosa* is a congenital skin condition in which large numbers of freckles appear in areas of skin exposed to the sun. With time and exposure to sunlight each year, the pigmentation becomes permanent and deeper. Ultimately atrophic spots appear, as well as wartlike excrescences that tend to ulcerate and eventually to become cancerous. Prophylactic removal of these lesions can prevent their progression to invasive, squamous cell cancers.

Pseudocancerous Lesions. A number of benign lesions occur on the face and eyelids. These usually are characterized by sudden onset and very rapid growth. In previous years many of these lesions were mistaken by clinicians and pathologists for squamous cell carcinoma, but subsequently they have been more fully studied and delineated. Principal among these lesions are keratoacanthoma, inverted follicular keratosis, pilomatrixoma, seborrheic keratosis, and pseudoepitheliomatous hyperplasia.

Other Benign Lesions of the Lids. Nevi commonly occur on the lids and may take a variety of forms. The dermal nevus usually occurs as the common mole found elsewhere on the skin. Others, however, may have a papillomatous or cystic pattern. These may be difficult to differentiate clinically from basal cell carcinoma or malignant melanomas. Whereas dermal nevi do not become malignant, junctional and compound nevi may undergo malignant changes.

Hemangiomas frequently are congenital lesions, several varieties of which are of particular significance to ophthalmologists (Plate 24E, F):

1. Nevus flammeus (port wine stain), an irregular blue-red patch of variable size, is

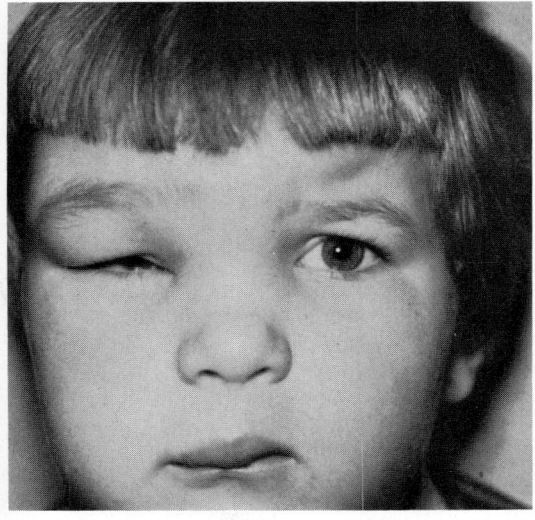

Figure 6-50 Lymphangioma of the lid.

formed by diffuse telangiectasia of mature vessels in the dermis. The lesion usually is permanent and no satisfactory treatment has been found.

2. Capillary hemangiomas are raised, soft red lesions which usually disappear spontaneously. They may sometimes present a frightening picture of rapid growth in the newborn.

3. Cavernous hemangiomas are lesions composed of simple endothelial-lined spaces larger than those present in capillary hemangiomas. They show no tendency for spontaneous involution, and are insensitive to irradiation. These lesions are commonly encountered in the orbit.

Hemangiomas may be accompanied by more extensive ocular and meningeal involvement (p. 179). *Lymphangiomas* also may involve the lids (Fig. 6-50).

External Tumors: The Conjunctiva and Cornea

Squamous Cell Carcinoma. Invasive, squamous cell carcinoma generally is observed near the limbus in older patients. These lesions rarely penetrate the sclera to extend intraocularly or to metastasize. Basal cell carcinoma of the conjunctiva is extremely rare.

Pseudocancerous Lesions and Carcinoma-in-Situ. Slowly growing opaque plaques occasionally are encountered at the limbus. Clinically these lesions usually follow a benign course. On histopathologic examination they rarely present unequivocal evidence of malignancy, although occasionally the microscopic picture may resemble that of Bowen's disease of the skin (squamous cell carcinoma-in-situ). In spite of the microscopic resemblance, these growths have none of the other characteristics of Bowen's disease of the skin. Carcinoma-in-situ at the limbus almost always can be treated by simple excision. Papillomas occasionally occur on the conjunctiva and also are treated by excision (Plate 24G).

Nevi. Nevi occur as pigmented and nonpigmented lesions on the bulbar conjunctiva and probably constitute the most common tumor of the conjunctiva. They usually are small, discrete, slightly elevated lesions. Nevi first become apparent in early childhood, but frequently enlarge or become more pigmented at or following puberty. Conjunctival nevi, usually of the junctional or compound type, are similar histopathologically to those in the skin. Nevi usually are excised for purposes of diagnosis; they cause irritation and may be cosmetically objectionable. Some authorities advise prophylactic removal of nevi to prevent malignant melanoma, although malignant change in nevi rarely occurs.

Acquired Melanosis. In this condition the conjunctiva acquires pigment insidiously in adult life. The melanosis appears as a flat and diffuse discoloration, ranging in color from tan or brown to black. The lesion characteristically spreads slowly and may regress spontaneously. Reese has termed this condition "precancerous melanosis" in view of its potential for progressing into a malignant melanoma. There is considerable controversy, however, regarding the histopathologic interpretation, prognosis, and treatment of these lesions.

Malignant Melanoma of the Conjunctiva. This rather rare lesion may arise from nevi, within areas of acquired melanosis, or *de novo* within apparently normal conjunctiva (Plate 24H, Figs. 6-51, 6-52). The management of these tumors is controversial, with simple excision, exenteration, and radiation therapy all having their advocates.

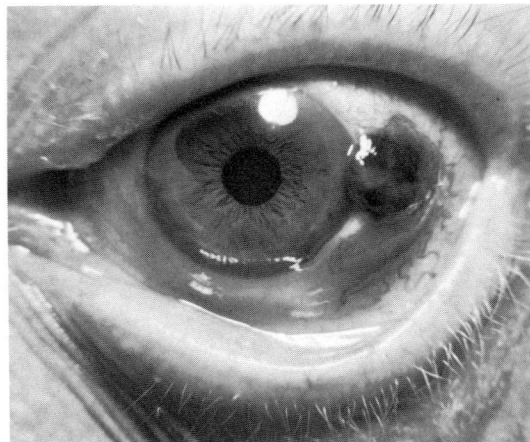

Figure 6-51 Large malignant melanoma of the conjunctiva.

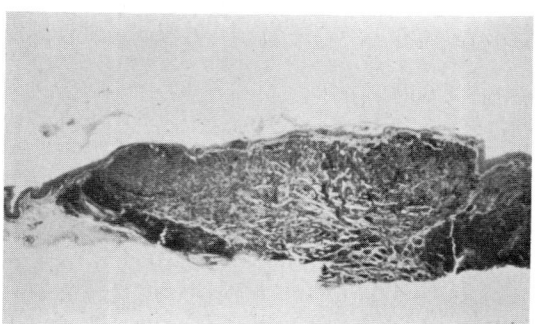

Figure 6-52 Low-power microscopic view of conjunctival malignant melanoma.

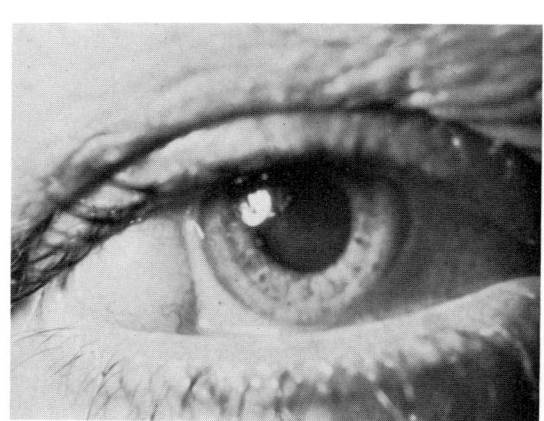

Figure 6-53 Dermal lipoma of the orbit.

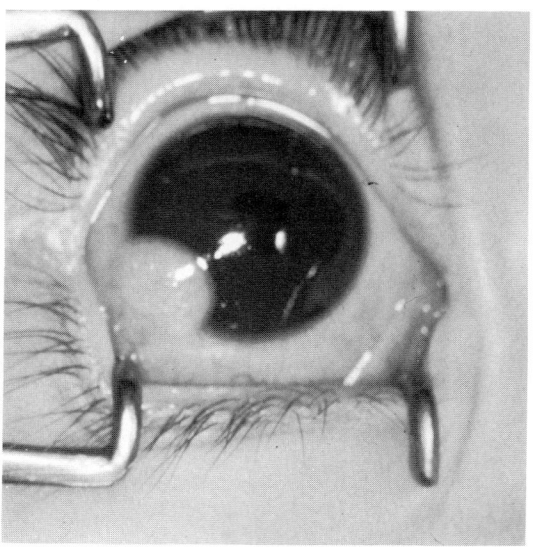

Figure 6-54 Limbal dermoid.

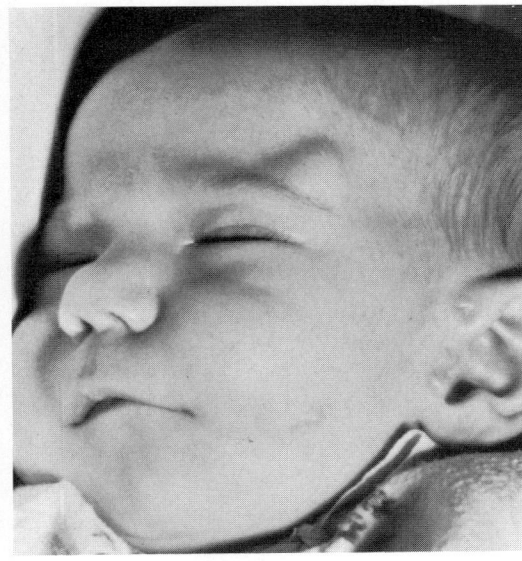

Figure 6-55 Dermoid attached to the superior temporal orbital rim (most common location).

Figure 6-56 Dermoid of the cornea.

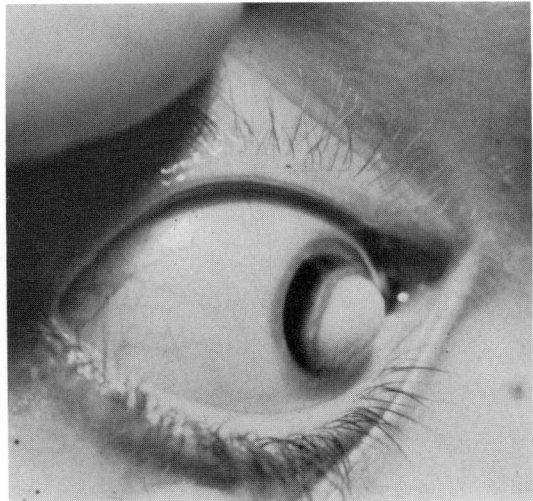

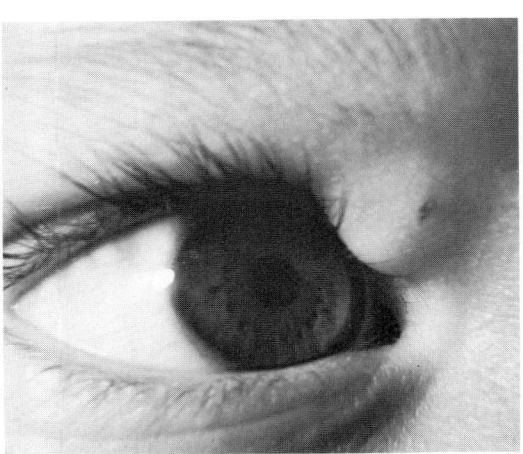

Figure 6-57 Dermoid of the lid.

Dermoids. These congenital tumors involve tissue of mesodermal and ectodermal origin (Figs. 6-53, 6-54). Dermoids appear as raised, circumscribed yellow growths. They generally are situated at the lower temporal limbus and involve the cornea, sclera, and bulbar conjunctiva. They may extend deeply into the posterior orbit, but these usually arise from the orbital rim (Fig. 6-55). Limbal dermoids are excised for cosmetic reasons. Occasionally, only the cornea, sclera, conjunctiva, or lid may be involved (Figs. 6-56, 6-57).

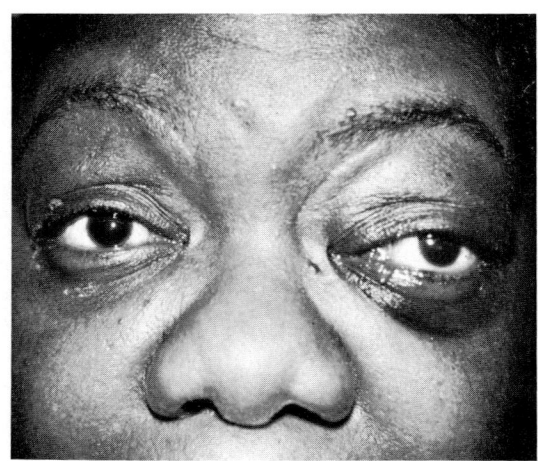

Figure 6-59   Pseudotumor of the left orbit.

Orbital Tumors

A wide spectrum of lesions invade the orbit (Figs. 6-58, 6-59). These range from benign dermoid cysts and hemangiomas to extremely malignant sarcomas and carcinomas. Certain inflammatory lesions, particularly pseudotumors may closely resemble neoplasms. The incidence of specific lesions depends considerably on the age group. Common ocular tumors in the pediatric age group include rhabdomyosarcoma, glioma of the optic nerve, der-

moid cysts, teratomas, metastatic neuroblastomas, and malignant lymphoid tumors. In adults the principal ones include lacrimal gland tumors, meningiomas, and metastatic carcinoma. Hemangiomas, lymphomas, and inflammatory pseudotumors occur with relative frequency in both children and adults. Orbital tumors manifest themselves as unilateral expanding lesions which cause proptosis. Consequently they must be differentiated from other orbital conditions presenting in a similar manner, such as endocrine ophthalmopathy, the histiocytoses, von Recklinghausen's disease, Paget's disease, and mucoceles. Helpful in diagnosis are various x-ray techniques, including the use of contrast media, radioactive scanning techniques, arteriography, venography, and ultrasonography. The definitive diagnosis of an expanding mass in the orbit depends upon histopathologic examination of the pathologic specimen. Often complete removal of the tumor is preferable to attempting biopsy. In some instances the extent of the tumor may make total excision impossible, and radiation or medical treatment must be resorted to.

Orbital Pseudotumor. This condition is one of the most common causes of unilateral exophthalmos. It may develop suddenly, insidiously, or run a course of months or years. The lesion may be diffuse or well localized. It may be palpable or firm, and adjacent to, or firmly fixed to, bone. Although the edema and lesion usually involve one eye first, the involve-

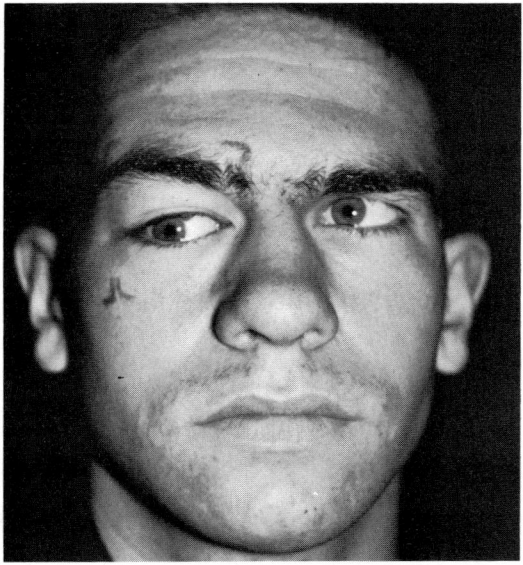

Figure 6-58   Ewing sarcoma metastatic to the right orbit with downward displacement of the globe.

ment often becomes bilateral. Congestion of the lids and conjunctiva may precede the appearance of exophthalmos or occur with it. Those cases that are characterized by limitation of ocular motility, in addition to exophthalmos and edema of the lids, are sometimes referred to as chronic orbital myositis. Biopsies are used to differentiate this condition from orbital neoplasms.

Certain additional clinical features help to differentiate them: pseudotumors occur most commonly in patients of middle or older age, while neoplasms frequently occur earlier; neoplasms almost invariably are unilateral; pseudotumors more frequently are associated with inflammatory signs; x-ray changes of the bone and orbit are common in neoplasms but are not seen frequently in pseudotumors.

Although pseudotumors of the orbit frequently resolve without treatment, regression may be hastened in some cases by x-ray therapy or corticosteroid treatment. In those unusual instances where vision is threatened, surgical excision and decompression may be necessary.

DEFICIENCY DISEASES

Dietary deficiency is a cause of ocular disease and loss of vision in many parts of the world, particularly in Africa and Asia. Vitamin deficiencies usually are multiple, with a combination of the ocular changes described below occurring.

Deficiency of Vitamin A

Vitamin A deficiency manifests itself in the early stages as night blindness (nyctalopia). The relation of this symptom to dietary deficiency was recognized by the ancient Egyptians, who advised ingestion of gull or fish livers as treatment. More severe and chronic deficiency of vitamin A results in xerophthalmia and keratomalacia.

Night Blindness. Vitamin A is intimately involved in the photochemistry of vision, specifically in the breakdown and resynthesis of rhodopsin. Night blindness due to vitamin A deficiency apparently occurs more often in males than in females and usually is observed in individuals less than 20 years of age. In the United States this disorder is common in a mild form, and the associated symptoms are an inability to see well at dusk, abnormally slow adjustment to the dim lights of a movie theater, and retarded recovery of vision after passing a car with strong headlights. Oral administration of vitamin A usually is effective in the treatment of this type of night blindness. It should be noted, however, that nyctalopia may be associated with cirrhosis of the liver and other conditions that interfere with absorption of fat. Night blindness also may occur as a hereditary and congenital defect, in pigmentary degenerations of the retina, and with changes in the retina in Oguchi's disease.

Xerophthalmia and Keratomalacia. Vitamin A deficiency causes xerosis, whose ocular complications are drying of the conjunctiva and cornea (xerophthalmia). Characteristically a foamy, triangular patch occurs on the equator of the conjunctiva just lateral to the cornea (Bitot's spot). The conjunctiva and cornea appear dry and lackluster, and meibomianitis frequently is present. The patient complains of a gritty feeling in the eyes and of photophobia. The principal histopathologic change is keratinization of the epithelium.

Keratomalacia occurs as a late stage of xerophthalmia. The cornea becomes soft and opaque; secondary infection, hypopyon, and perforating ulceration are common. In the early stages xerophthalmia regresses following treatment with vitamin A. Keratomalacia usually results in loss of the eye.

Deficiency of Vitamin B Complex

This and other avitaminoses, while not giving rise to the clear-cut ocular signs found with vitamin A deficiency, affect the eyes profoundly.

Vitamin B$_1$ (Thiamine). Deficiency of Vitamin B$_1$ is an etiologic factor in several disorders, including beriberi, Wernicke's encephalopathy, Korsakoff's syndrome, alcoholic neuritis, and polyneuritis of pregnancy. Ocular findings are dryness and inflammation of the conjunctiva, decreased sensitivity of the cornea, retrobulbar neuritis, optic atrophy, and ocular muscle paralyses.

Vitamin B₂ (Riboflavin and Nicotinic Acid)

PELLAGRA. The principal factor causing this disease is a severe deficiency of nicotinic acid (niacine) or its amide, along with their amino acid precursor, tryptophan. Pellagra is characterized by mental, neurologic, cutaneous, mucous membrane, and gastrointestinal symptoms. Optic neuritis, optic atrophy, retinitis, pupillary changes, and involvement of the extraocular muscles have been observed.

RIBOFLAVIN DEFICIENCY. This results in characteristic oral, cutaneous, and corneal lesions. The latter begin with the circumcorneal injection and subsequent proliferation and anastomosis of the limbal vessels, with the formation of loops and arcades. Corneal vascularization follows. Conjunctival irritation also may occur. The patient experiences burning of the eyes, photophobia, and dimness of vision.

Ocular Complications of Other Avitaminoses and Malnutrition

The ocular complications of vitamin B₁₂ deficiency (pernicious anemia) are discussed in the section on blood diseases (p. 234). Reduced levels of this vitamin also may be a factor in tobacco amblyopia. Severe deficiency of vitamin C (ascorbic acid) results in scurvy, a disease with hemorrhagic manifestations and abnormal osteoid and dentine formation. The characteristic ocular sign in infants or young children is proptosis. Insufficient vitamin C intake has been suggested as a cause of recurrent hemorrhages involving various parts of the eye. Ocular findings are not a significant part of rickets (vitamin D deficiency), although increased lacrimation, papilledema associated with tetany, and visual field changes have been described. When vitamin K has been administered during the late stages of pregnancy, it has been reported to re-

duce the incidence of retinal hemorrhages in the newborn. Deficiency of protein has been stated to be a predisposing factor to the formation of phlyctenules and also to be responsible, in part, for some instances of hypermetropia, presbyopia, diminished dark adaptation, and stye development. In animal experiments deficiency of certain essential amino acids results in corneal vascularization and lenticular opacities; similar changes in humans have not been demonstrated.

DEGENERATIVE DISEASES AND OCULAR CHANGES OF AGING

The eye undergoes constant change. In early life the normal changes of the eyes are in growth and development. Later, degenerative signs of age appear, some of which are common and expected. The term "senile" often is used clinically to describe certain of these degenerative changes in the elderly, as in "senile cataract" and "senile macular degeneration." This term, meant to denote that these changes are characteristic of old age, should not be used in the presence of the patient because of its dire connotations.

Many of the changes in the function and structure of the eye discussed in this section are not the usual or expected changes of aging. Some of these fit under the heading of *abiotrophies* — "the exceptional, progressive, anatomic and functional loss which may occur at any time during development or senescence." Some of the degenerations and abiotrophies may well be the result of allergy, infection or trauma, but their true nature is not recognized at the present time.

Anatomical Changes of Aging

In time the cornea flattens, giving rise to the onset or alteration of astigmatism. The flattening is more marked in the vertical meridian than in the horizontal meridian. Scleral thickness and rigidity increases, often with fat deposition that causes the sclera to appear more yellow. In older people the sclera sometimes thins just in front of the insertions of the lateral and

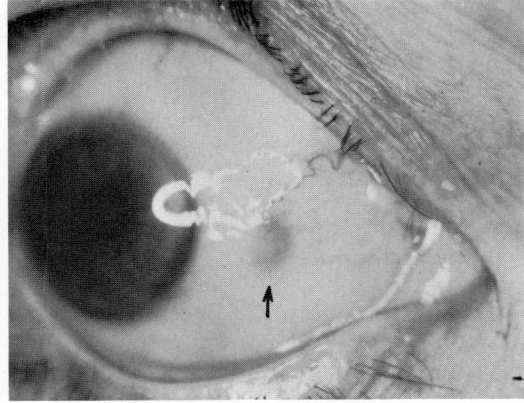

Figure 6-60 Senile hyaline plaque and thinning of the sclera.

visual fields, possibly the result of peripheral atrophic changes in the retina, is common.

Changes in the Eyelids and Lacrimal Apparatus

The lids of aged persons characteristically reveal wrinkled skin, enophthalmos, and slight ptosis. These changes result from loss of orbital fat, changes in elastic tissue, and decreased muscle tone. In elderly patients with chronic lid inflammation, entropion may occur (Fig. 6-61). The lid margin turns in and the lashes then irritate the conjunctiva and cornea. Two factors are involved: spasm of the orbicularis muscle fibers encircling the palpebral fissure and loss of tone of the skin, lid septum, and more peripheral portions of the orbicularis muscle. Atonic entropion may occur in the absence of chronic inflammation. Ectropion (Fig. 6-62) also is common. The lid margin is turned out and the palpebral conjunctiva exposed. Even mild degrees of entropion cause the lower punctum to fall away from the globe, producing epiphora and inflammation of the skin.

A redundancy of the skin of the upper lids (blepharochalasis) results from hypertrophy and loss of elasticity of the skin (Fig. 6-63). Xanthelasma palpebrarum, soft,

medial recti muscles, and dark choroid shows through in small areas. Benign lesions of calcium oxylate crystals may form in these areas (Fig. 6-60), but they require no treatment. They often are referred to as areas of *hyaline degeneration* or *senile hyaline plaques.* The connective tissue in the uveal tract becomes more marked and diffuse. The ciliary body thickens and its processes become hyalinized. Rigidity of the sphincter of the pupil and miosis occur secondary to the increased connective tissue present. The glasslike membranes of the eye thicken and develop wartlike excrescences, particularly at the periphery of Descemet's membrane and in Bruch's membrane (see Hassall-Henle bodies and drusen of the retina described in the following pages). Frequently the pigment epithelium atrophies, notably around the disc.

Functional Changes of Aging

With increasing age, one loses the ability to increase the curvature and thickness of the lens in order to see near objects distinctly (accommodation) and presbyopia occurs. Independent of presbyopia, however, visual acuity may decrease to some extent in the aged. Old people usually require strong illumination to attain their best visual acuity. This probably is related to the smaller size of their pupils and to the decreased transparency of the media. Cone sensitivity after dark adaptation is impaired. Concentric constriction of the

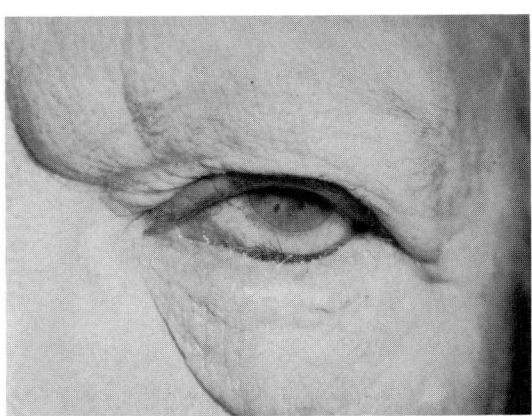

Figure 6-61 Spastic entropion.

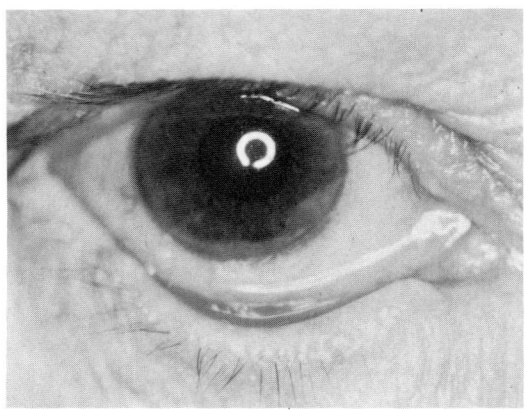

Figure 6-62 Ectropion due to relaxation of the lower lid.

yellow, slightly raised plaques on the eyelids, are frequently seen in normal individuals, particularly women, around the fifth decade of life. This condition occurs also with primary and secondary systemic lipid abnormality. The average age at which skin carcinomas occur is from 50 to 55 years, with a higher incidence in men than in women.

Decreased tear secretion commonly occurs with advancing years. If severe, this may result in inflammatory changes in the cornea and conjunctiva and the picture of keratoconjunctivitis sicca.

In elderly individuals the conjunctiva becomes thinner and more friable. Pinguecula, a yellow elevated area under the conjunctiva on either side of the cornea, frequently is seen in middle life or later (Fig. 6-64). The lesion is produced by hypertrophic, degenerated, connective tissue fibers. It may enlarge, becoming cystic or recurrently inflamed. Treatment usually is not indicated other than to reassure the patient, although occasionally pinguecula may be removed for cosmetic reasons.

Pterygium is a degenerative and hyperplastic process, the pathogenesis of which is not known (Figs. 6-65, 6-66). It consists of the encroachment of a fold of conjunctiva at the limbus onto the cornea. The pterygium is attached loosely to the cornea except at its apex where it is firmly adherent. It usually is raised, and ranges from pearly white to pink in color. In its early form it appears as a small growth resembling an insect wing, entering the cornea from the limbus for a few millimeters. It progresses slowly, tending in many cases to remain stationary for long periods of time or even indefinitely. If untreated, the membrane may cover most of the central cornea. Both eyes usually are affected, but the condition often appears first in one eye where it progresses rapidly. The symptoms may be recurrent irritation or loss of vision if the pupillary area becomes involved. Treatment is surgical exci-

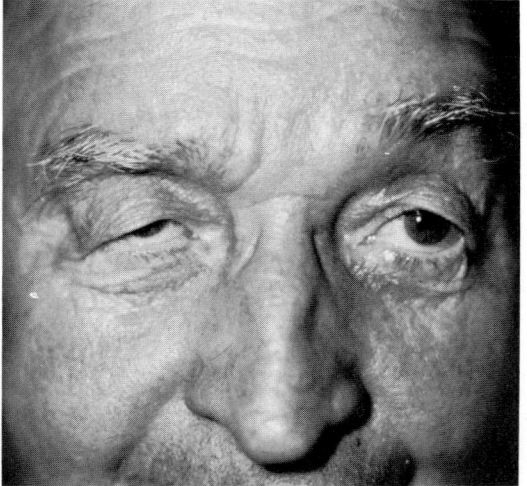

Figure 6-63 Blepharochalasis.

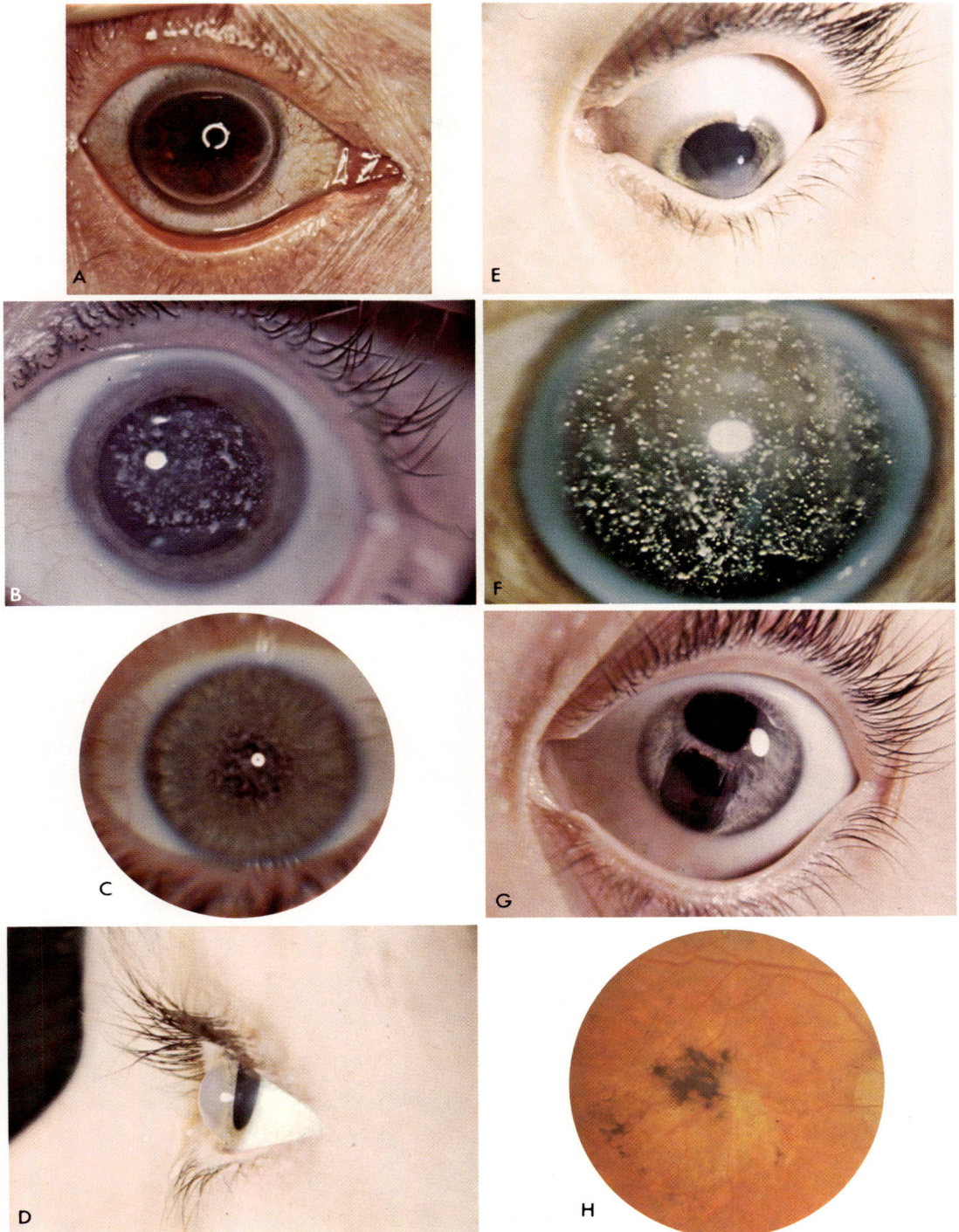

Plate 25 *(A)* Senile marginal degeneration. *(B)* Corneal dystrophy (granular type). *(C)* Corneal dystrophy (macular type). *(D)* Keratoconus with hydrops. *(E)* Frontal view of 25D. *(F)* Asteroid hyalitis. *(G)* Essential iris atrophy. *(H)* Senile macular degeneration is manifest by pigment dispersal and accumulation and retinal atrophy.

277

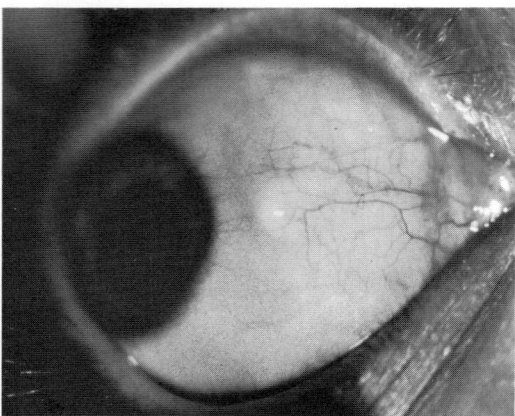

Figure 6-64 Pinguecula.

Figure 6-65 Early pterygium.

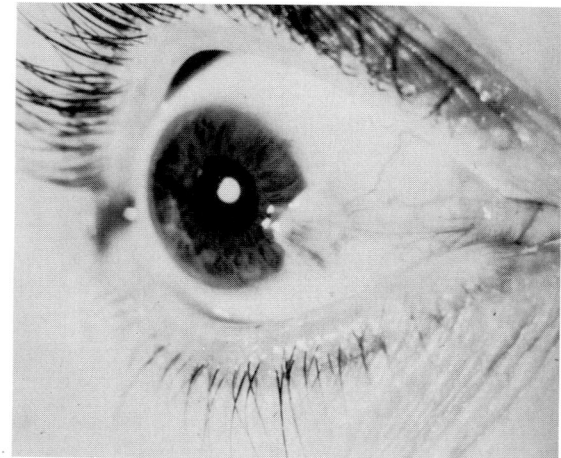

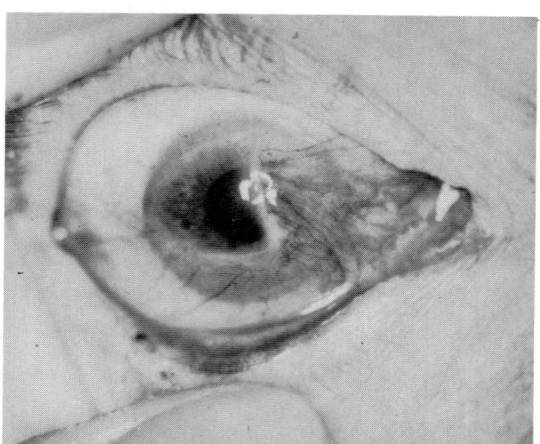

Figure 6-66 Pterygium encroaching on the pupil.

sion, sometimes accompanied by radiation. The condition may recur.

Changes in the Cornea

The cornea in the elderly generally has somewhat less luster and translucency than is seen in the young. Some dustlike opacities (cornea farinata), resulting from condensation in the stroma, frequently are seen in the deeper portions of the cornea with the slit lamp biomicroscope. Changes in the thickness and transparency of Bowman's and Descemet's membranes may result in a mosaic pattern, termed "crocodile shagreen."

Degenerative Processes of the Cornea. Arcus senilis, an opaque zone of lipoid infiltration near the corneal periphery, is the most frequent degenerative change of the cornea (Fig. 6-67). This usually begins as white arcs in the cornea superiorly and inferiorly, separated from the limbus by a narrow space of clear cornea. Eventually these arcs form a complete ring (circulus senilis). When present to a marked degree, the ring may take on a yellow color. This lesion never encroaches on the pupillary area and has no pathologic significance. It has been produced experimentally by feeding rabbits a diet rich in cholesterol. In elderly persons, however, it usually is unrelated to abnormal fat or lipid metabolism. An arcus similar in appearance to that just described is sometimes seen at birth or develops before or during middle age and is termed arcus juvenilis, or anterior embryotoxon.

Less common are *fatty degeneration* and *lipid keratopathy*, in which an accumulation of fats or lipids is visible in the cornea, and *hyaline degeneration* in which translucent, homogeneous, highly refractile substances are deposited in the cornea.

Hassall-Henle bodies are droplike excrescences of hyaline material, probably collagen, which can be seen with the slit lamp biomicroscope. They occur on the periphery of Descemet's membrane and project into the anterior chamber. The product of an aging change comparable to drusen of Bruch's membrane of the choroid, Hassall-Henle bodies usually do not interfere with vision. The *white limbus girdle of Vogt* is a crescent-shaped, lacy, white opacity occurring at the limbus in the interpalpebral area. It resembles an early, localized, band-shaped keratopathy whose histopathologic picture also is similar. The condition is benign and does not require treatment.

Senile marginal degeneration (superficial marginal keratitis of Fuchs) is an uncommon bilateral condition of unknown etiology occurring in people of middle age or over (Plate 25A). A gutter-like furrow gradually develops around the circumference of the cornea, usually without significant pain or inflammation. Commonly the central area of the cornea remains clear, and vision is not seriously affected.

Corneal Dystrophies. These disorders may be classified into groups according to the portion of the cornea primarily affected: the epithelium and Bowman's membrane, the stroma, the endothelium and Descemet's membrane.

Meesmann's corneal dystrophy is a dominantly inherited disorder in which large numbers of droplet-like opacities are distributed diffusely throughout the corneal epithelium and, occasionally, in Bowman's membrane. There is abnormal proliferation and degeneration of the epithelial cells with intracellular glycogen deposition. The disease is slowly progressive, but it is unusual for vision to be seriously impaired. No effective therapy is known. In *Cogan's microscopic cystic epithelial dystrophy*, small,

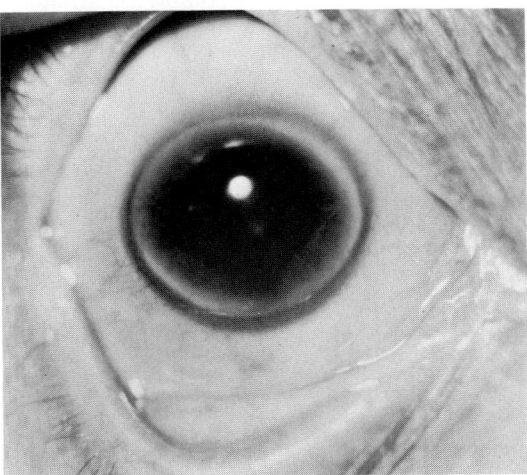

Figure 6-67 Arcus senilis.

gray opacities occur in the pupillary areas of both eyes. These are due to intraepithelial cysts containing keratinized debris and to the presence of reduplications of the basement membrane between the epithelial layers. Symptoms are minimal.

Three disorders involve primarily the stroma: granular, macular, and lattice dystrophies (Plate 25B, C). All three usually become manifest in the second decade of life, are hereditary, and are characterized by similar changes: bilateral, usually symmetrical, deposition of hyaline material in the superficial lamellae; degenerative changes of the superficial lamellae and Bowman's membrane; thickening of the epithelium; a slow progression with an absence of vascularization. The differentiating features are listed in Table 6-13. There is no known form of medical therapy. Penetrating keratoplasties have been performed successfully.

Salzmann's nodular dystrophy is an uncommon, nonfamilial, corneal disease occurring in patients with chronic keratitis, usually of the phlyctenular type. It is characterized clinically by the appearance of blue-white nodular opacities which protrude above the corneal surface. Histopathologically the nodules are thick, acellular plaques of hyalin located between the epithelium and Bowman's membrane. New lesions tend to occur intermittently in acute attacks. The disease may result in decreased vision, photophobia, lacrimation, and pain. Lamellar corneal grafting often is effective, but

no satisfactory medical treatment is available.

Keratoconus (conical cornea) is a condition, beginning about puberty and developing mainly in females, in which the apex of the cornea thins gradually and usually bilaterally (Plate 25D, E). The etiology is unknown, but its occurrence is related to hereditary factors. The presenting symptom is a reduction of the patient's vision which cannot be corrected with lenses. Early in the course of the disease the cornea does not look conical. Ophthalmoscopic examination with a high plus lens and retinoscopy, however, reveal a round, shadow-like reflex in the central part of the cornea instead of the usual even red reflex. The diagnosis of keratoconus is confirmed by the distorted reflex observed with a Placido's disc and abnormal keratometer readings. In more advanced stages, signs include the obvious cone-shaped cornea and indentation of the lower lid by the cornea. By slit lamp biomicroscopy, vertical lines are noted in the deep layers of the stroma; the corneal nerve fibers are increasingly visible; and in about 50 per cent of cases a yellow or green line is present around the base of the cone (Fleischer's ring). In advanced cases Bowman's membrane and Descemet's membrane rupture. Microscopically there is thinning of the tissue spaces between the corneal lamellae, fragmentation of the basement membrane of the corneal epithelium, fibrillation of Bowman's membrane, and folds or ruptures in Descemet's membrane. Contact lenses improve visual acuity in the early stages, but corneal transplantation is indicated when the corrected visual acuity is de-

TABLE 6-13 DIFFERENTIATING THE HEREDITARY DYSTROPHIES INVOLVING THE CORNEAL STROMA

Dystrophy	Synonyms	Type of Inheritance	Clinical Characteristics	Histopathologic Features
Granular	Groenouw I or Bucklers I	Dominant	Irregular, discrete, gray opacities occurring only in the central portion of the cornea	Lesions seen as focal areas of hyalin degeneration; stromal fibers appear granulated
Macular	Groenouw II or Bucklers II	Recessive	Many fine opacities; diffuse cloudiness of stroma between the lesions results in earliest and most severe impairment of vision of the three forms	Mucoid degeneration of the corneal lamellae
Lattice	Bucklers III or Biber-Haab-Dimmer	Dominant	Linear lesions having a filamentous interwoven appearance	Fusiform areas of hyalin degeneration and dense deposit of hyalin between epithelium and Bowman's membrane

creased to the point where it interferes with the normal activities of the patient. If transplantation is done before extreme corneal thinning occurs, the prognosis is excellent.

In *cornea guttata* excrescences of hyaline material involve the entire posterior surface of the cornea. The lesions resemble Hassall-Henle bodies; the latter, however, remain confined to the peripheral portion of Descemet's membrane. The changes of cornea guttata are most apparent by indirect illumination with the slit lamp biomicroscope. Cornea guttata may remain stationary or lead to the *combined dystrophy of Fuchs* in which there is edema of the stroma associated with, and probably caused by, pathologic changes in the epithelium and endothelium. In the more advanced forms of this latter dystrophy, epithelial bullae form, followed by vascularization and scarring. Corneal infection and glaucoma are additional, late complications. Some ophthalmologists advise penetrating keratoplasty at a relatively early stage of the disease.

Changes in the Vitreous

Detachment of the vitreous from the retina is a common change after middle life. On slit lamp examination this is seen as an optically empty space between the vitreous and the retina. Detachment from the area of the optic disc is recognized ophthalmoscopically as a dark, disc-sized ring in front of the disc. Symptoms of vitreous detachment are lightning flashes, a "ring" in the field of vision, and a sudden appearance of "spots" or "floaters." These symptoms gradually subside, and vision usually is not affected significantly. Vitreous detachment, however, may be associated with retinal tears and subsequent retinal detachment.

Liquefaction or *syneresis* of the vitreous body is a common aging change. Ophthalmoscopic examination reveals dotlike opacities, veil-like or membrane-like structures and strands floating in the vitreous. *Shrinkage* of the vitreous gel accompanies syneresis and may result in traction on the portions of the retina to which the vitreous remains attached. Such traction may play a role in retinal detachment. Associated symptoms are floaters and flashes of light. Vitreous traction on the retina has been cited also

as a cause of posterior pole edema in peripheral uveitis, following cataract extraction, and in central serous retinopathy.

Vitreous floaters or *muscae volitantes* refer to the commonly seen "spots before the eyes" that are a particularly frequent complaint of older persons and of patients with myopia. The floaters probably are fine aggregates of vitreous protein that occur as a degenerative change in the vitreous. The condition usually is innocuous.

Asteroid hyalitis are spherical and stellate opacities composed of calcium-containing lipid that are suspended in the vitreous (Plate 25F). They sometimes are called *"snowball opacities"* or *Benson's disease*. The condition usually is unilateral and is most frequent in older men. Presence of the opacities does not often give rise to symptoms. The opacities are attached to fibers of the vitreous and return to their original position following movement of the eye. It has been stated that asteroid hyalitis occurs more commonly in diabetics with hypercholesterolemia than in normal persons.

In *synchysis scintillans* the vitreous contains crystalline deposits composed primarily of cholesterol. The condition occurs after inflammation, chronic degeneration, trauma, and hemorrhage. It usually is associated with a fluid vitreous. In contrast to asteroid hyalitis, it often is seen in patients under 35 years of age and is generally bilateral. On examination, the crystals are noted to settle to a dependent position when there is no movement of the globe. There is no known effective treatment.

Changes in the Lens

The aging lens undergoes a number of morphologic and metabolic changes. The lens sutures become more complex; the size of the nucleus increases, with a relative decrease in the size of the cortical zone; the lens enlarges; accommodative power diminishes; the size of the zonular fibers decreases; and frequently the lens loses its transparency.

Senile cataracts usually are nuclear or cortical, with the latter progressing more rapidly than the former.

A *nuclear cataract* usually begins soon after the age of 40 as an extension of sclerosis of the nucleus of the lens. Yellow or brown pigment may be deposited. When very dark brown, the term *cataracta brunescens*, or *nigra*, is applied. Increasing optical density of the nucleus results in an increase in the refractive index and in myopia (sometimes termed "second sight," because the patient can read without glasses once more). This is a very slowly developing type of cataract, and it may be a number of years before a patient's vision is poor enough to justify an operation.

A *cortical cataract* manifests itself first as peripheral, wedge-shaped opacities ("water clefts") and as lamellar separations within the lens. The clefts extend into the pupillary area and are seen by focal illumination as radial gray or white bands. The separations, which evolve into peripheral pyramid-shaped opacities, are seen as concentric lines in the cortex. A *posterior subcapsular cortical cataract* or *cupuliform cataract* is an opacity in the posterior cortex just under the capsule. It usually is associated with a definite opacification within the posterior capsule. It is located centrally and, therefore, seriously affects vision very early, so that the lens often must be removed when most of it is still clear.

Immature or *incipient cataract* is incomplete. The lens is only slightly opaque, the lens cortex being, for the most part, clear. When the entire lens is completely opaque, the cataract is said to be mature. After a cataract is complete, the osmotic effect of degenerated lens protein may cause the lens to swell. When the lens is extremely swollen, the cataract is called *intumescent*. This type of cataract can lead to secondary angle closure (acute) glaucoma.

A *hypermature cataract* is one in which degraded protein molecules are absorbed or escape, leaving behind a shrunken yellow lens and wrinkled capsule. A *Morgagnian cataract* is a hypermature cataract in which the cortex has become completely liquefied and the nucleus, with its greater density, settles inferiorly within the intact lens capsule. Complete and hypermature cataracts present dangers to the eye such as spontaneous dislocation of the lens and phacolytic and angle closure glaucoma (p. 347).

Numerous *juvenile cataracts* of various types have been described as developing during infancy, childhood, and adolescence. These may be inherited, acquired, occur as an isolated finding, or as part of a systemic disorder.

Changes in the Iris and Ciliary Body

The characteristic histopathologic changes of the iris include stromal atrophy with resultant flattening of the iris, surface and obliteration of the iris crypts, and sclerosis of the sphincter muscle of the pupil.

Intraepithelial cysts frequently occur in the ciliary body and also are found in the iris. They are said to represent a separation of the two epithelial layers. Such cysts most often occur on the temporal side. They usually are bilateral and may be associated with similar cysts in the retina. Small intraepithelial cysts enlarge slowly, if at all, and are of no clinical significance. When larger, they may flatten the pupil with the involved sector not dilating as well as adjacent areas. The large cysts must be differentiated from tumors. Lesions in the ciliary body will usually transmit light. This contrasts with the transillumination picture of a melanoma or solid tumor. Intraepithelial cysts are best studied by gonioscopy.

Pupillary cysts may originate from an embryonic structure (the ring sinus of Szily) that has remained patent in the adult eye or from hyperplasia of the pigment epithelium around the pupil after long-term use of strong miotics.

Essential iris atrophy is a progressive disease of unknown etiology (Plate 25G). It is marked by a patchy degeneration and disappearance of the iris stroma followed by loss of the epithelium and holes in the iris. There is displacement of the pupil and eversion (ectropion) of the pupillary margin. The condition is accompanied by a severe form of glaucoma. Essential iris atrophy is a relatively rare disease that mostly affects women between 20 and 40 years of age. Gonioscopic examination shows adhesions of the iris to the trabecula, especially peripheral to the areas of iris atrophy.

Changes in the Choroid

Atrophy and *depigmentation* of the choroid occur in the aged. This is most common in the far periphery of the fundus but also is frequent in the peripapillary region. The red reflex (the red glow of the fundus due to the choriocapillaris) no longer is uniform, as it is in the young, and it may have a patchy, irregular appearance. Focal thickenings occur in Bruch's membrane (drusen of the retina or colloid bodies) and appear ophthalmoscopically as small, yellow dots scattered about the retina, particularly in the central area. Breaks may occur in Bruch's membrane, resulting in a clinical and histopathologic picture similar to angioid streaks. Sclerosis of the choroidal vessels from aging has been discussed previously (p. 248).

Primary choroidal sclerosis consists of atrophy or fibrous replacement of the muscular coat of the wall of the choroidal vessels. An uncommon diffuse disorder with a familial tendency, it is associated with secondary degenerative and pigmentary changes in the retina. It may be related to the tapetoretinal degenerations. On ophthalmoscopic examination one sees colloid bodies, pigment clumping and migration, and sheathing of the retinal veins. The choroidal vessels appear prominent through the atrophic overlying tissue. Primary choroidal sclerosis generally is divided into three types, depending on the clinical picture: diffuse or generalized choroidal sclerosis; peripapillary choroidal sclerosis (extending around the optic disc); central alveolar or macular sclerosis (situated at the macula or between the macula and the disc).

Changes in the Retina

Tapetoretinal Degeneration and Related Diseases. Retinitis pigmentosa, the most common and characteristic of this family of diseases, is discussed in the chapter on pediatric ophthalmology (p. 130), as are retinitis punctata albescens and fundus albipunctatus.

Oguchi's disease is a rare, recessive, hereditary form of night blindness that is seen on ophthalmoscopic examination as a gray-white discoloration of the fundus. When the patient is placed in the dark for a few hours, the fundus reverts to the normal red color. The discoloration gradually reappears on exposure to daylight. Most of the cases reported have occurred in Japanese people.

Choroideremia is an extremely uncommon sex-linked condition in which degeneration of the choroid, retinal pigment epithelium, and rod and cone layer occurs in affected males. Most frequently the onset is in the first decade, with the earliest symptom being night blindness. The condition is progressive in males and eventually results in blindness. On ophthalmoscopic examination one usually sees fine pigment mottling in the central area but coarse particles in the periphery. The pigment epithelium and choroid undergo progressive atrophy, particularly in the midperiphery, leading to exposure of the underlying sclera. The retinal vessels may slightly constrict; the disc is normal. Female carriers usually have no symptoms, but areas of pigmentation and depigmentation may be seen in the midperiphery. These changes are much less intense and more stationary than those in affected males (see p. 129).

Gyrate atrophy of the choroid and retina, a rare disease occurring in both sexes, is characterized by a patchy, progressive atrophy of the choroid and pigment epithelium of the retina. It usually begins in early childhood. Irregularly-shaped white areas of atrophy occur initially around the disc and macula but spread and become confluent. Areas of pigment stippling or clumping may also be seen. In this disease the fundus eventually can resemble that in choroideremia. The relationship of gyrate atrophy, choroideremia, and retinitis pigmentosa is not well understood.

Fundus flavimaculatus is a term recently introduced to describe a condition of a small group of patients in which multiple yellow or yellow-white, atrophic lesions are distributed throughout the posterior pole. Darkly pigmented lesions also may be present, similar to those seen in tapetoretinal degeneration. These changes, however, are not progressive, and there are no characteristic electroretinogram changes (p. 132).

Macular Degeneration. *Senile macular degeneration* commonly causes visual loss in the elderly (Plates 25*H*, 26*A*, *B*, *C*; Fig. 6-68). This is considered an acquired degenerative process. Sclerosis of the choriocapillaris has been suggested, but not proved, as its cause. Onset occurs about the sixth decade with gradual loss of vision. The condition almost always is bilateral, although at first only one eye usually is involved. Most often a fine stippling of pigment is seen in the macular area, with loss of the foveal reflex. Later there may be gross clumps of pigment and white spots resembling colloid bodies. Progression is gradual, but the end result usually is a dense central scotoma. Magnifiers, strong reading glasses, and telescopic lenses may be helpful. Patients should be reassured that the disease does not lead to blindness. Treatment with vitamins, vasodilators, retin, ascorbic acid, and low fat diets is not effective.

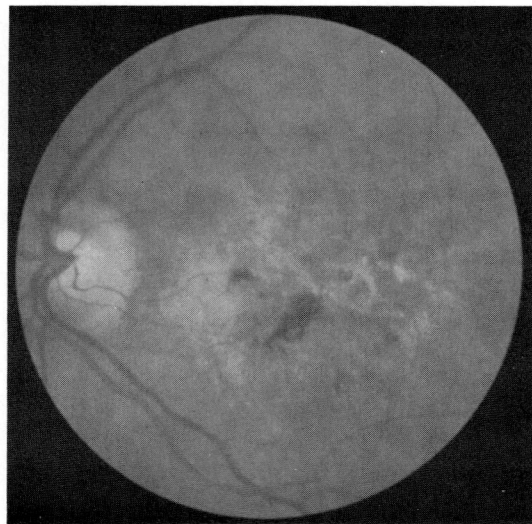

Figure 6-68 Senile macular degeneration; fellow eye of same patient as in Plate 25*H*.

An identical macular degeneration may occur in adults as an inherited disorder. Heredomacular degeneration in infants and children is considered in the chapter on pediatric ophthalmology (p. 132).

Disciform macular degeneration (Kuhnt-Junius disease) occurs in persons over 40 years of age. Initially a dark, sometimes black, round, raised area appears in or near the macular area (Plate 26*D*). This lesion apparently is an extravasation of blood between Bruch's membrane and the pigment epithelium. More superficial red hemorrhages usually occur at the margins of the dark areas. As the disease progresses, edema, exudation, and organization of recurrent hemorrhages result in a solid fibrotic mass involving the retina and choroid. This is seen ophthalmoscopically as a mottled dome-shaped elevation considerably beneath the level of the retinal vessels. The disorder is at first unilateral, but the other eye almost always becomes involved. Central vision decreases or is lost entirely. There is no treatment at the present time.

Circinate retinopathy is a form of macular degeneration in which large and small, yellow, sharply defined intraretinal exudates are seen in a circular or horseshoe arrangement around the macula (Plate 26*E*). Pigmentary changes or scarring, in addition to sclerosed choroidal vessels, may occur in the foveal area. This disorder is said to be most common in middle age, especially among women, but it usually is unrelated to systemic disease. Similar deposits may also develop secondary to other conditions such as diabetic retinopathy and chronic or recurrent central serous retinopathy.

Cystic degeneration of the macula is seen as a senile change, as a consequence of edema or inflammation, in myopia, and with vascular disease. A macular cyst is a sharply outlined, round, red defect about one quarter of a disc diameter in size. Often it is associated with a marked decrease in vision. Histologically, fluid-filled spaces are seen in the outer plexiform layer. The walls of a cyst may break down and a macular hole may form. These can be distinguished with certainty only by biomicroscopic examination. In contrast to other retinal holes, macular holes rarely are associated with retinal detachment. Degeneration of the macula may accompany changes in Bruch's

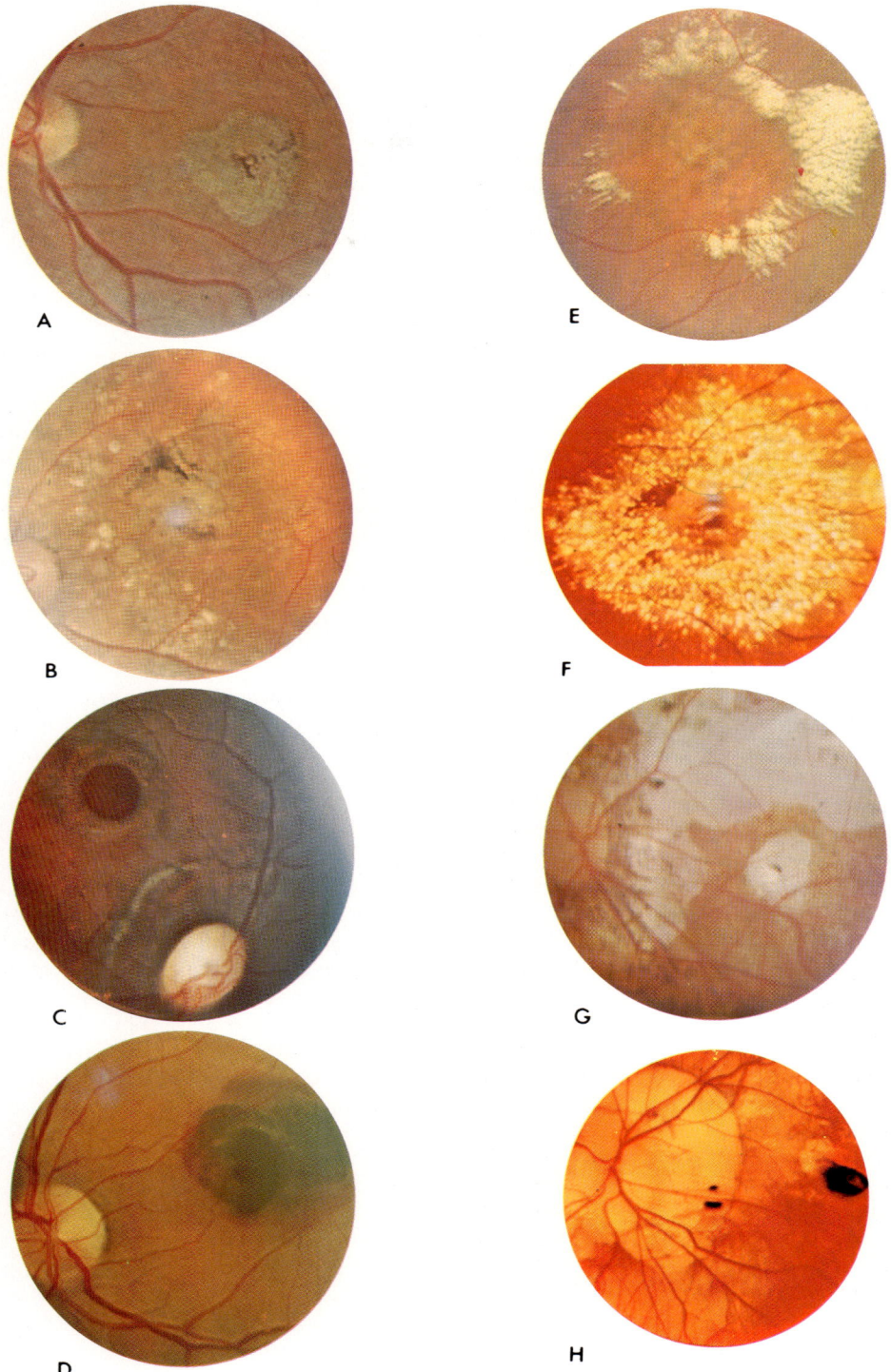

Plate 26 *(A)* Senile macular degeneration with pigment disturbance. *(B)* Senile macular degeneration with colloid bodies (drusen). *(C)* Senile macular degeneration with hole. *(D)* Deep retinal hemorrhage in early Kuhnt-Junius disease. *(E)* Circinate-type retinopathy. *(F)* Doyne's honeycomb degeneration. *(G)* Myopic degeneration. *(H)* Myopic degeneration with macular hemorrhage (Fuchs' black spot).

membrane colloid bodies, and Doyne's honeycomb choroiditis (Plate 26*F*).

Other Degenerative Retinal Conditions. *Lattice degeneration* is a sharply demarcated, circumferential lesion that is located at, or somewhat anterior to, the equator. It is characterized by an interconnecting network of fine white lines and usually is associated with numerous, round, punched-out areas of retinal thinning or actual retinal holes. There are strong vitreoretinal adhesions along the posterior margin of the lattice. Histopathologically lattice degeneration is seen as a sclerosis of retinal vessels associated with a pigmentary disturbance. The disease, which frequently is bilateral, affects about 6 per cent of persons over 10 years of age. It usually is a benign and asymptomatic condition, but in some instances tears develop along the margin of the lesion, causing retinal detachment.

Peripheral cystoid degeneration (Blessig's cysts; Iwanoff's cysts) appears to be a normal aging change generally found in the eyes of patients over 20 years of age. As these cysts gradually increase in size and number, they extend backward up to several millimeters into the retina from the ora serrata. On examination of the peripheral retina, one sees cysts that may be regularly arranged and closely packed to form red streaks or patches, with the greatest involvement on the temporal side. Occasionally the lesions appear as pink, gelatinous elevations, large enough to be distinguished individually. Histopathologically the cysts arise first in the outer plexiform layer, then eventually extend almost to the inner and outer limiting membranes of the retina.

Retinoschisis is a separation or splitting of the sensory retina into two layers. Of unknown etiology, this appears to be related to peripheral cystoid degeneration. In early stages one sees a flat, smooth elevation of the inner layers of the retina, the surface appearing gray-white and containing striations or white flecks. Retinoschisis may occur in any part of the retina, but appears characteristically in the lower, temporal periphery. The split usually occurs in the outer plexiform layer. The retinal blood vessels are in the inner layer of the split retina and often appear white peripherally, as if they were obliterated. In advanced form, retinoschisis appears as a smooth, convex, sharply outlined, transparent elevation. A peculiar reflection, which has been compared to the appearance of watered silk, is visible on the surface. It does not vary in shape or location with eye movements. Retinoschisis usually is benign, asymptomatic, and requires no treatment. If holes form in the internal and external walls, however, retinal detachment may result. Retinoschisis also may compromise vision by extending posteriorly where even the macula can be involved. Photocoagulation or surface diathermy has been used to prevent spread or retinal detachment. Juvenile retinoschisis is discussed elsewhere (p. 135).

Retinal Detachment. This abnormality usually occurs in patients over 45 years of age. It is more common in males (60 to 70 per cent), and in approximately 25 per cent of affected patients it may become bilateral. Detachments are more frequent in nearsighted (myopic) patients and occur in about 2 per cent of patients on whom cataract operations have been performed.

There are three major mechanisms by which separation of the neural retina from the pigment epithelium can occur:

1. Breaks or tears in the retina allow the escape of fluid from the vitreous into the subretinal space. The tears may be horseshoe-shaped, with a small, central flap or operculum, and they may be small and round. In other instances the retina may be torn from its insertion at the ora serrata (*dialysis* or *disinsertion*). These are seen in younger patients, usually from trauma, but also as a congenital defect. Blunt trauma and penetrating injuries of the globe may give rise to retinal holes. Patients frequently cite a history of trivial injuries and distant trauma, such as falls, but predisposing ocular changes usually can be found. Peripheral retinal degeneration, including peripheral cystoid degeneration, lattice degeneration, and retinoschisis, are factors leading to formation of retinal holes.

2. Fibrous bands in the vitreous or vitreous shrinkage may pull the retina forward from the pigment epithelium. Adhesions between the vitreous and retina may occur, with peripheral retinal degen-

of retinal holes. Organization of inflammatory exudates and hemorrhages in the vitreous may result in fibrous tissue formation and subsequent retinal detachment. Neovascularization of the retina may be followed by the formation of vascular strands extending out into the vitreous, and detachment may ensue. Contracture of a cyclitic membrane may have a similar result.

3. Subretinal fluid may accumulate from inflammation of the retina and choroid, disturbances in the retinal and choroidal circulation, and as part of the retinopathy of certain systemic diseases. These retinal detachments are exudative and not associated with retinal holes.

SIGNS AND SYMPTOMS OF RETINAL DETACHMENT. When the retina begins to detach, the patient complains of "floaters" or "spots" suddenly appearing before his eyes, and of recurrent flashes of light in a sector of the field corresponding to the detached retina. The patient notices a loss of vision or a cloud over that part of the field when the detachment is sufficiently extensive. This frequently comes on slowly and is described as a floating curtain or cloud in front of the eye.

On ophthalmoscopic examination the separated retina loses its pink color and appears gray and opaque with an indefinite margin. In a well advanced detachment, the separated area is ballooned out and often thrown into folds. The arterioles and venules lose their normal red color and appear almost black. In long-standing detachments the margin is defined sharply, and the detached retina is thin and transparent. When the detachment results from an inflammatory condition that has lifted up the retina, areas of choroiditis and many fresh vitreous opacities may be seen. On examination of the visual fields, a defect can be plotted corresponding to the portion of the retina that is detached.

Flat detachments are more difficult to diagnose because the retina projects only slightly forward from the pigment epithelium layer. The retinal vessels over a flat detachment darken and frequently change their course. Retinal striations caused by traction sometimes can be seen.

Binocular, indirect ophthalmoscopy frequently is invaluable in detecting retinal holes. Depression of the sclera in the region of the ora serrata during ophthalmoscopic examination is useful in bringing the retinal periphery into view. Slit lamp ophthalmoscopy is helpful in examining the retina as well as in evaluating the state of the vitreous. If the detachment is caused by a tumor, light will not come through the involved area when the retina is transilluminated. Because involvement frequently is bilateral, the fellow eye must be examined completely.

TREATMENT OF RETINAL DETACHMENT. This is discussed in the chapter on ocular surgery (p. 390). If the detachment is not treated, the entire retina usually becomes involved over a period of weeks or months, resulting in a blind eye.

Changes in the Optic Nerve

The optic disc is described by some authors as appearing ophthalmoscopically paler and flatter in the aged than in the young. Atherosclerotic changes frequently develop in the small vessels supplying the optic nerve and disc. Drusen of the optic disc (see Neuro-ophthalmology, p. 299) are considered by some to be an aging change. Histopathologically, arachnoidal cell nests, psammoma bodies in the arachnoid (spheroidal, acellular, laminated, hyaline structures laid down by meningothelial cells), and corpora amylacea (sphere-shaped, usually homogenous bodies in the nerve fiber tissue) are described as products of aging or of degenerative processes.

BIBLIOGRAPHY

Allergies

Blodi, F. C.: Sympathetic uveitis as an allergic phenomenon. Tr. Am. Acad. Ophth. 63:642, 1959.

Hogan, M. J., Kimura, S. J., and Thygeson, P.: Signs and symptoms of uveitis. I. Anterior uveitis. Am. J. Ophth. 47:155 (May issue, part 2), 1959.

Silverstein, A. M.: Uveal hypersensitivity reactions to protein antigens. *In* Maumenee, A. E., and Silverstein, A. M. (eds.): Immunopathology of Uveitis. Baltimore, Williams & Wilkins Co., 1964, pp. 209-220.

Theodore, F. H.: Bacterial allergy of the eye. Tr. Am. Acad. Ophth. 65:184, 1961.

Theodore, F. H., and Schlossman, A.: Ocular Allergy. Baltimore, Williams & Wilkins Co., 1958.

Wakesman, B. H.: Auto-immunization and the lesions of auto-immunity. Medicine *41*:93, 1962.

Witebsky, E., and Milgrom, F.: The nature of auto-sensitization with particular reference to the eye. *In* Maumenee, A. E., and Silverstein, A. M. (eds.): Immunopathology of Uveitis. Baltimore, Williams & Wilkins Co., 1964, pp. 196-208.

Infections

Allen, H. F., Burns, R. P., Gingrich, W. D., Givner, I., Key, S. N., Jr., Kimura, S. J., and Thygeson, P.: Infectious Diseases of the Conjunctiva and Cornea. Symposium of the New Orleans Academy of Ophthalmology. St. Louis, The C. V. Mosby Co., 1963.

Archer, D., and Bird, A.: Primary tuberculosis of the conjunctiva. Brit. J. Ophth. *51*:679, 1967.

Braley, A. E.: Acute herpetic keratoconjunctivitis. Am. J. Ophth. *43*:105, 1957.

Christensen, L., Beaman, H. W., and Allen, A.: Cytomegalic inclusion disease. Arch. Ophth. *57*:90, 1957.

Falls, H. F., and Giles, C. L.: The use of amphotericin B in selected cases of chorioretinitis. Am. J. Ophth. *49*:1288, 1960.

Ferry, A. P.: Cerebral mucormycosis (phycomycosis). Ocular findings and review of literature. Surv. Ophth. *6*:1, 1961.

Frenkel, J. K., and Jacobs, L.: Ocular toxoplasmosis. Arch. Ophth. *59*:260, 1958.

Hogan, M. J., Kimura, S. J., and Thygeson, P.: Pathology of herpes simplex keratoiritis. Tr. Am. Ophth. Soc. *61*:75, 1963.

Horsfall, F. L., Jr., and Tamm, I.: Viral and Rickettsial Infections of Man. 4th ed. Philadelphia, J. B. Lippincott Co., 1965.

Irvine, W. C., and Irvine, A. R., Jr.: Nematode endophthalmitis: Toxocara canis. Am. J. Ophth. *47*:185, 1959.

Jones, B. R.: Ocular syndrome of TRIC virus infection and their possible genital significance. Brit. J. Ven. Dis. *40*:3, 1964.

Kaufman, H. E.: Chemotherapy of herpes simplex keratitis. Invest. Ophth. *2*:504, 1963.

Kaufman, H., Swyers, J. S., and Lausch, R. N.: Corneal hypersensitivity to herpes simplex. Brit. J. Ophth. *51*:843, 1967.

MacCallan, A. F.: The epidemiology of trachoma. Brit. J. Ophth. *15*:369, 1931.

Maumenee, A. E. (ed.): Toxoplasmosis. Baltimore, Williams & Wilkins Co., 1962.

Mrinmay, G., Levy, P. M., and Leopold, I. H.: Therapy of toxoplasmosis uveitis. Am. J. Ophth. *59*:55, 1965.

Prendergast, J. J.: Ocular leprosy in the United States. Arch. Ophth. *23*:112, 1939.

Rodger, F. C.: The pathogenesis and pathology of ocular onchocerciosis. Am. J. Ophth. *49*:104, 1960.

Scheie, H. G.: Ocular changes associated with scrub typhus: A study of 451 patients. Arch. Ophth. *40*:245, 1948.

Scott, J. G.: Experience with live trachoma vaccine. Tr. Ophth. Soc. U. Kingdom *84*:615, 1964.

Swan, J. W., and Penn, R. F.: Scleritis following mumps. Am. J. Ophth. *53*:366, 1962.

Symposium, Viral keratoconjunctivitis. Am. J. Ophth. *43*:1, 1957.

Tanner, O. R.: Ocular manifestations of infectious mononucleosis. Arch. Ophth. *51*:229, 1954.

Thygeson, P., and Dawson, C.: Trachoma and follicular conjunctivitis in children. Arch. Ophth. *75*:3, 1966.

Thygeson, P.: Trachoma manual and atlas. Pub. Health Serv. Publ. No. 541, revised 1960.

Wilder, H. C.: Toxoplasma chorioretinitis in adults. Arch. Ophth. *48*:127, 1952.

Wilder, H. C.: Nematode endophthalmitis. Tr. Am. Acad. Ophth. *55*:99, 1950.

Woods, A. C.: Modern concepts of the etiology of uveitis. Am. J. Ophth. *50*:1170, 1960.

Heritable Diseases

Cogan, D. G., and Kuwabara, T.: Ocular pathology of cystinosis. Arch. Ophth. *63*:51, 1960.

Cogan, D. G., and Kuwabara, T.: Sphingolipidosis and the eye. Arch. Ophth. *79*:437, 1968.

Fonda, G.: Characteristics and low-vision corrections in albinism. Report of 161 patients. Arch. Ophth. *68*:754, 1962.

Goldberg, M. F., Maumenee, A. E., and McKusick, V. A.: Corneal dystrophies associated with abnormalities of mucopolysaccharide metabolism. Arch. Ophth. *74*:516, 1965.

Goldberg, M. F., and von Noorden, G. K.: Ophthalmologic findings in Wilson's hepatolenticular degeneration. Arch. Ophth. *75*:162, 1966.

Gutman, A. B.: Galactosemia. *In* Beeson, P. B., and McDermott, W. (eds.): Cecil-Loeb Textbook of Medicine. Philadelphia, W. B. Saunders Co., 1967.

Johnston, S. S.: Pupil-block glaucoma in homocystinuria. Br. J. Ophth. *52*:251, 1968.

Knox, W. E.: Phenylketonuria. *In* Stanbury, J. B., Wyngaarden, J. B., and Fredrickson, D. S. (eds.): The Metabolic Basis of Inherited Disease. New York, McGraw-Hill Co., 1960.

McKusick, V. A.: Heritable Disorders of Connective Tissue. 3rd ed. St. Louis, The C. V. Mosby Co., 1966.

Rones, B.: Ochronosis oculi in alkaptonuria. Am. J. Ophth. *49*:440, 1960.

Scheie, H. G., Hambrick, G. W., and Barness, L. A.: A newly recognized forme fruste of Hurler's disease (gargoylism). Am. J. Ophth. *53*:753, 1962.

Collagen Diseases

Anderson, B., Sr.: Ocular lesions in relapsing polychondritis and other rheumatoid syndromes. Am. J. Ophth. *64*:35, 1967.

Cogan, D. G.: Corneal scleral lesions in periarteritis nodosa and Wegener's granulomatosis. Tr. Am. Ophth. Soc. *53*:321, 1955.

Guyton, J. S.: Differential diagnosis of collagen disease. Arch. Ophth. *86*:563, 1956.

Manschot, W. A.: The eye in collagen diseases. Adv. Ophth. *11*:1, 1961.

Maumenee, A. E.: Ocular manifestations of collagen diseases. Arch. Ophth. *56*:557, 1956.

McKusick, V. A.: Heritable Disorders of Connective Tissue. 3rd ed. St. Louis, C. V. Mosby Co., 1966.

Nanjiani, M. R.: Ocular manifestations of polyarteritis nodosa. Brit. J. Ophth. *51*:696, 1967.

Percival, S. P. B.: Angioid streaks and elastorrhexis. Brit. J. Ophth. *52*:297, 1968.

Simmons, R. J., and Cogan, D. G.: Occult temporal arteritis. Arch. Ophth. 68:8, 1962.

Smith, M. E. and Zimmerman, L. E: Amyloidosis of the eyelid and conjunctiva. Arch. Ophth. 75:42, 1966.

Stafford, W. R., and Fine, B. S.: Amyloidosis of the cornea. Arch. Ophth. 75:53, 1966.

Vail, D. T.: Diffuse collagen diseases with ocular complications. Tr. Ophth. Soc. U. Kingdom 72:155, 1952.

Van der Hoeve, J.: Phakomatoses. Modern Trends in Ophthalmology. Vol 1. London, Butterworth, 1940, p. 124.

Blood Diseases

Alfano, J. E., and Roper, K. L.: Visual disturbances following acute blood loss. Am. J. Ophth. 38:817, 1954.

Allen. R. A., and Straatsma, B. R.: Ocular involvement in leukemia and allied diseases. Arch. Ophth. 66:490, 1961.

Chernoff, A. I.: The human hemoglobins in health and disease. New England J. Med. 253:322, 1955.

Francois, J., and Rabaey, M.: Corneal dystrophy and paraproteinemia. Am. J. Ophth. 52:895, 1962.

Geeraets, W. J., and Guerry, D., III.: Angioid streaks and sickle-cell disease. Am. J. Ophth. 49:450, 1960.

Goodman, G., von Sallmann, L., and Holland, M. G.: Ocular manifestations of sickle-cell disease. Arch. Ophth. 58:655, 1957.

Levine, R. A., and Kaplan, A. M.: The ophthalmoscopic findings in C + S disease. Am. J. Ophth. 59:37, 1965.

Mortada, A.: Bilateral exophthalmos and lymphoblastic aleukaemic leukaemia. Br. J. Ophth. 52:68, 1968.

Oglesby, R. B.: Corneal opacities in a patient with cryoglobulinemia and reticulohistiocytosis. Arch. Ophth. 65:63, 1961.

Wintrobe, M. M.: Clinical Hematology. 6th ed. Philadelphia, Lea & Febiger, 1967.

Cardiovascular Diseases

Ashton, N., and Harry, J.: The pathology of cotton wool spots and cytoid bodies in hypertensive retinopathy and other diseases. Tr. Ophth. Soc. U. Kingdom 83:91, 1963.

Duke-Elder, S., and Dorbee, J. N.: A System of Ophthalmology. Diseases of the Retina. Vol. X. St. Louis, The C. V. Mosby Co., 1967, p. 878.

Friedenwald, J. S.: Retinal and choroidal arteriosclerosis. In Ridley, F., and Sorsby, A. (eds.): Modern Trends in Ophthalmology. New York, Hoeber Medical Division, Harper & Row, 1940.

Harry, J., and Ashton, N.: The pathology of hypertensive retinopathy. Tr. Ophth. Soc. U. Kingdom 88:71, 1963.

Keith, N. M., Wagener, H. P., and Barker, N. W.: Some different types of essential hypertension: their course and prognosis. Am. J. M. Sc. 197:332, 1939.

Moses, C.: Atherosclerosis; Mechanisms as a Guide to Prevention. Philadelphia, Lea & Febiger, 1963.

Scheie, H. G.: Evaluation of ophthalmoscopic changes of hypertension and arteriolar sclerosis. Arch. Ophth. 49:117, 1953.

Seitz, R.: The Retinal Vessels. Translated by F. C. Blodi. St. Louis, The C. V. Mosby Co., 1964.

Wagener, H. P., and Keith, N. M.: Diffuse arteriolar disease with hypertension and the associated retinal lesions. Medicine 18:317, 1939.

Wise, G. N.: Arteriosclerosis secondary to retinal vein obstruction. Tr. Am. Ophth. Soc. 56:361, 1958.

Endocrine Diseases

Abrahamson, I. A., Sr., and Abrahamson, I. A., Jr.: Hypercarotenemia. Arch. Ophth. 68:4, 1962.

Adams, D. D.: The presence of an abnormal thyroid-stimulating hormone in the serum of some thyrotoxic patients. J. Clin. & Exper. Med. 18:699, 1958.

Ashton, N.: Diabetic microangiopathy. Advances Ophth. 8:1, 1958.

Cogan, D. G., Albright, F., and Bartter, F. C.: Hypercalcemia and band keratopathy. Arch. Ophth. 40:624, 1948.

Cogan, D. G., and Kuwabara, T.: Capillary shunts in the pathogenesis of diabetic retinopathy. Diabetes 12:293, 1963.

Day, R. M.: Ocular manifestations of thyroid disease. Arch. Ophth. 64:324, 1960.

Day, R. M., and Carroll, F. D.: Optic nerve involvement associated with thyroid dysfunction. Tr. Am. Ophth. Soc. 59:220, 1961.

Friedenwald, J. S.: A new approach to some problems of retinal vascular disease. Am. J. Ophth. 32:487, 1949.

Haddad, H.: Tonography and visual fields in endocrine exophthalmos. Am. J. Ophth. 64:63, 1967.

Hanno, H. A., and Weiss, D. I.: Hypoparathyroidism, pseudohypoparathyroidism and pseudo-pseudo-hypoparathyroidism. Arch. Ophth. 65:238, 1961.

Mulvaney, J. H.: The exophthalmos of hyperthyroidism. Am. J. Ophth. 27:589 (part I); 693 (part II); 820 (part III), 1944.

Rose, E.: The eye and the endocrines. Am. J. Ophth. 59:1, 1965.

Tassman, I.: Ocular changes in diabetes mellitus. Surv. Ophth. 12:299, 1956.

Werner, S. C.: The Thyroid: A Fundamental and Clinical Text. 2nd ed. New York, Hoeber Medical Division, Harper & Row, 1962.

Walsh, F. G., and Murray, R. G.: Ocular manifestations of disturbances in calcium metabolism. Am. J. Ophth. 36:1657, 1953.

Wyngaarden, J. B.: Gout. In Stanbury, J. B., Wyngaarden, J. B., and Fredrickson, D. S. (eds.): The Metabolic Basis of Inherited Disease. New York, McGraw-Hill Co., 1960.

Skin Diseases

Baehr, G., and Pollack, A. D.: Disseminated lupus erythematosus and diffuse scleroderma. J.A.M.A. 134:1169, 1947.

Bruce, G. H.: Retinitis in dermatomyositis. Tr. Am. Ophth. Soc. 36:282, 1938.

Horowitz, S.: Psoriasis vulgaria. Report on case showing skin, joint and eye lesions (keratitis psoriatica). Glasgow, M. J. 30:251, 1949.

Jay, B., Blach, R. K., and Wells, R. S.: Ocular manifestations of ichthyosis. Br. J. Ophth. 52:217, 1968.

Koch, F. L. P., and McGuire, W. P.: Acute disseminated lupus erythematosus. Am. J. Ophth. 29:1243, 1946.

Lever, W. F.: Histopathology of the Skin. 4th ed. Philadelphia, J. B. Lippincott Co., 1967.

McDonnald, C. E.: Neurodermatitis with cataract. Arch Ophth. *30*:767, 1963.

O'Brien, C. S., and Porter, W. C.: Glaucoma and nevus flammeus. Arch. Ophth. *9*:715, 1933.

Saebø, J.: Xeroderma pigmentosum with affection of the eye. Brit. J. Ophth. *32*:398, 1948.

Soll, S. N.: Eruptive fever with involvement of the respiratory tract, conjunctivitis, stomatitis and balanitis. Arch. Int. Med. *79*:475, 1947.

Sorsby, A., Roberts, J. A. F., and Brain, R. J.: Essential shrinkage of the conjunctiva in a hereditary affection allied to epidermolysis bullosa. Docum. Ophth. *5-6*:118, 1951.

Tumors

Boniuk, M. (ed.): Ocular and Adnexal Tumors: New and Controversial Aspects (Proceedings of an International Symposium). St. Louis, C. V. Mosby Co., 1964.

Dunphy, E. B., *et al.:* The diagnosis and management of intraocular melanomas; a symposium. Tr. Am. Acad. Ophth. *62*:517, 1958.

Ellsworth, R. M.: Treatment of retinoblastoma. Am. J. Ophth. *66*:49, 1968.

Ferry, A. P.: Lesions mistaken for malignant melanoma of the posterior uvea; a clinicopathologic analysis of 100 cases with ophthalmoscopically visible lesions. Arch. Ophth. *72*:463, 1964.

Hale, P. N., Allen, R. A., and Straatsma, B. R.: Benign melanomas of the choroid and ciliary body. Arch. Ophth. *74*:532, 1965.

Hogan, M. J., and Zimmerman, L. E.: Ophthalmic Pathology. 2nd ed. Philadelphia, W. B. Saunders Co., 1962.

Howard, G. M., and Ellsworth, R. M.: Differential diagnosis of retinoblastoma; a statistical survey of 500 children. Am. J. Ophth. *60*:610, 1965.

Reese, A. B.: Precancerous and cancerous melanosis. Am. J. Ophth. *61*:1272, 1966.

Reese, A. B.: Tumors of the Eye. 2nd ed. New York, Hoeber Medical Division, Harper & Row, 1963.

Reese, A. B., and Jones, I. S.: The differential diagnosis of malignant melanomas of the choroid. Arch. Ophth. *58*:477, 1957.

Reese, A. B., Jones, I. S., and Cooper, W. C.: Tumors of iris and ciliary body. Am. J. Ophth. *66*:173, 1968.

Willis, R. A.: Pathology of Tumours. 4th ed. London, Butterworth & Co., 1968.

Zimmerman, L. E.: Changing concepts concerning the malignancy of ocular tumors. Arch. Ophth. *78*:166, 1967.

Zimmerman, L. E. (ed.): Tumors of the Eye and Adnexa. International Ophthalmology Clinics. Vol. 2, No. 2. Boston, Little, Brown and Co., 1962.

Deficiency Diseases

Bicknell, F., and Prescott, F.: The Vitamins in Medicine. 3rd ed. London, Heinemann, 1953.

Bietti, G. B.: Ocular manifestations of vitamin deficiencies. *In* Sorsby, A. (ed.): Modern Trends in Ophthalmology. Vol. II. London, Paul B. Hoeber, Inc., 1947.

Blumenthal, C. J.: Nutritional keratitis. Proc. Nutritional Soc. *19*:92, 1960.

Goodman, L., and Gilman, A.: Pharmacologic Basis of Therapeutics. 3rd ed. New York, The Macmillan Co., 1965.

Heaton, J. M., McCormick, A. J. A., and Freeman, A. G.: Tobacco amblyopia: a clinical manifestation of vitamin B-12 deficiency. Lancet *2*:286, 1958.

Josephs, H. W., Baber, M., and Conn, H.: Studies in vitamin A: relation of blood level and adaptation to dim light and diet. Bulletin, Johns Hopkins Hospital *68*:357, 1941.

Kuming, B. S., and Politzer, W. M.: Xerophthalmia and protein malnutrition in Bantu children. Br. J. Ophth. *51*:649, 1967.

Livingston, P. C., Ridley, H., *et al.:* Discussion of ocular disturbances associated with malnutrition. Tr. Ophth. Soc. U. Kingdom *66*:19, 1946.

Nutrition reviews (1942 onward). Various articles on nutrition and the eye.

Rosenberg, H. R.: Chemistry and Physiology of the Vitamins. New York, Interscience Publishers, Inc., 1942.

Spillane, J. D.: Nutritional Disorders of the Nervous System. Edinburgh, Livingston, 1947.

Tassman, I. S.: Dietary deficiency and ocular disease (ophthalmologic review). Arch. Ophth. *8*:580, 1932.

Venkataswamy, G.: Ocular manifestations of vitamin A deficiency. Br. J. Ophth. *51*:854, 1967.

Venkataswamy, G.: Ocular manifestations of vitamin B-complex deficiency. Br. J. Ophth. *51*:749, 1967.

Walsh, F. B.: Clinical Neuro-ophthalmology. 2nd ed. Baltimore, Williams & Wilkins Co., 1957.

Yudkin, J.: Nutritional deficiency. *In* Sorsby, A. (ed.): Modern Ophthalmology. Vol. II, part 3, sec. 1. Washington, D. C., Butterworth, Inc., 1963.

Degenerative Diseases

Beren, C.: Aging process in eye and adnexa. Arch. Ophth. *29*:171, 1943.

Chi, H. H., Teng, C. C., and Katzin, H. M.: Histopathology of primary endothelial-epithelial dystrophy of the cornea. Am. J. Ophth. *45*:518, 1958.

Clark, W. B.: Hereditary and constitutional dystrophies of the cornea. Am. J. Ophth. *33*:692, 1950.

Cogan, D. G., and Kuwabara, T.: Arcus senilis: its pathology and histochemistry. Arch. Ophth. *61*:553, 1959.

Colloquia on Aging. CIBA Foundation. London, Churchill, 1955.

Fischer, F. B.: Senescence of the eye. *In* Sorsby, A., (ed.): Modern Trends in Ophthalmology. Vol. II. London, Butterworth, 1963.

Franceschetti, A., and Babel, J.: The heredofamilial degeneration of the cornea. Acta XVI. Concilium Ophthalmologicum (Britannia) 1951, pp. 245-285.

Goor, E. L.: Dystrophies of the cornea. Am. J. Ophth. *33*:674, 1950.

Jones, S. T., and Zimmerman, L. E.: Histopathologic differentiation of granular, macular and lattice dystrophies of the cornea. Am. J. Ophth. *51*:394, 1961.

Rones, B.: Senile changes and degenerations in the human eye. Am. J. Ophth. *21*:239, 1938.

Snell, A. C., and Irwin, R. S.: Hereditary deep dystrophy of the cornea. Am. J. Ophth. *45*:636, 1958.

Chapter Seven

NEURO-OPHTHALMOLOGY

Neuro-ophthalmology is the study of a wide array of conditions affecting the nerves and, by tradition, the muscles that serve the eye. Since either focal or disseminated conditions of nervous tissues may affect the visual system, much of neuro-ophthalmology is an integral part of neurology. Similarly, many conditions of neuro-ophthalmologic interest, such as unilateral exophthalmos, are part and parcel of general ophthalmology. Neuro-ophthalmology shares with general ophthalmology certain methods of examination, such as biomicroscopy and ophthalmoscopy, and also has several special techniques. Among these are study of the visual field, optico-kinetic nystagmus, and ophthalmodynamometry.

VISUAL FIELD EXAMINATION

A large proportion of patients referred for neuro-ophthalmologic examination require visual field examination. Frequently, abnormalities of the visual field are discovered in patients with unsuspected disease of the central nervous system. This examination is a formal way to measure visual function throughout the field of vision at some distances from the point of fixation. The visual field is divided into a central 30 degree sector and a remaining peripheral portion. One eye is examined at a time and the defects are plotted. Since the visual pathways have a constant, but complex, neuroanatomy and run at right angles to the major sensory and motor pathways of the brain, the pattern of involvement makes it possible to localize areas of disrupted function at various levels within the visual system. Such localization of the specific visual field defect often points to the underlying pathology.

The visual pathways originate in the ganglion cells and nerve fibers of the retina, which depart from the eye in the optic nerve. After passing out of the orbit by way of the optic foramen, the two optic nerves join to form the optic chiasm. In the chiasm there is a precise relationship between crossing and noncrossing fibers. From the chiasm the optic pathways take an arching course to the dorsal lateral geniculate body of the diencephalon and then split into two fillets, one going into the dorsal lateral geniculate body proper and the other continuing along the brachium of the superior colliculus to end in the superior colliculus. Originating from the dorsal lateral geniculate are secondary fibers that reach their terminus along the calcarine fissure of the occipital lobe by traveling in the visual radiation through portions of the temporal and parietal lobes.

The visual field can be measured with

instruments or by hand movements (confrontation). The most commonly used instruments are the arc perimeter (p. 425) and the tangent screen (Fig. 7-1). Patients with gross neurologic disease may not be able to provide the precise responses needed in tangent screen examinations. Many such patients, however, can cooperate sufficiently for a confrontation field, and the results can have considerable validity. To perform a confrontation examination, it is important for the patient to fixate an object straight ahead, usually some portion of the tester's anatomy. Serving as test objects are the hands or other objects moved in the periphery of the patient's visual field. Frequently it is of value to stimulate both half fields of vision at the same time, i.e., to stimulate the left and the right visual fields of the patient simultaneously to elicit minimal defects.

When a patient is able to cooperate in a more demanding examination, it is preferable to use a tangent screen. With a patch over one eye, the patient is asked to fixate a small, white object in the center of the tangent screen while seated 1 meter from it. Objects of varying size, usually 1 to 9 mm. in diameter and white surfaced, are brought into the patient's peripheral field of vision. As he identifies these objects serially, a given line of equal visual acuity, an isopter, can be defined. In most cases substantial information about the field of vision is gained from studying two or more isopters in each patient. To guarantee the adequacy of fixation, the blind spot (the projection of the optic nerve into the visual field) should be identified in every visual field examination. Central vision is tested by seeing whether or not the patient can properly appreciate small objects, usually 1 mm. in diameter, in the 5 to 10 degrees immediately about fixation.

VISUAL FIELD DEFECTS

Retinal and Choroidal Disease. Although visual field examination is used chiefly in neurologic disease affecting the optic nerve, the optic chiasm, and the retrochiasmal pathways, the examination is frequently of value in diseases of the retina. The visual field is a projection of retinal sensibility; the extent of a lesion that destroys that sensibility can be outlined. One such condition is retinitis pigmentosa, a hereditary degeneration of the retina in which the early complaint is night blindness. The characteristic visual field change is a scotoma 10 or more degrees away from fixation (Fig. 7-2), with the peripheral area beyond this ring or annular scotoma spared. A ring scotoma, which is an unusual field defect, is sufficiently characteristic of retinitis pigmentosa to help confirm or even suggest the diagnosis. Once the disease has been diagnosed, periodic visual field examinations help to document its slow progress.

Visual field defects also can accompany disease originating in the choroid that secondarily involves the retina, such as Jensen's disease or juxtapapillary choroiditis. In this condition a choroiditis occurs at or near the junction of the retina and the optic nerve. While the condition is

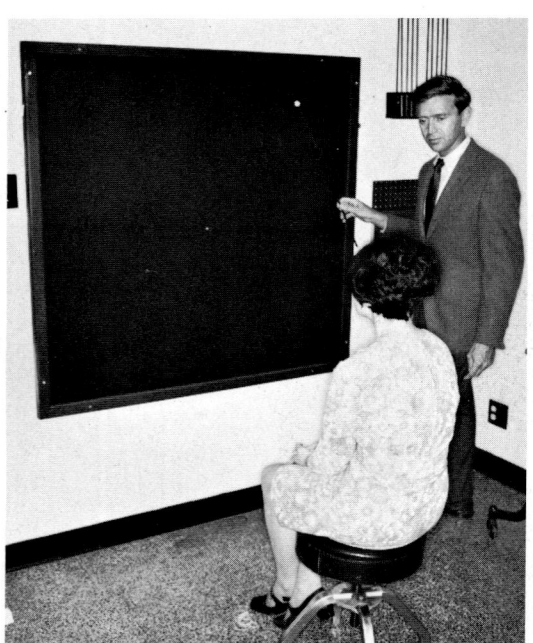

Figure 7-1 Tangent screen is used to test the central 30 degrees of the visual field. In general, examination by tangent screen is more precise than by arc perimeter. Tangent screen examination is of special value in the study of glaucoma defects and small defects in the central area.

Right Eye

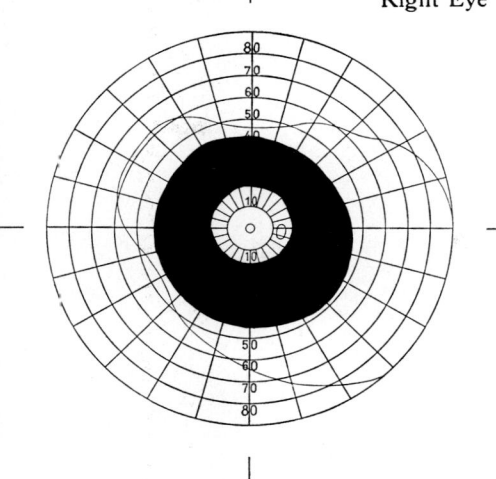

Figure 7-2 Ring scotoma characteristic of retinitis pigmentosa. Progress of this condition can be evaluated by periodic visual field examinations.

active the optic nerve fibers overlying the choroid cease to function, and a typical scotoma develops in the retina served by these nerve fibers. Since the pattern of nerve fiber distribution to the optic nerve from the retina is scimitar-shaped, an arcuate scotoma (Fig. 7-3) is commonly found.

Optic Nerve Disease. When the optic nerve is involved in a disease process, the most frequent visual field defect is central scotoma, the visual field equivalent of loss of central vision (Fig. 7-4). Within the optic nerve are both central and peripheral retinal nerve fibers, but those subserving the macular area (the central fibers) are most sensitive to a variety of deleterious conditions: trauma, malnutrition, pressure.

A central scotoma, although usually not specific, can at times suggest its cause by its form. For instance, in persons who use tobacco and alcohol heavily a particular type of scotoma described as centrocecal may occur between the blind spot and fixation. The patient notices first a relative loss of vision for red colors. Friends may appear falsely pale. Central vision may or may not be decreased substantially, but visual field examination reveals the greatest density of the scotoma in the area between the optic nerve and the fovea. The defect usually has a sloping border with areas of increased density toward its center.

Chiasmal Diseases. Study of the visual field is of considerable significance in tumors in the area of the optic chiasm. Be-

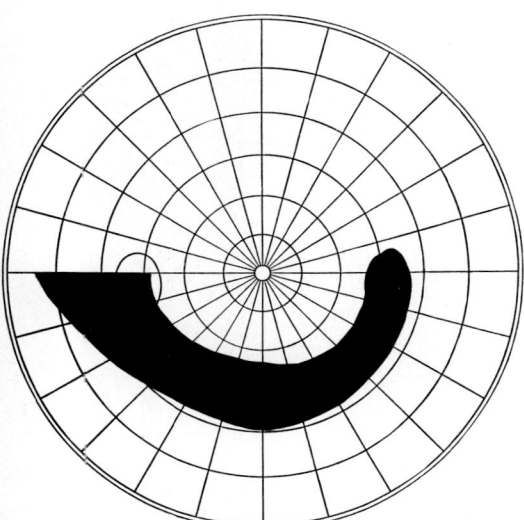

Figure 7-3 Record chart for tangent screen. An arcuate scotoma is found typically in juxtapapillary choroiditis and signifies a defect in transmission in the region of the optic disc.

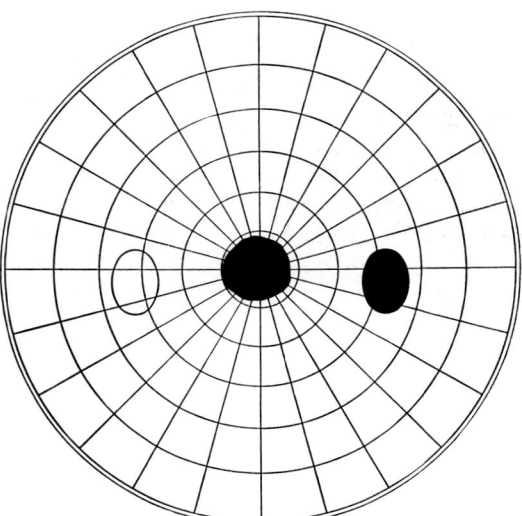

Figure 7-4 Record chart for tangent screen. Central visual acuity is severely compromised, and a large central scotoma is present. In some instances, a central scotoma may be minute and only be disclosed by careful examination.

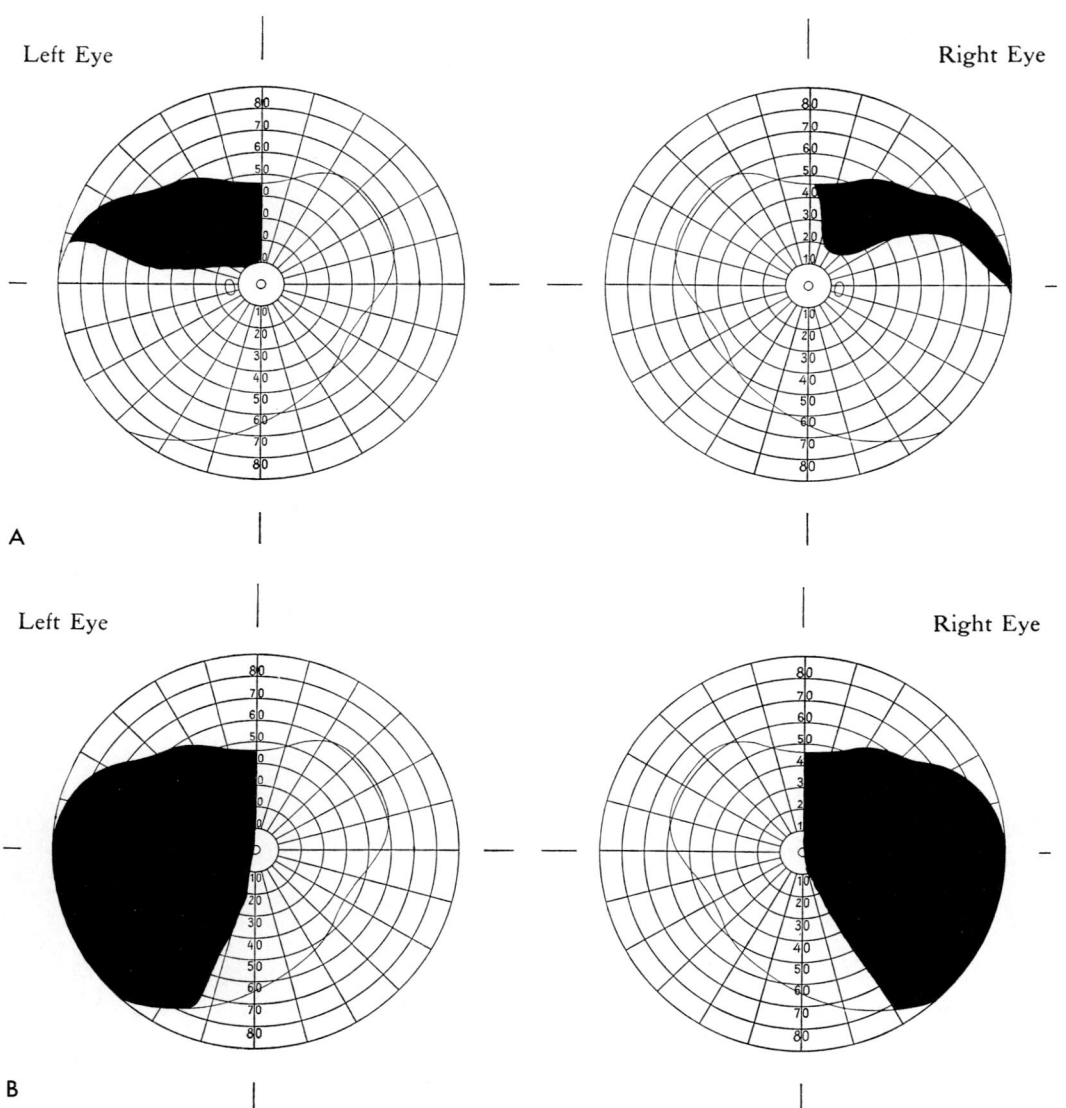

Figure 7-5 Representative sequence of visual field defects in untreated pituitary adenoma. *(A)* Upper bitemporal quadrantic field loss is seen when optic chiasm is first affected by tumor. *(B)* Further growth of tumor causes defect to increase and to include most or all of temporal visual field.

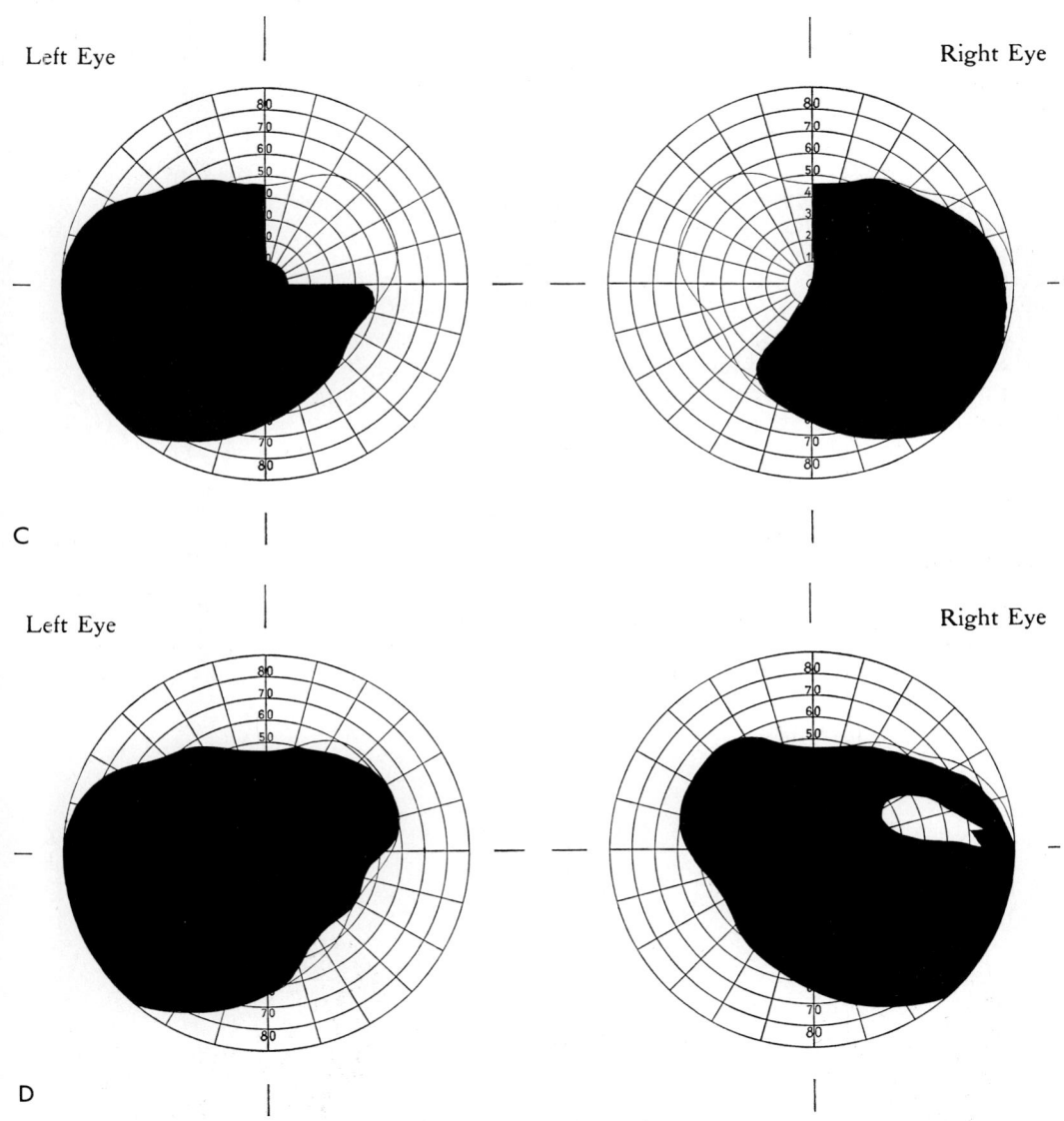

Figure 7-5 *Continued*

(C) After a period of relative stability, lower nasal fields are affected. *(D)* If still untreated, tumor obliterates useful vision and leaves a residual field.

cause of the neuroanatomy of the chiasmal decussation in which axons from nasal retina cross and fibers from temporal retina do not cross, it is possible to damage vision selectively in the temporal half of each visual field and to cause a bitemporal hemianopia.

Chromophobe adenoma of the pituitary gland, the most common lesion in adult life affecting the chiasm, follows in a characteristic sequence. As the tumor grows slowly upward and extends beyond the boundaries of the sella turcica, it presses upon the optic chiasm from beneath and thus first interrupts the lower nasal optic fibers that are represented in the visual field in the upper temporal region. At this stage a bitemporal quadrantanopia is present. With further growth, the tumor mass may compress all the crossing axons with loss of vision in the entire temporal field, leading to a complete bitemporal hemianopia. Even without any treatment, the visual field often is stable at this point for some time.

As the tumor grows, however, it next damages the superior temporal axons by compressing them against the overlying anterior cerebral arteries. Vision in the

inferior nasal field begins to fail, and if the growth of the tumor still is not checked, all sight finally is lost. Surgical extirpation of the tumor or x-irradiation to shrink the tumor mass can arrest and, in many cases, reverse this disastrous sequence by relieving the chiasmal compression. Once pressure is relieved, recovery often is substantial, its extent being related to the severity and duration of the chiasmal compression. It is several months before the full extent of recovery is known. Many cases depart from the usual pattern of symmetrical field loss, and it is possible for pituitary tumors to present with unilateral blindness or with a central scotoma. Figure 7-5A to D illustrates the common, progressive, bitemporal pattern of field loss with pituitary tumor.

Tumors other than pituitary adenomas can involve the chiasm. Craniopharyngioma in the young and meningioma or aneurysm of the circle of Willis in the adult can all give rise to bitemporal hemianopias. Craniopharyngiomas often are located above the chiasm; hence, early visual field loss can be found in the inferior temporal quadrants.

Retrochiasmal Lesions. Behind the optic chiasm, fibers from the left half of the visual field (the right half of each retina) pass and become intermingled on the right side of the brain. In keeping with the neuroanatomic principle that is demonstrated

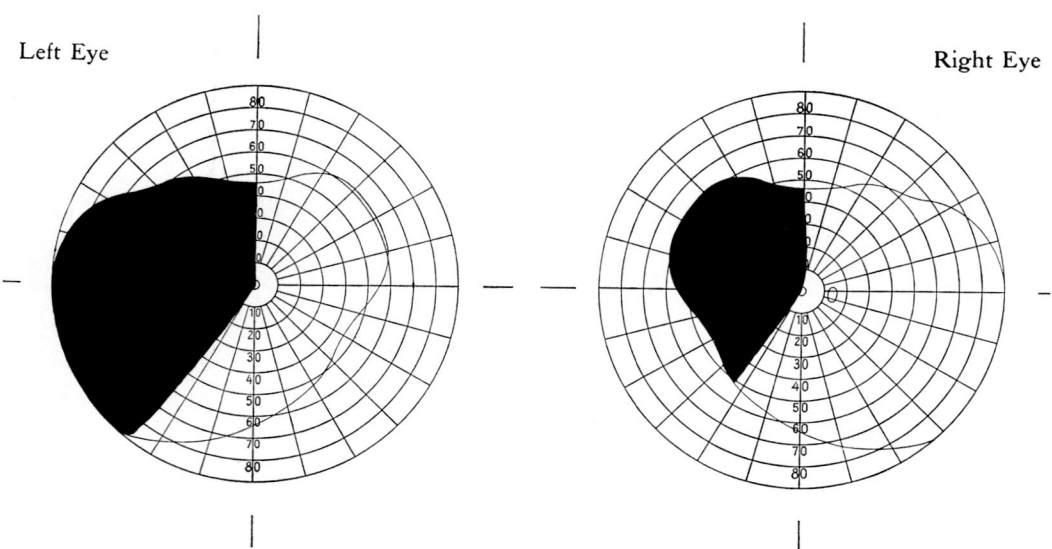

Left Eye   Right Eye

Figure 7-6 Finding a congruous, homonymous hemianopia suggests damage to retrochiasmal visual pathway in occipital lobe or in posterior parietal lobe.

by this left-right organization, lesions of the retrochiasmal pathway on one side lead to loss in the visual field on the other side, a condition called homonymous hemianopia. When the two visual fields suffer symmetrical loss of vision, the hemianopia is termed congruous (Fig. 7-6), and where there is marked asymmetry, incongruous (Fig. 7-7). In general, the more posteriorly the lesion is located in the visual pathway, the more congruous the field loss, for the two retinal fields become more perfectly overlapped as the visual fibers approach their terminus in the occipital lobe. Thus a lesion of the occipital lobe proper yields congruous visual field defects, whereas lesions in the temporal loop of the visual radiation or of the optic tract give incongruous visual field defects.

In addition, macular vision commonly is spared in homonymous hemianopias, even when the involvement is extensive. This sparing occurs so frequently that the phenomenon has received a distinctive name, macular sparing. Two explanations for its occurrence are the relatively large area in the visual pathways representing central vision, and a partial overlap of circulation between the middle and posterior cerebral arteries at the tips of the occipital lobes of the brain. Localizing homonymous hemianopia is aided greatly by the presence or absence of other signs. Specifically, the motor pathways from cerebrum to spinal cord frequently are involved by the same lesion that interferes with vision. Three common areas where such "half side" syndromes can occur are: where the optic tract crosses the cerebral peduncle; in the posterior part of the internal capsule; and in the parietal lobe. A lesion originating in the parietal lobe must be extensive to affect both the visual and motor systems, which are widely spread apart. Such extensive lesions often are accompanied by findings indicative of a parietal lobe syndrome, such as defects in simple calculation or in left-right orientation.

A bilateral homonymous hemianopia is rare, but possible. Most cases are secondary to multiple thromboses in the posterior circulation of the brain, usually of the posterior cerebral artery or its calcarine branches. On occasion the diagnosis is made in a patient with occlusion of the basilar artery, in which case a hemiplegia or a quadriplegia, slurred speech, vertigo, and diplopia also are frequently found. Thrombosis of the basilar artery can compromise circulation to the visual centers to such an extent that complete blindness results. Although he is blind, the pupillary reflexes of the patient are intact because the afferent limb of the pupillary pathway is entirely

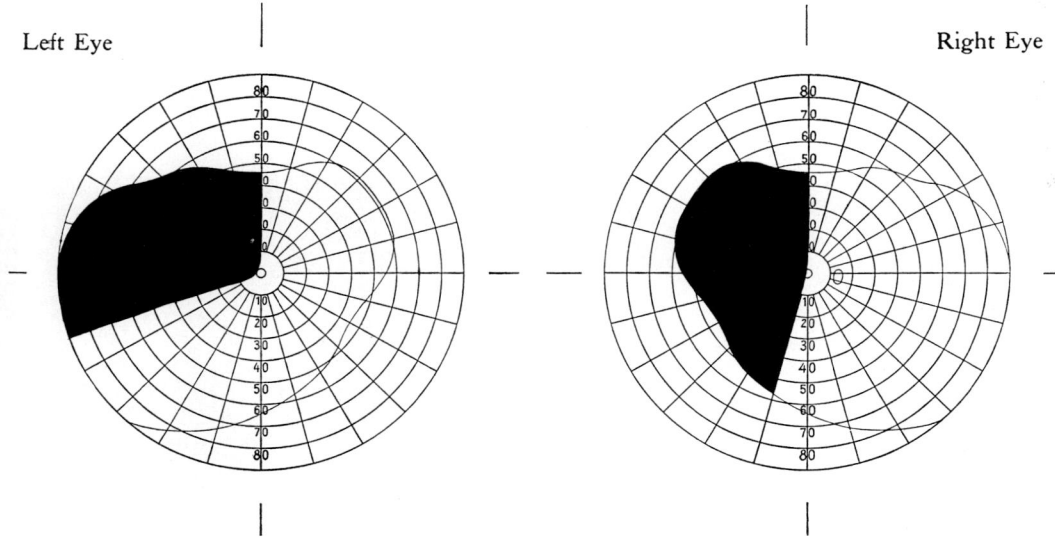

Left Eye   Right Eye

Figure 7-7 Incongruous hemianopic defects are more typical of interference with optic tract, or with visual radiations in the temporal lobe or anterior parietal lobe.

subcortical and does not go to the occipital cortex. When the pupillary reflexes in a blind patient are preserved, the lesion is localized to an area behind the dorsal lateral geniculate bodies, and the condition is called cortical blindness. This may occur in a reversible form after cranial trauma or an alcoholic debauch. In addition, angiographic studies of the vertebral circulation may be followed by temporary cortical visual loss.

Lesions in the visual sytem often give rise to visual hallucinations whose nature and location are of substantial diagnostic importance. Generally images arising from irritative lesions in the visual radiation of the temporal lobe are formed images. Those arising from irritative lesions in the occipital lobe are unformed images, such as jagged lines or flashing lights.

THE NORMAL OPTIC NERVE AND ITS VARIANTS

The intraocular portion of the optic nerve, called the optic disc or optic papilla, is the only portion of the central nervous system that can be visualized directly. When the optic nerve is diseased, changes in visual function may be rapid with loss of visual acuity, visual field, or both.

The ability to distinguish a normal optic disc from a pathologic disc depends on scrupulous examination and on experience. The range of "normal" is so wide that only many patients being observed repeatedly can lead to an appreciation of what constitutes a normal optic papilla. Plate 27*A* and *B* illustrates the most common attributes of a normal optic disc.

The main bundles of large axons from the ganglion cells of the retina reach the optic disc at its upper, lower, and nasal borders. Their great density contributes to a distinct difference in color when compared with the temporal border of the disc, which receives the fine fibers from the foveal area. This differential distribution of size and density of nerve bundles leads naturally to contrast in definition of mar-

gins between the two sides of the disc. On the nasal side the preponderance of large nerve fibers gives a pink color to the disc and often contributes to a somewhat blurred appearance of the margins. On the temporal border the more delicate central nerve fiber bundles result in a substantially less pink color and sharper, better defined margins. Since the color of the disc is related largely to the fine capillary network accompanying the nerve fibers rather than to the color of the nerve fibers themselves, the disc often is pale in anemia. Optic disc pallor also is seen in the newborn and in infants. Only with the passage of years does the optic disc attain its normal color.

In addition to the wide range of normal appearances, there are many congenital variants of the optic nerve. The importance of knowing these variants is related more to the confusion and misdiagnosis resulting from their inadequate recognition than to their effects on vision.

Variants of the Optic Nerve

Glial Veil. Figure 7-8 shows a characteristic form of glial veil. Just anterior to and on the surface of the optic disc is an irregular, gray membrane, usually not as large as that illustrated, which blocks a full view of the optic disc structure. When of lesser degree than pictured, it tends to be centered near the nasal aspect of the physiologic cup. Glial veil is due to a persistence of glial elements. These sheath the embryonic hyaloid artery and then normally resorb. The condition is benign, stable, and of no pathologic significance.

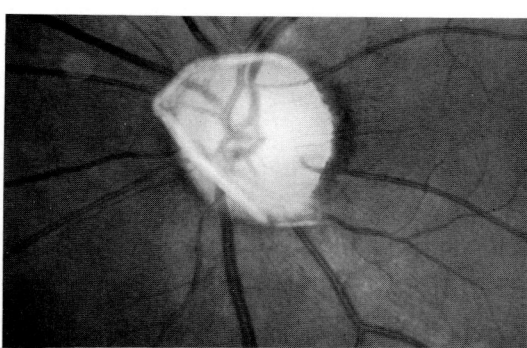

Figure 7-8 Glial veil. Gray membrane hides optic disc from view. This minor anomaly is of no pathologic significance.

Medullated Nerve Fibers. For optimum transmission of light to the more deeply placed photoreceptors, the nerve fiber fascicles of the retina need to be transparent. To make this possible, myelinization of the optic nerve fibers in the normal eye ceases abruptly at the cribriform plate through which the optic nerve enters the eye. Occasionally myelinization proceeds beyond the cribriform plate into the eye, presenting a vivid contrast to what is seen normally. A white patch of fibers may extend a variable, but usually short, distance beyond the optic disc onto the face of the retina, ending in a feathered edge as myelinated and unmyelinated fibers intermingle (Plate 27C). These opaque fibers obscure the blood vessels that run in the nerve fiber layer as they approach the optic disc. At times the myelinization can be so extensive as to interfere with vision. This results in an enlarged blind spot. The dramatic and unusual appearance of myelinated nerve fibers makes this an easy condition to recognize. Occasionally, isolated patches of medullation are seen in areas of retina away from the optic nerve and may present more of a diagnostic problem. Here also the feathered or tufted border usually gives away the condition.

Drusen or Hyaline Bodies of the Optic Disc. Drusen are highly refractile granular bodies found on the optic disc or deep within its substance (Fig. 7-9). When they are superficial, their glistening, irregular appearance is so characteristic that a trained observer can recognize them instantly. When they are beneath the surface of the disc, they are more subtle. The papilla may appear to be raised and to have blurred margins, leading to confusion with papilledema. (Since drusen tend to become more superficial with age, buried drusen usually occur in children.) An examiner can seek evidence of an irregular, elevated disc margin or hyaline-like bodies within the disc by transillumination with the ophthalmoscope beam. There are further aids in differentiating buried drusen from papilledema: the frequent simultaneous occurrences of anomalous presentation of blood vessels on the disc; the lack of hyperemia of the disc tissue; and the normal appearance of the retina immediately adjacent to the optic disc. Observing parents or siblings frequently is of value because many times the condition

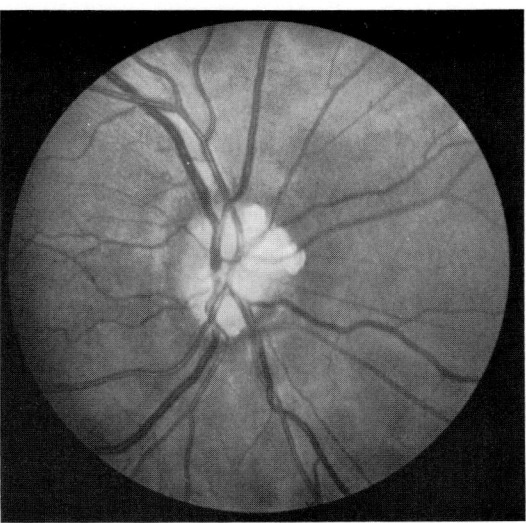

Figure 7-9 Drusen or hyaline bodies of optic disc. Characteristic presentation of glistening hyaline bodies of optic disc. They must be searched for by careful ophthalmoscopy in any instance of suspected papilledema. In children, hyaline bodies may be buried in nerve head substance and show up only on transillumination of the optic disc.

is familial. Other than causing confusion with papilledema, the condition is seldom of any importance. At times the hyaline bodies lead to nerve fiber damage with consequent visual field defects, usually arcuate in nature. Association with neurologic disease, although reported, is uncommon.

Hypoplasia of the Optic Disc. Although this unilateral defect in the formation of the optic nerve is uncommon, it is of some importance because vision is often very poor. The eyes may be straight or there may be a strabismus. If they are straight, reduced vision in one eye often is discovered on routine school examination. A large visual field defect may accompany this condition. Diagnosis awaits recognition by the examining physician of the characteristic small appearance of the optic disc (Plate 27D). Early diagnosis often spares the child unnecessary examination and unwarranted treatment.

Pseudoneuritis. Frequently in small, hyperopic eyes the relatively small diameter of the scleral foramen causes the optic nerve fibers to heap up as they traverse it.

Plate 27 (A) Normal optic disc. Disc has a clearly visible physiologic cup surrounded by a broad rim of pink neural tissue. Note lesser density of pink coloration on temporal border of disc. (See arrow.) Central retinal artery and vein can be seen to branch and leave disc. There is considerable normal variation in this branching pattern.

(B) Normal optic disc. Temporal border is paler and more sharply defined than nasal border. Demarcation between disc and surrounding retina is harder to see than in 27A, owing to a less pigmented retina and the lack of pigment ring. Note normal pink color of disc tissue and the branching pattern of central retinal artery and vein.

(C) Myelinated nerve fibers. Myelinization of nerve fibers on and about the optic disc. Normal disc structure is obscured. Branches of central retinal artery are hidden from view by opaque nerve fibers. Note tufted or fibrillar manner in which myelinated fibers merge into normal transparent fibers of retina.

(D) Hypoplasia of optic disc. Nerve head appears small and lacks its normal oval or round shape, owing to a marked reduction in diameter.

(E) Early papilledema. Optic disc is elevated and its margins are blurred. Small vessels of disc are engorged, and a flame-shaped hemorrhage is present at the lower pole. No spontaneous venous pulsations were visible.

(F) Fully developed papilledema with a pronounced hemorrhagic component. Veins are engorged, the physiologic cup is largely filled in, and edema extends into peripapillary retina.

(G) Fully developed papilledema in malignant hypertension. In addition to marked elevation and engorgement of optic disc, the macula lutea and peripheral retina contain multiple hemorrhages and exudates. Marked involvement of peripheral arteriolar tree usually serves to differentiate papilledema in severe hypertension from that associated with increased intracranial pressure.

(H) Papilledema secondary to leukemic infiltration of optic nerve meninges. Patient had no signs of increased intracranial pressure; optic disc of contralateral eye was normal. Note small, round hemorrhages of different sizes some distance from optic disc.

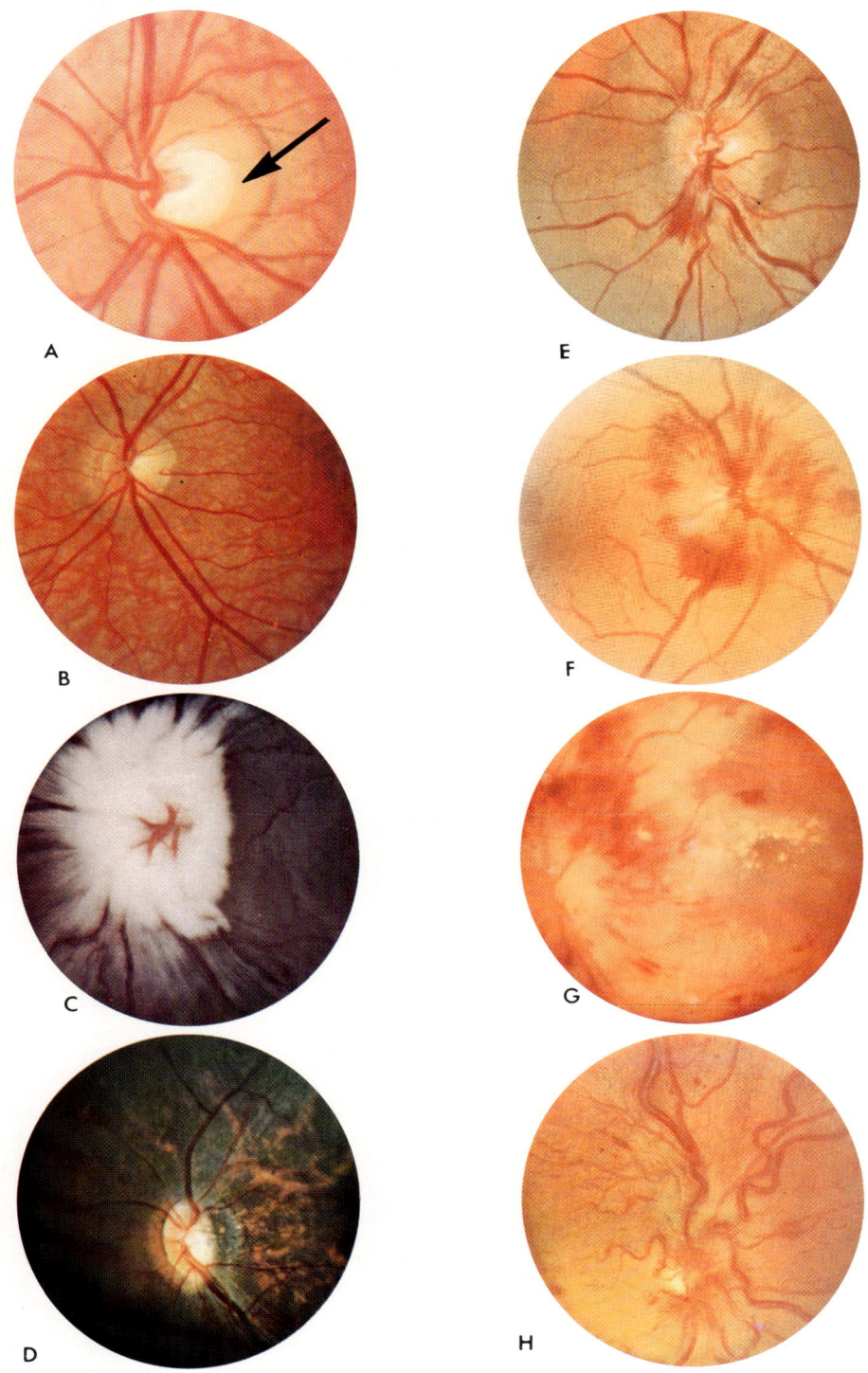

An elevated disc is seen on ophthalmoscopy with its margins completely blurred. Superficially the disc resembles papilledema and may be confused with it. The absence of edema in the peripapillary retina, the absence of hemorrhages or exudates, the presence of normal venous pulsations, and the lack of engorgement of the disc distinguish this anomaly from true papilledema.

PAPILLEDEMA

Papilledema, which is also called choked disc, signifies edema of the optic nerve head, usually as the result of raised intracranial pressure. Despite visible swelling, there is no inflammation. Visual impulses pass from retina to optic nerve unimpeded. Good visual function is thus preserved and serves to distinguish a choked disc from an optic disc affected by inflammation or toxins (p. 304).

Since papilledema usually calls forth a series of painful and even dangerous procedures, diagnosis should be made only after stringent criteria have been met. Specifically, the examiner should be familiar with the various anomalies and with the wide range of normal appearances of the optic disc. In almost all circumstances there is time for an experienced observer to evaluate the optic discs carefully before judging whether or not papilledema is present. In some instances he may be wise to defer judgment because at times even trained observers are unable to say with certainty, especially in the early stages of increased intracranial pressure, whether or not minor changes in a disc represent incipient papilledema. Repeated examinations generally lead to a sound diagnosis in a matter of days or weeks.

The nature of the development of papilledema makes early diagnosis difficult. A choked disc develops from a normal disc by barely perceptible stages. With increased intracranial pressure there is at first a turgescence of the veins and a slight blurring and protrusion of the disc margin, most marked at the upper and lower poles and on the nasal side. Engorgement of

TABLE 7-1   SIGNS OF PAPILLEDEMA

1. Blurred margins of disc.
2. Elevation of disc—number of diopters.
3. Enlargement of the veins—dilated and tortuous.
4. Loss of spontaneous venous pulsation.
5. Deflection of vessels over edge of disc.
6. Hemorrhages—flame-shaped on or near disc.
7. Reddish discoloration.
8. Few exudates.
9. Folds in retina, edema in retina.
10. Bilateral.
11. Transitory obscuration of vision—advanced cases.

the capillary network of the optic disc leads to an enhanced red coloration. Normal, spontaneous, venous pulsations cease. None of these changes alone warrants the diagnosis of choked optic disc, but if on repeated examinations they are found in increasing degree and in combination, the existence of papilledema is likely (Table 7-1). Progression is the key to diagnosis in incipient papilledema. When hemorrhages, usually linear or flame-shaped, appear on or about the optic disc in company with the above findings, papilledema can be considered to exist with some certainty (Plate 27E). Once established, papilledema often progresses, and the entire optic disc becomes measurably elevated.* As the optic disc juts farther forward with still greater swelling, the physiologic cup is entirely filled in (Plate 27F), large vessels on the disc may be buried in the edematous mass, and the peripapillary retina is infiltrated with edema and thrown into folds that run parallel with the disc border. Edema can extend into the retina as far as the region of the macula lutea, leading to the formation of a star figure.

The rate at which papilledema develops is proportional to the height of intracranial pressure. When extreme intracranial pressures come on in a relatively short time, such as in acute meningococcal meningitis, papil-

---

*Optic disc elevation may be roughly gauged by setting the ophthalmoscope on a high plus setting, then turning toward the minus until a vessel becomes visible on the face of the optic disc. The reading is noted, a vessel of similar orientation is sought in the peripapillary retina, and the reading is again noted. The difference between the two readings indicates the approximate elevation of the optic nerve head. It is essential that the two vessels sighted be directed in the same meridian; otherwise the refraction of the patient can obscure the findings.

ledema may occur in a matter of four or five hours. Generally, with the increased intracranial pressure in brain tumors, papilledema develops over a period of weeks.

Despite substantial study, the pathogenesis of papilledema is still unclear. Prominent among the explanations are blocked drainage of fluids from the eye, forced entrance of fluids from the subarachnoid space, venous engorgement with failure of venous return, and local edema as part of a cerebral edema. At times it appears that one or another of these pathogenetic mechanisms may be paramount. Often several are operative simultaneously.

The pathology of papilledema is the pathology of edema itself with the individual nerve fibers of the nerve head swollen and spread apart from one another. Small blood vessels, as noted clinically, are engorged, and at times there are areas of focal necrosis within the disc. In prolonged, high-grade papilledema, glial cells proliferate and a marked gliotic reaction gains increasing importance. Severe, secondary, optic atrophy and loss of vision may result.

Most commonly papilledema is accompanied by increased intracranial pressure from an intracranial tumor in which the pressure of the cerebrospinal fluid exceeds 200 mm. of water. Subdural hematoma and cerebral abscess lead to the same result. Location of the tumor mass also is important. Owing to the internal hydrocephalus they cause, tumors in the posterior fossa and cerebellar tumors give papilledema more frequently than tumors more anteriorly placed. Extradural lesions, such as pituitary tumors or chordoma, rarely lead to papilledema.

In infants whose sutures are open, papilledema usually does not occur with increased intracranial pressure. The sutures in most instances bulge and the skull enlarges allowing sufficient decompression to prevent the development of papilledema. Whether or not papilledema occurs in infants depends on the absolute pressure, the type of blockage of flow, the expansibility of the sutures, and the rate at which the increased intracranial pressure occurs. In children papilledema occurs readily when the sutures are closed and intracranial pressure rises. Papilledema also occurs in children whose sutures close early, as in craniostenosis, and in whom intracranial pressure rises because of the normal growth of the brain.

Papilledema is common in acute meningitis, and the increased intracranial pressure makes meningitis much more dangerous than it would otherwise be. When possible, a spinal tap should be done in acute meningitis by a neurologist or neurosurgeon, and adequate emergency care should be immediately available. In all cases of suspected meningitis, it is mandatory to visualize the optic disc before proceeding to special studies.

In the differential diagnosis of papilledema, systemic and ocular causes must be considered. Swelling of the optic disc often accompanies hypertension in its more malignant phases (Plate 27G). Even without a history of high blood pressure or evidence of hypertension from general physical examination, the extreme changes in the arterial tree on funduscopic examination and the amount of retinal edema and hemorrhage found in the periphery give solid clues to the pathogenesis. Papilledema also may be seen in severe toxemia of pregnancy and with the hypertension of Kimmelstiel-Wilson or other renal diseases. It is noteworthy that exudative phenomena in the retina are often severe with renal disease.

A variety of other conditions can lead to edema of the nerve head (Table 7-2). Venous stasis can lead to a swollen optic disc, preceding or accompanying central retinal vein thrombosis. In children, vitamin A intoxication and lead poisoning must be considered in the differential diagnosis. Cystic fibrosis with associated pulmonary disease and even pulmonary disease itself can cause the optic disc to swell. In these instances there is a direct relationship between the level of carbon dioxide in the blood and the papilledema. The height of papilledema may often be titrated inversely to the level of carbon dioxide pressure. Occasionally, a long-term treatment with steroids in nephrotic and asthmatic children also can lead to edema of the optic disc.

In addition, papilledema may be found in anemia, either that of sudden onset as

TABLE 7-2 CAUSES OF PAPILLEDEMA

I. Increased intracranial pressure
  A. Brain tumors (particularly those below the tentorium)
    Tumors of the fourth ventricle and cerebellum in children; meningioma of the middle and anterior cranial fossa; pinealoma; craniopharyngiomas; metastatic tumors
  B. Pseudotumor cerebri
  C. Brain abscesses, especially temporal lobe
  D. Subarachnoid hemorrhage, usually secondary to a rupture of an intracranial aneurysm
  E. Subdural hematoma
  F. Hydrocephalus
  G. Craniostenosis
  H. Meningitis
  I. Arachnoidal adhesions with internal hydrocephalus
II. Orbital conditions
  A. Tumors of the optic nerve
  B. Congestive thyroid exophthalmos
III. Ocular conditions
  A. Acute glaucoma
  B. Hypotony
    1. Penetrating wounds
    2. Intraocular surgery
    3. Uveitis
IV. Systemic disorders
  A. Malignant hypertension
  B. Blood dyscrasias
  C. Anemia
  D. Massive blood loss
  E. Pulmonary emphysema
  F. Pulmonary insufficiency associated with cystic fibrosis of the pancreas
  G. Infectious polyneuritis (Guillain-Barré syndrome)
  H. Poliomyelitis
  I. Hypoparathyroidism in children
V. Toxic factors
  A. Methyl alcohol
  B. Carbon dioxide poisoning
  C. Lead poisoning

after massive gastrointestinal bleeding, or in the chronic anemias. In the latter the hemoglobin level usually is well below 10 gm. and swelling of the optic disc is moderate.

Any orbital condition that compresses the optic nerve and the globe can cause the optic disc to swell. Thus papilledema often is found in conditions as diverse as malignant exophthalmos and leukemic infiltration of the meninges of the optic nerve (Plate 27*H*).

An atrophic nerve head either lacks disc tissue or has gliosis, both of which limit the expression of disc edema; papilledema rarely occurs in the presence of optic atrophy. Choked disc often is less apparent in the flat disc of myopia than in the small, heaped-up disc of hyperopia.

Prognosis of Papilledema. The prognosis of papilledema is intimately associated with the condition causing it. As the pathologic condition is corrected, or at least its effects on intracranial pressure lessened, papilledema regresses. When intracranial pressure is brought to normal, papilledema subsides by degrees in the ensuing weeks. All signs that the optic disc was ever swollen may have disappeared within two months. If the edema was longstanding and of high degree, the nerve head may appear somewhat pale. However, a return to a normal or a near normal disc appearance is only possible if the intracranial pressure can be brought down to tolerable levels. In the higher grades of chronic papilledema (Plate 28*A*), transient obscurations of vision, momentary episodes of blurred or decreased vision lasting seconds (in contrast to the episodic visual loss lasting minutes found in carotid artery disease), often are reported. More worrisome are the changes in the periphery of the visual field which often are the first signs of impending visual loss. These early changes are of sufficient importance to warrant repeated, careful examination of the peripheral visual field. Loss of peripheral visual field in chronic papilledema generally is considered an indication for neurosurgical intervention to relieve the increased intracranial pressure. The source of the visual loss in chronic papilledema is the marked glial reaction that develops in the optic disc. Once begun, this glial proliferation can lead to blindness, and every effort usually is made to relieve papilledema before such an unfortunate circumstance occurs.

OPTIC NEURITIS

Optic neuritis is a general term describing loss of vision, usually acute, with disease of the optic nerve. Although the term implies inflammation, its use is sufficiently broad to include visual loss from metabolic, toxic, and demyelinating conditions. The course of optic nerve lesions in these categories is different enough to warrant separate descriptions of several of the common presentations.

Optic neuritis usually occurs in unilateral episodes having a characteristic clinical course. The patient experiences acute onset of blurred vision in one eye that often is accompanied by marked pain or discomfort on movement or palpation of the globe. Decreased visual acuity and a central scotoma (often best shown by using colored test objects) are found on examination.

The optic disc appears normal or closely resembles the disc seen in the lower grades of papilledema with blurred margins, hemorrhages, exudates, and moderate elevation (Plate 28B). The similarities and differences between papilledema and optic neuritis affecting the optic disc (papillitis) are listed in Table 7-3.

The classification of optic neuritis depends on the site of involvement. When the pathologic process extends beyond the optic disc to involve the retina, it is called neuroretinitis. When the optic disc appears normal the condition is called retrobulbar neuritis, and when the optic disc is swollen and hyperemic the term papillitis is used.

For a first attack of optic neuritis either at or behind the papilla, the prognosis is favorable, but it is somewhat better for the retrobulbar variety. The course of the disease often is typical. After a precipitous decline, vision remains stable for a short time and then begins to improve, usually within three weeks of onset. With disappearance of the central scotoma and recovery of normal visual acuity, improvement may be complete. Some residual visual field defect often remains and the optic disc gradually becomes somewhat paler on the affected side. The pallor may be focal or general.

TABLE 7-3 DIFFERENTIATION OF PAPILLEDEMA FROM PAPILLITIS

Indication	Papilledema	Papillitis
Visual acuity	Normal	Decreased
Visual field	Enlarged blind spot	Central scotoma
Venous pulsations	Absent	Present
Pain on eye motion	Absent	Present
Disc elevation	May be >2D	<2D

Demyelinating Diseases. Multiple sclerosis is present or will develop in about 25 per cent of patients with optic neuritis. A large percentage of the other 75 per cent do not have and will not develop other manifestations of multiple sclerosis. Many have what for practical purposes is an idiopathic, self-limited malady. Whether it is a local variant of multiple sclerosis or an independent condition is not known.

In patients who have had multiple sclerosis with optic neuritis, the optic nerve shows profound changes when examined pathologically. Dominating the picture are focal areas of axonal demyelinization and gliotic plaques, and in early lesions phagocytic cells distended with ingested myelin frequently are seen. In acute attacks of optic neuritis the efficacy of treatment is unproved, and studies of the effectiveness are extremely difficult because of the nature of the underlying condition with its extreme exacerbations and remissions. Normally, systemic steroids are given, and the bulk of medical opinion holds that their use is worthwhile.

Care must be taken to ensure that demyelinating disease in optic neuritis is not diagnosed erroneously. Despite the clearcut clinical picture outlined above, many cases are atypical. In patients over 40 years of age, vascular disease must be considered carefully. In patients over 55 years of age, special attention should be given to the possibility of the presence of temporal arteritis. At times neoplasms may simulate optic neuritis even to the extent of vision improving temporarily with steroid treatment. The characteristic upsweep of visual acuity in acute optic neuritis is what differentiates it from neoplasm. Without this characteristic improvement a tumor must be considered likely, for it usually causes progressive and relentless visual loss.

Neuromyelitis optica, or Devic's disease, is a bilateral optic neuritis which can be devastating to the optic nerve, and which is accompanied by transverse myelitis. The combination often is considered a variant of multiple sclerosis, but it is sufficiently distinct to warrant clinical recognition. As in the demyelinating diseases already de-

Plate 28   *(A)* Chronic atrophic papilledema. Glial proliferation in this chronically edematous disc gives it a fluffy appearance and threatens vision. Such patients often complain of momentary obscurations of vision. Note horizontal retinal folds between disc and fovea centralis.

(B) Papillitis. Optic disc margins are blurred, and both hemorrhages and exudates are present. Vision was severely compromised, and a central scotoma was found on examination of the visual field.

(C) Juxtapapillary chorioretinitis. Details of optic disc are obscured by inflammatory reaction in vitreous. After treatment with steroids, inflammation resolved and a chorioretinitic lesion at inferior pole of optic disc became visible. Note deep hemorrhage in lower half of picture.

(D) Primary optic atrophy. Optic disc margins are clearly defined and lamina cribrosa is visible. Disc substance has largely disappeared.

(E) Secondary optic atrophy. Marked glial reaction followed acute papillitis. Optic disc margins are obscured by gliosis, and physiologic cup is filled in. Contrast with 28*D*.

(F) Optic atrophy after occlusion of central retinal artery. Total pallor of optic disc followed acute closure of central retinal artery. Branches of central retinal artery are irregularly sheathed. A small patch of new vessels (neovascularization) has formed at lower temporal border of disc (arrow).

(G) Temporal pallor. After attack of retrobulbar neuritis, temporal portion of optic disc becomes increasingly pale. Because temporal portion of optic disc normally is pale, evidence of visual field loss or visual acuity loss is required before temporal pallor can be diagnosed.

(H) Horner's syndrome with heterochromia of iris. Ptosis and miosis on right make diagnosis of Horner's syndrome straightforward. A lighter colored iris on same side is strong evidence that condition was present at birth or shortly after.

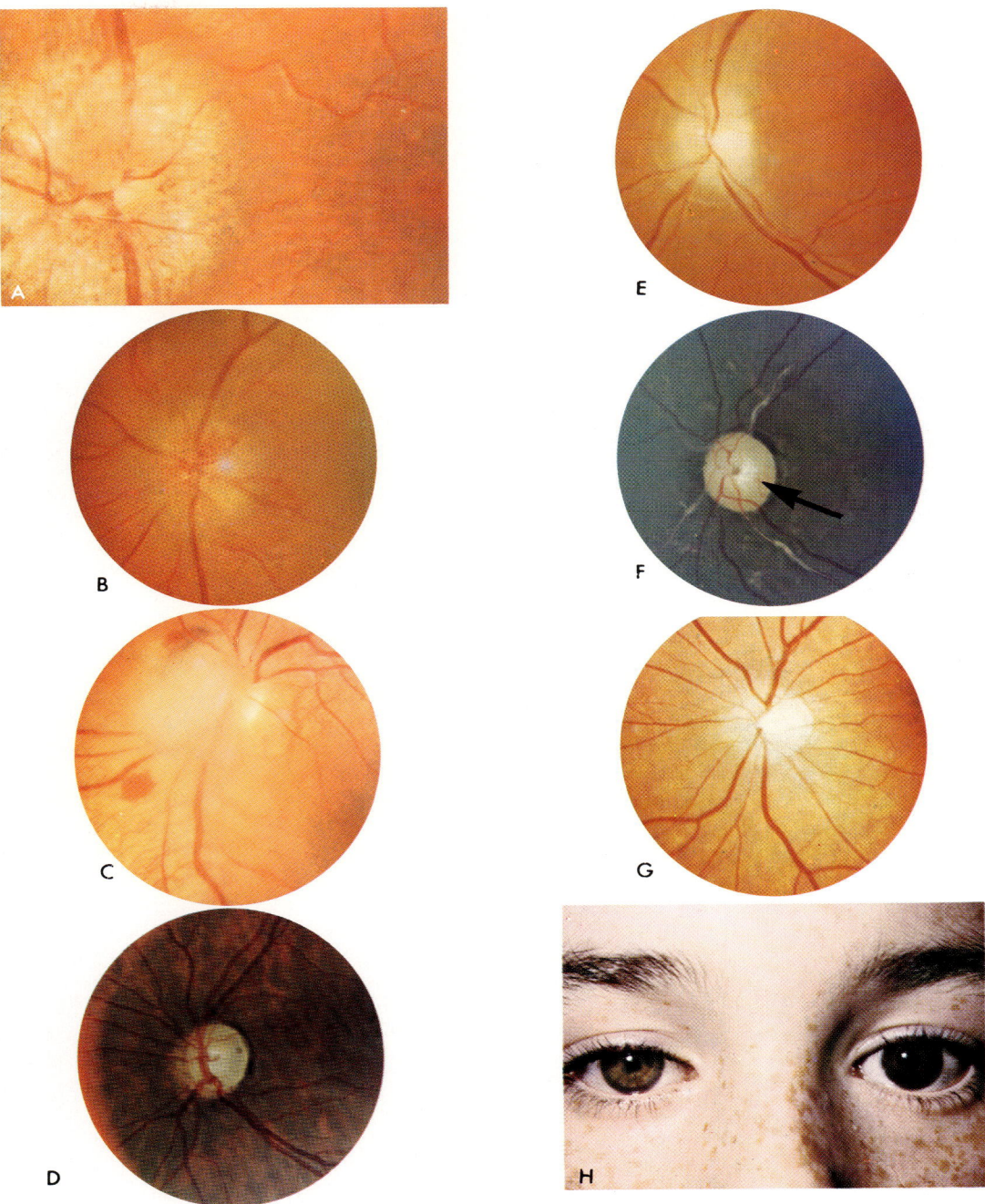

scribed, the condition rapidly approaches a nadir from which improvement then begins. During the acute phase of the illness the spinal cord is so extensively involved that the patient often dies.

In addition to multiple sclerosis and Devic's disease, in both of which normal myelin is destroyed, there are states in which myelin formation is defective as a result of an inborn error of metabolism. Termed leukodystrophies, these conditions do not affect the visual system distinctively. Rather, the visual pathways take part in a general breakdown of central nervous system tissue.

Inflammations. A form of optic neuritis also occurs in some inflammatory conditions. It has been described following most of the viral illnesses of childhood (mumps, measles, influenza), in herpes zoster infection of the gasserian ganglion, and in Behçet's disease (p. 18). Optic neuritis also can be part of any general involvement of the central nervous system (encephalitis) or of its coverings (meningitis). The optic nerve is involved frequently in neurosyphilis, especially in its cerebral meningeal and parenchymatous forms, and rarely is affected by tuberculosis.

Optic neuritis uncommonly results from a contiguous spread of inflammation. Formerly sinus disease and infected teeth were thought to cause optic neuritis, but in patients who have severe and well recognized sinus infections the optic nerve rarely is affected.

Inflammation within the eye also can cause optic neuritis. A clear example is found in juxtapapillary choroiditis, or Jensen's disease as it often is called. In this condition an inflammatory site in the choroid adjacent to the optic disc leads to swelling and hyperemia of the contiguous portion of the disc, a focal optic neuritis (Plate 28C). The function of the retinal nerve fibers overlying the lesion and of the affected portion of the optic disc is disturbed, resulting in visual loss. This focal involvement of the nerve fiber layer and the optic disc usually has an arcuate scotoma as its counterpart in the visual field (Fig. 7-3). As the primary condition is brought under control, the scotoma frequently disappears.

In severe thyrotropic exophthalmos, vision may be endangered, owing to exposure of the cornea or to involvement of the optic nerve. Characteristically. the visual field shows central scotomas and the fundi are normal. Vision usually improves as the basic condition is brought under control, but exceptions occur. Papilledema is not common during the course of this disease. When it occurs, however, a less favorable prognosis is indicated. Systemic steroid therapy usually is helpful.

Metabolic Disorders. Optic neuritis is uncommon in metabolic conditions, but it has been reported on rare occasions in diabetes mellitus. It has been found also in some cases of pernicious anemia where it is bilateral and occurs preponderantly in males. Loss of vision is substantial and the field loss usually is centrocecal. With proper replacement therapy, vision improves, often to levels of near normal. There appears to be a synergism between pernicious anemia and tobacco that is deleterious to the optic nerve, for the optic neuritis of pernicious anemia occurs predominantly, if not solely, in smokers. This has led to speculation that the optic neuritis occasionally seen in smokers who do not have pernicious anemia could be related to an effect of components of tobacco smoke, such as cyanide or nicotine, on vitamin B_{12} metabolism.

The evidence is clear that extreme dietary deficiencies may affect the optic nerve. During World War II and the Korean War, bilateral visual loss was reported in American prisoners of war who were subjected for long periods to an inadequate diet. Generally prisoners who ate 1000 calories a day or less, with little thiamine content in that pitiful dole, experienced visual difficulty. Visual loss was central and there was little or no recovery when adequate nutrition was again available. Similarly, general deterioration of vision has been reported in West Indian children whose diets were inadequate. In these instances vision usually improved when dietary supplements were available.

Hereditary Optic Neuritis (Leber's Disease)

This is a devastating and little understood form of optic neuritis that occurs predominantly in postpubertal males. Vision declines precipitously within a relatively brief time. Often the loss is asymmetric in onset, first in one eye, then in the other. In nearly all cases central vision is involved selectively, resulting in large central scotomas. On ophthalmoscopic examination the condition can present as a papillitis with the disc edematous and elevated a diopter or two, or as retrobulbar neuritis with a normal appearance to the optic disc. Leber's disease differs from the optic neuritis seen with multiple sclerosis in that it is bilateral, familial, nonrecurrent, and does not undergo remissions. Once present, the central scotomas do not disappear, and vision is permanently impaired. Despite the availability of several family trees, study of genetic patterns has failed to define the mode of transmission. Several authors have recommended therapy with ACTH; it appears to be of some, but limited, value.

Toxic Amblyopias

Although toxic amblyopias generally are considered a type of optic neuritis, the exact site in the visual pathway most sensitive to drugs is not known. Digitalis is typical of compounds that cause reversible toxic amblyopia. First described by Withering in 1785, the ocular manifestations of digitalis toxicity are blurred vision and altered color perception. Objects may appear to be covered with snow or to be colored green, blue, or yellow, with yellow vision (xanthopsia) the most common. Visual acuity can decline substantially, with a central scotoma present on the visual field examination. Cessation or decrease of digitalis therapy generally results in amelioration of the visual defect. Xanthopsia also has been reported on rare occasions in patients taking chlorothiazide (Diuril). Since many cardiac patients are treated with both digitalis and chlorothiazide, it is well to remember that either may be the source of the patient's xanthopsia.

Trimethadione (Tridione), a drug often used in treating petit mal seizures, may lead to brightness-related visual loss (hemeralopia). In dim light the patients have normal vision, but in bright light a precipitous drop in acuity occurs and the patients often are dazzled.

The antibiotics streptomycin and chloramphenicol have been reported to cause optic neuritis as have several sulfonamide compounds. While these instances appear to be uncommon, it is important to stop therapy with any of these substances at the first sign of visual loss.

Optic neuritis also has been associated with the use of DL-penicillamine in Wilson's disease. In this instance the penicillamine apparently disturbs the normal metabolism of pyridoxine. Supplemental pyridoxine reverses the situation and restores vision. Heavy metals, such as arsenic and thallium, may be toxic to the optic nerve. With the advent of antibiotics the use of arsenicals decreased, as did reports on their toxic effects. Thallium, however, is used at times in the local treatment of ringworm or as a rat poison and is extremely toxic. Frequently ingested by children, it can affect both the peripheral and the central nervous system, leading to peripheral neuritis and an encephalitis that often includes an optic neuritis. Loss of hair is characteristic of this condition and often points up the correct diagnosis.

A less clearly understood but more common condition is tobacco-alcohol amblyopia (p. 293). The frequent association of smoking and drinking in patients with this type of centrocecal visual loss is responsible for the hyphenated name. Under certain circumstances, however, either tobacco or alcohol can cause this condition. Tobacco-alcohol amblyopia starts with a decreased appreciation of color, especially red, followed by moderate loss of visual acuity. Although there may be marked asymmetry of involvement, both eyes are affected. In the early stages of the disease, ophthalmoscopic examination generally is normal, and the diagnosis is made when a characteristic centrocecal visual field defect is found in which the scotoma between the fixation point and blind spot has areas of more dense visual loss, often called nuclei. The existence of these nuclei together with a history of prolonged, excessive use of tobacco and alcohol make the diagnosis likely. Improvement generally follows abstention from alcohol and tobacco together with adequate nutrition. Because visual loss occasionally is associated with pernicious anemia in smokers, it is wise to rule out this condition.

At times chronic alcoholics undergo an acute, relatively short-lived amaurosis (blindness) for which no sound pathologic basis has been established. During such a period pupillary reflexes are intact, indicating a cortical blindness. The condition clears completely within 24 hours if no further alcohol is ingested.

Much more grave are the effects of methyl alcohol poisoning on the optic nerve. Although methanol usually is drunk as bootleg whisky or denatured alcohol, it also can pass rapidly through the skin; e.g., poisoning has been reported in workers exposed to high concentrations of methanol in paints. Onset of symptoms usually is delayed 8 to 40 hours, after which headache, abdominal pains, restlessness, and loss of vision are followed in severe cases by coma and death.

The initial visual complaint of methanol poisoning is hazy or blurred vision. In clear distinction to ethanol amaurosis, the pupils become less reactive to light as vision is lost. On ophthalmoscopic examination the optic discs are hyperemic, and retinal edema is present in more severe cases. When vision deteriorates, the optic nerve loses substance and becomes pale within two months. In acute cases bicarbonate solutions are administered to regulate acidosis. Treatment often is unsatisfactory. Some authors recommend the administration of ethanol on the theory that it slows the formation of toxic products from the already ingested methanol. Corticosteroids are of little value.

Prognosis is good if visual complaints are absent for the first two days. When vision is severely affected and retinal edema is present, permanent visual loss is to be expected. Since it is often biphasic, with an initial amaurosis that first lessens and then increases permanently, favorable prognostication for apparent visual improvement early in the course of the disease is dangerous.

Optic neuritis can also result from allergy. Although rare, its occurrence has been documented in susceptible patients who have eaten pork, chocolate, or turkey, who have been stung by a bee, or who have poison ivy dermatitis. If possible, these hazards must be scrupulously avoided by individuals with such allergies.

OPTIC ATROPHY

The diagnosis of optic atrophy is based on appearance and function. The optic disc is pale to ophthalmoscopic examination and visual performance is deficient. Deficient vision can be manifested by loss of visual field, loss of visual acuity, or a combination of the two. Without a change in vision, the diagnosis of optic atrophy is not tenable, save in special instances. This is particularly true in infants and children whose normal optic disc is pale. Optic atrophy follows any condition in which retinal ganglion cells or their axons are destroyed, or the axons of the ganglion cells are transected anywhere between their source in the retina and their termination in the dorsal lateral geniculate body and the superior colliculus. Such an interruption leads to the death of these cells and the gradual disappearance of their axons and cell bodies.

Since the optic nerve may have a different appearance in each condition listed in the following sections, optic atrophy is best described for each separately. There is, however, one overriding, descriptive classification that applies to all atrophic discs based on their general appearance.

An atrophic disc that has sharp margins, enlarged physiologic cup, enhanced visibility of the lamina cribrosa, and a white color is said to have undergone primary optic atrophy (Plate 28D). An atrophic disc that has blurred margins, poor visibility of the lamina cribrosa, filling-in of the physiologic cup, and gray-white glial tissue on its surface and along its blood vessels is said to have undergone secondary optic atrophy (Plate 28E). In both types, the number of small blood vessels visible on the face of the disc decreases. The terms primary and secondary optic atrophy are used widely in ophthalmology.

Atrophy in Ocular Diseases. Optic atrophy after retinal disease, often called consecutive atrophy, occurs in characteristic form in retinitis pigmentosa. The disc is slightly yellow, the physiologic cup is not visible, and the retinal arterioles are markedly narrow. The equatorial region of the eye contains pigmentary deposits. Congenital syphilis may produce a pigmentary retinopathy with consecutive optic atrophy that resembles retinitis pigmentosa, but in which the pigment usually is more dispersed. A combination of pale optic disc and narrowed retinal arterioles is seen also after central retinal artery occlusion (Plate 28F). New vessel formation (neovascularization) or marked sheathing of the arterioles supports the diagnosis of old arterial occlusion, as does a history of sudden unilateral loss of vision. Atrophy of the optic nerve need not be total. With focal inflammation (as in Jensen's disease), the corresponding portion of the optic disc may atrophy.

Atrophy Secondary to Papilledema or Papillitis. Chronic papilledema and papillitis are leading causes of optic atrophy in which a marked proliferation of glial elements fills in the physiologic cup, masks the lamina cribrosa, and renders the disc margins indistinct. In chronic papilledema the edema and the stasis slowly call forth this glial reaction. In papillitis a comparable but much more rapid sequence takes place. The end stage of each is remarkably similar and neither is reversible. In papilledema these changes can be prevented by relieving the increased intracranial pressure before the glial reaction is extreme. When chronic papilledema regresses, it is possible in succeeding months for the disc either to become indistinguishable from a normal one or to resemble closely a disc with primary optic atrophy.

Primary Optic Atrophy with Tabes Dorsalis and/or Retrobulbar Neuritis. Tabes dorsalis is a prototype of primary optic atrophy. In this disease damage to the optic nerve axons adjacent to the chiasm is followed by slow degeneration of their axons at the optic disc. The physiologic cup enlarges and the lamina cribrosa becomes visible. Loss of nerve fibers and regression of the vascular net that normally serves them lead to increasing pallor of the optic disc and to increasing distinctness of its margins. When these patients are checked for an Argyll Robertson pupil, their visual acuity should be known. Lack of pupillary response to

light in a nearly blind patient obviously does not indicate pupillary abnormality. The diagnosis of an Argyll Robertson pupil is not valid in tabetic patients who have marked optic atrophy.

As mentioned previously, retrobulbar neuritis can be followed by optic atrophy affecting the entire optic disc or only a portion of it. Retrobulbar neuritis in multiple sclerosis often involves central vision selectively. The nerve fibers serving central vision, the papillomacular bundle, may atrophy. This leads to an optic atrophy limited to the temporal portion of the optic disc through which the papillomacular bundle enters. This selective involvement can lead to a selective optic atrophy called temporal pallor (Plate 28G). Often this is the only stigmata remaining after an attack of retrobulbar neuritis. It is difficult to diagnose because the temporal border in a healthy optic disc normally is somewhat paler (it contains finer axons with a less dense vascular supply) than the other regions of the optic disc. As in other types of optic atrophy, the term is best reserved for instances when a definite field defect, such as a central scotoma, can be demonstrated.

Atrophy with Intracranial Lesions. Whether or not optic atrophy develops with intracranial pathologic conditions depends on the location and nature of the lesion and on the presence or absence of increased intracranial pressure. Lesions affecting the visual pathways but not raising intracranial pressure, e.g., a pituitary adenoma, lead to simple (primary) optic atrophy. Generally the farther the lesion is from the eye, the longer it takes for optic disc pallor to be noticeable. In occipital lobe lesions that affect a secondary neuron, the pallor of the optic disc may not be observable for years, if at all. In contrast, lesions of the optic nerve may lead to optic disc pallor in a matter of weeks.

Increased intracranial pressure complicates the situation, for if the papilledema itself is of sufficient magnitude it can lead to optic atrophy as already discussed (p. 300). Thus with intracranial pathologic change visual loss can result either from direct effect on the visual pathways by a lesion, or through the indirect mechanism of an edematous optic disc becoming atrophic.

Atrophy with Toxins. Optic atrophy from the ingestion of toxins may be primary or secondary. Many toxic substances change the optic disc in a characteristic fashion. Methanol, which may cause either a primary or a secondary optic atrophy, often leads to a primary optic atrophy in which the disc tissue for practical purposes disappears and a large area of lamina cribrosa is apparent. After quinine poisoning, the disc margins generally are sharp. Quinine optic atrophy, however, is characterized by extremely narrow retinal arterioles and by unexpectedly good vision in an eye with a pale disc.

Atrophy in Glaucoma. In glaucoma the cupping of the optic disc and the loss of the visual field are evidences of optic atrophy. Glaucoma cupping usually is differentiated from other types of optic atrophy by the nasal displacement of the blood vessels and the backward bowing of the lamina cribrosa. At times glaucoma optic atrophy is difficult to distinguish from primary forms of optic atrophy in which the blood vessels are naturally to the nasal side of the optic disc.

OPHTHALMODYNAMOMETRY

Cerebrovascular Disease

In recent years, interest in and knowledge of cerebrovascular disease has upsurged. The concept of the focal atheromatous process has been popularized and carotid artery disease has been differentiated from disease of its intracranial branches. Careful pathologic studies, arteriograms of the neck vessels, and results gained in the surgical treatment of carotid artery thrombosis have all supported the distinction of intracranial from extracranial vascular disease.

Since the ophthalmic artery is the first major branch of the carotid artery above the bifurcation of the internal and external carotid in the neck, the pressure in the ophthalmic artery or its branches is related to carotid pressure. The pressure in the ophthalmic artery may be judged approximately from the pressure of its derivative, the central retinal artery, which is visible on the face of the optic disc. Compression of the eye by a simple technique can serve as an approximate measure of the pressure of the central retinal artery. The pressure needed to cause the normally nonpulsative arterioles on the disc to collapse with diastole may be equated with the diastolic pressure in the vessel, and the pressure needed to obliterate the pulse entirely may be equated with systolic pressure.

No claim is made that the pressures measured by a special instrument, the ophthalmodynamometer (Fig. 7-10), represent the true perfusion pressure of the vessel. Several significant factors, among them variability of intraocular pressure and of scleral rigidity, preclude such a claim. Rather, it is important to compare readings from the two eyes, with variation of 15 per cent or greater considered significant when the test is done by an experienced observer. Such a difference suggests reduced perfusion on the side of the lower pressure.

Positive results usually are more important than negative ones. Collateral circulation may develop to return the readings to normal over a period of time. Serial readings taken after known occlusion, as after carotid ligation for arteriovenous fistula, can be used to judge development of collateral circulation. Similarly, serial readings can be used to evaluate the success of reconstructive or replacement therapy in carotid occlusive disease.

The technique for ophthalmodynamometry is straightforward and can be readily mastered after a brief instruction period and some practice.* The physician should have sufficient skill with the ophthalmoscope to keep a clear view of the optic disc while the instrument is applied to the eye. A topical anesthetic should be used to prevent discomfort, and the pupil should be dilated to achieve adequate visualization of the optic disc, especially in the elderly. Care must be taken to apply the plunger at the

---

*For details of the technique read Toole, J. F. and Patel, A. N.: Cerebrovascular Disorders, New York, McGraw-Hill Book Co., 1967, pp. 65–69.

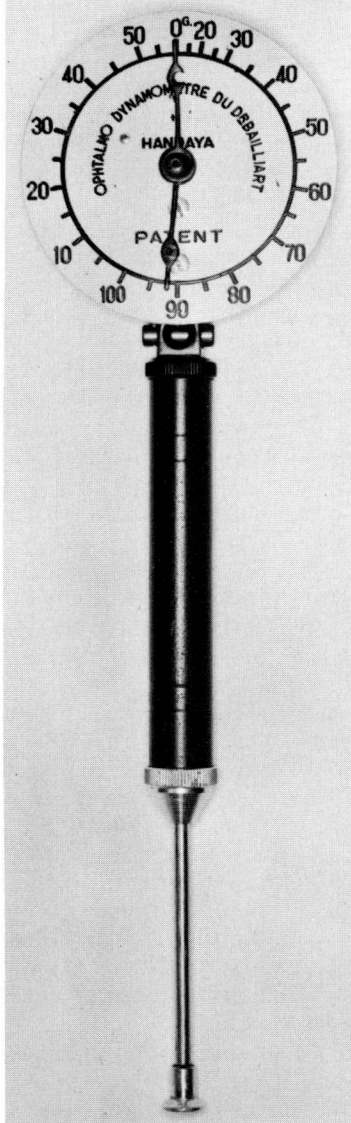

Figure 7-10 Ophthalmodynamometer. Footplate is applied to temporal side of eye while branches of central retinal artery on the optic disc are viewed with an ophthalmoscope. As pressure is applied, visible pulsations of these arterioles begin (diastolic pressure). When pressure on globe is increased sufficiently, pulsations cease (systolic pressure). For details on use of instrument see text.

same rate of speed to each eye. If systolic pressure is being measured, it is not wise to keep the artery closed off for more than a few seconds. The test may be applied at the bedside and often can aid in emergency diagnosis of cerebrovascular disease. The chief contraindications are ocular; e.g.,

ophthalmodynamometry should not be done after eye surgery or without direct ophthalmologic consultation in patients with a history of retinal detachment.

Occlusive Vascular Disease

Eye signs figure prominently in vascular disease of the brain. In recent years improved arteriographic techniques have greatly enhanced the accuracy of diagnosis, allowing superior correlation of the effect of lesions in intracranial blood vessels on ocular function. In addition, as surgical techniques have been developed to replace sections of the carotid arteries, the differentiation of large vessel disease from smaller vessel disease has taken on increased importance. Vascular diseases of the brain that lead to infarction, particularly thrombosis and embolism, are relatively common. The signs and symptoms resulting from blockage of some vessels are characteristic.

Common or Internal Carotid Artery. The ophthalmic artery is the first major branch of the carotid artery after it enters the cranium. In a young person a slow closing of the lumen of the carotid artery in the neck usually causes no visible effect on vision because the circle of Willis continues to supply the ophthalmic artery. In an older person, however, the collateral circulation is more limited and less responsive. Partial occlusion of the carotid artery (Fig. 7-11) often leads to fleeting attacks of unilateral blindness, usually called amaurosis fugax, associated with a contralateral weakness. Ophthalmodynamometry may give some indication of the relative perfusion pressures to the two eyes. Even when the attack is over, grossly unequal readings frequently will indicate a deficient perfusion to the side with the lower pressure.

At times complete blockage of the carotid artery causes no symptoms. This is especially true if the blockage is slow in onset and if the rest of the major vessels are functioning well. More often, however, the blockage causes signs and symptoms of cerebral infarction. When the ophthalmic artery is involved, sudden blindness occurs;

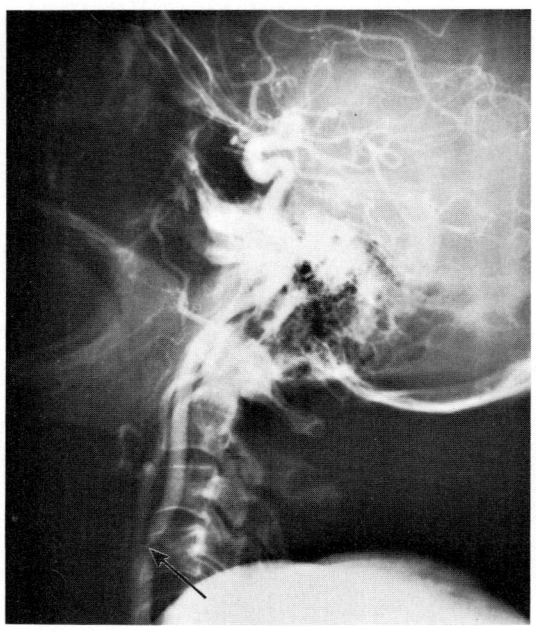

Figure 7-11 Stenosis of internal carotid artery. Arteriogram demonstrates a marked stenosis (arrow) of internal carotid as it originates from common carotid artery. (Courtesy of Mark Mishkin, M.D.)

the characteristic ophthalmoscopic picture of central retinal artery occlusion may follow, its onset depending on local collateral supply. Occasionally the ophthalmic artery is spared, but the visual pathway is damaged behind the chiasm, with a resultant homonymous hemianopia manifest in the opposite side of the visual field.

Basilar Insufficiency and Thrombosis. Complete, sudden thrombosis of the basilar artery leads to loss of consciousness and causes death in a matter of hours or days. Through its paramedian and circumflex branches the basilar artery supplies blood to the motor and autonomic nerves of the eye. Through its terminal branches, the posterior cerebral arteries, it supplies blood to the posterior optic radiation and visual cortex. Thus, when blood flow through the basilar artery fails, diplopia and blindness may be associated with major signs of brain stem and long tract involvement. Differences in collateral circulation lead to considerable variability in the clinical picture.

As collaterals increase their function, initial, severe signs often disappear in an hour or less. Failure of basilar circulation results in a multitude of syndromes; in the visual system loss of vision and diplopia, with third nerve palsy, predominate. The pupil may be dilated or miotic, depending on whether the Edinger-Westphal nuclei or the sympathetic tracts are involved. Nystagmus occurs when the vestibular nuclei or their major pathways are damaged.

Anterior Choroidal Artery and Middle Cerebral Artery. These two vessels can be described together because the visual effects of thrombosis are the same for each. Both have branches supplying portions of the optic tract and of the optic radiation. When blood flow through either artery is stopped, homonymous hemianopia, hemiplegia, and hemianesthesia result. Generally occlusion of the anterior choroidal artery is less serious, for most often the patient retains consciousness and his symptoms clear more rapidly than in occlusion of the middle cerebral artery.

Posterior Cerebral Artery. Each posterior cerebral artery supplies blood to the posterior optic radiation and to the occipital lobe. Between the territories of the posterior cerebral and middle cerebral arteries a small but significant area of terminal overlap exists. The overlap is in the projection area of central vision and is thought to explain why central vision often is spared when the posterior cerebral artery fails to supply an adequate amount of blood to the occipital lobe.

Carotid Cavernous Fistula. Carotid cavernous fistula, usually the result of trauma, leads to progressive and characteristic ocular signs. Headache and a roaring sound in the head (bruit) are followed by protrusion of one or both globes. The proptosis or exophthalmos is readily differentiated from most other forms of exophthalmos in that it usually is pulsatile, the pulsations of the globe being synchronous with the pulse. The bruit is the direct result of blood rushing at high pressure from the carotid artery into the cavernous sinus. Pressure and flow within the cavernous sinus rise and are transmitted to its tributaries. By their proximity the ophthalmic veins figure prominently. They are grossly dilated, and the carotid pulse transmitted through them causes visible ocular pulsations. Not only do the veins of the orbit swell and push the eye forward, but the veins of the anterior part of the globe also are engorged and present a typical appearance reminiscent of a caput medusae. A form of secondary glaucoma from the increased venous pressure often is present.

As viewed ophthalmoscopically, the retinal veins are dilated and tortuous, and the optic disc commonly demonstrates mild papilledema. Cranial nerves three, four, and six frequently are involved, and palsies of the muscles served by them occur with regularity. A history of trauma to the head followed by pulsating exophthalmos and a bruit are virtually pathognomonic. Demonstration of the fistula by arteriography (Fig. 7-12) confirms the diagnosis and often aids the surgeon in planning therapy. A wide choice of treatment, none of which is entirely satisfactory, is available. Arteriography itself may be the therapy for thrombosis; the fistula site occasionally closes after the procedure. Some fistulae spontaneously cure by a thrombotic process. Many cases are treated by application of a clamp about the internal or common carotid. The clamp has a screw arrangement that allows the arterial lumen to be occluded in a graded fashion. Sufficient time is taken to allow collateral circulation to build up to compensate for the diminished perfusion before the flow is totally stopped. When the vessel is occluded, flow through the fistula often decreases dramatically, with a consequent lessening of symptoms.

Vascular Disease

Arteritis. Temporal arteritis is being recognized increasingly as a cause of blindness in patients over 50 years of age. The findings vary widely from person to person, but in most the presentation is characteristic. Weeks of poor appetite, lassitude, and low grade fever usually are accompanied by constant pain over the distribution of the temporal artery. The temporal artery is knobby and tender to palpation, and the area overlying it is painfully sensitive to light touch. Over a third of untreated patients lose their vision, owing to occlusion of the arterial supply to one or both eyes. The presentation is so variable that the condition should be suspected in any person

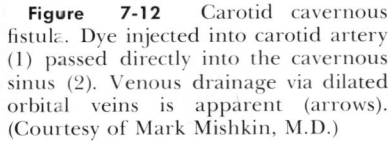

Figure 7-12 Carotid cavernous fistula. Dye injected into carotid artery (1) passed directly into the cavernous sinus (2). Venous drainage via dilated orbital veins is apparent (arrows). (Courtesy of Mark Mishkin, M.D.)

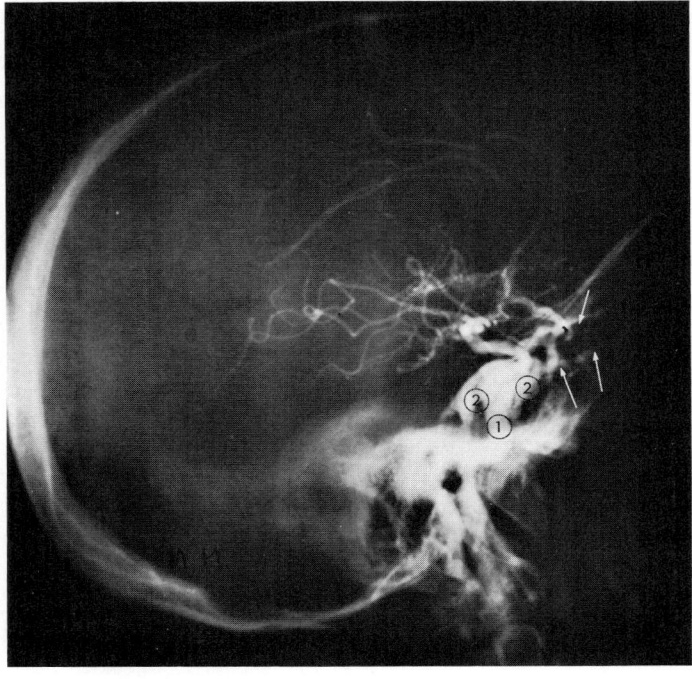

over 50 years of age who has sudden, unexplained visual loss. The ocular findings depend on the location and nature of the arterial closure. The closer the stoppage is to the eye, the more likely the typical ophthalmoscopic picture will be that of acute occlusion of the central retinal artery. Often no ophthalmoscopic findings are seen at the time of visual loss.

An increase in the sedimentation rate of blood supports the diagnosis. Final confirmation is obtained by temporal artery biopsy. Pathologically, the intima and media of the temporal artery break down and are replaced by granulomatous, inflammatory tissue containing giant cells (giant cell arteritis).

In most cases high doses of steroids (up to 60 mg. prednisone daily) need to be used for as long as a six-month period. They probably arrest the manifestations of the disease while the underlying condition runs its self-limited course. Steroids often are effective in halting the progress of the condition, but they are of no avail in returning visual function that is already lost; once blind, the patient is permanently blind. In a patient with the clinical picture described above, it is imperative to obtain a sedimentation rate and to begin treatment promptly. Temporal artery biopsy, which can be done later, is still reliable after steroid therapy is underway.

Aneurysm. Aneurysms of the intracranial vessels comprising the circle of Willis (Fig. 7-13) can cause manifold symptoms. By their size and location they can cause visual field defects or cranial nerve palsies. Rupture of an intracranial aneurysm can announce itself with headache, followed by coma and death. With subarachnoid bleeding it is common to see subhyaloid hemorrhages that receive their name after their preretinal location. Most saccular aneurysms involve the eye only at the time of rupture, being "silent" until then. In a minority of cases an unruptured aneurysm compresses a motor nerve to the eye or interferes with the primary visual pathway. Aneurysm in any one location presents a great variation in signs and symptoms; nevertheless, location is an important distinguishing characteristic of these vascular anomalies.

When located beneath the anterior clinoid process, aneurysms of the carotid artery often press against the ophthalmic division of the trigeminal nerve and cause pain referred into the orbit. Corneal sensation in that eye may be normal or reduced. In addition, paresis (usually partial, but sometimes total) of the oculomotor nerve often is seen. Major involvement of the pupil commonly serves to differentiate the third nerve paresis found with aneurysm from the spontaneous oculomotor palsy

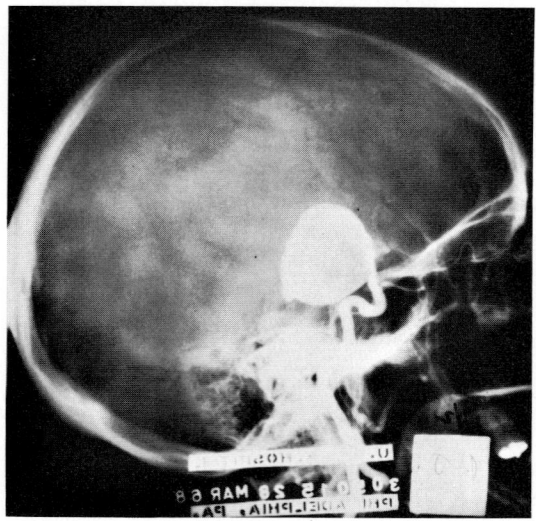

Figure 7-13 Giant aneurysm arising from region of bifurcation of internal carotid artery. This aneurysm compressed visual radiations in the temporal lobe, causing an incongruous hemianopia to the contralateral side. (Courtesy of Mark Mishkin, M.D.)

often seen with diabetes mellitus in which the pupil is spared. Infraclinoid aneurysm usually does not affect the optic nerve, and vision is normal.

In contrast to infraclinoid aneurysms, supraclinoid aneurysms, in keeping with their proximity to the visual pathways, frequently cause defects in the visual field. When the aneurysm is anteriorly placed, the optic nerve may be the site of maximum compression, with blindness and optic atrophy ensuing. In other locations pressure on the chiasm can produce a bitemporal field defect simulating that found with pituitary tumor. An accompanying paresis of the oculomotor nerve often distinguishes aneurysm from pituitary tumor in which nerve palsies are unusual.

Aneurysms occur in many locations on the circle of Willis, with a marked predilection for points of bifurcation or areas where embryonic arteries have resorbed. The aneurysmal mass may act as a tumor, compressing neighboring nervous tissue with the signs and symptoms appropriate to that location.

Where the aneurysm has been treated successfully, the prognosis for vision in the presence of visual field defects is variable and depends on the duration and extent of the visual loss. Oculomotor palsies usually clear up in a short time. After a patient has recovered from third nerve palsy, an unusual syndrome may be found in which inappropriate lid or pupillary movements coincide with ocular movements. Termed the pseudo-von Graefe's sign (see description, p. 250), this phenomenon is attributed to misdirection of regenerating oculomotor nerve fibers. The most common result is lid elevation when adduction is attempted: it is assumed that fibers intended for the medial rectus have by chance innervated the levator of the lid. In keeping with physiologic laws, the lid then droops on abduction. When the pupil is involved, it usually dilates with adduction. Once established, the condition is permanent and indicates a recovered third nerve palsy.

Subarachnoid hemorrhage is the most feared result of intracranial aneurysm, and its general signs of stiff neck, headache, convulsion, and coma are familiar to the neurologist. The most common ocular findings in subarachnoid hemorrhage, as already mentioned, are oculomotor palsy and subhyaloid hemorrhages, which are preretinal and large. When the patient is erect for any length of time, the blood elements settle and the hemorrhage assumes a boat shape. Hemorrhages of this type are believed to occur secondary to rapid compression of venous drainage of the retina by the precipitous rise in intracranial pressure that occurs after rupture of intracranial aneurysm. The prognosis for resorption of the hemorrhage and for renewal of oculomotor function is good if the aneurysm can be treated successfully.

NEURO-OPHTHALMOLOGY OF TUMORS

Optic Glioma. Optic gliomas are slow-growing, intrinsic tumors of the optic nerve or of the optic chiasm usually occurring between the second and sixth years of life. Visual loss is the first symptom, but in younger children strabismus may develop before the poor vision is discovered. If the glioma is bilateral, vision deteriorates so markedly that the child may bump into large objects. Older children frequently complain first of decreasing vision. As the tumor grows, proptosis develops. This is nonpulsatile and irreducible, but there is no pain. The optic disc may be swollen or atrophic. Loss of ocular movement is a late manifestation. When located in the chiasm, the tumor may involve the hypothalamus and occasionally may lead to a syndrome characterized by hypersomnia, polydipsia, and polyuria. More often, obesity and mild eunuchoidism are present. Because optic nerve glioma frequently is associated with von Recklinghausen's disease (neurofibromatosis), other associated signs, such as cafe au lait spots, should be sought in any child with unexplained optic atrophy, especially if it is unilateral. An optic glioma causes the optic foramen to enlarge concentrically to give a characteristic and virtually pathognomonic x-ray appearance (Fig. 7-14). Patients undergo x-irradiation or surgery, depending upon the site and extent of the tumor. Prognosis is favorable when the tumor involves only the optic nerve, but unfavorable when it involves the chiasm.

Pituitary Tumor. Tumors of the anterior lobe of the pituitary gland occur characteristically in the middle years of life. They usually are classified chromophobic, chromophilic, and basophilic by the staining quality of their cells. Classification based on cell type has won wide acceptance since each type (with occasional exception) presents a different clinical syndrome. All three types are benign; carcinoma of the pituitary is rare.

Chromophobe adenomas, the most common of the three, are nonsecretory and produce symptoms through pressure on other tissues and displacement. When still within the sella turcica, chromophobe adenomas often produce frontal headache. As normal pituitary tissue is compressed, panhypopituitarism insidiously appears. If the tumor continues to grow, the sella enlarges, its wall erodes and the mass rises through the dorsum sellae to impinge on the optic chiasm. The chief sign of chiasmal interference is visual loss. This loss typically first appears in the upper temporal (Fig. 7-5) field of each eye, frequently giving no symptoms. If the tumor is not treated, the field loss progresses until the inferior temporal fields are lost and temporal field blindness is complete in each eye. If allowed to progress further, the inferior visual fields on the nasal side of each visual field are encroached upon; finally, the superior nasal field is lost and blindness results.

Not all pituitary adenomas produce typical, symmetrical, bitemporal field loss, because the nature of the visual field defect depends on the growth pattern of the tumor, the anatomical localization of the optic chiasm in relation to the dorsum sellae (several distinct relationships are possible), and the relationship of the chiasm to the neighboring blood vessels. Most common among the alternative patterns of visual field loss are a dense central scotoma with a unilateral optic atrophy or central bitemporal field defects. It is unusual, but possible, for pituitary tumor to affect the motor nerves to the eye. Papilledema is uncommon enough to render the diagnosis suspect when it is present. In most cases

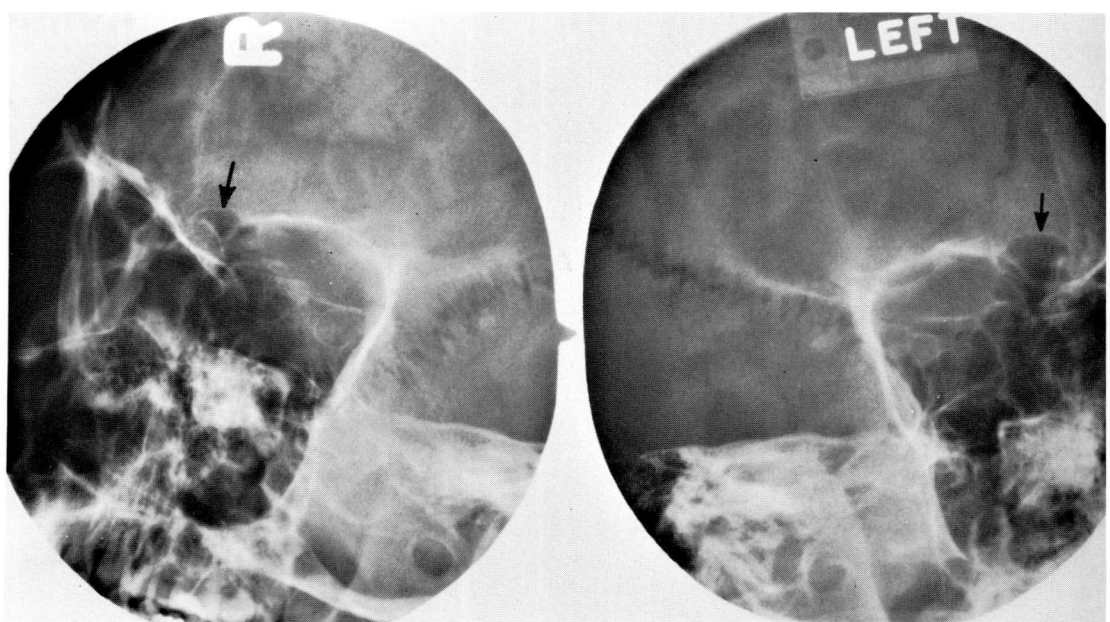

Figure 7-14   Glioma of optic nerve. Concentric enlargement of optic foramen on the left (see arrows) is apparent when radiographs are compared. (Courtesy of Norman Leeds, M.D.)

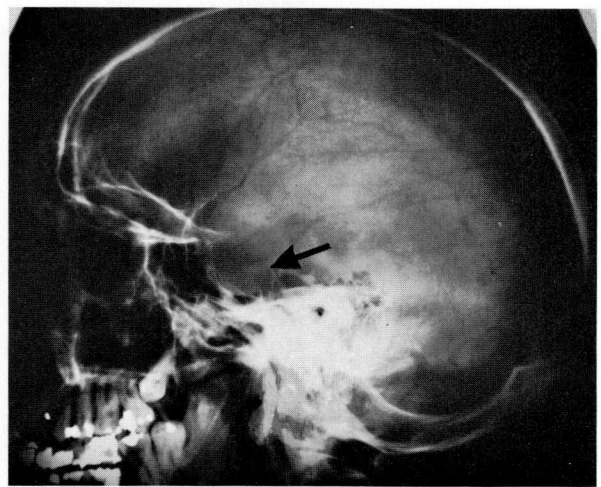

Figure 7-15 Sella turcica is eroded greatly by gradually enlarging chromophobe adenoma. Arrow indicates posterior clinoid processes that are virtually destroyed. (Courtesy of Mark Mishkin, M.D.)

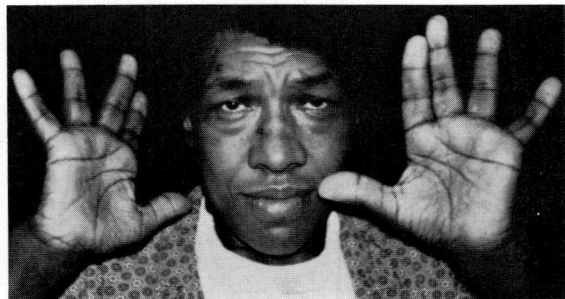

Figure 7-16 Acromegaly. Clinical diagnosis of acromegaly was made in this patient who gave a history of gradual enlargement and coarsening of her facial features, hands, and feet. On visual field examination, an upper bitemporal defect, as in Figure 7-5A, was found.

definitive diagnosis follows study of skull films. In these, enlargement of the pituitary fossa and erosion of the sella turcica signal pituitary tumor (Fig. 7-15). Occasionally craniopharyngioma, meningioma, or aneurysm may invade the sella and mimic a pituitary tumor.

Chromophilic tumors of the pituitary gland secrete excessive amounts of growth hormone. In childhood this excessive secretion leads to overgrowth of the long bones and to gigantism. In adult life the hands, feet, and skull enlarge, and the soft tissues of the face are typically gross. Chromophilic and chromophobic tumors impinge on the chiasm in similar ways. The clinical differentiation between the two is based on the presence or absence of the effects of excess growth hormone. The clinical appearance of an acromegalic is so characteristic that the diagnosis often is suspected as the patient crosses the office threshold (Fig. 7-16).

The third tumor of the pituitary, the basophilic, is small, remains confined to the sella, and rarely affects vision. The signs and symptoms of Cushing's syndrome usually lead to biochemical tests to aid in its diagnosis.

Pituitary tumor is treated either by radiation or surgery, the choice depending on technical factors. With successful treatment it is common for vision to improve and for the visual field defect, as measured by tangent screen examination, to lessen gradually over many months. Vision may improve even when the optic disc is pale. The more severe and longstanding the visual loss, the greater the likelihood it will be permanent.

Meningiomas. Meningiomas of the sphenoid wing usually are classified according to their distance from the midline. Such a classification is clinically useful since the behavior of these tumors and their symptoms vary considerably with location. Like pituitary tumors, they occur in middle life and have a higher incidence in women.

Tumors of the inner one third of the sphenoid ridge give substantial evidence of their presence. Their proximity to the optic nerve where it joins the optic chiasm leads to early visual symptoms that vary with the exact location of the lesion. Generally the patient complains of hazy vision in one eye, and visual field examination reveals a unilateral nasal or temporal hemianopic defect, or a central scotoma. Early ophthalmoscopic examination may show a normal disc. Later, optic atrophy or papilledema is common. A group of signs, the superior orbital fissure syndrome, originate from interference with structures passing through the superior orbital fissure. All of the motor nerves to the eye pass through that fissure and are easily compressed by meningiomas in the region. As a result, any combination of muscle palsies may be found, but abducens palsy is the most common. The pupil and the oculomotor nerve frequently are involved, resulting in a unilateral, dilated, nonreactive pupil. When the branches of the fifth nerve passing through the superior orbital fissure are affected, corneal sensation is deficient and sensation in the upper lid also may be diminished. Exophthalmos, usually mild, occurs when the tumor invades the orbit through the superior orbital fissure or when venous drainage to or in the cavernous sinus is partially blocked (Fig. 7-17). The diagnosis of meningioma of the sphenoid wing often is suspected on clinical grounds. X-rays of the skull may reveal osteoma formation at the site of attachment of the tumor or show evidence of bony erosion (Fig. 7-

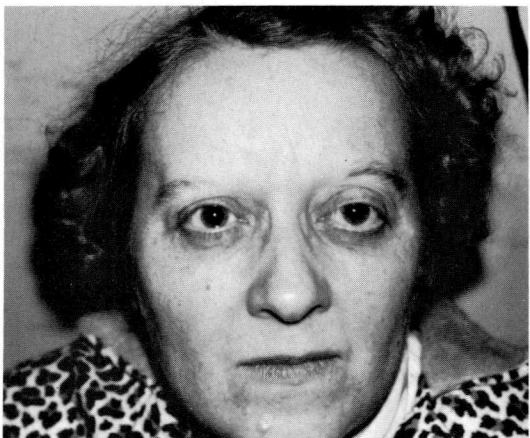

Figure 7-17 Unilateral exophthalmos with meningioma of sphenoid wing. Left eye is 3 mm. farther forward than the right. Patient complained of frequent headaches; x-ray disclosed typical findings of meningioma of sphenoid wing. (See Figure 7-18.)

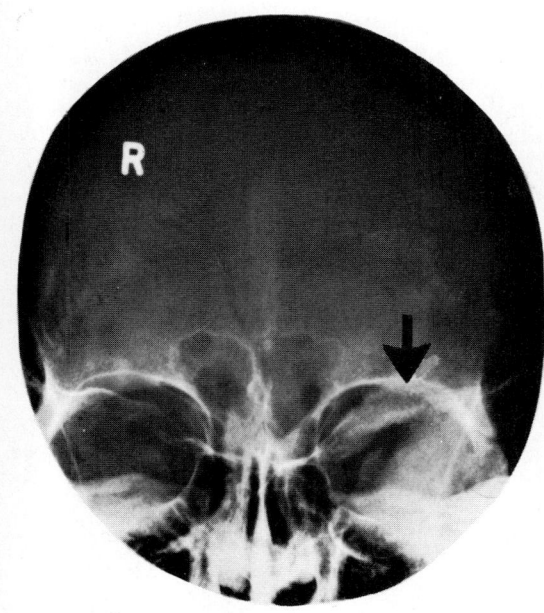

Figure 7-18 Meningioma of lesser wing of the sphenoid bone. Unilateral exophthalmos and headache brought this patient to a physician. Skull x-ray demonstrates hyperostosis (arrow), commonly produced by meningiomas. (Courtesy of Mark Mishkin, M.D.)

18). In most cases, however, diagnosis depends on an arteriographic study which, in a typical case, shows a tumor stain or cloud and displacement of arteries at the base. In many instances a feeder vessel originates from the ophthalmic artery.

If the tumor is not discovered before the onset of general symptoms, such as headache, the patient may be found to have an atrophic nerve head on the side of the tumor and papilledema on the contralateral side. This combination usually is called the Foster-Kennedy syndrome, and, although rare, it is widely recognized.

In their early stages, tumors of the middle third of the sphenoid ridge cause considerably less general or ocular symptomatology than those of the inner third. When sufficiently grown, these tumors also lead to multiple oculomotor palsies by compressing the nerves to the eye, to unilateral exophthalmos, and to loss of vision.

From the outer third of the sphenoid ridge arises meningioma-en-plaque, a form of meningioma that differs materially from those already described. It is a diffuse and invasive tumor that is not truly local. Clinically the temple is full on the side of the lesion and exophthalmos is

progressive. Later the bony reaction damages the optic nerve and vision is lost. For unknown reasons the condition occurs predominantly in women. Treatment of these meningiomas is surgical, for they do not respond to x-irradiation. The smaller tumors may be entirely resected or partially removed if access is limited. Since these tumors usually are slow growing, even a partial resection often results in substantial alleviation of symptoms for long periods of time.

Cerebellopontine Angle Tumor. The common tumor of the cerebellopontine angle is the acoustic neuroma. It originates from Schwann cells, usually occurs in middle life, and is of equal incidence in both sexes. Although not invasive, the tumor causes considerable harm by stretching and compressing neighboring structures.

Deafness, gradual in onset, is the first symptom. As the trigeminal nerve is affected slowly, corneal sensation diminishes, and the patient often complains of paresthesias about the face. Partial facial palsy is frequent. Later the combination of poor lid closure (lagophthalmos) and decreased corneal sensation can lead to corneal ulceration. Nystagmus and a cerebellar form of ataxia are present in a high percentage of cases. Abducens palsy also may be found, either as a direct result of tumor compression or secondary to increased intracranial pressure. More extensive signs, either cranial nerve or brain stem, are found with larger tumors. Since papilledema may be present or absent, it contributes little to the differential diagnosis.

Unilateral involvement of a combination of the fifth, sixth, seventh, and eighth cranial nerves points strongly to a lesion in the cerebellopontine angle. X-ray examination often reveals an enlarged, internal auditory meatus. A significant percentage of acoustic neuromas are associated with von Recklinghausen's disease, so stigmata of that condition should be sought. Treatment is surgical. Facial palsy frequently follows surgery, and corneal exposure can become a serious problem. Usually it is necessary to sew the lids together (tarsorrhaphy) on the side of the tumor to protect the cornea against exposure and consequent ulceration. As facial nerve function improves, the lids can be reopened quite simply.

Pinealoma. Tumors of the pineal gland are uncommon. They usually occur between the first and third decades of life and have manifold ocular signs. Their progress is characteristic. Occlusion of the aqueduct of Sylvius by the tumor mass leads to internal hydrocephalus with headache and papilledema. Pressure on the roof of the midbrain is followed by a syndrome, first described by Parinaud, which includes limitation of vertical gaze, usually involving elevation but also possibly depression; preservation of horizontal eye movements; loss of convergence; and pupillary disturbances (the pupils usually are dilated and non-responsive, but they may be miotic). Unilateral lid retraction and palsies of the muscles served by the third cranial nerve frequently are found. Destruction of normal pineal parenchyma and hypothalamic seeding of the tumor produce marked changes in endocrine status. X-irradiation of these radio-sensitive tumors often results in dramatic improvement with complete remission of eye signs, but such remissions often are short-lived.

Craniopharyngioma. These tumors of the epithelial remnants of Rathke's pouch occur predominantly in children and are located along the pituitary stalk. They may have an infrasellar position, but are more commonly suprasellar. They differ from pituitary tumors in the younger average age of those afflicted and in the course of the visual field loss. In keeping with their usual location above the chiasm, the first field defects are inferotemporal and usually are much more asymmetric than those seen with pituitary adenoma. The tumor often involves the third ventricle directly, causing internal hydrocephalus and papilledema. The papilledema is often severe and is succeeded by secondary optic atrophy if pressure is not relieved. Since the optic nerve is subject to atrophy from compression of its axons behind the optic foramina and from secondary changes on the disc itself, combinations of atrophy and papilledema are possible.

The presence of bitemporal visual field defects in a child with papilledema suggests craniopharyngioma. In addition, the proximity of the hypothalamus to the pituitary gland leads frequently to signs such as loss of secondary sex characteristics, polyuria, and polydipsia.

The clinical course is irregular, with periods of stability or even of improvement followed by further deterioration. Finding typical suprasellar calcifications on skull x-rays greatly aids in making the diagnosis. Treatment is surgical, but usually is not satisfactory.

Pseudotumor Cerebri. Occurring mainly in obese, young females, pseudotumor cerebri is a common and inadequately understood syndrome whose chief components are headache, papilledema secondary to increased intracranial pressure, and lack of diagnostic findings when the patients are fully examined in the hospital. Headache, the initial complaint, often is accompanied by dizziness. The degree of papilledema varies. The disc signs often are so minimal that it is impossible to differentiate them from a normal variant. When there are no hemorrhages or exudates and only minimal blurring of the disc margins, concentric peripapillary folds and the presence or absence of venous pulsations should be looked for. Visual fields are normal except for blind spot enlargement due to the swollen optic disc. When double vision is present, it most often is secondary to sixth nerve palsy, although the third nerve may be involved. The chief danger is visual loss secondary to chronic papilledema. During the illness visual function must be continually monitored by serial examination of both visual acuity and visual field. A deleterious change in either makes it mandatory to bring down the intracranial pressure to more tolerable levels. Treatment with systemic steroids and repeated spinal taps often accomplish this satisfactorily; if they do not, a subtemporal decompression usually is done. In a majority of cases, drastic measures are not required; rather, the condition follows a benign course and gradually resolves. Careful clinical studies have done little to explain the pathogenesis of this condition. It is postulated that interference with drainage through the venous sinuses at the base of the skull is responsible for the elevated intracranial pressure.

Disorders of the myoneural junction or of the muscle itself may affect the extraocular muscles, limiting the movements of one or both eyes. Eye muscles frequently are involved in myasthenia gravis and in the hereditary dystrophies, myotonic dystrophy, and ocular myopathy, but they are spared in the limb or pelvic girdle types of muscle dystrophy.

Myasthenia Gravis. Myasthenia gravis, the chief signs of which are weakness and excessive fatigability of skeletal muscles, presents with eye signs in approximately 50 per cent of cases. Generally the disease is held to represent a defect of unknown etiology which interferes with transmission of impulses through the myoneural junction. This neuromuscular transmission defect often is found in association with hypertrophy or tumor of the thymus gland. The connection between the two is unknown.

Ptosis and diplopia, which are more severe late in the day and which lessen with rest, are the first ocular symptoms. Usually bilateral, the condition is often asymmetric (Fig. 7-19), and the extent of involvement can vary widely from day to day or week to week. Any of the eye muscles can be affected, but those that rotate the globe upward often are the first. Myasthenia gravis usually is a widespread condition, but in some instances it is confined entirely to the extraocular muscles. The smooth muscles within the eye are spared, and pupillary and accommodation reflexes are normal. When ptosis is found with weakened facial musculature, the combination gives rise to a characteristic appearance, often termed the myasthenic facies.

The diagnosis of myasthenia gravis is made by the characteristic appearance of the patient and from the history of increased severity of weakness on exercise. It is confirmed by demonstrating excess fatigability and then improved strength when anti-acetylcholinesterase agents are administered. For the eye, fatigability often may be demonstrated by bringing out a ptosis through repetitive eyelid closure that was barely apparent before.

Anticholinesterase compounds, such as Tensilon (edrophonium) or Neostigmine, increase muscle power in this condition and their administration constitutes a necessary diagnostic test. A ptotic lid is excellent to observe during testing as it is usually a sensitive indicator. In the absence of visible response to these agents, myasthenia gravis is difficult to diagnose. In recent years myasthenic-like syndromes have been reported in association with malignant tumors of the lung, pancreas, and some other organs. In contrast to myasthenia gravis, these conditions spare the muscles of the eye and respond poorly to anticholinesterase agents. Treatment of myasthenia gravis by continued administration of anticholinesterase agents is less efficacious for the eye muscles than for muscles located elsewhere in the body.

Myotonic Dystrophy. Myotonic dystrophy is an hereditary muscle dystrophy that involves several other organ systems as well. Myotonia, a condition of abnormally slow muscle relaxation, is found in combination with progressive dystrophy of musculature of the face and of the distal limbs. Additionally, testicle atrophy in males, early baldness, cataracts, and a high incidence of feeblemindedness testify to its general nature. Quite distinctive cataracts are often

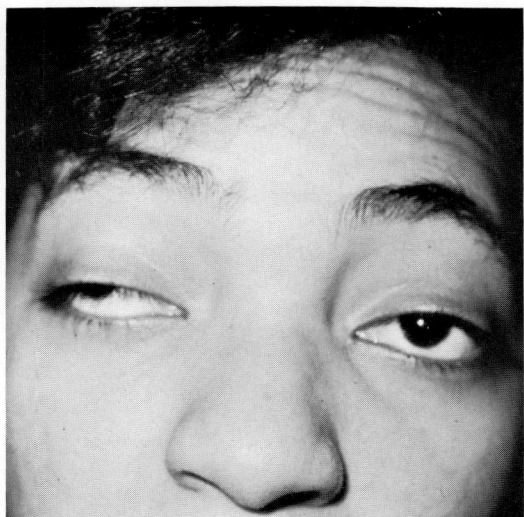

Figure 7-19 Eye findings in myasthenia gravis. Bilateral ptosis and limitation of ocular movements are present. Note how patient's eyebrows are raised as he attempts to substitute action of frontalis muscle for that of levator of the lid.

present which contain iridescent dots in the anterior and posterior cortex as seen by slit lamp examination.

Bilateral ptosis, in combination with weakness of the orbicularis oculi, is frequent. In the later stages eyelid closure may be limited, leading to corneal exposure and ulceration from infrequent and insufficient closure during the day or night. Involvement of the extraocular muscles varies. When they are affected, it is usually symmetrically, and such muscle involvement may lead to bilateral, total, external ophthalmoplegia in which the eyes appear frozen in place. It is more usual for a small but definite range of movement to be retained. When eye movements are restricted by the myopathy, the normal, protective Bell's phenomenon is lacking. This, in combination with deficient lid closure from myopathy of the orbicularis oculi, leads inexorably to chronic ulceration of the lower half of the cornea. In such a circumstance it is necessary to create lid adhesions to allow the cornea to heal and to protect it from further exposure. At times the nature of the disease is not properly understood and the patient is subjected to surgical procedures for drooping lids. This is especially true if ptosis was the complaint that brought him to the physician in the first place. Elevation of the lids in patients who do not exhibit Bell's phenomenon and have poor lid closure is fraught with danger and may lead to loss of the eye from corneal ulceration.

Ocular Myopathy. Ocular myopathy is an hereditary, slowly progressive, ocular muscle dystrophy that is bilaterally symmetrical and begins in childhood. Ptosis and restriction of gaze movements (Fig. 7-20) slowly increase as time passes. To compensate partly for the ptotic lids, the eyebrows are held in an elevated position. When facial musculature also is involved, the unusual combination of ptosis and poor lid closure with exposure of the inferior half of the cornea is found, just as in myotonia dystrophica. Occasionally, ocular myopathy may be associated with weakness of the pharyngeal muscles or the shoulder girdle muscles. As with myotonia dystrophica, the condition is more widespread than is

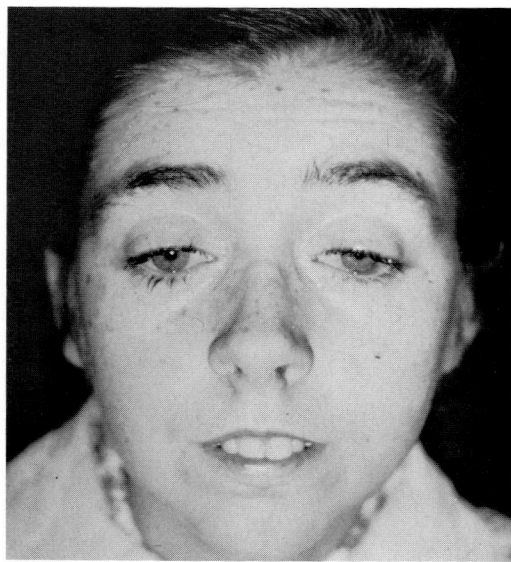

Figure 7-20 Ocular myopathy. Patient is unable either to open or to close eyes fully, owing to ptosis and poor lid closure. Antibiotic ointments were necessary to prevent corneal ulceration from exposure. Note how eyebrows are elevated in an attempt to raise the lids as in Figure 7-19, illustrating myasthenia gravis.

immediately apparent. In ocular myopathy, abnormalities of cardiac conduction, either with right bundle branch block or atrioventricular block, are common. An electrocardiogram should be part of the diagnostic workup of any patient with ocular myopathy. Ocular myopathy differs from myotonic dystrophy not only in the lack of myotonia, but by the presence of a clear lens. In addition, a characteristic pigmentary degeneration of the retina often accompanies ocular myopathy.

Generally treatment of ocular myopathy is supportive. When the condition is confined to the ocular muscles it does not limit the patient, who may pursue a normal life. Since frequently there is a family history of ocular myopathy and the gene appears to be dominant, the implications of parenthood need be discussed with any patient with this condition.

NYSTAGMUS

Nystagmus (involuntary to and fro eye movements) is the ocular manifestation of irregular motor impulses to the extraocular muscles. Nystagmus occurs in several characteristic forms; the most common are aptly named pendular and jerk.

Jerk nystagmus has two phases, a slow or physiologic phase in one direction and a rapid corrective motion (a jerk) in the other direction. By convention the direction of the rapid corrective movement is used to describe the direction of the nystagmus. In pendular nystagmus the eye undergoes oscillations with no apparent change in velocity in different directions. The distinction between pendular and jerk nystagmus is of considerable clinical importance since each type means something different.

Jerk Nystagmus. Jerk nystagmus may be physiologic or pathologic, depending upon the cause. It is part of normal function when the vestibular apparatus undergoes stimulation through calorics or through rotation of the head. In such instances the nystagmus expresses excessive stimulation of a normal physiologic system. It may be used profitably to test the integrity of that system, with such tests playing a major part in evaluation of labyrinthine and vestibular nerve functions.

Eyes will reposition themselves with a jerk motion after following serially presented objects to one side. This phenomenon, often called railway nystagmus, can be elicited simply by having a subject watch a rotating drum on which vertical stripes are painted (Fig. 7-21). The eyes follow the moving bars in a slow phase and then undergo a rapid correction toward the direction from which the bars are coming. This type of physiologic nystagmus, called opticokinetic nystagmus, has been studied extensively. Two valuable clinical uses have been developed for it. It can be used to measure the resolving power or visual acuity of the eye objectively by presenting a series of drums each of whose vertical bars are smaller in width. This graded testing situation is especially useful when subjective tests are not possible, such as in the testing of visual acuity in young children.

Opticokinetic nystagmus has also been of value in differential localization of lesions causing homonymous hemianopia. Lesions of the parieto-occipital region frequently diminish the opticokinetic response as the drum turns toward the normal side. In contrast, after a lesion of the optic tract, even one severe enough to give a complete homonymous hemianopia, the response is

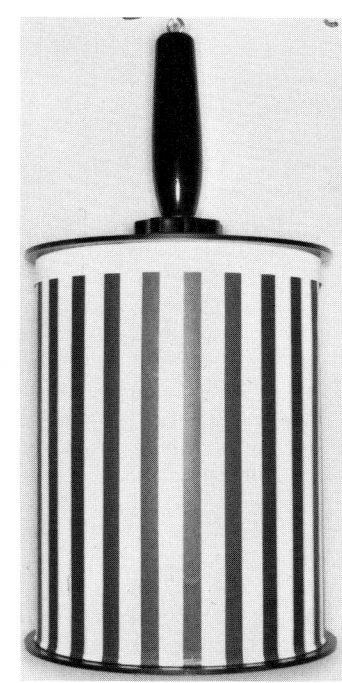

Figure 7-21 Opticokinetic drum. Opticokinetic nystagmus is elicited in normal patients when eyes fix on vertical stripes of drum rotating before them.

equal to the rotating drum whether it turns to the left or the right.

Opticokinetic nystagmus also may aid in discovering malingerers. It is difficult to have full faith in a claim of blindness when the eyes follow the rotating stripes of an opticokinetic drum. Without special equipment the presence of opticokinetic nystagmus is not valid proof against claims of diminished vision. The stripes of the standard opticokinetic nystagmus drum are broad enough to be visible with severely diminished central acuity.

Jerk nystagmus is a constant accompaniment of acute labyrinthitis with sudden onset and severe symptoms. The patient experiences vertigo, nausea, and vomiting. His hearing is preserved. The nystagmus is horizontal or rotary and has a fast component to the side opposite the affected labyrinth. Severe symptoms decline over a period of days or weeks, and the nystagmus gradually disappears. Acute labyrinthitis must be differentiated from Meniere's disease, in which attacks of vertigo are recurrent and short-lived and in which hearing loss is present.

Nystagmus of central origin occurs most often with lesions of the brain stem or cerebellum. In contrast to the abrupt beginning of labyrinthine nystagmus, the onset in central nystagmus often is insidious, and vertigo is either less bothersome or absent. In the production of nystagmus the pathologic nature of the lesion is less important than its location. Diseases of the vestibular nuclei are more apt to cause nystagmus than are other lesions in the brain stem.

Nystagmus is prominent in multiple sclerosis, which frequently is accompanied by focal demyelinated areas in the vestibular nuclei or their connections. In addition, when multiple sclerosis involves the medial longitudinal fasciculus, a characteristic, usually bilateral, syndrome called internuclear ophthalmoplegia is produced (p. 334). When horizontal gaze movements are attempted in the syndrome, adduction is limited or absent. Abduction is accompanied by coarse nystagmus. When a lesser nystagmus in the eye attempting adduction accompanies the coarse nystagmus of the abducting eye, the discrepancy in amplitude between the two eyes defines the condition. Vascular lesions, especially in hypertensive persons, are another frequent cause of central nystagmus. Both occlusion of the posterior inferior cerebellar artery and thrombosis of the paramedian penetrating vessels can interfere with the optomotor reflexes and lead to nystagmus. Also, lesions in the posterior fossa affect the cerebellum and often produce nystagmus. When of cerebellar origin, nystagmus varies remarkably with head position and can be vertical, horizontal, or rotatory. At times it is not possible to differentiate cerebellar nystagmus from lesions of vestibular nuclei.

Alcohol intoxication, barbiturates, Dilantin, and inflammation of the brain in encephalitis also can lead to central nystagmus. Nystagmus that follows ingestion of toxic amounts of a drug ordinarily relents as the drug is metabolized. Malnutrition complicates the picture in chronic alcoholism, frequently necessitating general supportive measurements including vitamin supplements before the nystagmus relents.

Pendular Nystagmus. Defective vision in the first years of life is the most common cause of pendular nystagmus. Several of the conditions leading to this type of ocular nystagmus are listed as follows:

1. Optic atrophy
2. Congenital anomalies of the optic disc—coloboma
3. Albinism
4. Bilateral macular lesions
5. Congenital cataract
6. High astigmatism
7. Corneal opacification

In each condition an incomplete or defective set of visual impulses is transmitted to the brain, preventing the development of the normal fixation reflexes, and pendular nystagmus of ocular derivation occurs. If vision is lost after the second year of life, ocular nystagmus develops in a partial or abortive form. If vision is lost in adulthood, the eyes often are stable.

In addition, two clinical entities, congenital nystagmus and spasmus nutans in which the eyes apparently are normal, have pendular nystagmus as a major sign. In congenital nystagmus the abnormal ocular movements are noted shortly after birth. The oscillations are pendular over a rather narrow range of gaze positions and are jerky elsewhere. Since the movements diminish visual acuity, the patient adopts the position in which they are of least magnitude in order to attain the clearest vision possible. Frequently the position is an eccentric one, with the head turned habitually. A child who rejects attempts to have him hold his head straight (which increases the nystagmus) erroneously may be thought to have torticollis. When the position of least nystagmus is at an extreme gaze position with marked head turning, the eye muscles in some instances may be reset on the globe to bring the point of least nystagmus to a more forward position. The cause of congenital nystagmus is unknown. There are family histories that clearly demonstrate several generations having this condition, but most cases are sporadic. The nystagmus continues for a lifetime and visual acuity is never normal. Many of these patients, however, adapt remarkably and do much better in the world than simple measurements of visual acuity would suggest. This is especially true in near work and reading.

The spasmus nutans form of pendular nystagmus is found in children with normal eyes. The history is usually straightforward. An apparently normal child develops a rapid, shimmering, pendular nystagmus at approximately 6 months of age. This nystagmus often is accompanied by torticollis and head nodding. Movements of the two eyes may be asymmetric in magnitude (at times it may appear that only one eye is moving). Spasmus nutans is without known cause and of no pathologic significance. It is self-limited and usually disappears after two to three months, but on rare occasions it can last for years. At times it is difficult to differentiate from congenital nystagmus, which also can present head nodding, and the date of onset may not be clearly known. In such instances the course of the condition often makes the diagnosis more clear.

THE PUPIL

Trauma. Ocular trauma often leaves a dilated, nonreactive pupil. Traumatic iridoplegia, as this condition is called, is usually transitory, but can be permanent. A tear of the iris sphincter muscle frequently accompanies the trauma and can be recognized by a characteristic V-shaped notching of the pupillary rim, which is seen with a slit lamp.

In some cases the iris musculature remains functional, but the lens subluxates. When the lens is loose it fails to support the iris, causing the iris to quiver on movement. Such shimmering or iridodonesis usually is visible to the naked eye. Irido-

donesis frequently is present after cataract extraction. At times iridodonesis occurs in normal eyes, especially in the large eye of the myope.

Infections. The iris reacts to infections and inflammations. Whenever the anterior segment of the eye is inflamed, as in iritis, the pupil becomes small owing to spasm of the sphincter pupillae, and its reactions to light and accommodation are diminished in amplitude. Photophobia is common. An inflamed iris responds to atropine and dilates, unless the inflammation has caused secondary changes with formation of adhesions (synechiae). Some viral infections, such as herpes zoster, can involve the iris so extensively that an actual iridoplegia supervenes and the pupil is nonreactive.

In syphilis several types of pupillary change can be found, the most common being the Argyll Robertson pupil. The pupils are small, often pinpoint; they react not at all to light, react briskly to accommodation, and dilate poorly following instillation of mydriatics (see Table 7-4). The dissociation of the reactions to light and accommodation distinguishes this condition. Pupils that have a dissociation of light and accommodation reactions and are not pinpoint are frequently seen in juvenile paresis, whereas the complete Argyll Robertson pupil is more often described in tabes dorsalis. Since a complete Argyll Robertson pupil often is premonitory to tabes dorsalis, it remains an important diagnostic sign.

Despite widespread, longstanding recognition of the Argyll Robertson pupil, the actual pathologic condition is not known. With recently improved diagnostic tech-

TABLE 7-4   COMPARISON BETWEEN THE PUPILLARY DISORDERS

Test	Argyll Robertson Pupil (Usually bilateral)	Tonic Pupil (Usually unilateral)
Light reaction	Absent	Usually decreased
Near reaction	Present and brisk	Present and delayed
Pupil size—ordinary room light	Small	Large
Dilatation to mydriatics	Poor	Good
Sensitivity to 2.5 per cent Mecholyl	Usually none	Present

niques, the luetic basis of Argyll Robertson pupil is being proved with even greater frequency in patients in whom it formerly was only suspected. Differential diagnosis is limited. Argyll Robertson–like pupils have been reported in herpes zoster, in pinealoma, and in other tumors in the region of the collicular plate, and rarely in diabetes mellitus. The diagnosis of Argyll Robertson pupil can be especially difficult in elderly patients whose pupils normally are somewhat miotic and are poorly reactive. Frequently it is diagnosed mistakenly in patients who have had long-term miotic therapy for glaucoma and whose pupils react poorly to any drugs because of the atrophy that follows prolonged drug use.

Since a blind eye will not react to light, but will react to accommodation, the diagnosis of Argyll Robertson pupil is reserved for sighted eyes to avoid confusion and misdiagnosis.

Tonic Pupil. It is important to differentiate the Argyll Robertson pupil, which is virtually pathognomonic of central nervous system lues, from tonic pupil, a benign disorder of pupillary motility without systemic implications. Characteristically tonic pupil has a decreased or absent light reflex, a slow or delayed contraction to near vision, and a slow or delayed redilatation phase. Unlike the Argyll Robertson pupil, the tonic pupil is usually unilateral and dilates well to mydriatics. The two conditions are compared in Table 7-4. In normal room light, the tonic pupil is not pinpoint, but is usually larger than its fellow normal pupil. Accommodation may be slowed measurably, and the knee and ankle reflexes may be depressed. The serology is negative. Because of its benign nature, no pathologic studies are available to define the lesions responsible. The tonic pupil, however, is supersensitive to parasympathomimetic drugs, thus making tenable a theory of peripheral denervation. The supersensitivity to parasympathomimetics constitutes the basis of a useful clinical test in which fresh, 2.5 per cent methacholine (Mecholyl) solution is instilled in both the normal and the affected eye. Generally, 2.5 per cent Mecholyl is too dilute to cause the normal pupil to constrict, but a significant miosis in 30 minutes in the

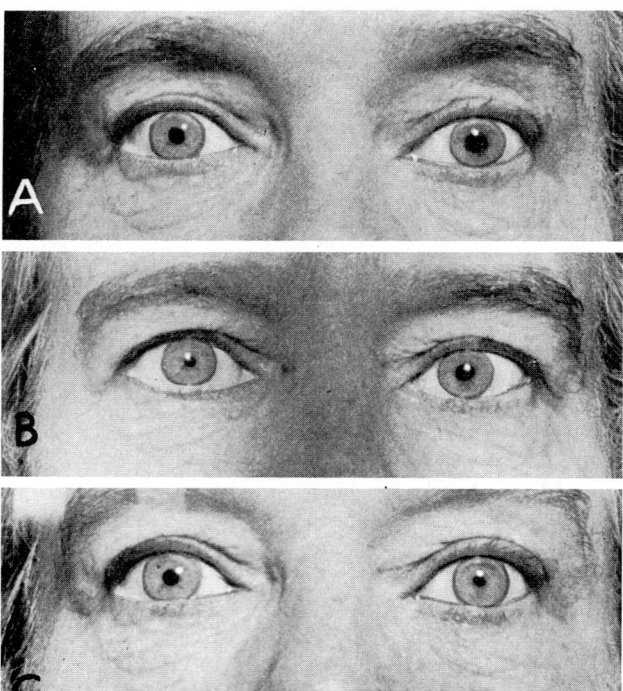

Figure 7-22 Patient with tonic left pupil. *(A)* Appearance of pupils as patient looks into infinity before instillation of Mecholyl. *(B)* Size of pupils on convergence. *(C)* Constriction of left pupil one-half hour after instillation of Mecholyl. (Scheie: *Arch. Ophth.* *24*:1940.)

tonic pupil usually is accepted as evidence of supersensitivity and as a capstone to diagnosis (Fig. 7-22). Once established, a tonic pupil lasts the lifetime of the patient as does the supersensitivity to cholinergic drugs. Accommodation may be lost for a time and then return.

Horner's Syndrome

Horner's syndrome is a denervation syndrome in which the sympathetic nervous supply to the eye has been lost. The pupil is miotic and the lid ptotic. The fibers that supply the sweat glands separate from the fibers that supply the pupil and the smooth muscles of the lid just after the superior cervical ganglion is reached in the neck. Thus if the sympathetic supply is cut in the middle cranial fossa or more anteriorly, a dissociated condition results in which sweating on the ipsilateral side of the face persists, while ptosis and miosis are evident. In contrast, involvement of the sympathetic innervation at or below the superior cervical ganglion results in a complete Horner's syndrome, in which ipsilateral loss of sweating (anhydrosis) accompanies ptosis and miosis. Many descriptions of Horner's syndrome include enophthalmos as one of its components. Enophthalmos, in most cases, is apparent because of the ptosis, but when the location of the globes is accurately measured, it is found not to be real. Occasionally, however, there is a small amount of enophthalmos in Horner's syndrome. Although usually not noted, the ocular tension on the denervated side is often a few millimeters of mercury less than on the normal side.

Horner's syndrome may follow a lesion anywhere along the long route of the sympathetic fibers through the brain stem, out from the spinal cord, up to the neck, along the carotid sheath, and forward in the middle cranial fossa to the orbit. There is no known crossing of these fibers. Lesions at any level from the hypothalamus down lead to ipsilateral change. In the brain stem vascular thromboses often affect the sympathetic pathways; outside the spinal cord the most common cause of Horner's syndrome is carcinoma of the lung, especially an apical tumor; the sudden onset of the syndrome in an adult male makes a roent-

genogram of the chest mandatory. Among other causes of Horner's syndrome is unintentional injury to the sympathetic chain during carotid arteriography. The permanent sympathetic denervation that can follow birth injury is responsible for a failure of normal pigmentation to develop in the iris, resulting in heterochromia, with the iris on the denervated side lighter in color (Plate 28H).

OCULAR MOTOR NERVES

The Third Nerve. The third nerve contains somatic motor fibers to supply the inferior rectus, the inferior oblique, the superior rectus, the medial rectus, the levator of the lid, and, in addition, visceral motor (parasympathetic) fibers to the iris sphincter and ciliary muscles. Selective loss of autonomic innervation to the intraocular structures may occur with sparing of the innervation to the extraocular muscles (a condition usually called internal ophthalmoplegia). Conversely the extraocular muscles may be afflicted with palsy, with sparing of the iris sphincter and ciliary muscles (external ophthalmoplegia). Loss of all third nerve function (total oculomotor ophthalmoplegia) results in ptosis, outward deviation of the eye, a dilated and non-

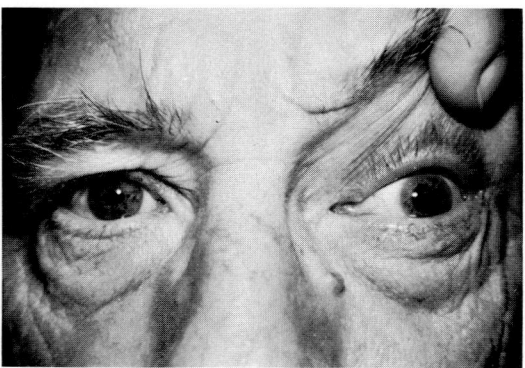

Figure 7-23 Complete third nerve palsy. Ptotic left lid is elevated to show exotropic eye. Pupil is dilated and nonreactive to light or accommodation. The eye can be neither elevated nor adducted.

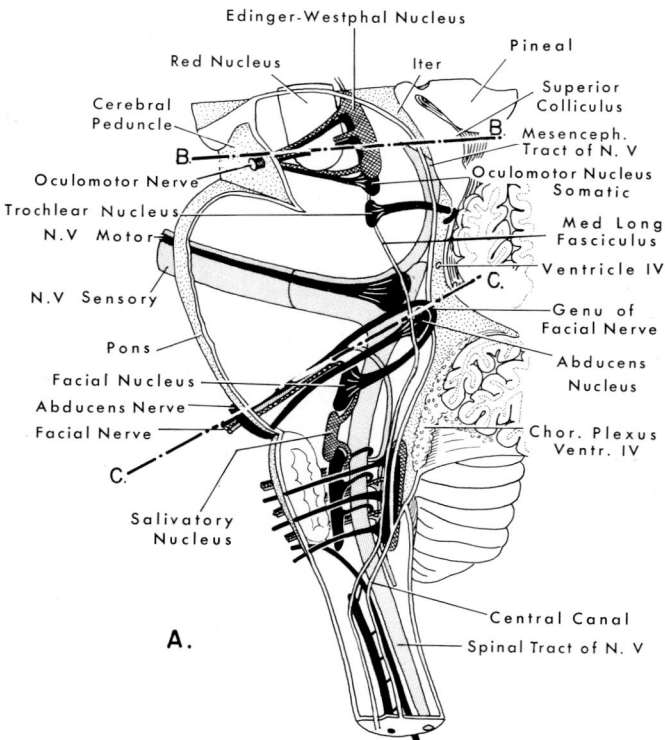

Figure 7-24   Relation of ocular motor nuclei to other brain stem structures as illustrated in schematic diagrams. *(A)* Sagittal view. Note long pathway of medial longitudinal fasciculus, which plays important role in control of horizontal eye movement. Curious dorsal arching course of fourth nerve contrasts with simpler path of its neighbor, the third nerve. Complex relation between abducens nucleus and facial nerve fibers is illustrated also in *C.*

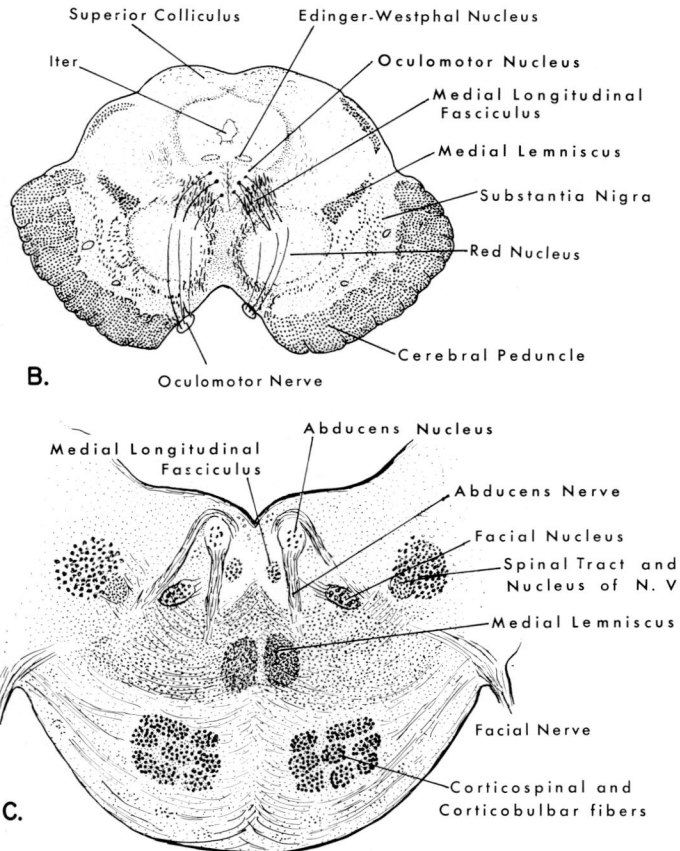

Figure 7-24 *Continued.*

(B) Note pathway followed by oculomotor nerve fibers through red nucleus. Also note their proximity to cerebral peduncles as they emerge from brain stem. An understanding of these anatomical relations helps in an understanding of the nature of common brain stem syndromes.

(C) Abducens nucleus sends fibers ventrally. These fibers pass near the medial longitudinal fasciculus, the medial lemniscus, and the corticospinal pathway before they leave the pons.

reactive pupil, and complete loss of accommodation (Fig. 7-23).

In an oculomotor palsy topical localization depends largely on the presence or absence of associated findings. Lesions within the substance of the midbrain are most often vascular and give additional signs of neurologic involvement, e.g., when the third nerve is affected in its passage through the red nucleus a tremor of the contralateral limbs accompanies the oculomotor palsy (Benedikt's syndrome) (Fig. 7-24A, B). If the lesion is extensive enough to involve the medial lemniscus, a contralateral hemianesthesia is superimposed. A combination of third nerve palsy and contralateral hemiplegia (Weber's syndrome) is often described as a result of thrombosis of small vessels to the cerebral peduncle at the base of the midbrain (Fig. 7-24B). Since the oculomotor nerve passes near the peduncle as many independent fillets, it is common for the resulting third nerve palsy to be incomplete. The interruption to the corticospinal motor pathways is supranuclear and high enough to involve the innervation to the tongue and face. Just outside the brain stem the third nerve may be affected by relatively diffuse processes such as tuberculous meningitis. Improved public health measures, however, have made central nervous system tuberculosis a rare disease.

The most common conditions to affect the third nerve as it passes from the midbrain to the eye are aneurysm, diabetes mellitus, and tumor. Intracranial aneurysm can lead to third nerve palsy either in its "silent" phase or when subarachnoid bleeding occurs. In both instances the pupil usually is dilated. In diabetes mellitus it is common to have the painful, rather sudden onset of an oculomotor palsy with sparing of the pupil. Diabetics with third nerve palsy are often managed conservatively because many of them are beyond the age when neurosurgery would be contemplated, even if an aneurysm were to be found. They usually recover with few sequelae. In succeeding years, however, it is not uncommon for another cranial nerve, either the third on the opposite side or one of the sixth nerves, suddenly to become paretic.

Tumors in the region of the cavernous sinus, either primary or metastatic, often cause third nerve palsy. Gradual onset and involvement of neighboring structures often aids in their differential diagnosis. As they progress, a cavernous sinus syndrome is produced. In its complete form this syndrome comprises paresis of cranial nerves three, four, and six, loss of sensation over the distribution of the trigeminal nerve's first and second divisions, and exophthalmos.

It is wise to suspect the use of a mydriatic, such as atropine, in a patient with internal ophthalmoplegia who is otherwise healthy. A simple and effective clinical test is the application of a single drop of 1 per cent pilocarpine solution; this will not affect the pupil after a mydriatic, but it will constrict the denervated iris.

When a patient with increased intracranial pressure develops a unilateral, dilated pupil, it is an early sign of uncal herniation. This constitutes a neurosurgical emergency, for the internal ophthalmoplegia presages external ophthalmoplegia and neurological decompensation.

The Fourth Nerve. The superior oblique muscle, which plays an important role in rotating the eye down and in to the reading position, is innervated solely by the fourth cranial nerve. Isolated palsies are infrequent. When present, paralysis of the superior oblique leads to double vision in which the images of the two eyes are tilted with respect to one another. Such torsional diplopia is considerably more annoying than the simple horizontal displacement of images found with paralyses of horizontally acting muscles. It is common for these patients, especially children, to avoid the field of action of the paretic superior oblique muscle by tilting the head toward the opposite shoulder, thereby substituting an ocular torticollis (wry neck) for the annoying diplopia. Such signs, however, are not universally found. An adult with a fresh superior oblique palsy usually complains of blurred vision, which is his way of describing double vision.

Owing to the unusual decussation of the trochlear nerve fibers in the anterior medullary velum, a tumor in this region can result in bilateral fourth nerve palsy (Fig. 7-24). The decussation of the fibers of the trochlear nerve also lays a rational groundwork for an ipsilateral third nerve palsy and a contralateral fourth nerve palsy. This occurs when a single, one-sided lesion damages the contiguous oculomotor and trochlear cell columns at the junction of the midbrain and the pons. Lesions in and around the cavernous sinus usually cause paresis of the superior oblique. This is associated with paresis of the ipsilateral third and/or sixth nerves. Lastly, the superior oblique function depends on the fragile mechanical arrangement of a long tendon to the superior oblique muscle acting through a pulley fixed to the bone on the medial wall of the orbit. Dislocation of the pulley by trauma, especially by a gouge in boxing or by sinus surgery, will result in an apparent superior oblique palsy in which the muscle is healthy but cannot act for lack of mechanical advantage.

The Sixth Nerve. The abducens nerve innervates a single ocular muscle, the lateral rectus, which abducts the eye. Paresis of this muscle results in horizontal diplopia that is maximal when an attempt is made to turn the eye into its field of action and absent when the eye is turned away from its field of action (Fig. 7-25). Consequently, it is common for a patient with a unilateral, sixth-nerve paresis to avoid diplopia by turning his head toward the

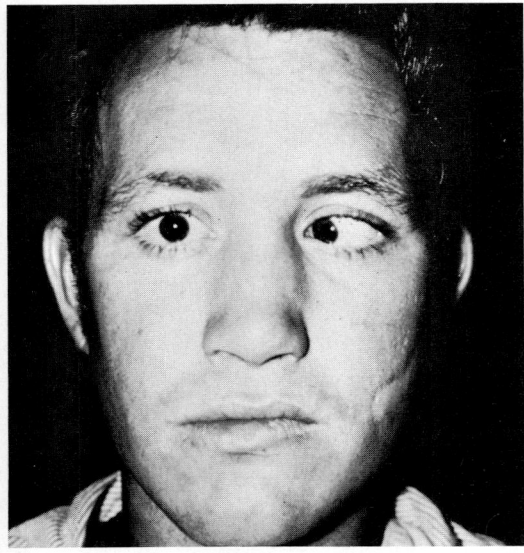

Figure 7-25 Abducens nerve palsy. Left eye could not be brought outward further than midline. In straight ahead gaze, eye is turned inward by unopposed tonus of intact medial rectus muscle.

side of the paretic muscle, which takes the eye through the action of the normal medial rectus out of the field of action of the paretic lateral rectus.

The abducens nerve is distinguished among the cranial nerves by its length and by its hazardous pathway from the brain stem to the orbit. It is especially susceptible to damage when the intracranial pressure is elevated, and, although common, its failure in such instances either unilaterally or bilaterally has no localizing value. Localization is only possible when an abducens palsy occurs with associated signs. Within the pons, the nucleus of the abducens is intimately related to the looping course of the facial nerve fibers. When an artery supplying the paramedian area of the lower pons occludes, the result can be paralysis of both the sixth and seventh nerves and a crossed hemiplegia (Millard-Gubler syndrome); both cranial nerves and the corticospinal pathways are affected. At the same level a lesion at the base may spare the facial nerve but involve the abducens nerve and the corticospinal tract, leading to an abducens palsy on one side and a hemiplegia on the other side. Palsy of eye muscles in association with a contralateral hemiplegia makes it possible for the level involved to be estimated accurately. The abducens nerve emerges from the brain stem at the junction of the pons and medulla, turns abruptly upward, and remains close to the brain stem until it bends forward under the petrosphenoid ligament (Gruber's ligament) to enter the middle cranial fossa.

Before the advent of antibiotics, middle ear infections frequently spread into the petrous bone, involving the overlying meninges and the nearby fifth and sixth cranial nerves. Pain, often referred to the eye, and diplopia due to the sixth nerve palsy (Gradenigo's syndrome) often preceded cerebral abscess or lateral sinus thrombosis. Today, when this now rare syndrome occurs, it usually disappears with the administration of high dosages of antibiotics without sequelae. Within the cavernous sinus the sixth nerve is affected frequently by pathologic processes, such as cavernous sinus thrombosis, tumor, or aneurysm, but the involvement offers few distinctive features. Generally, when cavernous sinus lesions affect the sixth nerve, they also involve cranial nerves 3, 4, or 5. Lesions at the superior orbital fissure commonly affect the sixth nerve and are also localized by the associated involvement of other neighboring cranial nerves.

As mentioned previously (p. 163), congenital defects in the formation or function of the lateral rectus muscle can lead to the erroneous diagnosis of sixth nerve palsy. This is especially true in Duane's syndrome (p. 164). When the lateral rectus appears to be weakened, myasthenia gravis and thyrotropic exophthalmos should be sought, since its function is often deficient in these conditions.

Supranuclear Lesions

Characteristically, supranuclear lesions in the ocular motor system affect both eyes and typically involve conjugate gaze movements, allowing the globes to remain aligned in parallel. Lesions in a single motor nerve to the eye or in its nucleus affect the motions of a single eye and lead to malalignment of the globes. Thus lesions in the cortex and in the subcortical motor pathways result in conjugate deviations of the eyes, deviations that are not accompanied by diplopia in that the eyes are still in parallel. In cortical lesions the direction in which the eyes turn depends both on the location and on the nature of the lesion. Irritative foci in either the frontal or the occipital eye fields turn the eyes toward the opposite side. It is common, for instance, to find adversive, conjugate deviation of the eyes during epileptic seizures. In contrast, when destructive lesions involve the cortical gaze centers, the eyes turn toward the side of the lesion.

In the unconscious patient deviation toward the side of the lesion often aids in ascertaining laterality. When a patient is conscious, he may experience difficulty in attempting to rotate his eyes into the contralateral field of gaze; in fact, he may not be able to gaze in the contralateral direc-

tion. In less severe cases, he simply may have difficulty sustaining a lateral gaze position. As a practical matter, patients with a horizontal gaze paresis are commonly thought to be uncooperative in a routine examination. Generally when a patient is unable to follow an object into a certain gaze position, he simply states that he can see it, all the while keeping his gaze fixed straight ahead. The presence of a gaze paresis becomes apparent when, with constant urging, the patient fails to turn his eyes in one direction, whereas he readily turns them in the other.

Within the brain stem the gaze mechanisms for vertical and horizontal gaze are separate. Vertical gaze often is disturbed in lesions at or above the superior colliculi (Fig. 7-24), resulting in a clinical syndrome first delineated by Parinaud. Loss of upward and downward gaze frequently is accompanied in this syndrome by absence of convergence and by abnormal pupillary reactions. With relief of pressure, as when a pinealoma shrinks after treatment by x-irradiation, the entire syndrome can disappear.

Lesions within the substance of the pons often play havoc with the horizontal gaze mechanism that operates through the medial longitudinal fasciculus (Fig. 7-24A, B, C). Such lesions result in a syndrome in which horizontal eye movements are disconjugate. This syndrome is called internuclear ophthalmoplegia because the pathologic process interrupts the medial longitudinal fasciculus between the third nerve nucleus in the midbrain and the sixth nerve nucleus in the lower pons. It is discovered when an attempt is made to gaze laterally; the eye that should move into the adducted position does not, and the eye that should abduct does, but it undergoes coarse nystagmus in so doing. Although a similar coarse-abduction nystagmus can be seen in sixth nerve paresis, the combination of paresis of adduction and abduction nystagmus is distinctive. The fact that convergence usually is preserved indicates that the supranuclear connections, and not the nucleus itself, have led to failure of the medial rectus muscle. Multiple sclerosis is commonly present in bilateral cases, whereas in unilateral cases involvement, usually vascular in origin, is seen with unusual frequency in hypertensives. Once established, the syndrome tends to be permanent.

BIBLIOGRAPHY

Cogan, D. G.: Neurology of the Ocular Muscles. 2nd ed. Springfield, Ill., Charles C Thomas, 1956.

Cogan, D. G.: Neurology of the Visual System. Springfield, Ill., Charles C Thomas, 1966.

Ford, F. R.: Diseases of the Nervous System in Infancy, Childhood and Adolescence. 5th ed. Springfield, Ill., Charles C Thomas, 1966.

Hoyt, W. F., and Beeston, D.: The Ocular Fundus in Neurological Disease. St. Louis, The C. V. Mosby Co., 1966.

Kearns, T. P.: Neuro-ophthalmology. Arch. Ophth. 79:87, 1968.

Kestenbaum, A.: Clinical Methods of Neuro-ophthalmologic Examination. 2nd ed. New York, Grune & Stratton, 1961.

Lombardi, G.: Radiology in Neuro-ophthalmology. Baltimore, Williams & Wilkins Co., 1967.

Lowenfeld, I.: Mechanisms of reflex dilatation of the pupil. Docum. Ophth. 12:185, 1958.

Merritt, H. H.: Textbook of Neurology. Philadelphia, Lea & Febiger, 1967.

Toole, J. F., and Patel, A. N.: Cerebrovascular Disorders. New York, McGraw-Hill Book Co., 1967.

Strong, O. S., and Elwyn, A.: Human Neuroanatomy. 5th ed. R. C. Truex and M. B. Carpenter (eds.). Baltimore, Williams & Wilkins Co., 1964.

Walsh, F. B. and Hoyt, W. F.: Clinical Neuro-ophthalmology. 3rd ed. Baltimore, Williams & Wilkins Co., 1969.

Chapter Eight

GLAUCOMA

Glaucoma is a common cause (approximately 15 per cent) of blindness in adults in the United States. Recent surveys indicate that at least one in every 40 individuals over 40 years of age has the disease.

Blindness from glaucoma can be prevented by present-day medicine and surgery with early recognition and treatment. Every physician should be aware of the disease and understand something of present-day concepts. He should be well informed about its symptoms and constantly alert for its possible presence.

In glaucoma the intraocular pressure is elevated to a dangerous level. The glaucomatous eye might be compared to an overly inflated basketball in which pressure is transmitted equally to all parts. Since the optic nerve is highly vulnerable to damage by increased intraocular pressure, loss of vision results.

The relatively constant flow of aqueous humor into and out of the eye normally maintains intraocular pressure at 20 mm. Hg or somewhat less (Plate 29*A*). Aqueous humor, both a secretory product and a filtrate, is formed just behind the iris by the ciliary body. The substance then flows forward between the iris and the lens, through the pupillary space, and into the anterior chamber from which it escapes into the venous system of the body through a specialized drainage apparatus at the periphery of the chamber (p. 70). Upon leaving the eye, aqueous humor traverses the trabecula, flows through the canal of Schlemm, and then enters the venous system via the aqueous veins. Control mechanisms, as yet hypothetical, probably affect the rate of production and escape of aqueous from the eye. These neurogenic, enzymatic, and hormonal mechanisms have all been postulated.

Increased intraocular pressure could result from obstruction (increased resistance) to outflow from the eye, increased rate of formation of aqueous humor, or increased osmolality of the aqueous with retention of fluid within the eye. The first is probably the chief cause of primary glaucoma, but hypersecretion of aqueous occasionally is another cause. Many different causes of obstruction will be uncovered, and their precise location within the drainage apparatus will undoubtedly be determined.

CLASSIFICATION OF GLAUCOMA

Glaucoma is generally divided into two broad groups, primary and secondary. By definition, primary glaucoma is unrelated to other ocular disease. Secondary glaucoma occurs as a consequence of another recognizable ocular abnormality or disease,

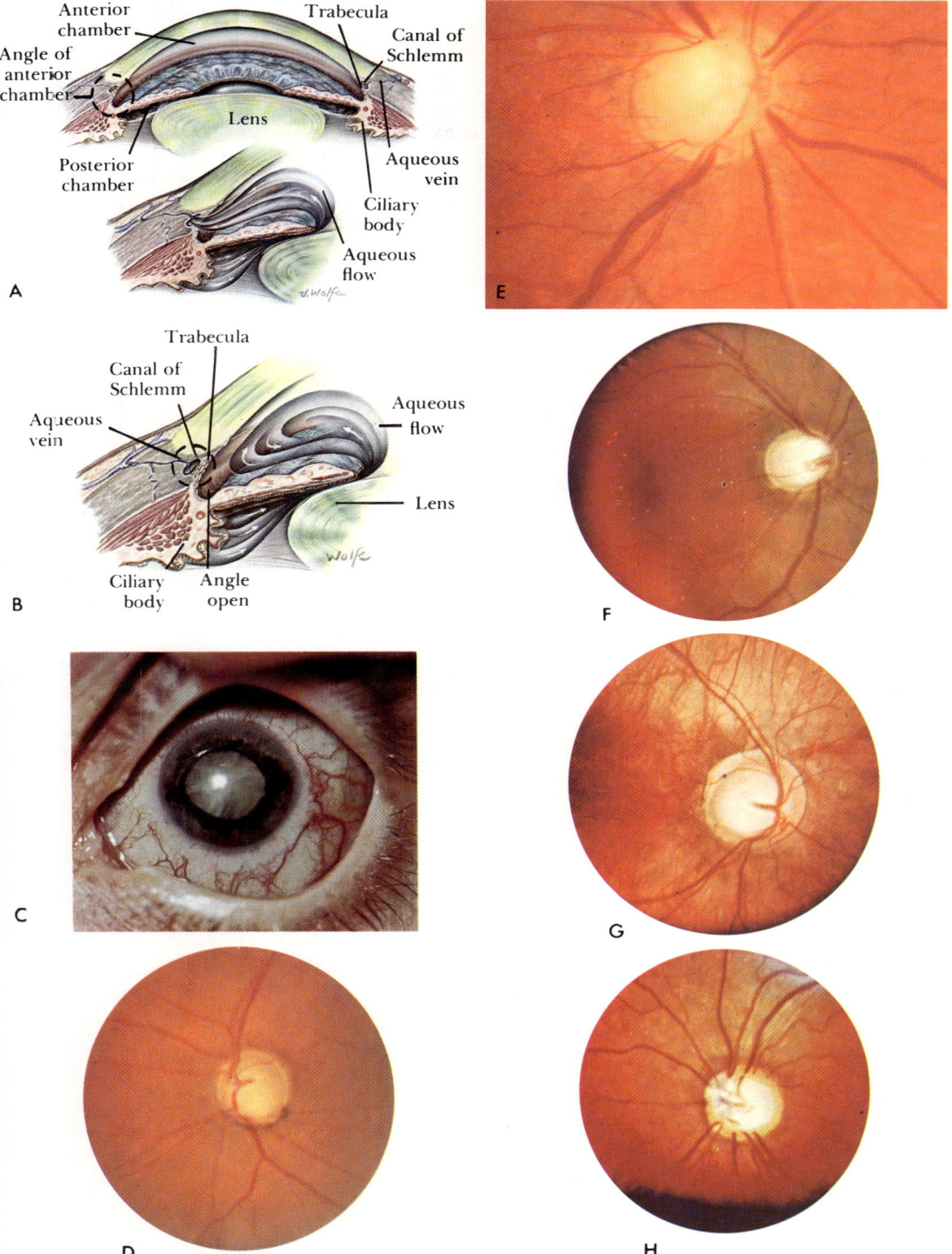

Plate 29 *(A)* Drawing that shows flow of aqueous from ciliary body leaving eye through the trabecula and canal of Schlemm via a normal open, wide angle. *(B)* Chronic simple glaucoma. Arrows indicate obstruction to aqueous outflow in angle wall. *(C)* Dilated vessels of caput medusa with advanced glaucoma. *(D)* Early glaucoma cupping. *(E)* Moderate glaucoma cupping. *(F)* Moderately advanced glaucoma cupping. *(G)* Advanced glaucoma cupping. *(H)* Very advanced glaucoma cupping with atrophy.

such as intraocular tumor, inflammation, vascular disorder, or injury.

The following simple classification of glaucoma is suggested:

I. Primary glaucoma
   A. Glaucoma in the adult
      1. Chronic simple (open, wide angle) glaucoma
      2. Narrow angle (angle closure, iris block) glaucoma
   B. Congenital glaucoma
      1. Juvenile
      2. Infantile
   C. Absolute glaucoma
II. Secondary glaucoma

PRIMARY GLAUCOMA

Primary glaucoma can occur at any time in life from in utero to old age. The adult form, occurring in individuals over 30 years of age, may be acute or chronic. Chronic simple glaucoma occurs much more frequently than acute glaucoma, but the incidence of both increases significantly after 40 years of age. Each is a separate entity requiring different management.

Congenital glaucoma, sometimes defined as glaucoma occurring in individuals under 30 years of age, is separable into infantile and juvenile types. Its incidence is much lower than that of glaucoma of older individuals. Infantile glaucoma may be fully developed and present characteristic signs at birth, or it may develop at any time up to 2 or 3 years of age. The characteristic signs of the disease result from the inability of the fibrous coats (cornea and sclera) of the infant eye to withstand increased intraocular pressure. The eyeball, therefore, enlarges, sometimes dramatically (buphthalmos).

Juvenile glaucoma occurs in older children and in young adults up to 30 years of age whose eyeballs no longer grossly enlarge. The age limit and the terminology are designated for several reasons: a congenital origin, or predisposition, seems likely in this age group; the term calls attention to the possible presence of glaucoma in children and young adults at ages when it often is overlooked; and the surgical management and response of these age groups are somewhat different from that of individuals over 30 years of age.

Absolute glaucoma is an entity only by definition. The term is applied to any eye, usually a painful one, which is blind as a result of glaucoma of any type or from any cause.

Primary Glaucoma in the Adult

Our present day knowledge of primary glaucoma has stemmed largely from gonioscopic and tonographic studies of aqueous outflow. Gonioscopy, widely used only recently, permits visualization of the angle of the anterior chamber and the trabecula. Such observations enable the ophthalmologist to separate glaucoma into two types and to recognize them clinically: chronic simple (open, wide angle) glaucoma, characterized by an open angle and a chronic, insidious course; and narrow angle (angle closure, iris block, acute congestive) glaucoma, characterized by a very narrow or closed angle and episodes of high intraocular pressure associated with acute congestive attacks that cause pain and blurred vision. Not only are two types recognizable, but also the treatment for each is quite different. Chronic simple glaucoma should be managed by medicine whenever possible; narrow angle glaucoma should be treated primarily by surgery.

CHRONIC SIMPLE (OPEN, WIDE ANGLE) GLAUCOMA

Mechanism. In chronic simple glaucoma the angle is open and, as shown by gonioscopy, the aqueous is in free contact with the trabecula (Plate 29B). Since, as shown by tonography, increased resistance to aqueous outflow is the cause of elevated intraocular pressure, the obstruction must be located within the drainage apparatus itself at one or more of the following sites: the trabecula, the canal of Schlemm, or the aqueous veins that lead from the canal into the venous system. The degree of obstruction generally is related to the elevation in intraocular pressure.

Diagnosis. Diagnosing chronic simple

TABLE 8-1   STEPS IN THE DIAGNOSIS OF WIDE
ANGLE (CHRONIC SIMPLE) GLAUCOMA

1. Symptoms: usually none or minimal.
2. Visual acuity: normal until disease is advanced.
3. External examination: few changes.
4. Ophthalmoscopic examination: normal to markedly cupped disc.
5. Slit lamp examination: negative.
6. Tension: elevated.
7. Gonioscopic examination: variable angle depths.
8. Visual fields: normal to typical defects of glaucoma.
9. Provocative tests—water drinking: positive in 82 per cent.
10. Tonographic studies: diminished aqueous outflow.

glaucoma presents many challenges because the disease evokes few symptoms and may progress slowly to blindness without causing discomfort. Early diagnosis, which is essential to prevent visual loss, requires the physician to be highly suspicious and always alert to the possibility of the disease. Although the incidence increases rapidly in patients over 40 years of age, its occurrence at any time in life must be kept in mind. Meticulous, complete, ocular examinations are essential, and repeated observations and prolonged follow-up may be necessary for adequate evaluation. The following routine examination and diagnostic tests are suggested (Table 8-1).

HISTORY.   Chronic simple glaucoma presents few symptoms. Occasionally a patient may experience dull headaches when the pressure is high. Fluctuations in pressure are characteristic, but they usually are not marked and occur gradually. Diurnal variations of a few millimeters of mercury, with elevations during the night and early morning hours, have been used for diagnostic purposes. High and rather rapid rises in intraocular pressure, however, may occur after the patient has taken large amounts of fluid. At such times edema of the corneal epithelium may give blurred vision and a rainbow effect or halo around lights. This is especially true of young individuals with glaucoma because their intraocular pressure tends to be more labile with rapid rises and falls. The course, however, usually is painless, and visual loss may be so gradual that the patient is unaware of any difficulty until marked visual loss has occurred. A family history is of great importance because of hereditary disposition.

VISUAL ACUITY.   Visual acuity is of little or no diagnostic value because central vision (central visual field) is preserved until blindness is imminent.

EXTERNAL EXAMINATION.   The eye appears normal to external inspection unless the disease is far advanced. Pupillary contraction, then, may be poor due to atrophy of the pupillary musculature, and the episcleral vessels (caput medusae) may be dilated (Plate 29C).

OPHTHALMOSCOPIC EXAMINATION.   Ideally, the diagnosis should be made before glaucoma cupping and atrophy of the optic nerve appear. Although cupping is not an early diagnostic sign, it is characteristic (Plate 29D to H). The optic nerve is vulnerable to pressure owing partly to its blood supply, which comes from the arterial circle of Haller-Zinn, and partly to the weak structure of the lamina cribrosa of the sclera, through which the optic nerve passes. Cupping and optic atrophy result from outward bowing of the lamina cribrosa and from damage to the optic nerve fibers (Fig. 8-1A, B). The nerve fibers are particularly vulnerable at the upper and lower poles of the optic nerve and characteristic visual field defects develop.

Glaucoma cupping begins with enlargement of the physiologic blind spot. This progresses temporally, above and below, causing the normal pink rim of optic nerve between the cup and the disc margin to disappear gradually. As the cup enlarges it also deepens and the retinal vessels can be seen to break sharply at the disc border where they descend into the cup. Also, the central retinal artery and vein are displaced nasally. Simultaneously, the optic nerve becomes increasingly pale (atrophic).

Early in the disease, the optic nerve may be normal or the nerve head may show only minimal cupping. Any suggestive cup, however, should be considered glaucomatous until the disease can be excluded. Visual field studies should be done to search for defects typical of glaucoma.

SLIT LAMP BIOMICROSCOPIC EXAMINATION.   Examination of the eye by this means is of little help in the early diagnosis of chronic simple glaucoma, but it is essential in differentiating primary glaucoma

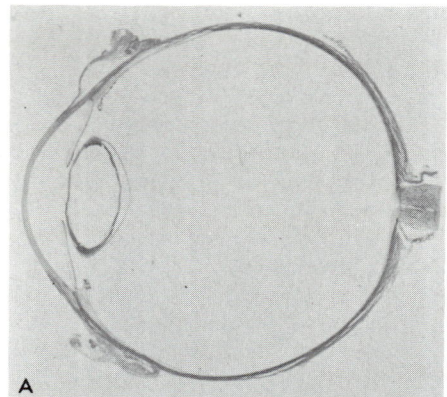

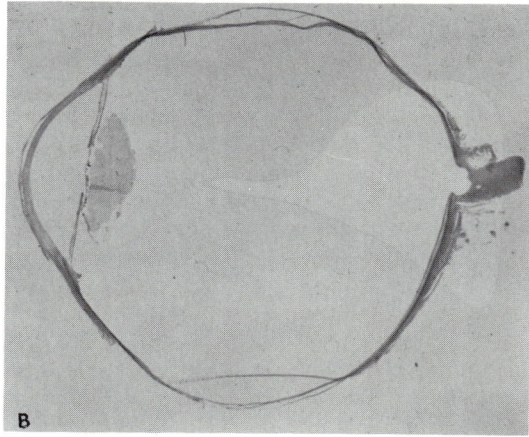

Figure 8-1 Photographs of microscopic sagittal section of eye. *(A)* Normal optic nerve head without cupping. *(B)* Normal optic nerve head with cupping.

from secondary glaucoma, including pigmentary glaucoma, glaucoma associated with pseudoexfoliation of the lens capsule, uveitis, and other conditions (p. 419).

TONOMETRY. Tonometry measures intraocular pressure and is the single most important test for diagnosing chronic simple glaucoma. It should be a routine part of each ophthalmologic examination. The two most commonly used tonometers are the Schiötz and the Goldmann (Fig. 8-2*A*, *B*). Since each must be applied to the cornea, topical instillation anesthesia is needed. Ophthaine is very satisfactory and quick acting, but any good surface anesthetic such as tetracaine HCl is acceptable.

Schiötz Indentation Tonometer. This is the most popular tonometer because it is relatively inexpensive, readily available, easy to use, and durable. It is accurate and highly satisfactory for everyday clinical use.

The instrument is applied to the anesthetized cornea with the patient's head in a horizontal position. The intraocular pressure is measured indirectly and depends upon how deeply the plunger of the tonometer indents the cornea. The softer the eye, the greater the indentation and the higher the scale reading on the tonometer. The harder the eye, the less the indentation and the lower the reading. A calibration table is then used to convert the scale reading into mm. Hg of intraocular pressure.

Goldmann Applanation Tonometer. This tonometer is attached to a slit lamp biomicroscope, and the pressure is measured

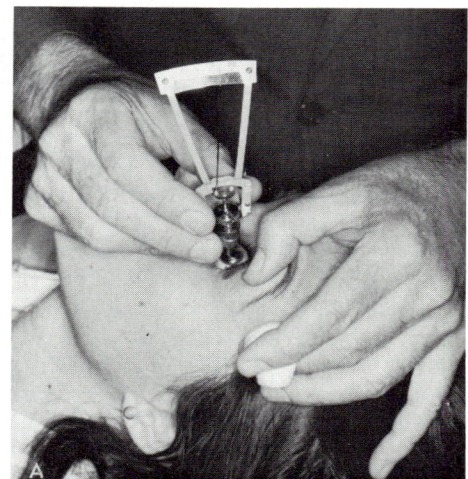

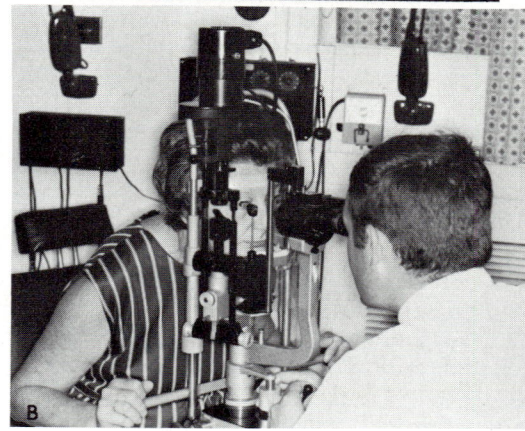

Figure 8-2 Measurement of intraocular pressure. *(A)* Schiötz tonometer. *(B)* Applanation tonometer.

as in slit lamp biomicroscopy with the patient in an upright position. The intraocular pressure is determined by measuring the force needed to flatten an area of the cornea 3.06 mm. in diameter. The Goldmann tonometer is more accurate than the Schiötz, but it is somewhat more difficult to use and it is more time-consuming. It is the choice, however, for clinical research and to verify or check a Schiötz reading that may seem at variance with the clinical picture. Since the Schiötz instrument relies upon the pressure required for indentation, it may give false high or low measurements of intraocular pressure in the occasional eye whose corneal-scleral rigidity is greater or less than normal.

Although normal intraocular pressure is 20 mm. Hg or less, as with all physiologic measurements variations occur from individual to individual and from day to day. Also, the ability of a given eye to withstand a given level of intraocular pressure may not be the same. A borderline elevation in pressure, therefore, may be normal for one individual, whereas for another the eye may not tolerate pressures well within the normal range.

The term "low tension glaucoma" has been applied to the eye that develops characteristic optic nerve and visual field changes of glaucoma but whose pressure readings are normal repeatedly. Thus to diagnose glaucoma on borderline pressure readings alone can be erroneous. Intraocular pressure readings of 21 mm. Hg or more, however, should be regarded with suspicion, and the patient should be studied carefully and followed.

GONIOSCOPIC EXAMINATION. Gonioscopic examination (p. 436) should be done after tonometry, because the gonioscopic lens exerts significant external pressure upon the globe and lowers the intraocular pressure (Fig. 8-3A, B). If done before tonometry, therefore, low pressure readings will result. Gonioscopy should be done whenever glaucoma is suspected or if the angle of the anterior chamber is found to be narrow on slit lamp biomicroscopic examination. This is of the utmost importance in separating chronic simple from narrow angle glaucoma, but it does not help to diagnose chronic simple glaucoma because of the normal angle of the anterior chamber. Gonioscopy is important also as a supplement to slit lamp bio-

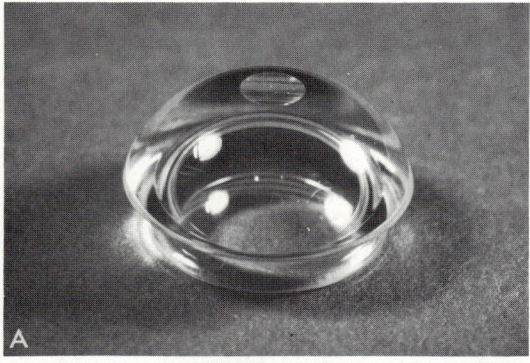
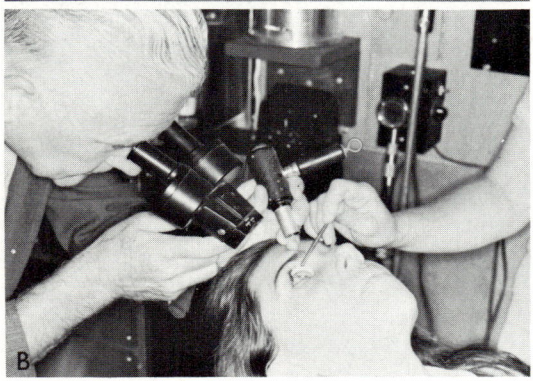

Figure 8-3 Gonioscopy. (A) Koeppe gonioscopic lens for study of contour and depth of angle. (B) Gonioscopic examination.

microscopic examination in differentiating primary glaucoma from the secondary glaucomas which often show angle abnormalities. Angle depth always should be evaluated. Although the angle is open in chronic simple glaucoma, the depth may range from wide open to very narrow, as in the normal population.

PERIMETRY. Any patient with a suspiciously cupped optic nerve should have his visual fields examined. True glaucoma cupping and optic atrophy give characteristic arcuate or nerve-fiber bundle defects that rarely are seen without cupping, although a surprising amount of cupping may occur at times with no demonstrable visual field defect. Even when the diagnosis is obvious without them, however, visual field examinations should be done repeatedly to follow the progress of the disease and for effective treatment.

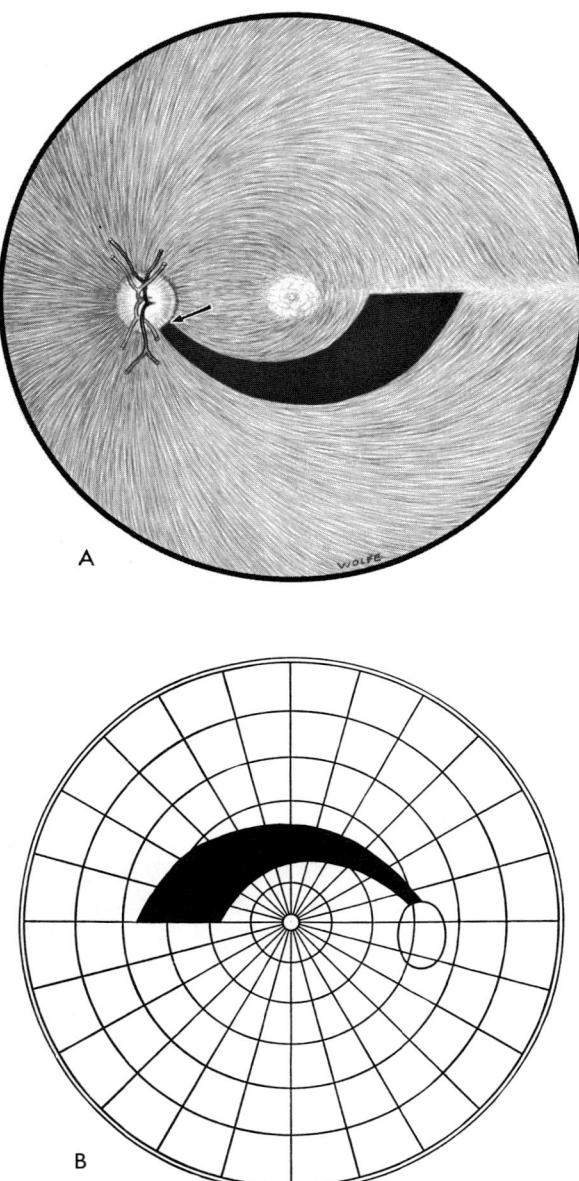

Figure 8-4 Visual fields in glaucoma.

(A) Lesion interrupting arcuate fibers at lower pole of optic nerve (arrow).
(B) Superior arcuate visual field defect from lesion in *A*; typical of glaucoma.

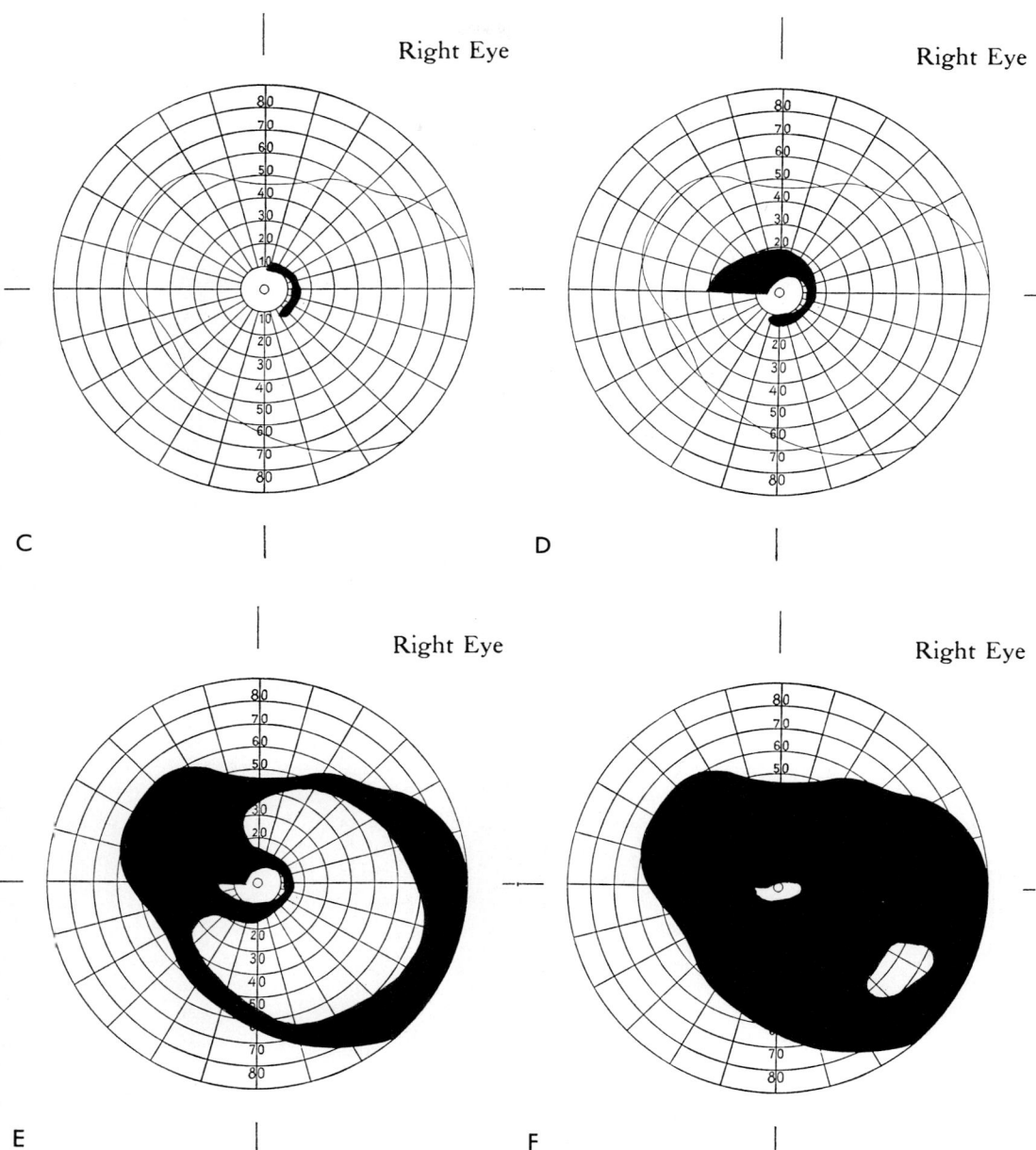

Figure 8-4 *Continued*

(C) Glaucoma defect arching upward and downward from blind spot (right eye).
(D) Arcuate nerve fiber bundle defect superiorly; partial defect inferiorly (right eye).
(E) Defects arching above and below fixation to meet in a nasal step (right eye).
(F) Loss of entire field except small areas centrally and temporally (right eye).

Advanced visual field defects may extend to the periphery of the field, but early defects are detected in the central 30 degrees that can be studied on the tangent screen at 1 meter with 1 or 2 mm. white test objects.

The arcuate nerve fibers that supply the superior and inferior temporal quadrants of the retina are the first to be damaged by increased intraocular pressure (Fig. 8-4A). They originate from the ganglion cells of the entire temporal area of the retina and run to the upper and lower poles of the optic nerves along an archlike course that sweeps around the macula above and below. The longest fibers come from ganglion cells above and below the horizontal raphe, a line on the 180 degree meridian that begins at a point adjacent to the macula temporally and extends to the periphery of the retina. The shortest fibers arise near the disc. Visual field defects in glaucoma may extend from the upper and lower poles of the physiologic blind spot to the horizontal raphe, depending upon the degree of damage to the arcuate nerve fibers (Fig. 8-4B to F).

Usually the initial visual field defect is enlargement of the blind spot, which may occur at the upper or lower pole, or both. This is termed "winging of the blind spot" or Seidel's sign. As the defect increases, it extends along the path of the arcuate nerve fibers and results in the classic arcuate or nerve-fiber bundle scotoma. When complete, such a scotoma extends superiorly or inferiorly from the blind spot arching around the macula and ending in a straight line on the horizontal raphe of the nasal side of the field, corresponding to the temporal raphe in the retina (Bjerrum's scotoma). If it occurs either above or below, corresponding localized cupping can be seen at the upper or lower pole of the disc. If it develops above and below simultaneously, a ring scotoma is present around the macula. The steplike visual field defect at the horizontal raphe is called the Roenne step.

As the disease progresses, so does destruction of vision. Macular vision, however, is retained until the disease is far advanced; thus patients frequently are unaware of visual loss until they are practically blind.

Even after loss of central vision, however, a residual portion of the temporal field frequently may be retained. Some conditions such as pituitary tumors, tabes dorsalis, and coloboma of the optic nerve can produce visual field defects suggestive of glaucoma.

PROVOCATIVE TESTS. These should be done on all patients whose ocular findings suggest chronic simple glaucoma. Among the most popular tests are the water drinking (done alone or in combination with tonography [Becker]) and the use of locally applied corticosteroids.

Water Drinking. This test (also called water provocative) probably is the most widely used. It depends upon the simple procedure of flooding the tissues with water to cause an increased flow of aqueous through the eye. The patient comes to the office in the morning after having taken nothing to eat or drink after midnight and having been instructed to discontinue at least two days beforehand any medication for glaucoma that he may have been taking. After his intraocular pressure is recorded, he drinks one liter of water within five minutes. Subsequently the pressure is recorded at 20-minute intervals for at least one hour. If the eye is glaucomatous, the pressure rises from increased resistance to aqueous outflow. A rise of 8 mm. Hg or more is significant. In patients with known glaucoma, the test is positive more than 80 per cent of the time, but like all provocative tests it is more reliable in severe glaucoma than in mild.

Tonography. This diagnostic test is based on the principle that pressure on the normal eyeball forces aqueous humor from the eye and results in reduced intraocular pressure. The less the resistance to aqueous outflow, the greater the escape of aqueous from the eye, and hence the greater the fall in intraocular pressure.

The plunger of the electronic tonometer of known weight is placed upon the eye, and the pressure is recorded continuously for four minutes by a galvanometer. Initial and final pressures are read from the tracing, and the coefficient of facility of aqueous humor outflow is calculated. Outflow is measured in cubic millimeters (cu. mm.) of aqueous humor per mm. Hg of intraocular pressure. Values of 0.11 cu. mm. or less almost always are indicative of glaucoma; those of 0.16 cu. mm. or less are suggestive.

The technique for tonography is somewhat difficult to master and has several sources of inherent error. Like the water drinking test, it is most reliable in severe, well established glaucoma. In mild and borderline cases the variability is greater and the reliability less.

When combined with the water provocative test, tonography is done 45 minutes after the intake of water. It is possible that the water itself may lead to a lower coefficient of outflow by increasing resistance to aqueous outflow. Theoretically, the combined tests are more searching than either done alone.

Corticosteroids. In some individuals, particularly those with glaucoma or glaucoma-predisposed eyes, corticosteroids cause increased resistance to aqueous outflow, with a resultant rise in pressure. Betamethasone, 1 per cent, instilled four times daily for three weeks, has been used as a provocative test (Becker). This can induce rises in intraocular pressure in seemingly normal eyes of relatives of glaucoma patients and even in eyes of others with no family background of glaucoma. Whether or not these individuals really will develop clinical glaucoma at a subsequent time still is not known.

Treatment. The treatment of chronic simple glaucoma is primarily medical. Surgery is advised only if adequate medical therapy fails to control the disease. Operations not only can be accompanied by serious complications, but they also fail to control intraocular pressure adequately in 10 to 15 per cent of eyes. Most procedures for chronic simple glaucoma create a fistula through the corneoscleral wall to provide a channel for aqueous to drain into the potential space beneath the conjunctiva and Tenon's capsule (p. 386). Such operations can lead to cataract formation at the time of operation or even years later, and to complications such as infection and hemorrhage. Infections such as conjunctivitis may permit pathogenic organisms to traverse the fistula to enter the eye itself. Hypotony of the eyeball with edema of the posterior pole of the eye and loss of vision may ensue. Endophthalmitis may occur at any time after surgery.

If, in spite of maximum medical therapy, the optic nerve continues to be damaged, surgery should be advised. A nonfunctioning optic nerve cannot be restored, but such complications as cataracts ensuing from surgery can be dealt with and infection treated with antibiotics.

Effectiveness of medical therapy is evaluated by repeated tonometry, visual field examinations, and inspection of the optic nerves. A truly uncontrolled intraocular pressure, increased cupping of the optic nerve, and increasing visual field defects are indications for surgery. Medical treatment lowers intraocular pressure by increasing the facility of aqueous outflow through the use of miotics and by inhibiting aqueous formation through the use of carbonic anhydrase inhibitors or epinephrine preparations.

INCREASING AQUEOUS OUTFLOW WITH MIOTICS. Miotics are of two types: parasympathomimetic (cholinergic) and anticholinesterase (Tables 8-2, 8-3). Pilocarpine nitrate, a cholinergic in 1 to 4 per cent solutions, is the most commonly used miotic agent. Therapy is started with weak solutions, and the strength is increased if the intraocular pressure is not controlled adequately (at levels of 20 mm. Hg or below). A frequently employed anticholinesterase is phospholine iodide, although phospholine can have toxic effects by lowering the body levels of cholinesterase accompanied by gastrointestinal symptoms. The prolonged effect permits its use only once daily or even less often, and it never need be used more than twice a day. Physostigmine, or eserine, is not as commonly used because it causes an irritative follicular conjunctivitis.

How miotic agents reduce the intraocular pressure of chronic simple glaucoma is obscure. When the pupillary and ciliary musculature contract, however, they exert a pull on the scleral spur and the trabecula which probably decreases resistance to outflow through the trabecula and permits aqueous to enter the canal of Schlemm with greater facility.

Drugs such as pilocarpine usually are well tolerated, but if a patient has incipient cataracts, he may find the marked blurring of vision from a small pupil intolerable.

TABLE 8-2 PARASYMPATHOMIMETIC (CHOLINERGIC) AGENTS

Miotic	Dose
Acetylcholine—effect transient	Not used clinically
Methacholine (Mecholyl, acetyl-beta-methylcholine chloride)—effect transient; occasionally used for acute, narrow angle glaucoma	10 to 20% q. 5 to 10 mins.
Carbachol (Carcholin, Doryl, carbamyl chloride)	¾ to 4% q. 4 to 8 hrs.
Pilocarpine (hydrochloride or nitrate)	½ to 10% q. 4 to 6 hrs.

(After Becker and Shaffer, 1965.)

TABLE 8-3 ANTICHOLINESTERASE DRUGS

Miotic	Dose
Physostigmine (eserine)—tends to produce conjunctival irritation and allergy	¼ to 1% q. 4 to 6 hrs.
Prostigmin bromide (neostigmine)—not widely used	3 to 5% q. 4 to 6 hrs.
Isoflurophate (Floropryl, DFP)	0.01 to 0.1%; longlasting—use once or twice daily or even every other day
Echothiophate (Phospholine Iodide)	0.06 to 0.25%; longlasting—use once or twice daily or even every other day
Demecarium bromide (Humorsol, BC-48, Tosmilen)	0.06 to 1.0%; longlasting—use once or twice daily or even every other day

(After Becker and Shaffer, 1965.)

TABLE 8-4 CARBONIC ANHYDRASE INHIBITORS

Substance	Dose
Acetazolamide (Diamox)	125 to 500 mg. q. 4 to 12 hrs. 5 to 10 mg./kg. q. 4 to 6 hrs. (infants) 250 mg. in 2.5 ml. distilled H_2O, i.v. or i.m.
Methazolamide (Neptazane)	50 to 100 mg. q. 8 hrs.
Dichlorphenamide (Daranide)	50 to 200 mg. q. 6 to 8 hrs.
Ethoxzolamide (Cardrase)	50 to 250 mg. q. 4 to 8 hrs.

(After Becker and Shaffer, 1965.)

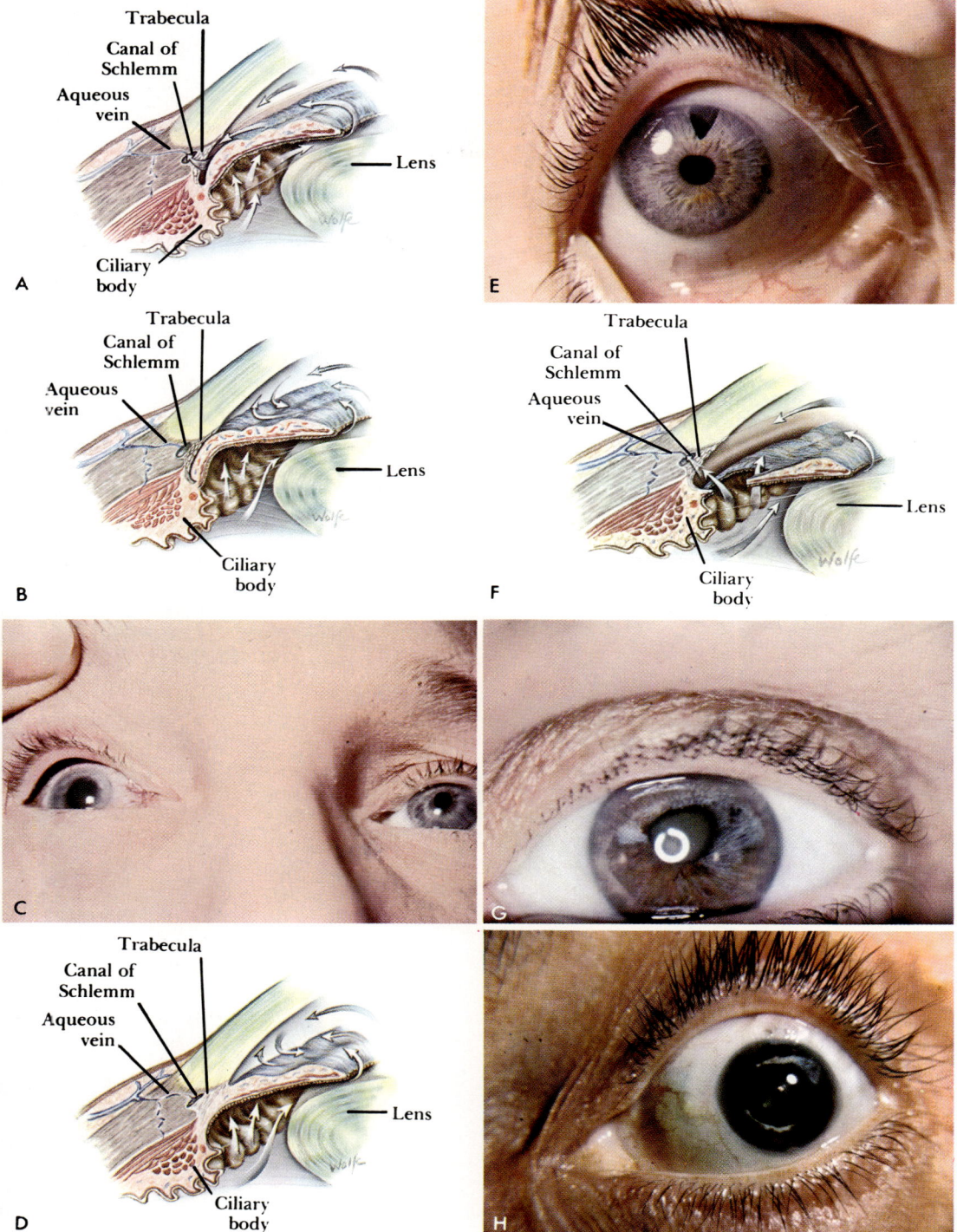

Plate 30 Narrow angle glaucoma. *(A)* Interval, or preglaucoma, phase with narrow angle, but with normal aqueous outflow and no synechiae. *(B)* Acute congestive (iris block) phase; iris against trabecula, but no synechiae formation. *(C)* Photograph of eye in acute congestive phase showing semidilated pupil and red eye. *(D)* Chronic narrow angle phase; iris root adherent to trabecula. Result of fulminating or repeated acute attacks. *(E)* Photograph of eye after peripheral iridectomy for early narrow angle glaucoma. *(F)* Chamber deepens after peripheral iridectomy; aqueous flows through peripheral iridectomy into anterior chamber. *(G)* Iris atrophy with narrow angle glaucoma, following single acute attack. *(H)* Iris atrophy with narrow angle glaucoma, following irreversible acute attack (chronic phase).

347

Strong miotic agents such as phospholine iodide and diisopropyl phosphorofluoridate (DFP) cause even more severe blurring and considerable discomfort. They also may produce iris cysts arising near the pupillary border and partially obscuring it. Some observers have suggested that phospholine iodide may cause cataracts. In young people marked artificial myopia due to spasm of accommodation may result from any miotic agent. If possible, strong miotics should be used only at bedtime so that most of their ill effects will have worn off by morning.

Epinephrine applied locally is believed by some to facilitate aqueous humor outflow in addition to decreasing aqueous formation. In certain patients, it lowers tension dramatically. It should be used only once daily because it tends to cause marked conjunctival irritation. Even if used every other day, it still may help to lower pressure, and the danger of irritation is reduced.

INHIBITING AQUEOUS PRODUCTION

Carbonic Anhydrase Inhibitors (Table 8-4). Carbonic anhydrase is essential to aqueous formation. It is found in the ciliary body, but the mechanism by which it assists aqueous formation is not understood. Carbonic anhydrase inhibitors reduce the rate of aqueous production by the ciliary body. Acetazolamide (Diamox) is the most widely used, but several similarly acting substances are available. Although Diamox takes effect within one to two hours after being administered, its effect lasts for only six to eight hours, so it must be given repeatedly. It can be administered intravenously, but it usually is taken orally in doses as great as 250 mg. four times daily. Diamox Sequels, which have a prolonged action, can be given instead of tablets once or twice daily. Carbonic anhydrase inhibitors can have serious systemic side effects that have led to reservations about their use for long-term therapy. Paresthesias and numbness of extremities, loss of appetite, agranulocytosis and renal calculi can result. Mental depression can be profound.

Since epinephrine probably reduces aqueous production as well as increasing the outflow, it can be used as an adjunct to therapy.

Cardiac Glycosides. These substances have a tension-lowering effect when given systemically, but as yet they rarely have been used in the treatment of glaucoma.

Follow-up. All patients who are started on treatment for chronic simple glaucoma should be seen as frequently as necessary until fully regulated and at three- to six-month intervals thereafter. At each visit the intraocular pressure should be taken and the optic nerve inspected. Visual fields should be examined at least once a year, or more often if increased cupping of the optic nerve warrants or if control of intraocular pressure is poor. Whenever a patient who is receiving maximal medical treatment shows signs of poor control of pressure and loss of visual field, surgery should be advised without delay. The operations most commonly used are iridencleisis, corneoscleral trephination (Elliott), posterior sclerotomy, and iridectomy with scleral cautery.

NARROW ANGLE (IRIS BLOCK, ANGLE CLOSURE, ACUTE CONGESTIVE) GLAUCOMA

Mechanism. Narrow angle glaucoma occurs in eyes whose anterior chamber angle is extremely narrow, so that at times contact of the iris with the trabecula may obstruct the outflow of aqueous (angle closure, iris block). The intraocular pressure then rapidly elevates and causes the acute congestive attacks which characterize the disease. Such narrow-angled eyes behave normally until the angle closes from contact of the iris with the trabecula. Tonography shows that until obstruction occurs, aqueous humor enters and leaves at a normal rate. The underlying cause of this disease is narrowness of the angle.

The iris might be compared to a rubber dam floating in a water-filled sink with a screen over its drainpipe. When flow of water carries the rubber dam into contact with the drain, water no longer can flow from the sink. A head of pressure builds up as water accumulates in the sink behind the dam. This is analagous to what happens in angle closure glaucoma when the iris comes into contact with the trabecula overlying the canal of Schlemm and prevents the escape of aqueous.

A narrow anterior chamber angle is a combination of anatomic and functional factors. The anatomic factor is attributed to an anterior position of the lens-iris dia-phragm, probably hereditary. The functional factor is in the form of a physiologic iris bombé which occurs from resistance to aqueous flow from the posterior to the anterior chamber over the area of contact between the posterior surface of the iris and the anterior surface of the lens. This resistance causes the iris to bow forward. When a portion of the periphery of the iris is excised (peripheral iridectomy), a direct channel is formed through the iris for the aqueous to flow into the anterior chamber. As a result the iris surface flattens and the angle of the anterior chamber widens, a phenomenon that can be confirmed by gonioscopy.

Although the underlying cause of narrow angle glaucoma is well known, the factors precipitating acute attacks are not well understood. Pupillary dilatation is one factor. The sphincter iridis relaxes and allows the iris root to sag forward and close the angle. Stress and excitement may increase aqueous flow which could increase the physiologic bombé, setting off an acute attack.

Classification of Narrow Angle Glaucoma. Narrow angle glaucoma comprises three phases:

1. *Preglaucoma and interval phases.* These are more or less identical. Preglaucoma occurs in a patient who has a very narrow angle but has no symptoms of glaucoma (Plate 30A). Although the intraocular pressure is normal, it can be made to rise by provoking pupillary dilatation.

Interval glaucoma is found in a patient who has had a known acute attack of glaucoma or whose history suggests one. As with preglaucoma the intraocular pressure is normal between attacks, although it can be made to rise by pupillary dilatation, and the angle is very narrow. The eye with a narrow angle that yields positive results in a dilatation test must be considered to be glaucomatous even though the pressure is normal at other times.

2. *Acute congestive (iris block, angle closure) phase.* During this phase the angle is closed completely by contact between the iris and the trabecula (Plate 30B, C). The pressure is elevated. With proper medical therapy angle closure (iris block) is reversible. If not relieved in 48 to 72 hours, however, adhesions develop between the iris root and

GLAUCOMA 349

the trabecula that cannot be relieved, and chronic, narrow angle glaucoma ensues.

3. *Chronic narrow angle (iris block, angle closure) phase.* This type of glaucoma may develop as an outgrowth of a fulminating attack that cannot be relieved or that is neglected; repeated, mild, acute attacks with slowly increasing synechiae; and slowly progressive elevation of intraocular pressure, probably due to subclinical acute attacks that give no symptoms but during which synechiae gradually increase. As a result the angle is closed permanently by adhesion of the iris to the trabecula (Plate 30D).

Diagnosis. Early diagnosis is essential because surgery done at an early stage nearly always is successful. Although formerly the most serious type, narrow angle glaucoma now carries a most favorable prognosis if peripheral iridectomy is done before adhesions (chronic, narrow angle phase) develop (Plate 30E, F). The prognosis also has improved because of such recent additions to therapy as Diamox and hyperosmotic agents. These nearly always control an acute attack and allow iridectomy to be done safely during the interval phase.

The incidence of glaucoma is higher in females than in males. A family history should always be sought because heredity is important. Narrow angle glaucoma may be easy or difficult to diagnose depending somewhat upon the phase (Table 8-5). A complete ocular examination, including gonioscopy, is essential.

PREGLAUCOMA AND INTERVAL PHASES. A patient at the preglaucoma phase shows no symptoms relating to glaucoma, but one at the interval glaucoma phase may have a history suggestive of acute glaucoma or known acute attacks. Classic symptoms include ocular discomfort, attacks of blurred vision, and halos around lights. Discomfort may be marked or only a dull headache, usually localized around the eye. Halos result from edema of the corneal epithelium and often occur at times when pupils tend to dilate as in the semidarkness of the movie theater. These signs and symptoms usually subside after a few minutes in a lighted room when the pupil constricts. Emotional upsets may also be a predisposing factor. Occasionally a patient notices that discomfort disappears while he sleeps, which is when the pupil is miotic.

When these patients come to the ophthalmologist for examination, they are free of symptoms. The only positive finding may be a shallow anterior chamber. Segmental atrophy of the iris stroma and even of the pigment layer may be present and most marked near the pupillary border (Plate 30G, H). In the preglaucoma and interval phases, the optic nerve is normal because the eyes have not been subjected to long periods of elevated pressure.

On routine eye examination the usual method used to detect narrow angles is by slit lamp biomicroscope. The periphery of the anterior chamber always should be inspected by a very thin beam from the instrument being slowly moved from the central area toward the angle (Fig. 8-5A, B). When the angle is narrow, the iris can be seen very close to the inner surface of the periphery of the cornea. Gonioscopy then confirms this finding. Routine tonometry is not helpful in the diagnosis of either preglaucoma or interval glaucoma because the intraocular pressure is normal. Visual fields also are normal, reflecting the healthy state of the optic nerves.

Provocative tests should be done to determine whether or not the angle can be closed and a rise in pressure induced. Pupillary dilatation, which relaxes the sphincter pupillae, allows the iris root to bow forward and close the angle. Aqueous cannot escape from the eye. Tonography reveals marked impairment of outflow (Fig. 8-6A, B). The hazards of the test should be explained to the patient, and he should be told that he may have symptoms of acute congestive glaucoma. The possibility exists that the pressure cannot be controlled, but the hazards are very small with present-day therapeutic methods. The importance of

TABLE 8-5   DIAGNOSIS OF NARROW ANGLE GLAUCOMA

Signs	Interval or Preglaucoma Phase	Acute Congestive Phase	Chronic Phase
Symptoms	None; blurring of vision; halos around lights	Severe	Mild to severe
Visual acuity	Normal	Depressed	Normal to severe loss
External examination	Shallow chamber; iris atrophy±*	Shallow chamber; signs of acute glaucoma; iris atrophy±	Shallow chamber; congestive signs; iris atrophy
Ophthalmoscopic examination	Normal optic nerve	Usually normal	Normal to severe atrophy or cupping
Slit lamp examination	Possible sector iris atrophy; narrow angles	Sector iris atrophy±; epithelial edema; aqueous flare; narrow angles	Iris atrophy
Intraocular pressure	Normal	Markedly elevated	Usually markedly elevated
Gonioscopic examination	Very narrow or optically closed angle	Closed angle	Closed angle (adhesions)
Visual fields	Normal	Normal to slight constriction	Normal to extreme glaucomatous damage
Provocative tests: dark room, mydriatic agents	Usually positive	Unnecessary	Unnecessary
Tonographic studies	Normal aqueous outflow	Diminished aqueous outflow	Diminished aqueous outflow

*+ = yes; − = no

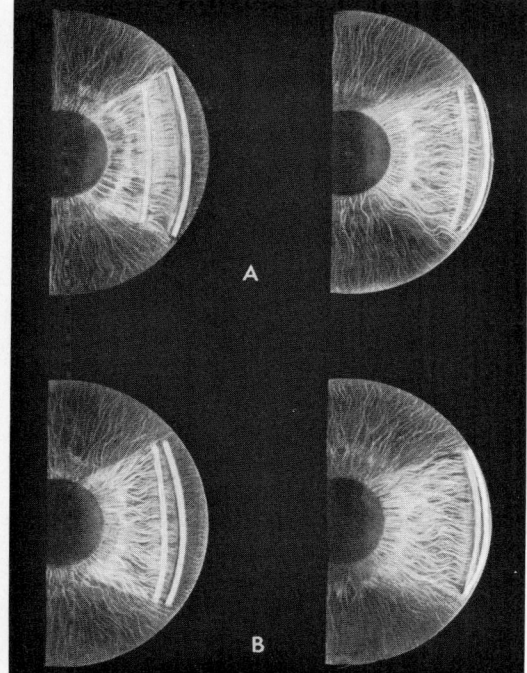

Figure 8-5 Slit lamp appearance with *(A)* normal and *(B)* shallow angles.

taken promptly because usually it falls rapidly when the patient is brought into the light and the pupil constricts. If discomfort is noticed during the test, the pressure should be taken before one hour. If the pressure rises significantly, miotic medication should be given to reduce it.

Chemical Mydriasis Tests. Several different mydriatic agents may be used, including eucatropine, 5 per cent; mydriacyl, 1 per cent; and homatropine, 2 per cent. Drops are instilled twice in each eye five minutes apart, and the intraocular pressure is recorded at 20-minute intervals for one and onehalf hours. Chemical tests are advantageous because gonioscopy can be done to confirm angle closure should the pressure rise. If the angle remains open by gonioscopy after a rise in pressure, chronic simple glaucoma should be suspected, because pupillary dilatation can have the reverse effect of miotics on the trabecula, increasing resistance to aqueous outflow with a resultant rise in pressure.

A pressure rise of 8 mm. or more is considered positive, but much higher elevations are characteristic of narrow angle glaucoma. The pupil should be constricted promptly with physostigmine, 0.5 per cent. This usually produces prompt miosis and

establishing the diagnosis far outweighs the small danger involved. Two types of pupillary dilatation tests are available:

Darkroom Test. The patient is placed in a dark room for one hour. At the end of this time the intraocular pressure should be

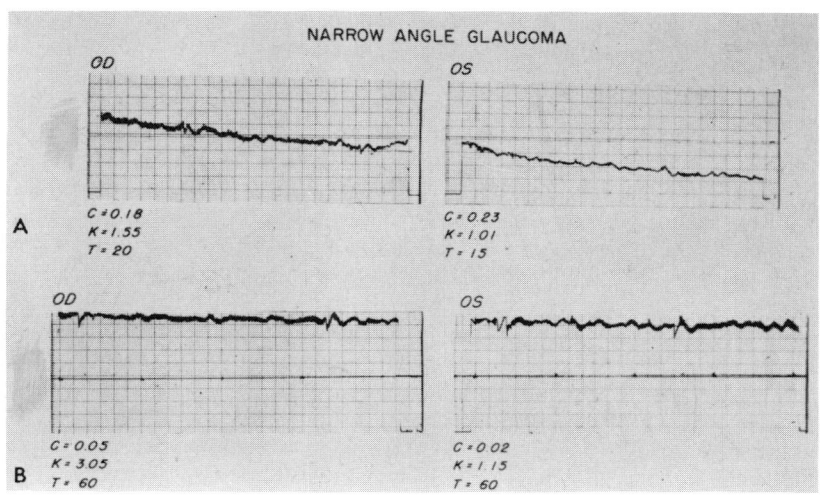

Figure 8-6 Tonographic tracings illustrating outflow of aqueous in narrow angle glaucoma. *(A)* Normal outflow during preglaucoma phase. *(B)* Marked diminution in outflow during acute congestive phase.

is more effective than pilocarpine for neutralizing a chemical mydriatic test. If the pupil does not constrict and the intraocular pressure continues to rise, Diamox should be given as well as urea or glycerol. After the pressure has been controlled, pilocarpine should be prescribed for use four times daily for the following two days. A mydriatic agent may have a prolonged effect and cause secondary pupillary dilatation after the effect of the miotic wears off in about six to eight hours. When a patient is exposed to the hazards of a mydriasis test, whether or not the test is positive, he should be kept under observation until the pupil constricts.

A positive mydriasis test is highly significant, but a negative test can be misleading. Patients whose mydriasis tests are negative often suffer attacks of acute congestive glaucoma in the near or distant future. They should be informed of this possibility if their angles are sufficiently narrow to warrant concern. They should be familiarized with the symptoms of acute glaucoma so that they will seek help promptly if an acute attack should ensue. If negative, a mydriasis test should be repeated from time to time.

ACUTE CONGESTIVE (IRIS BLOCK, ANGLE CLOSURE) PHASE. A typical attack of acute congestive glaucoma should be easy to diagnose. Severe pain in the eye, regional headache, and blurred vision dominate the picture. Gastrointestinal symptoms sometimes mask the acute glaucoma. Severe nausea and vomiting caused by the vagus reflex may obscure the ocular symptoms and result in a false diagnosis of an acute abdominal condition such as gall bladder disease. Acute glaucoma also can be overlooked easily in the patient who has had abdominal surgery. Pre- or postoperative medication, such as atropine, which dilates the pupil, may be a precipitating factor. Ocular pain and inflammation in a patient after general surgery are most commonly due to acute congestive glaucoma or a corneal abrasion resulting from mechanical injury or from an irritative anesthetic agent.

Blurred vision during acute glaucoma results from edema of the corneal epithelium, as well as from depressed function of the retina and optic nerve. External examination reveals a shallow anterior chamber, an edematous cornea, and a red, inflamed eye, often with edematous conjunctiva. The pupil is semidilated and constricts poorly to all stimuli. The phenomena probably are due to compression of the iris musculature and to diminished blood supply, especially to the sphincter area of the iris. The vessels that enter the iris from the major arterial circle of the ciliary body are compressed with the root of the iris by aqueous attempting to traverse the trabecula to enter the canal of Schlemm. Interruption of blood supply leads to a sector type atrophy of the iris stroma and, at times, of the epithelial layers. Atrophy becomes more marked as the pupillary border is approached. Such areas of atrophy are indicative of previous acute attacks of glaucoma and can be of diagnostic help. Corneal haze often makes ophthalmoscopic, slit lamp biomicroscopic, and gonioscopic examinations difficult. Usually the cornea can be cleared sufficiently for examination by the instillation of glycerin, a hygroscopic agent. The optic nerve characteristically is normal, and visual field tests are not helpful. If the attack is prolonged and severe, or if attacks have been repeated, atrophy and cupping rarely may have occurred.

Narrow angle glaucoma is suggested by slit lamp biomicroscopy, but gonioscopic examination eliminates any doubt and almost always reveals a narrow angle in the fellow eye. An aqueous flare is present which, with redness of the eye, can mistakenly lead to a diagnosis of glaucoma secondary to inflammation. A closed angle, however, weighs heavily toward narrow angle glaucoma. Slit lamp biomicroscopy may reveal small, anterior, subcapsular, lens opacities (glaukomflecken) of previous acute attacks. Tonometry reveals a markedly elevated intraocular pressure, so provocative tests are unnecessary.

CHRONIC NARROW ANGLE (ANGLE CLOSURE) PHASE. Chronic narrow angle glaucoma may have either very mild or severe symptoms. The diagnosis is obvious when it follows an unrelieved attack of acute congestive glaucoma, for the classic signs of acute congestive glaucoma (red eye, hazy cornea, usually marked iris atrophy, shallow anterior chamber, and closed angle) are still present. Chronic narrow angle glaucoma also may result from repeated mild attacks of acute congestive glaucoma which cause little or no congestion and irritation, and from the pressure gradually rising because synechiae have increased with each attack. Finally, chronic narrow angle glaucoma may develop from slowly progressive angle closure with no clinical episodes of acute glaucoma. The situation simulates chronic simple glaucoma from which it may be difficult to differentiate. Each may have a very narrow angle and elevated tension with cupping of the optic nerve and visual field defects.

Treatment. Treatment of narrow angle glaucoma is primarily surgical. The diagnosis should be made early so that a peripheral iridectomy can be done before synechiae form. Medical therapy should be employed only to terminate an acute attack or to prevent one until an operation is feasible. If angle closure has developed, medical therapy should be given a trial, but usually it is unsuccessful.

PREGLAUCOMA AND INTERVAL PHASES. In these phases peripheral iridectomy is highly effective and should be performed as soon as possible (Plate 30*E, F*). This simple, safe procedure deepens the angle, and subsequent pupillary dilatation causes no rise in pressure. Medical treatment should be used only until surgery can be arranged or if the patient is too ill or debilitated. Pilocarpine, 1 per cent, is instilled four times daily. The patient should always use it at dusk and before watching movies. Strong miotics such as phospholine iodide should be avoided because marked pupillary constriction increases the resistance to aqueous flow between the iris and the lens, which aggravates the physiologic iris bombé and possibly precipitates an acute congestive attack.

ACUTE CONGESTIVE PHASE. An attack of acute congestive glaucoma should be controlled by medical therapy whenever possible. Peripheral iridectomy subsequently should be done as soon as possible to avoid the hazard of operating when the intraocular pressure is high during a later acute attack (Plate 30*E, F*). The following medical measures are utilized more or less simultaneously.

Miotic Agents (p. 345). By constricting the pupil, miotic agents retract the iris from the corneoscleral wall to reopen the angle and allow aqueous to escape. If the acute attack has been present for several hours, the pupillary musculature may be inert and unable to respond to miotics. Pilocarpine, 1 per cent, or eserine, 0.5 per cent, are the most commonly used. Eserine is more effective because it inactivates cholinesterase, permitting acetylcholine to accumulate in the tissues. Pilocarpine should not be used initially because it occupies the motor end plate and partially blocks the effect of acetylcholine, the physiologic and more potent substance. Eserine should be instilled every few minutes for a half hour and then alternated at 15 minute intervals with pilocarpine. Strong miotic agents such as Floropryl, Humorsol and phospholine iodide are dangerous and should be avoided. Miotics always should be instilled in the fellow eye to avoid the danger of an acute attack.

Carbonic Anhydrase Inhibitors (See Table 8-4). These substances are important in the treatment of acute congestive glaucoma. Diamox, the most widely used, should be given immediately by mouth in a dose of 500 mg. and repeated with 250 mg. every four hours. If the patient is nauseated, the same amounts can be given intravenously.

Hyperosmotic Agents. The use of hyperosmotic agents such as glycerol, urea, and mannitol has enabled the ophthalmologist to relieve almost all acute attacks of glaucoma. Glycerol is advantageous because it is safe and can be given in an ophthalmologist's office. It is given by mouth in a dose of approximately 1 ml./kg. body weight in 50 per cent solution. Mannitol, less commonly used, is given in similar dosage, but must be administered intravenously.

With the use of such combined therapy, the intraocular pressure usually falls within 30 minutes to an hour. Miotics should be continued at least four times daily and the angle assessed by gonioscopy. If the use of miotics maintains normal intraocular pressure, only a simple peripheral iridectomy should be done. Attacks of acute glaucoma almost certainly will recur if not operated. If the acute attack has been severe and if synechiae are causing consistently elevated intraocular pressure, even when the patient is on miotics, iridencleisis or iridectomy with scleral cautery may be necessary. If the need for a filtering operation is questioned, then a peripheral iridectomy may be done because it is simple and there are few complications. Even if iridectomy fails to control the intraocular pressure because of synechiae, it prevents future acute attacks and medical therapy even may be effective. A filtering operation can be done later if needed.

CHRONIC NARROW ANGLE (CONGESTIVE) PHASE. Chronic congestive glaucoma responds poorly to medical treatment. Since the angle is closed by synechiae, a filtering operation, usually an iridencleisis or an iridectomy with scleral cautery, is indicated to prevent further deterioration of the eye.

Congenital Glaucoma

Congenital glaucoma can be defined as glaucoma occurring in individuals up to 30 years of age (p. 338).

JUVENILE GLAUCOMA

The upper and lower age limits given for juvenile glaucoma are arbitrary. There seems little doubt that glaucoma occurring at age 25 can have the same origin and run the same course as glaucoma at 35 or 40. The same probably is true at the lower age limit of 2 to 3 years, the approximate time when the eyeball ceases to enlarge as a result of increased intraocular pressure. This age, however, varies: little or no enlargement occurs in some three-year-olds, but significant enlargement occurs in others. The mechanisms of the glaucoma can be the same, but the resultant clinical picture depends on the ability of the cornea and sclera to withstand increased intraocular pressure.

Juvenile glaucoma runs the insidious course of chronic simple glaucoma and presents the same diagnostic problems; the diagnosis can be more challenging because the presence of glaucoma often is not suspected in younger age groups. Too often the disease is discovered only after marked glaucoma cupping and severe visual loss have occurred. Unfortunately, glaucoma cupping may be atypical in young persons, especially in the presence of myopia. The cup tends to be shallow and broad.

In general, glaucoma is more severe in the juvenile age group, and the intraocular pressure tends to be more labile with greater day-to-day variations. Rapid rises in pressure with halos are more frequent than in chronic simple glaucoma of older persons. All children and young adults with rapidly progressive myopia should be suspected of having glaucoma. Myopia probably is aggravated by the effect of elevated pressure on the somewhat distensible sclera and cornea of young people.

The methods of diagnosing juvenile glaucoma and chronic simple glaucoma are identical. Congenital anomalies, such as posterior embryotoxon (Axenfeld's syndrome), aniridia, spherophakia, congenital dislocation of the lens, neurofibromatosis, Sturge-Weber syndrome, and signs of pigment dispersion in the form of Krukenberg's spindle, often are associated with glaucoma and should alert the ophthalmologist. Glaucoma may occur at any time in life in patients having these anomalies.

Treatment. Surgery usually is necessary for juvenile glaucoma because response to medical therapy almost invariably is poor. Even those who seemingly do well on medical treatment, however, hardly can expect it to preserve their vision for a lifetime. Miotics cause spasm of accommodation with discomfort and blurred vision due to artificial myopia, so the youthful and often irresponsible patient tends to use them unfaithfully. Nevertheless, an adequate medical regimen should be given a thorough trial.

Weak solutions of phospholine iodide, 0.06 per cent, have a prolonged effect that results in a more or less constant refractive change throughout the day. This can be corrected by spectacles. Phospholine iodide is tolerated better than pilocarpine, which must be used three or four times daily and causes episodic spasm of accommodation and artificial myopia after each instillation. The symptoms disappear in one or two hours but recur with each instillation to the great inconvenience of the patient. Epinephrine is useful in controlling pressure and may be used when the disease is mild or as a supplement to miotic therapy. Carbonic anhydrase inhibitors have little value because it is not likely that they could be continued safely for a long period of time.

Indications for surgery are similar to those for chronic simple glaucoma and include progressive cupping of the optic nerve and loss of visual field. It is obvious, however, that a young person with poorly controlled intraocular pressure and a long life ahead should undergo surgery. Filtering procedures such as goniopuncture usually are done.

Goniopuncture consists of making a small perforation in the angle wall. It is simple and safe to perform and is accompanied by few operative or postoperative complications. The eye retains its normal appearance and its function is undisturbed. This procedure, repeated once or twice, is successful in about 50 per cent of eyes. If it fails, more conventional but more hazardous procedures, such as iridencleisis, trephination, iridectomy with scleral cautery, and various types of sclerectomy, should be utilized.

INFANTILE GLAUCOMA

Infantile glaucoma may be primary or secondary to other ocular congenital anomalies and diseases, such as ocular inflammation and tumors. Infantile glaucoma accounts for approximately 5 per cent of blindness among persons in schools for the blind in this country, much of which could have been prevented by early diagnosis and proper management.

Mechanism. Infantile glaucoma is an autosomal recessive disease that is thought to result from an imperfect drainage mechanism related to incomplete cleavage of the periphery of the uveal tract from the corneoscleral wall. The uveal portion of the iris meshwork and the meridional muscle fibers of the ciliary body seem to insert into the trabecular area, at times as far forward as Schwalbe's line; thus aqueous outflow is impaired. Other mechanisms are involved in the different types of secondary infantile glaucoma.

Diagnosis. Early diagnosis is essential because present-day surgical techniques, utilized early, can control the pressure and arrest the disease in at least 80 per cent of eyes. If not successfully operated upon, the eyes enlarge progressively until profound visual loss and eventual blindness occur. As in glaucoma of the adult, damage is permanent.

In approximately one third of patients, the disease occurs in utero and typical signs are present at birth. Enlarged eyes (buphthalmos) and hazy corneas make the diagnosis obvious to the obstetrician and pediatrician. Since damage to the eye and impaired development have occurred in utero, the visual prognosis, even with control of pressure, is much poorer than in the two thirds of infants in whom the disease develops after birth. Insurmountable amblyopia is common, particularly in the eye that shows more severe involvement if the disease is asymmetrical.

Early diagnosis of infantile glaucoma that develops after birth can be as difficult as diagnosis of chronic simple glaucoma in the adult. Ophthalmologists and pediatricians should be familiar with the earliest signs of infantile glaucoma and constantly alert to its possibility, even though the disease is rare in any individual practice. Most of the following diagnostic signs stem from the vulnerability of the cornea and sclera to elevated intraocular pressure:

PHOTOPHOBIA, BLEPHAROSPASM, AND TEARING. These are the commonest initial signs of infantile glaucoma and call the attention of the mother or pediatrician to the disease. When unexplained photophobia and tearing are present during the child's first two or three years of life, infantile glaucoma should always be excluded. These symptoms probably result from early corneal edema and accompanying corneal irritation. Occasionally congenital obstruction of the nasolacrimal apparatus, a common cause of tearing in the first year of life, may be diagnosed erroneously as glaucoma. No photophobia is present; however, the tear ducts are obstructed.

CORNEAL HAZE. Initially, subepithelial and epithelial edema causes a mild but definite milky corneal haze (Fig. 8-7). If the stroma also becomes edematous, the corneal opacity is more marked, and the

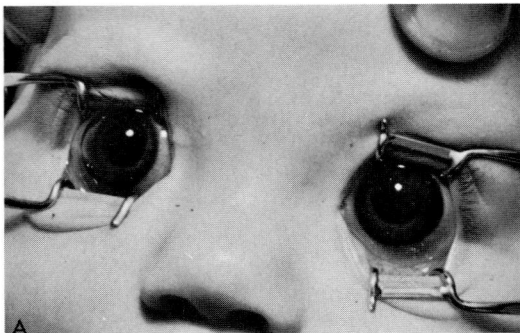

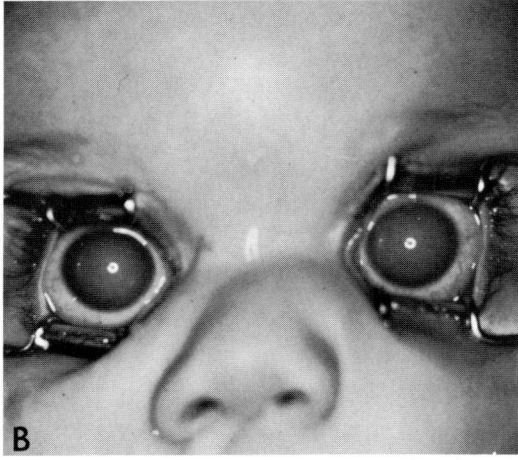

Figure 8-7 Congenital glaucoma. *(A)* Enlargement of corneas. *(B)* Enlargement of corneas with corneal haze.

cornea may resemble scleral tissue. Corneal haze usually clears dramatically following successful surgery, but if edema of the stroma has been severe and persistent, a permanent cicatrix and opacity may have developed.

ENLARGEMENT OF THE CORNEA. Shortly after onset of corneal haze or coincident with it, the entire eyeball, including the cornea, enlarges progressively until the corneal diameter may measure 18 mm. or more (Fig. 8-7). The greatest stretching and thinning takes place at the limbus, where the globe may rupture from some trivial trauma as the child becomes older. Corneal diameter measurement is important in the diagnosis even though the disease can occur in microphthalmic eyes. Any corneal diameter over 12 mm., or one that is increasing, should be regarded with suspicion.

RUPTURES IN DESCEMET'S MEMBRANE. Descemet's membrane is less elastic than the cornea and sclera, so corneal enlargement places it under tension. Linear ruptures may occur that can be horizontal and sinuous, branching or single, or that even can encircle the cornea within the limbus. If aqueous diffuses into the corneal stroma along the course of the ruptures, it causes localized corneal edema and opacity that, at times, is generalized. The edema clears after tension normalizes, but the edges of Descemet's membrane that have retracted along the sites of the ruptures remain visible as parallel hyaline-like lines that can be seen throughout life with a slit lamp biomicroscope or an ophthalmoscope. They may cause irregular astigmatism and distorted vision. Corneal haze and rupture of Descemet's membrane can occur in infants as a result of birth trauma inflicted by the obstetrical forceps. Almost invariably the condition is unilateral and the intraocular pressure is normal.

CUPPING OF THE OPTIC NERVE. Cupping of the optic nerve is not of great diagnostic importance. It is valuable in following patients postoperatively when increasing cupping indicates poor control of pressure.

ELEVATED INTRAOCULAR PRESSURE. When infantile glaucoma is suspected, the intraocular pressure should be measured and the eye examined completely with the child under general anesthesia. Deep general anesthesia is necessary for accurate tonometry, and great judgment is required to evaluate the results. Ocular changes caused by infantile glaucoma often are more severe than the pressure would indicate.

Significant variations from day to day and even from one time of day to another can cause erroneous tonometry values. False high readings can result from light anesthesia or an inadequate airway. Without other objective signs of infantile glaucoma, surgery always should be deferred and the pressure measured a few days later. Finding normal pressure should not lead to false security, for it may have been measured at its lowest ebb. Dehydration from fluids being withheld in preparation for anesthesia may result in low pressure readings. Barbiturates given preoperatively and certain anesthetic agents also lower intraocular pressure. Low readings might come, theoretically, from a thin cornea and a large corneal diameter.

TONOGRAPHY. Tonography is of less value in diagnosing infantile glaucoma than in diagnosing the adult type. The technique is difficult and the results in an anesthetized child are uncertain.

GONIOSCOPY. Although gonioscopy is an essential preoperative study, it is of little value in diagnosing infantile glaucoma. It is valuable, however, in excluding the associated anomalies such as Axenfeld's syndrome, aniridia, nevoxanthoendothelioma and others. Opinions differ as to whether or not the angle of the eye with infantile glaucoma presents a characteristic appearance. If it does, the characteristics are rather nebulous and, therefore, of little value in establishing the diagnosis. The apex of the angle of most infants is poorly developed, so in a child with unilateral infantile glaucoma the angle of each eye may seem identical. If the affected eye is enlarged, rather characteristic segmentation or palisading of the pigment stroma at the periphery of the iris is seen. This probably results from secondary enlargement of the eye and stretching of the base of the iris. It also can be seen in high myopia.

In infantile glaucoma the angle of the anterior chamber is open and the canal of Schlemm is in its normal position anterior to the scleral spur. In at least 90 per cent of eyes, the canal fills with blood when the jugular veins are compressed, which indicates that absence of the canal is not the cause of increased intraocular pressure. In advanced infantile glaucoma, however, when the limbal tissues are markedly stretched and distorted, the canal of Schlemm does not fill with blood. It probably has been obliterated.

Differential Diagnosis. Many conditions simulate infantile glaucoma and must always be excluded. The most common are megalocornea, high myopia, congenital idiopathic edema of the cornea, rubella keratitis, corneal injury during birth with ruptures of Descemet's membrane and corneal edema, corneal lipoidosis, cystinosis, and the mucopolysaccharidoses (MPS) that are associated with corneal opacity. The latter include Hurler's syndrome (MPS 1),

Hunter's syndrome (MPS 2), Sanfilippo's syndrome (MPS 3), Morquio's syndrome (MPS 4), Scheie's syndrome (MPS 5), and Maroteaux-Lamy's syndrome (MPS 6).

Differentiation may require examination and measurement of corneal diameter and intraocular pressure. Specific studies must be ordered as indicated. This is true, for example, in differentiating mucopolysaccharidoses from infantile glaucoma secondary to causes such as uveitis. Retinoblastoma always should be kept in mind because it is not an unusual cause of elevated intraocular pressure. Careful ocular examination under general anesthesia usually establishes the diagnosis.

Treatment. Surgery should be prompt. Medical treatment is of no value for it only permits the eye to deteriorate. Goniotomy, alone or combined with goniopuncture, is the procedure of choice. The operation will control intraocular pressure in 80 to 85 per cent of uncomplicated eyes, and where goniotomy fails, iridectomy with scleral cautery can control the pressure in about half the eyes. The prognosis for a good visual result is best when the disease develops in infants from three to six months of age, and who, at the time of surgery, show little ocular enlargement or damage. In children born with obvious signs of infantile glaucoma, especially if other anomalies such as aniridia are present, the prognosis is much poorer.

Once the pressure is controlled, the long-term prognosis is excellent. Some patients have been followed for 20 years or longer with good vision and a seemingly permanent cure. They should be followed carefully throughout their lives, however, because of possible recurrences, although these are rare after six months. The uninvolved eye should be followed particularly carefully because a predisposition to glaucoma must be assumed. Later complications may occur, especially in large eyes, where injury from relatively trivial trauma may lead to rupture, retinal detachment, or intraocular hemorrhage. Late edema of the cornea may occur secondary to ruptures of Descemet's membrane and subsequent defects in the corneal endothelium. The need for early diagnosis and prompt surgery is emphasized.

ASSOCIATED ANOMALIES

Numerous ocular and systemic anomalies may be associated with congenital glaucoma. (See chapter on Pediatric Ophthalmology.) All patients with these anomalies should be observed carefully for glaucoma because it may begin at any time in life:

I. Local ocular anomalies
   A. Iridocorneal dysgenesis (anterior chamber cleavage syndrome)
      1. Posterior embryotoxon of Axenfeld
      2. Rieger's syndrome
         a. Hypoplasia of the anterior stromal leaf of the iris
         b. Iridotrabecular adhesions
         c. Posterior embryotoxon (Axenfeld)
   B. Essential iris atrophy
   C. Aniridia
   D. Pigmentary glaucoma
   E. Megalocornea
   F. Microcornea
   G. Microphthalmia
   H. Spherophakia (microphakia)
   I. Myopia
   J. Retinitis pigmentosa
   K. Glaucoma secondary to local ocular disease
II. Systemic conditions with associated glaucoma
   A. Phakomatoses
      1. Neurofibromatosis (von Recklinghausen's)
      2. Encephalotrigeminal angiomatosis of Sturge-Weber
   B. Heritable disorders of connective tissue
      1. Marfan's syndrome
      2. Homocystinuria
      3. Hurler's syndrome (MPS 1)
   C. Lowe's syndrome
   D. Pierre Robin syndrome
   E. Hallerman-Streiff syndrome
   F. Chromosomal disorders
      1. Turner's syndrome
      2. 16-18 Trisomy
      3. 13-15 Trisomy
      4. Down's syndrome (mongolism)

   G. Oculodentodigital syndrome
   H. Dyscraniopygophalangeo (Ullrich's syndrome)
   I. Congenital melanosis oculi
   J. Juvenile xanthogranuloma
   K. Idiopathic infantile hypoglycemia
   L. Congenital rubella syndrome

SECONDARY GLAUCOMA

Glaucoma that can be attributed to associated ocular disease or abnormality is termed secondary glaucoma. It includes glaucoma occurring with uveitis, intraocular tumors, trauma, hemorrhage, changes in the lens, congenital anomalies, and glaucoma from the effects of certain medications such as steroids and many other causes. Only a few are reviewed in this chapter (pp. 359 and 360).

Mechanisms. The most important mechanism is increased resistance to aqueous outflow, although others play a part in causing increased intraocular pressure. Sources of resistance may be located in the trabecular meshwork or the canal of Schlemm and may even involve the aqueous veins. The trabecula can become obstructed by various inflammatory cells, red blood cells, protein of plasmoid aqueous, lens material, and pigment (Krukenberg's spindle). Contusion injury to the trabecula often causes delayed fibrotic changes, atrophy, and hyalinization, with obstruction to aqueous outflow. Access of aqueous to the trabecula may be prevented by synechiae (angle closure), which develop following an empty or shallow anterior chamber, complicating surgery, or perforating injury. Choroidal detachment often is a factor. Angle closure also may occur with pupillary block and iris bombé when the periphery of the iris comes in contact with, and later adheres to, the trabecular area. Aqueous veins probably are compressed during an inflammatory process such as herpes zoster ophthalmicus, which causes edema of the sclera and, later, cicatricial changes. Hypersecretion of aqueous probably occurs with inflammatory glaucoma when hypertonic aqueous (increased protein in the aqueous) with fluid retention also may be a factor.

Treatment. If the pupillary block is promptly relieved by iris transfixion or iridectomy, the angle will reopen. If synechiae have formed and the iris has permanently adhered to the trabecula, iridectomy no longer opens the angle and the iris must be freed by cyclodialysis.

Common Types of Secondary Glaucoma

Corticosteroid Induced Glaucoma. Prolonged use of corticosteroid medications instilled locally can result in increased intraocular pressure, probably from changes that the medications produce in the trabecula. The condition simulates chronic simple glaucoma and can progress to glaucoma cupping and visual loss. This type of glaucoma usually subsides after corticosteroid therapy has been discontinued, but it has been reported to persist. Occasionally a patient may have had preexisting mild, chronic, simple glaucoma aggravated by corticosteroid therapy. Apparently the incidence of glaucoma secondary to such therapy is higher in patients with a family history of chronic simple glaucoma.

Whenever a patient has an elevated intraocular pressure, he should be asked if he is using corticosteroids. A patient whose intraocular pressure has been elevated while using corticosteroids should be considered a "glaucoma suspect." Corticosteroids should be discontinued at least a month before the diagnosis of primary glaucoma is made. In practice, topical corticosteroid therapy should be used only under careful supervision with intraocular pressure measured repeatedly. At times it may be desirable to continue the therapy even though the intraocular pressure is elevated, but antiglaucoma drugs should be used. In general the corticosteroids that do not cause elevated intraocular pressure should be employed. Recent studies indicate that hydroxymethylprogesterone, 1 per cent (Medrysone) is a corticosteroid to fulfill these qualifications.

Some of the corticosteroids that cause an increase in pressure are betamethasone, prednisolone, dexamethasone, hydrocortisone, and triamcinolone. Dexamethasone seems to cause the highest rise in pressure per dose. The following is a list of drugs containing these corticosteroids:

1. *Prednisolone:* Blephamide, Isopto-cetapred, Metimyd, Neo-Delta-Cortef, Neo-Deltef, Neo-Hydeltrasal, Predmycin, Sulfapred, Vasocidin, Hydeltrasol, Isopto-Prednisolone, Prednefrin, and Metreton.

2. *Dexamethasone:* Neo-Decadron, Decadron, and Isopto-Maxidex.

3. *Hydrocortisone:* Chloromycetin with hydrocortisone, Cortisporin, Isopto P-H-N, Neo-Cortef, Neo-Polycin, Ophthocort, Terra-Cortril, Cortril, Hydrocortone, Isopto-Sterofim, and Optef.

4. *Triamcinolone:* Neo-Aristocort.

Lens-induced Glaucoma. Glaucoma of lenticular origin is frequent. Complete or partial dislocation of the lens may cause elevated pressure and can occur spontaneously with many conditions, including Marfan's syndrome, cystinuria, and hypermature cataract. This last condition with marked swelling of the lens (intumescence) also can cause the angle of the anterior chamber to narrow and finally close. Hypermaturity of the lens can cause phacolytic glaucoma also.

Although rare, glaucoma secondary to exfoliation of the lens occurs with glass-blowers' cataract. Pseudoexfoliation of the lens capsule, an entity of obscure etiology, frequently is associated with glaucoma. Exfoliated lens capsule material or a precipitate from the aqueous humor results in a frosted appearance of the pupillary border. Particles resembling dandruff can be seen on the trabecula. These particles and pigment that has migrated from the pupillary border of the iris probably obstruct aqueous outflow.

On slit lamp biomicroscopic examination the lens has a characteristic appearance. The pupillary area of the anterior lens capsule usually has a central, disclike, frosted opacity on its anterior surface. Outside the pupillary zone is a peripheral area of clear capsule. With wide dilatation of the pupil, a more peripheral frosted zone of the lens can be seen that continues on to the zonular fibers.

Glaucoma and Retinal Detachment. Occasionally glaucoma occurs with some retinal detachment, but the possibility of a previous, probably long-forgotten, contusion of the eyeball always should be excluded. Gonioscopy should be done to exclude contusion angle deformity, indicative of an old injury.

Glaucoma Secondary to Intraocular Tumors. The following mechanisms can be implicated when glaucoma occurs secondary to intraocular tumors: volume occupied by the tumor, irritation by toxic products liberated by the tumor, and angle closure as the tumor occupies more space and pushes the iris forward.

Pigmentary Glaucoma. Glaucoma occurs in about 40 per cent of eyes with Krukenberg's spindle and marked pigmentation of the trabecula. The pigment is derived from an unexplained atrophy of the epithelial layers of the iris. When a transilluminating light is placed upon the sclera, the periphery of the iris transilluminates. Presumably the pigment obstructs outflow channels through the trabecula and causes the intraocular pressure to rise. The condition is a recessive characteristic. Pigmentary glaucoma runs a chronic simple course and is treated identically. Although the use of local corticosteroids is apt to aggravate it, pigmentary glaucoma often shows a dramatic response to Levo-epinephrine applications.

Essential Atrophy of the Iris. The causes of essential atrophy of the iris are uncertain. Pathologic changes appear to be related directly to multiple occlusions of iris vessels. Normally the iris has a rich blood supply with a major circle supplying the ciliary portion, the lesser circle of the pupillary zone, and the rich anastomotic network in between. In essential atrophy of the iris, the lumens of the smaller arteries and capillaries markedly reduce in diameter. Complete occlusions are located adjacent to areas of iris atrophy and occur in vessels that had supplied these areas. It is not known what causes arterial occlusion.

Epithelial Ingrowth. Epithelial ingrowth occurs after intraocular surgical procedures or penetrating wounds where wound healing is poor. A remaining fistular tract permits conjunctival epithelium to grow into the anterior chamber, to obstruct the trabecula, and occasionally to give rise to a pupillary block. Irradiation, removal of the cells by curettage and excision, and cryosurgery have been advised. None is satisfactory. The best treatment is prevention by meticulous surgery and good wound closure.

BIBLIOGRAPHY

Ballintine, E. J.: Glaucoma. Arch. Ophth. 76:869, 1966.

Becker, B., and Friedenwald, J. S.: Clinical aqueous outflow. Arch. Ophth. 50:557, 1953.

Becker, B., and Shaffer, R. N.: Diagnosis and Therapy of the Glaucomas. St. Louis, The C. V. Mosby Co., 1965.

Chandler, P. A.: Narrow angle glaucoma. Arch. Ophth. 47:695, 1952.

Goldmann, H.: Problems in present-day glaucoma research. In Streiff, E. B., and Babel, E. (eds.): Modern Problems in Ophthalmology. Vol. 1. Basel, S. Karger AG, 1957.

Goldmann, H.: Abflussdruck, Minutenvolumen und Widerstand der Kammerwasserströmung des Menschen. Docum. Ophth. 5-6:278, 1951.

Grant, W. M.: Physiological and pharmacological influences upon intraocular pressure. Pharmacol. Rev. 7:143, 1955.

Grant, W. M.: Tonographic method for measuring the facility and rate of aqueous flow in human eyes. Arch. Ophth. 44:204, 1950.

Haas, J. S. (Chairman): Symposium, the secondary glaucomas. National Society for the Prevention of Blindness, 1964.

Kolker, A. E., Becker, B., and Mills, D. W.: Intraocular pressure and visual fields: effects of corticosteroids. Arch. Ophth. 72:772, 1964.

Kronfeld, P. C., et al.: Tonography symposium. Tr. Am. Acad. Ophth. 65:133, 1961.

Newell, F. W. (ed.): Glaucoma: transactions of the first, second, third, fourth and fifth conferences. New York, Josiah Macy, Jr., Foundation, 1956-60.

Scheie, H. G.: Goniopuncture: an evaluation after eleven years. Arch. Ophth. 65:38, 1961.

Scheie, H. G.: The management of infantile glaucoma. Arch. Ophth. 62:35, 1959.

Sugar, H. S.: The Glaucomas. New York, Paul B. Hoeber, Inc., 1957.

Symposium on Glaucoma. Tr. New Orleans Acad. of Ophth. St. Louis, The C. V. Mosby Co., 1967.

Theobold, G. D.: Pseudoexfoliation of the lens capsule: relation to "true" exfoliation of the lens capsule as reported in the literature and role in the production of glaucoma capsulocuticulare. Am. J. Ophth. 37:1, 1954.

Wolff, S. M., and Zimmerman, L. E.: Chronic secondary glaucoma associated with the retrodisplacement of iris root and deepening of the anterior chamber angle secondary to contusion. Am. J. Ophth. 54:547, 1962.

Chapter Nine

OCULAR INJURIES

All physicians, especially those concerned with trauma, should be familiar with the treatment of the injured eye and adnexa. Since the dramatic appearance of a serious eye injury may mask injury elsewhere, however, the general condition of a patient always should be assessed for possible intracranial or other associated injury.

Ocular injuries require immediate and definitive treatment. The first person available, whether physician, nurse, or layman, most often renders immediate treatment. It is mainly prophylactic and directed towards preventing further injury and future complications. Usually the ophthalmologist sees the patient only after referral for definitive treatment.

The eye is vulnerable to trauma, but it has a highly developed protective mechanism. The bony orbital rim wards off and prevents many mechanical injuries, and the orbital contents cushion the effect of direct blows. The eyelashes and eyelids are highly sensitive and quickly close reflexly through visual, mechanical, and other stimuli. Simultaneously the eyes rotate upward beneath the upper lids (Bell's phenomenon) to protect the cornea. When the eye is irritated, lacrimal secretion greatly increases. Protective goggles and shatterproof safety lenses have been extremely helpful, but frequently they are not available or not used.

BURNS

Chemical. Chemical burns of the eye are not unusual in industry or in the home (Plate 31*A* to *E*). Regardless of the nature of the chemical, immediate, copious irrigation is of the utmost importance. If no other means is available, the entire face should be submerged in a container of tap water and the eyes opened and closed continuously. If no container is available, the face and eyes may be held beneath a faucet. Sterility should be temporarily ignored. It is more essential for the chemical to be diluted and washed away as quickly as possible. Citric and boric acids are advised for alkali burns; sodium bicarbonate for acid burns. Five per cent ammonium tartrate is said to dissolve particles of lime that may have become imbedded in the conjunctiva. Industrial workers usually are instructed on the management of chemical burns of the eye. After first-aid therapy, patients should be referred to an ophthalmologist.

If the cornea is involved, or if the burn is due to alkali, the ophthalmologist usually sends the patient to a hospital. Initially an alkali burn may appear innocuous, but alkali penetrates and softens the tissue and further release of hydroxyl ions causes the injury to progress. Only after three or four days, or even longer, does its true extent become apparent. Acid, on the other hand, is neutralized quickly by the tissues, which permits the extent of the injury to be determined immediately.

Irrigation should be repeated at 15 to 30 minute intervals or done continuously by polyethylene tubing inserted through the lid. If the eye appears seriously injured, atropine should be instilled. Local and systemic application of antibiotics and steroids helps prevent secondary infection and tissue scarring. With scarring, the conjunctival cul-de-sacs may be shortened and the eyelids become adherent to the globe (symblepharon). Freeing the conjunctival adhesions by a glass rod or spatula is advised. Occasionally corneal ulceration may progress to perforation. At times this may be prevented by a protective conjunctival flap or corneal transplant. If a chemical injury causes severe iridocyclitis, secondary glaucoma may result.

Thermal. Although the blink reflex protects the eye itself from thermal burn injury, the cornea should be inspected as a safety measure. Late effects of contracture of the eyelids can be serious. The eyelids may be injured by flash burns and fiery explosions such as happen in airplane accidents and certain industrial accidents. Burns of the lids nearly always are associated with facial burns, so a plastic surgeon usually co-manages them with the ophthalmologist. Some surgeons cover the eyelids with sterile dressings and antibiotic ointments. Others prefer to leave the burned areas exposed or to use pressure dressings. At any sign of lid contracture beginning eversion (ectropion), lid adhesions should be created (tarsorrhaphy). Skin grafting may be necessary to prevent severe contracture and exposure of the eye. Full thickness grafts can be taken from the upper eyelid of the fellow eye (if uninjured), the supraclavicular or infraclavicular areas, the inner aspect of the forearm, or from behind the ear.

Radiation. The type and severity of radiation injury to the eye depends on the wavelength of the radiant energy and the degree of exposure. Ultraviolet radiation is absorbed largely by the cornea. Injuries to operating room and nursing personnel occur from accidental or careless exposure to ultraviolet lamps. Patients also may include mountain climbers afflicted with snow blindness and arc welders. Symptoms start three to six hours following exposure with extreme discomfort. The eyes water, burn, and feel full of sand. Objective findings usually are limited to punctate staining of the cornea. Rarely is the cornea scarred permanently. Associated burns of the face and eyelids are the rule. The average patient is well and comfortable within 10 to 15 hours after instillation of local anesthetics and antibiotics.

Radiant energy from the sun (eclipse blindness) (Plate 31F), an atomic bomb, a laser, or a photocoagulator may cause burns of the choroid and retina. Edema of the retina in the macular region follows the initial injury and often is bilateral. A tiny hole in the fovea results in a small, but permanent, central scotoma. Although the scotoma annoys the patient, his visual acuity usually is good. The iris may absorb infrared radiation that increases the temperature of the tissue and causes cataractous changes.

Therapeutic use of roentgen and beta radiation, or accidental exposure to it from inadequately protected diagnostic equipment, and injuries from atomic irradiation, can cause cataracts that are indistinguishable from the ordinary posterior subcapsular type. They usually progress to completion and require surgery. Signs of injury, however, may not appear for several years after exposure. Seen ophthalmoscopically, the characteristic feature is a posterior, subcapsular, doughnut-shaped lens opacity. This is sharply demarcated anteriorly and has a bivalve configuration when viewed with the slit lamp. The uveal tract may show inflammatory changes and even be accompanied by secondary glaucoma at times. The retina and optic nerve are quite resistant to radiation.

MECHANICAL INJURIES

When an eye is injured severely, both eyes should be covered with sterile dressings to immobilize the injured one and to prevent further injury. If no bandages are

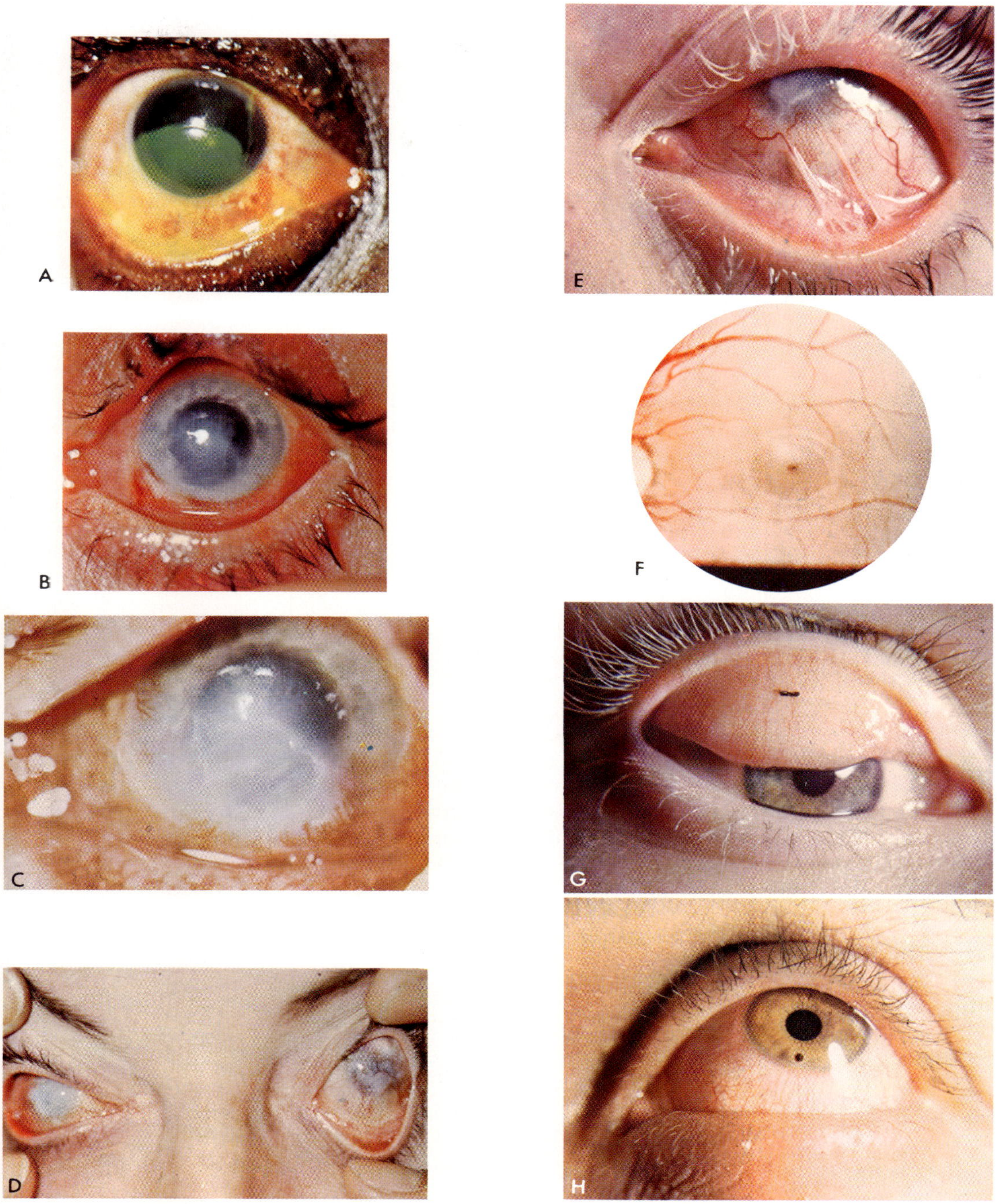

Plate 31 *(A)* Acute alkali burn of eye with fluorescein staining of cornea. *(B)* Acute alkali burn with corneal damage. *(C)* Same patient as shown in 31*B*. Corneal damage shows progression in picture taken at one month interval. *(D)* Bilateral alkali burn with late corneal scarring and vascularization. *(E)* Symblepharon, corneal scarring, and vascularization following alkali burn of eye. *(F)* Eclipse burn of macula. *(G)* Conjunctival foreign body beneath upper lid. *(H)* Metallic foreign body on lower aspect of cornea.

available, a clean handkerchief will suffice. Manipulation of the eye, such as to remove blood clots or foreign bodies, should not be attempted, because a simple wound could be converted into one with extensively herniated ocular contents (Fig. 9-1). Detailed examination should be deferred until the patient is under the care of an ophthalmologist. If possible, the patient should be moved by litter.

To facilitate inspection, lighting should be adequate and local anesthetics should be instilled gently into the eye. If a laceration of the eyeball is suspected, the facial muscles should be paralyzed (facial akinesia) by procaine injection into the facial nerve over the neck of the mandible. This prevents the lid from closing in response to pain and the ocular contents from extruding. Unless the injury obviously is too severe, the visual acuity should be recorded before any manipulation is done or medication given, because the physician is immediately medicolegally responsible. A patient who may have been unaware of poor vision before treatment may later assume that all visual loss in the injured eye is attributed to the injury or to the treatment. Preexisting amblyopia and even presbyopia have been causes of litigation.

After extensive eyelid laceration or avulsion, the eye should be protected by whatever means available. Simple dressings,

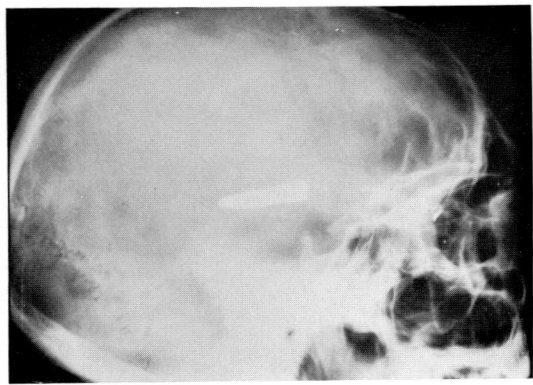

Figure 9-2 Bullet within brain, having entered through lid. No neurologic symptoms when admitted; subsequent intracranial hemorrhage with loss of consciousness. Life saved by immediate surgical intervention.

using copious amounts of petrolatum, may suffice, or a Buller's shield may be used.

The general condition of the patient should be ascertained and associated bodily injuries properly attended to, such as splinting an injured extremity and recognizing and managing shock. The orbital margins should be palpated to detect irregularities or defects. Emphysema of tissues indicates fracture or penetration into a sinus, usually the ethmoid. A fracture through the apex of the orbit with damage to the optic nerve or hemorrhage into the optic nerve sheath may cause unexplained loss of vision. Diplopia suggests a fracture (blowout) of the orbital floor or injury to the extraocular muscles or to their nerve supply. Enophthalmos is another diagnostic sign of orbital floor fracture, but it may be masked by orbital edema or hemorrhage that actually causes proptosis. Whenever a fracture is suspected, careful roentgen studies, including body section and Waters view films, should be made of the orbit. Intracranial involvement often occurs with mechanical injuries to the eye and adnexa (Fig. 9-2).

LACERATIONS OF THE EYELID

The need for correct management of ocular injuries is well illustrated in caring for injuries to the eyelids (Fig. 9-3). Intracranial injury and involvement of adjacent structures should always be suspected be-

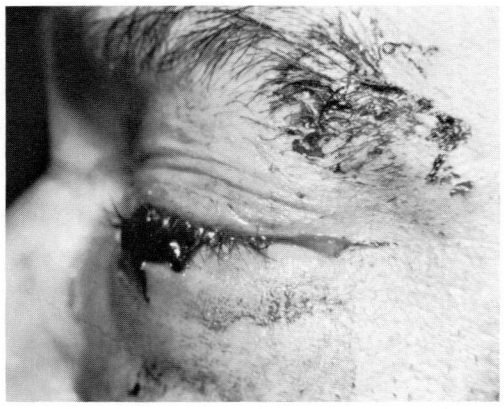

Figure 9-1 Injured eye which could be damaged further by removal of clotted blood.

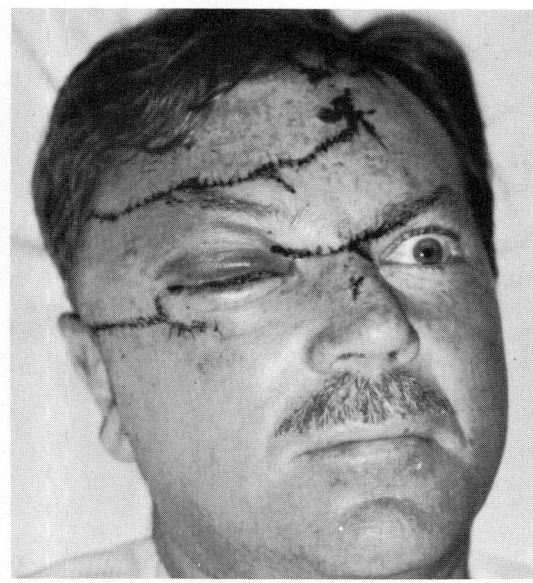

Figure 9-3 Lacerations of face and lid; examination of eye revealed severe ocular injuries.

cause the walls of the orbit are very thin. Whenever doubt exists, careful roentgen examinations should be done as soon as the patient is admitted to a hospital. Missiles, knives, tree branches, coat hangers, pencils, and other objects (some relatively blunt) have been known to injure deeper structures seriously.

Certain basic principles are important in the repair of lid lacerations. Proper care may prevent severe deformity requiring months of plastic surgery. The excellent blood supply of the lids minimizes tissue necrosis and the danger of infection and permits primary closure. Antibiotics rarely are necessary. The laceration should be cleansed with sterile saline solution, but if the amount of dirt is extensive, a cleansing agent such as tincture of green soap may be used. Large particles should be removed from the injured area by forceps. The excellent vascularity makes debridement unnecessary. Furthermore, excision might result in permanent deformity with need for extensive plastic reconstruction because eyelid tissue is limited.

To repair lacerations requires an awareness of certain details of lid anatomy. The eyelid has two easily separated layers: anterior and posterior. The gray line of the intermarginal portion of the eyelid marks the junction of the two layers. The anterior is made up of skin, subcutaneous tissue, orbicularis muscle, the lash follicles, and their associated glands. The posterior (inner) layer consists of the tarsal plate, the levator muscle, and the conjunctiva. The tarsal plate, a flat structure of dense fibrous connective tissue that is lined by the conjunctiva, forms the basis for most surgical techniques used in the repair of extensive lacerations or reconstruction of the eyelids.

Superficial lacerations, parallel to the lid margin, may not require closure, especially if they are small and within a lid fold. With larger lacerations and separated wound edges, simple, interrupted 6-0 black silk sutures may be used. A deeper, more extensive laceration that involves the orbicularis muscle fibers or one that is perpendicular or irregular requires careful closure, because the wound edges retract and tend to heal with unsightly scars. Prior to skin suture, the orbicularis muscle fibers should be approximated carefully with 5-0 plain catgut. If the lacerations are horizontal across the upper lid, they may sever the levator palpebralis muscle and cause complete ptosis. Their repair requires prompt, meticulous attention and should be done by an experienced ophthalmologist.

An injury that divides the entire thickness of the eyelid and extends through the lid margin presents special problems. Encircling the palpebral fissure and running parallel to the lid margin are the bundles of the orbicularis muscle of both eyelids. When these fibers are cut, they immediately contract, causing marked separation of the wound edges. If repair is deferred for more than a week, the muscle fibers also undergo fibrosis. This may result in notching of the lid margin (coloboma). Fibrosis also causes the edematous tarsal plate to thicken and shrink (Fig. 9-4). What may have been an intact eyelid, therefore, except for the laceration site, is converted into two nubbins of connective tissue, one medial and other lateral. Since they cannot be approximated, regardless of the type of dissection, extensive reconstructive surgery becomes necessary. If not promptly repaired, even a small laceration forms a notch, with loss of

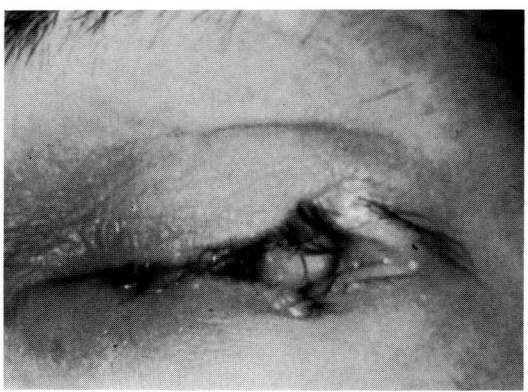

Figure 9-4 Shrinkage and fibrosis of lids with resultant notching, following untreated laceration through lid margin.

continuity and tearing due to malfunction of the lid margin. If repair is not meticulous, lashes may become misdirected, grow against the cornea and cause discomfort and often corneal ulceration. Healing usually follows prompt, careful repair.

Several techniques are available for repair of lacerations that extend through the lid margin, but simple approximation is preferred by this author. The severed wound edges are approximated accurately and held by interrupted sutures placed separately through the inner and outer layers of the lid. Irregular edges of the wound can be evened by excision with as little tissue as possible removed. It may be helpful to shape the opposing edges of the tarsal plate in a slightly concave manner so that when they are approximated, a slight pouting (overcorrection) of the lid margin results.

With the firm tarsal plate as a foundation, the cut edges of the tarsus are approximated carefully by three or four mild, 6-0 chromic catgut sutures. The edges of the lid margin (intermarginal space) must be meticulously aligned. To insure accurate approximation and to avoid any possible inversion of lashes, a fine 6-0 silk suture is placed through the gray line of the intermarginal space on each side of the laceration. The catgut sutures are placed through the cut edges of the tarsal plate from the inside. When tied, the knots are within the

lid substance where they are absorbed without abrading the cornea. Finally the orbicularis muscle and skin are closed with interrupted 6-0 silk sutures, and a gentle pressure dressing is applied. This method of closure may be used following the loss of lid margin tissue due to injury or after removing tumors with a wedge of tissue through the lid margin. Even large defects may be closed by an incision made through the lateral canthus (canthotomy) and the adjacent skin undermined to relieve tension. At times, when large portions of the eyelid are destroyed, reconstruction or extensive grafting is required.

Lacerations or tears through the canalicular portion of the lid (medial to the lacrimal puncta) involve the canaliculi. This is the weakest portion of the lid and is the site of tears from blunt trauma, as when one's eyelid catches on a nail or a tree branch, or, as can happen in sports such as basketball, even on a fingernail. Prompt reconstruction prevents permanent tearing. Canalicular tears or lacerations of the lower lid are more serious than those of the upper lid because the lower canaliculi are largely responsible for conducting tears to the lacrimal sac and nose (Fig. 9-5). Medial repair is more difficult than repair of lateral lacerations because the canaliculus must be restored and the adjacent tissues are soft and areolar. The medial canthal ligament is

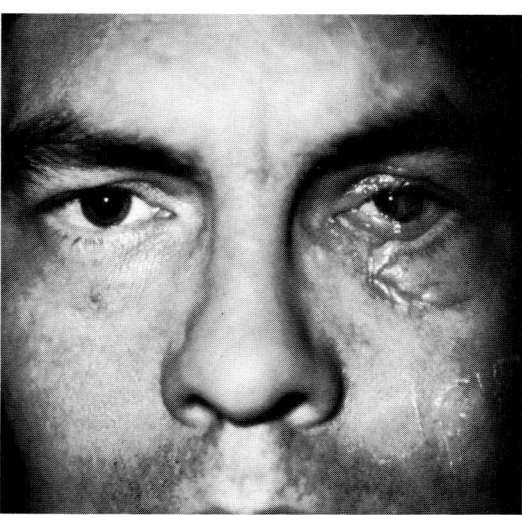

Figure 9-5 Laceration involving canalicular part of lower lid with subsequent contracture and shrinkage to half the length of the lid. Permanent tearing resulted.

difficult to identify, gives little support to the wound even when sutured, and inadequately withstands the pull of the orbicularis muscle. Thus the wound edges and the cut ends of the canaliculi separate, with resultant closure of the canaliculi.

An excellent method of treatment is to prepare a new canaliculus by dissecting a 5 or 6 mm. strip of tarsus from the medial end of the inferior border of the lower tarsal plate or the superior border of the upper tarsal plate. This is prepared as a pedicle flap that remains attached to the medial border of the tarsal plate. The flap is sutured to the anterior lacrimal crest as a substitute for the canthal ligament. Excellent support is provided for the lid. To insure patency of the duct, a polyethylene tube is inserted through the punctum and torn ends of the canaliculus, and the tissues adjacent to the laceration or tear are sutured. The tube is allowed to remain in place for approximately two weeks.

FOREIGN BODIES

Conjunctival. Frequently conjunctival foreign bodies lodge beneath the upper lid in the concavity of the tarsal plate (Plate 31G). The patient can remove these by grasping the lashes of the upper lid and pulling the lid down over the lower one. Gentle pressure upon the lid as it retracts to its normal position permits the lashes of the lower lid to brush away the foreign body. If the patient is unsuccessful in doing this, he may consult a physician. The lower lid should be everted and the foreign body removed by a stream of saline or wiped off with a moistened applicator. Foreign bodies rarely lodge in the upper or lower cul-de-sacs. In the lower, they are easily found and removed by irrigation or an applicator. In the upper, the lid may need to be doubly everted for them to be seen. A loose lash occasionally may find its way into the upper or lower punctum, or more rarely, within a meibomian gland and cause a foreign body sensation. Unless one is aware of this possibility, the lash easily can be overlooked. Once found, however, it can be removed readily with a cilia forceps or hemostat.

After a conjunctival foreign body has

been removed, relief usually is immediate, but discomfort may persist if the cornea has been scratched. As a precaution, whenever a patient complains of a foreign body sensation, fluorescein should be instilled, because the cornea stains at the site of a foreign body. If an abrasion is present, local antibiotics should be prescribed prophylactically. The patient should be told that he will have discomfort until healing occurs, which usually is a matter of hours, but could be a day or two.

Corneal. When a foreign body is found in the conjunctiva, the cornea also should be inspected carefully, for foreign bodies are common on the surface of the cornea (Plate 31H). Since the cornea is very sensitive, considerable discomfort is the rule, although occasionally there may be little distress. The patient usually complains of a foreign body beneath the upper lid because movement of the lid margin over the corneal foreign body causes pain. The cornea should be inspected by focal illumination from a penlight or other appropriate light source. As the light is moved slowly from the sclera to the limbus, the foreign body reflects light rays from the corneal surface (scleral scatter). A binocular loupe is essential for visualizing small foreign bodies. For a detailed examination by an ophthalmologist, a slit lamp and a corneal microscope should be used. Also helpful is the instillation of fluorescein to stain the foreign body site.

The technique for removing corneal foreign bodies depends upon skill and available facilities. For any manipulation of the cornea, a local anesthetic such as tetracaine hydrochloride, 0.5 to 1 per cent, should be instilled. Irrigation, however, can be done safely without anesthetizing and always should be attempted first because mechanical removal usually causes some additional corneal trauma. A fine, forceful stream of saline can be directed toward the foreign body from an atomizer irrigator or from a hypodermic syringe with a fine needle, e.g., No. 27, all of which should be sterilized. If a general physician or nurse cannot remove the foreign body by irrigation, he or she may wish to use an applicator moistened with saline. This procedure, however, may remove considerable corneal epithelium. If mechanical removal is necessary, the patient usually should be referred to an ophthalmologist, who with the aid of a slit lamp or corneal microscope can remove the object with a pointed knife needle or fine hypodermic needle. This technique causes the least possible corneal injury. When the foreign body is iron or is pigmented such as cigarette ash, the corneal site may be stained. Often it appears ringlike. The stained, devitalized tissue should be removed because it becomes an irritant and leads to infection. The ring may be removed by a knife needle used under magnification, although some physicians prefer to use a spud or fine dental burr.

No dressing is needed after the foreign body and pigment have been removed. Local antibiotics such as Chloromycetin or Neosporin drops should be prescribed for hourly use, since every corneal foreign body leaves an abrasion that is subject to infection. The foreign body itself may carry virulent particles. Patching the eye prevents the instillation of antibiotics and is associated with a rise in the conjunctival bacterial count. Because of the danger of infection, the patient should be seen each day and the cornea stained with fluorescein until healing occurs. If the injury or subsequent infection involves Bowman's membrane, scarring occurs, and even small corneal scars in the pupillary area can distort vision.

Intraocular. The presence of intraocular foreign bodies usually is not suspected, so they commonly are overlooked and roentgen studies are neglected. The presence of an intraocular foreign body must be excluded, however, whenever an eye appears to have a laceration or penetrating injury, large or small. A careful history should be taken to determine the patient's activities when the injury was incurred. Also, the type work his co-workers were doing is important because a metallic chip, for instance, can enter the eye from a considerable distance.

When small, high velocity fragments enter the eye, especially through the sclera, almost no symptoms may be present, and it may be several years before they do appear. The more sensitive cornea, however, simulates foreign body sensation when the eyelid moves over the site of injury. If the iris is involved and the lens capsule perforated, a painful iritis may result, and soon after, blurred vision occurs from lenticular haze (traumatic cataract). An intraocular foreign body should be sought carefully with a slit lamp and corneal microscope. The path of the foreign body often can be traced through the cornea with an underlying hole in the iris and injury to the lens. Tiny intraocular foreign bodies cause little more than a microscopic tract through the cornea. Whenever a hole in the iris is suspected, however, the pupil should be dilated to expose the lens to view and permit examination for possible passage of a foreign body. Any hemorrhagic area in the conjunctiva should be suspected as the point of entrance of a foreign body.

If small foreign bodies remain in the eye, they may cause it to be lost from hemorrhage, infection, or detached retina. A large (over 5 mm.) foreign body that enters the eye with force usually disrupts it markedly with severe bleeding, injury to the lens, and corneal and vitreous loss. Enucleation, which usually is necessary, should not be done before intracranial involvement is excluded. Aside from the damage that a foreign body causes, the great danger is purulent infection, since practically all foreign bodies must be assumed to be contaminated. Broad spectrum antibiotics, therefore, should be used prophylactically in full clinical dosage.

An intraocular foreign body may be seen with an ophthalmoscope (Plate 32A). Frequently, however, its presence can be confirmed only by roentgen examination, which always should be done in suspicious cases (Figs. 9-6, 9-7), especially if the media are hazy, as they are with traumatic cataract or intraocular hemorrhage. Special bone-free and fluoroscopic techniques have been devised. Once the diagnosis is established, or whenever real doubt exists about intraocular foreign bodies being present, the patient should be referred to an ophthalmic surgeon.

An intraocular foreign body may be localized in several ways. Roentgen pictures taken with a Comberg contact lens placed

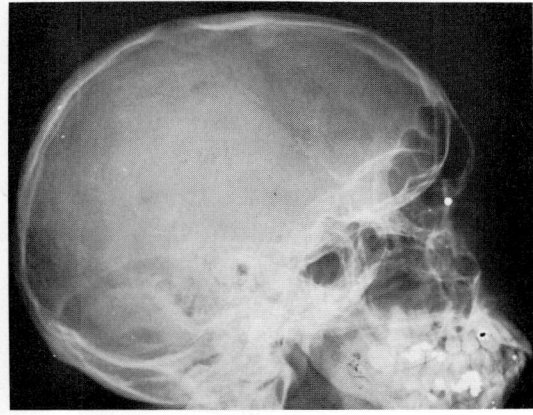

Figure 9-6 Radiopaque foreign body in region of eye (lateral view).

on the cornea can be helpful. A study of the relationship between the foreign body and the four lead dots of that lens permits rather accurate localization. The Sweet technique is a popular method based on mathematical calculations from roentgen pictures of the eye taken from different angles. Particularly helpful to the operation is the Berman electronic localizer that indicates placing of the scleral incision so that the magnet is applied directly over the

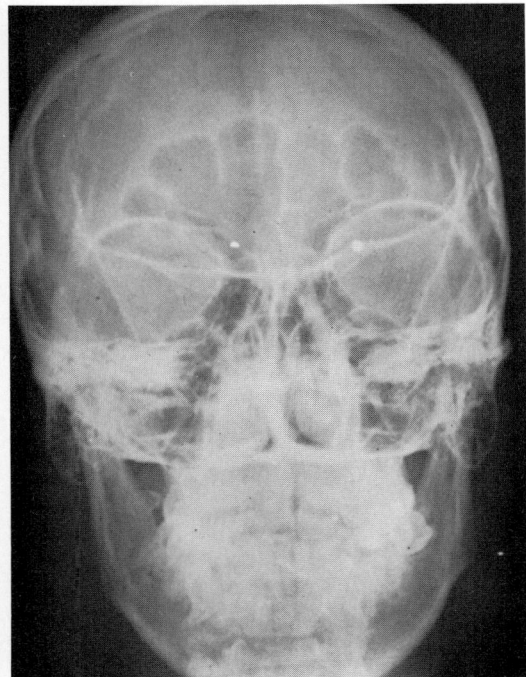

Figure 9-7 Same foreign body as in Figure 9-6 (anterior-posterior view).

metallic object. It is also of value in distinguishing magnetic from nonmagnetic foreign bodies.

Generally, unless the foreign body is readily accessible in the anterior chamber, only magnetic (nickel and iron) foreign bodies should be removed. Serious ocular damage usually results from any attempt to remove nonmagnetic foreign bodies from the posterior portion of the eye.

Magnetic foreign bodies in the anterior chamber should be removed through a limbal incision. If they are posterior to the lens, they should be removed through the sclera. Foreign bodies in the anterior vitreous should be removed through the pars plana of the ciliary body where the two retinal layers are fused, which minimizes the danger of retinal detachment. When the foreign bodies are more posterior, the incision should be made as near to the foreign body as possible. The sclera is incised carefully by a scratch to, but not through, the choroid. A magnetic field is used to pull the foreign body through the intact retina and choroid. To insure the smallest opening possible, the long axis of the body should be kept parallel to the magnet. Diathermy, cryosurgery, or light coagulation should be used around the site of the removal to seal the hole and to prevent retinal detachment. Systemic antibiotics should be continued until danger of infection is past.

Although the eye may survive the introduction of pieces of iron or copper, late irritative changes occur. Small particles may slowly be absorbed without damage to the eye, but usually it deteriorates. Iron oxidizes and combines with the ocular tissues (siderosis) (Plate 32*B*), causing irritation (uveitis) and gradual loss of the eye. Clinically the iris has a brown appearance that indicates ferrous staining, and a yellow-brown cataract usually is present. Histologically the iron can be demonstrated easily by the Prussian blue reaction. The iron is found within epithelial structures (corneal, iris, ciliary body, lens, and retinal pigment epithelium), the iris dilator muscle, and sensory retina. Anterior subcapsular cataracts and retinal degeneration and gliosis also are seen. Effects on the aqueous outflow pathways (sclerosis) may result in glaucoma. Copper, even more than iron, is irritating and toxic to the eye (a condition called chalcosis) and causes problems similar to those of siderosis. In addition to uveitis, a characteristic sunflower-like cataract develops. No satisfactory histochemical test is available to demonstrate copper intraocularly.

The eye may tolerate inert material such as lead, stainless steel, glass, aluminum, and certain types of plastics. Organic matter, however, such as wood and plant material, usually causes an overwhelming purulent panophthalmitis, and the eye is lost in a very few days.

INJURIES OF THE CONJUNCTIVA

Lacerations or tears of the bulbar conjunctiva may occur without injury to the eyelids or to the eyeball itself. Management of lacerations of the tarsal conjunctiva is discussed under lacerations of the eyelids (p. 364). Serious damage to the eye itself, especially laceration of the sclera or the presence of an intraocular foreign body, should be excluded. Localized edema and chemosis occur and the conjunctival defect stains with fluorescein. A tear more than 5 to 6 mm. long usually requires sutures. Administration of local antibiotics is advisable, and visual acuity should be recorded.

ABRASIONS AND SUPERFICIAL LACERATIONS OF THE CORNEA

Corneal abrasion is common, but diagnosis depends on the patient's account of the injury. If possible, the cornea should be inspected under magnification and stained with fluorescein, which will show the abraded areas as bright green. Antibiotic solutions should be used locally. Infection is a hazard, especially following injuries from highly contaminated objects such as vegetable matter and fingernails.

Increasingly severe pain and a gray opacity (infiltrate) at the site of the abrasion are signals of the infection. Vision may be lost from ensuing corneal opacity or from subsequent perforation of the cornea following destruction of corneal tissue. Corneal injuries usually heal rapidly without scarring if Bowman's membrane or the corneal stroma is not involved. In the absence of opacification, if the corneal surface is rendered irregular, impaired vision may result.

Corneal abrasions may heal with an unhealthy or inadequate base that results in "recurrent corneal erosion." In this syndrome, the epithelium remains loosely attached to the area of the previous injury. Several weeks or months later, the patient experiences photophobia and foreign body sensation when awakening at night or early in the morning. Loose epithelial cells which peel off with resultant break of the continuity of the corneal surface cause the discomfort. This can be demonstrated by fluorescein staining. Examination may reveal minute, gray-white dots within the epithelium. The dots can be seen with a slit lamp or corneal microscope and when the patient is symptom-free. Recovery from "recurrent corneal erosion" may be spontaneous, but if attacks are repeated, the condition can be cured by cauterization of the affected area with half-strength tincture of iodine.

PERFORATING INJURIES OF THE EYEBALL

General Management. Management of perforating injuries of the eyeball requires great judgment. Every effort should be made to prevent further injury than that caused by the initial trauma. Once a perforating injury is suspected, both eyes should be covered and detailed examination postponed. No attempts should be made to remove blood clots that might be protruding through the lids. Careful examination of the eyes should be deferred until done by an ophthalmologist with anesthesia, facial akinesia (procaine injection of the seventh nerve) to prevent squeezing of the lids, and good light, adequately magnified. Detailed examination may be deferred until

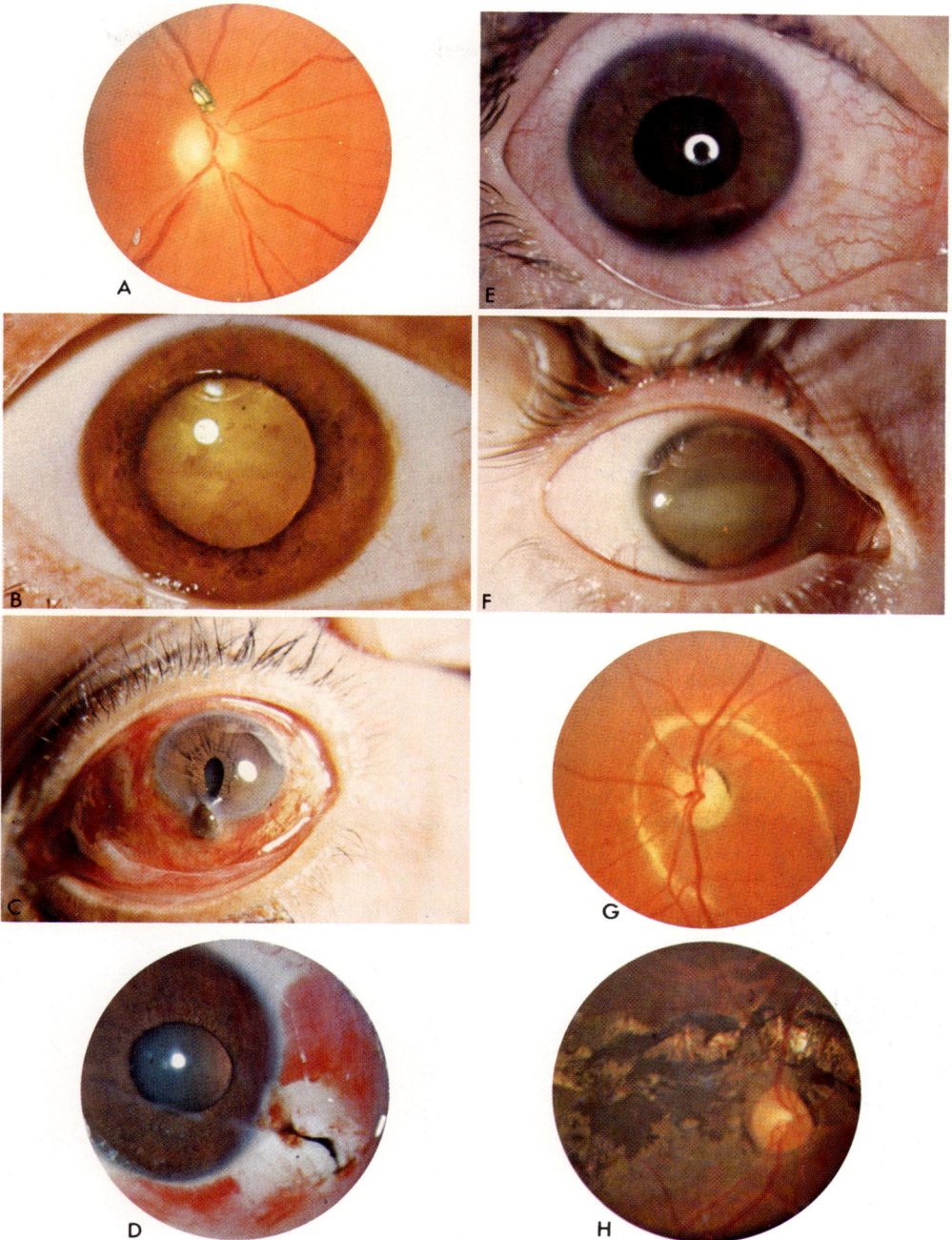

Plate 32 *(A)* Intraocular grenade fragment in vitreous anterior to optic nerve. *(B)* Siderosis with discoloration of iris and lens. *(C)* Corneal laceration with prolapsed iris. *(D)* Radial scleral laceration perpendicular to limbus with good prognosis. *(E)* Partial hyphema resulting from contusion of globe. *(F)* Blood staining of cornea following contusion, anterior chamber hemorrhage, and secondary glaucoma. *(G)* Choroidal rupture evident as a linear, crescent-shaped, white line concentric to disc. *(H)* Chorioretinal atrophy and pigment disturbance following contusion of globe.

the ophthalmic surgeon is ready to carry out surgical repair. If an ophthalmologist is not available for some time, atropine instillation usually is advisable to forestall traumatic iridocyclitis. Infection, once started, is difficult to control and rapidly destroys vision. Broad spectrum chemotherapy or antibiotic therapy, therefore, should be instituted as soon as possible. After any allergies have been determined, full therapeutic doses of streptomycin and penicillin given intramuscularly are in order. A booster dose of tetanus toxoid should be considered. Either local or systemic steroids, or both, are helpful in preventing or treating reactions to trauma.

Large, jagged wounds accompanied by extensive vitreous hemorrhage, with vitreous loss, usually require the eye to be enucleated, including extrusion of the lens or prolapse of the ciliary body. This need not be done immediately because infection rarely is a problem and there is little danger of hemorrhage or shock. Furthermore, the possibility of intracranial injury should be excluded by careful observation of the patient and by roentgen studies, especially if a sharp, pointed object or a high velocity fragment is involved (Figs. 9-8, 9-9, 9-10). Delaying enucleation a day or so reassures the patient that every attempt is being made to save the eye. Such assurance is a psychological help. Whenever doubt exists about the need to remove an eye, another ophthalmologist should be consulted.

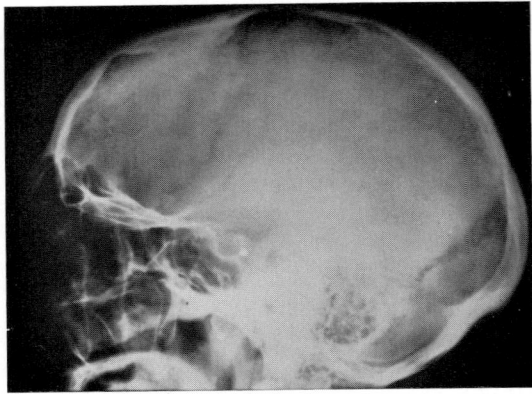

Figure 9-9 Shotgun pellet adjacent to carotid artery (lateral view) (same patient as in Figure 9-8).

If enucleation is not indicated clearly and is delayed, sympathetic ophthalmia becomes a grave consideration beginning two weeks after the injury and becomes most dangerous from the fourth to the twelfth week. Fortunately, the need for enucleation usually becomes apparent in two weeks, so an injured eye can be observed safely for that time. Then any doubtful eye should be observed carefully for at least a year. In 80 per cent of affected patients the disease occurs during the first three months.

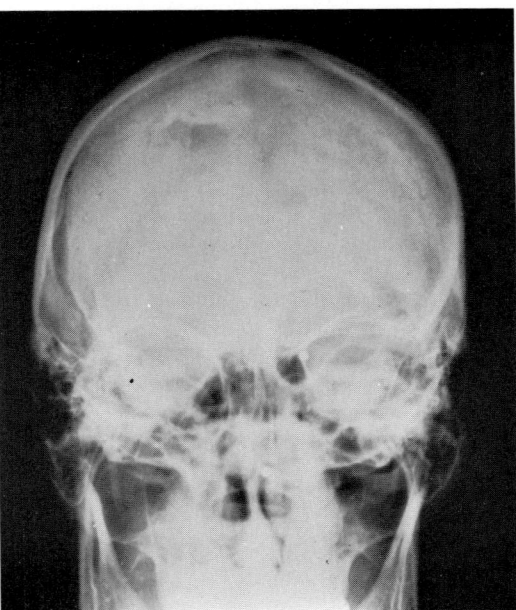

Figure 9-10 Same foreign body as in Figure 9-8 (anterior-posterior view).

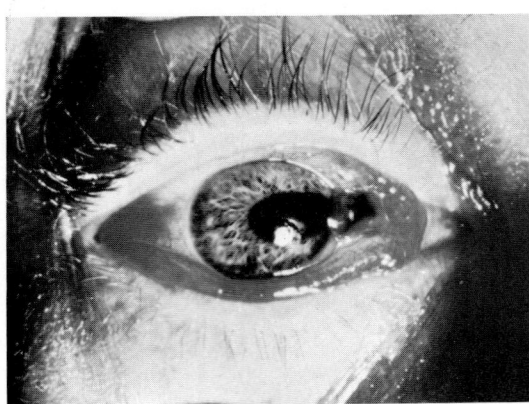

Figure 9-8 Shotgun injury with iris prolapse.

Sympathetic Ophthalmia. This is a bilateral, granulomatous uveitis that may follow any surgical or traumatic perforations involving the uveal tract (Fig. 9-11). The incidence is not high, but the disease must always be kept in mind because of its tragic results. It is thought to be an allergy to the patient's own uveal pigment. Histologically, sympathetic uveitis is characterized by a chronic granulomatous, inflammatory infiltrate of the uveal tract with sparing of the choriocapillaris (Fig. 9-12). Epithelioid cells within the infiltrate characteristically may phagocytize melanin granules. Dalen-Fuchs nodules (tubercles of epithelioid cells between Bruch's membrane and retinal pigment epithelium) may be found. It is prone to occur in an injured eye when subacute inflammation persists and uveal tissue is incarcerated in the wound, especially if associated with intraocular foreign bodies. If such an eye develops hypotony, it should be enucleated. Sympathetic ophthalmia in one eye leads to photophobia and inflammatory signs with blurring of vision in the other eye. The course may be relatively mild and indolent or overwhelming, with rapid blindness. Once the disease is established, ACTH and steroid therapy can be helpful, but the results usually are dismal. The best prevention, therefore, is to enucleate a dangerously injured eye.

Corneal Lacerations. Many factors influence the management of corneal lacerations: type, location, and size of the wound; the presence or absence of a foreign body; associated lens injury (traumatic cataract);

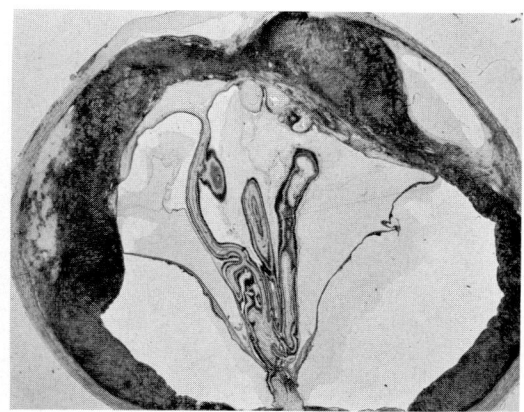

Figure 9-12 Histopathologic section of eye with sympathetic uveitis, showing characteristic massive inflammatory infiltrate of the uveal tract.

and intraocular hemorrhage. Exceptionally small corneal lacerations with no herniation (prolapse) of iris tissue may be left unsutured, but a gentle pressure dressing leads to smooth healing. Atropine or pilocarpine may be used to retract the iris from the wound, depending upon its location. Appositional corneal sutures employing 8-0 silk or 7-0 mild chromic catgut on wedged or fine sharp needles should be used to close large wounds.

Corneal lacerations often are accompanied by intraocular damage. Most ophthalmic surgeons excise the prolapsed iris (Plate 32C), closing the corneal wound as described above. The use of antibiotics lessens the chance of infection, permits simple replacement of the iris, and avoids excision of a sector of the iris, thereby producing better functional and cosmetic results. If associated with severe lens injury, repair of an iris prolapse may be delayed as long as two or three days to allow aqueous to digest the lens. The delay permits linear extraction or aspiration of the lens material through the corneal wound at the time of repair. The iris can be freed readily from the lips of the wound after such a short time. If the iris prolapse is cared for immediately, however, and the wound sutured, the lens material becomes highly irritative and predisposes to phaco-anaphylactic endophthalmitis and second-

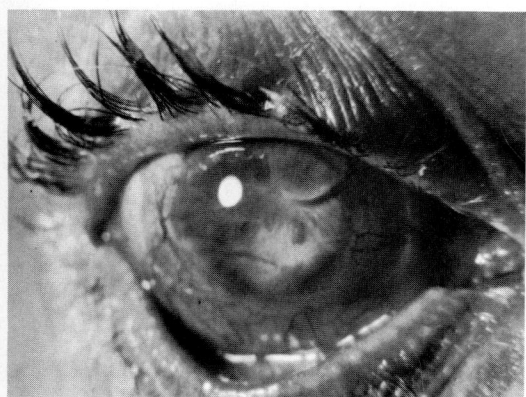

Figure 9-11 Sympathetic ophthalmia occurring following perforation.

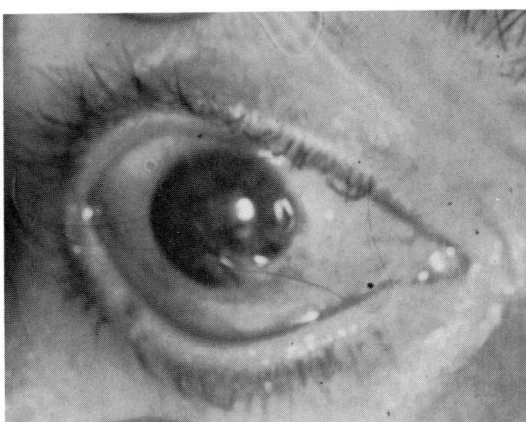

Figure 9-13 Perforating injury of eye with corneal laceration and traumatic cataract. After repair of cornea, lens material caused progressive iridocyclitis, which was relieved by aspiration of the cataract.

ary glaucoma (Fig. 9-13). Histologically phacoanaphylactic endophthalmitis is characterized by a zonal type of chronic, granulomatous, inflammatory infiltrate. The subsequent lens-iris reaction makes it difficult to remove the lens from the eye without damaging the iris. These complications and delayed recovery may not be attributed to the irritative lens material when the clinical picture already is obscured by the trauma of the original injury plus the further insult of the operative repair. If the injured lens is not removed, however, the eye may be lost.

Scleral Lacerations. The prognosis for wounds through the sclera into the ciliary body must always be guarded because of intraocular hemorrhage and associated injury to the lens, iris, retina, and vitreous body (Plate 32D). The outlook is best in clean wounds where little or no hemorrhage or vitreous disturbance has occurred. A clean wound perpendicular to the limbus bleeds less than a jagged wound or one parallel with the limbus, because the blood supply of the ciliary body runs in an anterior-posterior direction with the vessels parallel to one another.

Scleral lacerations should be closed with interrupted 7-0 mild chromic catgut sutures after prolapsed uveal tissue has been ex-

cised. The conjunctiva and Tenon's capsule also must be sutured. If the laceration is posterior to the ciliary body, the sclera should be treated with diathermy or cryotherapy to prevent retinal detachment.

CONTUSION OF THE EYEBALL

The primary effect of severe blunt force on the globe may be local injury at the site of impact from energy suddenly being dispersed throughout a closed system. The aqueous, which is a major center of force, can drive the iris diaphragm posteriorly, causing tears of the iris root, or into the ciliary body, giving the appearance of "recessed angle" (contusion angle deformity). Traumatic cyclodialysis (separation of the ciliary body from the sclera) rarely occurs. Severe anterior chamber hemorrhage with all of its complications often accompanies such tears. Contrecoup injury occurs to the posterior portions of the eyes. Contusions of the eyeball may result by transmission of energy when adjacent tissues are struck by

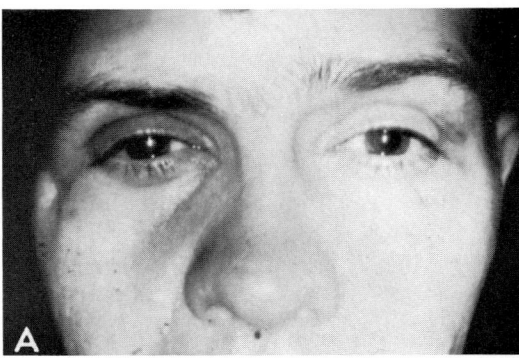

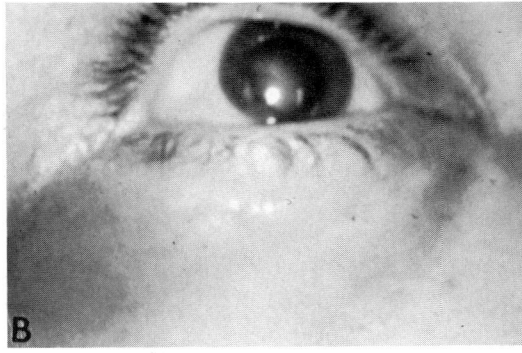

Figure 9-14(A), (B) Injury to zygomatic area resulting in severe contusion to eyeball from transmitted energy.

a high velocity missile such as a shell fragment (Fig. 9-14A, B). The eye may be damaged from the direct effect of the immediate mechanical injury or from other factors such as alterations of the neurovascular system. Marked pressure ischemia usually occurs initially followed by post-traumatic dilatation, hyperemia, and intraocular hemorrhage. Many of the effects upon ocular tissues are not clearly understood. Several types of ocular injury are associated with blunt trauma.

Hyphema. This is a common and extremely serious result of ocular contusion in which there is hemorrhaging into the anterior chamber, usually from tears of the ciliary body and iris (Plate 32E). Reflex hyperemia of the iris and ciliary body contributes to delayed hemorrhage and recurrent bleeding, which occurs from the third to fifth day. Patients with hyphema should be admitted to a hospital, sedated heavily, and kept on strict bedrest. Both eyes should be patched to provide immobility. Systemic and local steroids help to prevent recurrent bleeding by reducing irritation and hyperemia. It probably is more logical to use mydriatics than miotics, because they help put the eye at rest and prevent hyperemia. Diamox may help to avert rises in intraocular pressure.

In most partial hyphema cases, the blood is absorbed spontaneously. Massive bleeding may occur at the time of injury or during the following two weeks, and it may cause secondary glaucoma and blood staining of the cornea with loss of vision or even loss of an eye. The anterior chamber fills with dark, clotted blood (blackball hemorrhage). Blood staining almost always occurs as a result of increased pressure that forces blood pigment into corneal stroma (Plate 32F). Vision is not impaired unless the blow causes retinal damage.

Treatment in the past has not been satisfactory. Attempts at irrigation and mechanical removal of the clotted blood often are discouraging because the clot is indistinguishable from the delicate iris to which it firmly adheres. Removing the clot may injure the lens and cause avulsion of the iris or further bleeding. Fibrinolysin, which dissolves the clot, has proved helpful for irrigation, but it should be used only if the intraocular pressure is elevated and the anterior chamber is filled with blood. Urea administered intravenously and glycerol lower the intraocular pressure temporarily and may hasten absorption of the hemorrhage. They should be tried at least once or twice before fibrinolysin is used.

After the hyphema clears, contusion angle deformity commonly is seen by gonioscopy. The drainage mechanism of the angle of the anterior chamber may be injured seriously and result in chronic glaucoma with early onset, or it may not be revealed for months or years later. The course is similar to chronic simple glaucoma and treatment should be the same.

Traumatic Iridocyclitis. A severe form of this condition may follow trauma by blunt force. It results from vascular and tissue damage with histamine release, vasodilatation, and development of inflammatory signs. Minute tears in the lens capsule may allow small amounts of irritative lens material and uveal pigment to be liberated. Atropine used locally and steroids used orally and systemically usually resolve the iridocyclitis promptly. Occasionally an indolent endophthalmitis results in eventual loss of the globe.

Rupture of the Iris Sphincter. Trauma by blunt force also may cause single or multiple ruptures of the sphincter pupillae muscle. The pupil enlarges and irregular, small notches appear along the pupillary border at the site of the ruptures. The pupil constricts abnormally to light.

Iridodialysis. This condition, which is another result from trauma by blunt force,

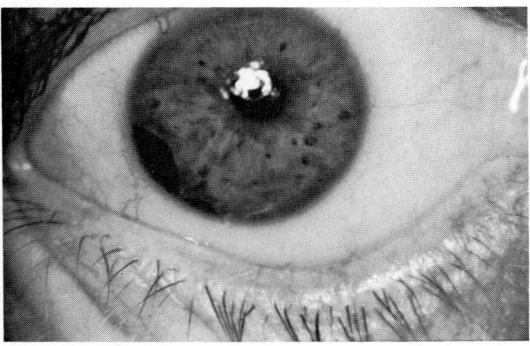

Figure 9-15 Iridodialysis caused by blunt trauma to the eye.

appears as an accessory pupil at the iris root (Fig. 9-15). It is caused by the easy tearing of the weak attachment of the iris to the ciliary body. Occasional diplopia is the only symptom. Holes in the iris at any location, whether the result of surgery or trauma, are permanent, because the iris has no capacity for self-repair. No treatment is indicated.

Injury to the Lens. Injury to the eyeball by blunt force may result in cataract formation years later. A characteristic flower-like bruise appears in the deep layers of the cortex (Fig. 9-16). If the lens capsule ruptures, a cataract may develop rapidly with a great deal of lens material in the anterior chamber (Fig. 9-17). In youngsters the cataract may be absorbed spontaneously, but usually the lens material must be removed by aspiration or linear extraction because of secondary glaucoma or irritation to the eye. Partial dislocation of the lens (subluxation) or complete dislocation (luxation) is not unusual. When this occurs, the zonule ruptures and vitreous may herniate forward into the anterior chamber around the edge of the lens. This type of injury often is associated with hyphema and contusion angle deformity. The displaced lens also may become cataractous years later.

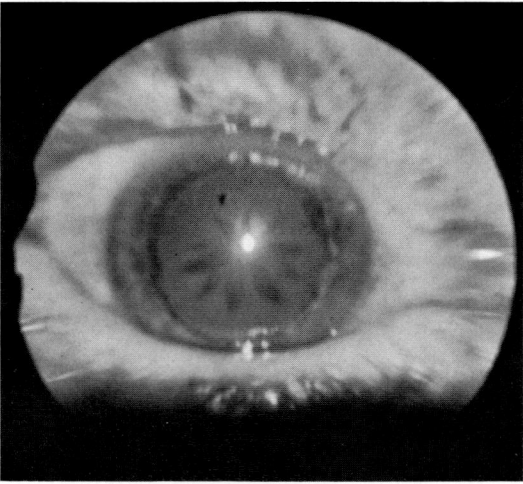

Figure 9-16 Flower-like cataract of ocular contusion.

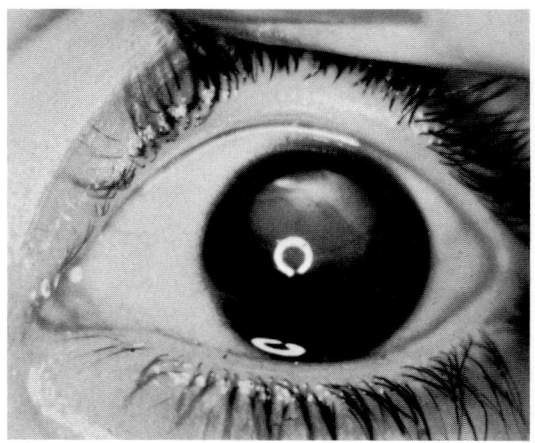

Figure 9-17 Traumatic cataract due to rupture of lens capsule caused by blunt injury to the eye.

Injuries to the Choroid and Retina. Contusions of the globe may injure the choroid and retina extensively. Ruptures of the choroid may be seen immediately or may be obscured by hemorrhage, becoming visible only after the blood has been absorbed. Hemorrhage into the choroid may be massive, pushing the choroid forward and producing a dark globular area resembling choroidal detachment seen after surgery. A choroidal rupture usually appears as a linear, crescent-shaped white area because the sclera is visible through the rupture (Plate 32G). Usually the ruptures are at the posterior pole of the eye and parallel to the disc border, but often they are between the disc and macula, through the macula itself, temporal to the macula, or even encircling the optic nerve. If the macular area of the retina is injured, vision is lost. Extensive edema of the choroid and retina may occur with or without retinal hemorrhage. Extensive chorioretinal atrophy may follow hemorrhage and edema of the choroid after retinal trauma. Large areas of the fundus may be involved and show marked pigmentary disturbance (Plate 32H), polycystic changes of the macular region and solitary macular cysts or holes. Trauma caused by blunt force is a common cause of peripheral retinal cysts, holes, and disinsertion (separation of the retina from the ciliary body) with ensuing retinal detachment. Chorioretinal damage was a common cause of profound loss of vision during World War II and resulted from direct blows to the eyes or indirect trauma to tissues near the eye.

Commotio Retinae. This frequently is seen in association with blunt injury to the eye and is due to a contrecoup effect. Extensive retinal edema is present, often associated with retinal hemorrhage. The retina, particularly the macular region, has a pale white edematous appearance. The periphery of the retina may show similar patches of edema, probably depending upon the nature and location of the injury and whether maximum force is direct or contrecoup. Cystoid degeneration of the macula and hole formation may occur immediately or months or years later.

Fat Emboli. These may occur when the long bones are fractured. Histologically they appear as lipid material within the lumen of small vessels. This can be demonstrated by special stains such as oil red O performed on frozen sections.

Purtscher's Retinopathy. This condition follows crushing injuries to the chest. It is characterized by edema of the retina with hemorrhages. Histologically it may be similar to fat emboli. Lipid material plugs up tiny vessels and may escape into the surrounding retinal tissue.

Glaucoma Secondary to Ocular Injuries. Secondary glaucoma may result from contusion of the eyeball. Numerous mechanisms are involved, such as severe anterior chamber hemorrhage, extensive synechiae that close the angle, severe angle contusion deformity, traumatic cyclodialysis or lens injury. The lens can precipitate glaucoma in several ways: a partially or completely dislocated lens can irritate the ciliary body, cause iridocyclitis, and dislocate anteriorly into the anterior chamber. Since the lens and iris form a valve-like mechanism, the aqueous cannot enter the anterior chamber to escape from the eye. Glaucoma also can result from allergy to lens material (phacoanaphylactic endophthalmitis). Liquefied lens proteins may leak through the intact capsule of a cataractous lens and set up an inflammatory reaction. The inflammatory cells and protein block the trabecula and cause glaucoma (phacolytic glaucoma). The inflammatory reaction is purely macrophagic (histiocytic), with the macrophages engulfing the liquefied lens protein and, along with free lens motion, mechanically blocking the aqueous outflow

pathways. Osmotic and irritative factors also may play a role. A hypermature, traumatic cataract may become swollen and push the iris forward to cause angle closure glaucoma. Vasomotor pressure combined with hypotony also may result in glaucoma and may alternate in the same eye. In elevating the protein content of the aqueous, traumatic iridocyclitis can contribute to secondary glaucoma.

Rupture of the Eyeball. Severe blunt injury can rupture the eyeball, usually at the equator. Since repair rarely is possible, the eye often must be removed. Hypotony and massive hemorrhage into the vitreous are diagnostic signs. The intraocular pressure can be elevated, however, and the signs masked because of massive vitreous hemorrhage and associated edema of the orbital tissues. Superior ruptures occasionally can be seen when the upper lid is retracted. When doubt about the rupture exists, the sclera should be inspected through a conjunctival incision. Sympathetic ophthalmia always is a danger.

ORBITAL INJURIES

Blunt force or penetrating objects may cause orbital fractures. The orbital rim is composed of rather massive, heavy bone. The walls of the orbit behind the rim, particularly the orbital floor (roof of the maxillary sinus) and the inner wall (lamina papyracea of the ethmoid) are thin and especially vulnerable to fracture. Following any severe injury about the eye, the orbital rim should be palpated. When any doubt exists about the injury, roentgen studies should be obtained. Fractured dislocation of the zygomatic bone and arch with facial deformity and depression of the cheekbone is common. The external canthus appears lowered. An otolaryngologist or maxillofacial surgeon usually treats these fractures by replacing the broken fragments through an incision at the posterior portion of the zygomatic arch. The bone then is elevated into place either with a periosteal elevator inserted into the temporalis muscle fossa or with a special toothed clamp that grasps the arch. Early correction is advised. Fractures through the superior orbital rim often extend into the cranial cavity and frontal sinus. Cerebral spinal fluid leak, meningitis, and brain abscess can occur. Fractures through the medial orbital rim and nose may shear off the nasolacrimal duct and close it permanently with consequent tearing. Fractures through the inferior orbital rim and those involving the zygomatic arch often are associated with depressed fractures of the orbital floor.

When trauma occurs from blunt force direct to the eye, the classic blowout fracture results (Figs. 9-18, 9-19). The weakest part of the orbit, the floor, is depressed into the maxillary sinus, but the orbital rim remains intact. The intraorbital pressure rises sharply. The soft orbital contents herniate into the opening, and they include the inferior rectus and inferior oblique muscles. These become trapped at the fracture site, and diplopia results on upward and downward gaze.

Any patient who has had a direct injury should be tested for diplopia. This also may result from injury to branches of the third, fourth, or sixth nerves, or to injury to the

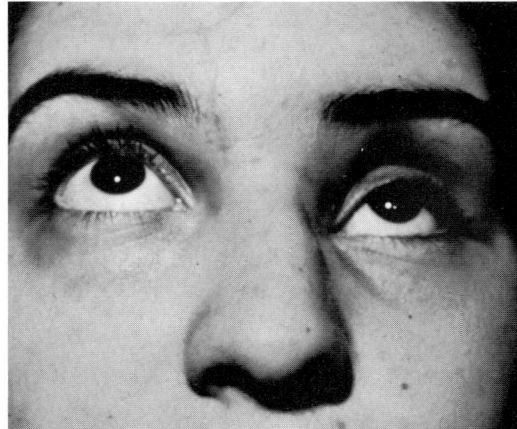

Figure 9-19 Limitation of upward gaze of left eye in the same patient as Figure 9-18.

trochlea of the superior oblique muscle at the upper medial aspect of the orbit. When doubt exists as to the cause of the diplopia, an exploratory incision should be made through the lower lid and the orbital floor exposed.

Enophthalmos is a diagnostic sign of blowout fracture, but it can be misleading because orbital hemorrhage and edema may cause exophthalmos that persists for days after the injury. Blowout fractures should be repaired as soon as possible by the Caldwell-Luc approach or by an incision through the lower lid to expose the orbital floor. After the herniated tissues are freed from the fracture site, the defect is covered with a sheet of plastic material or by a bone

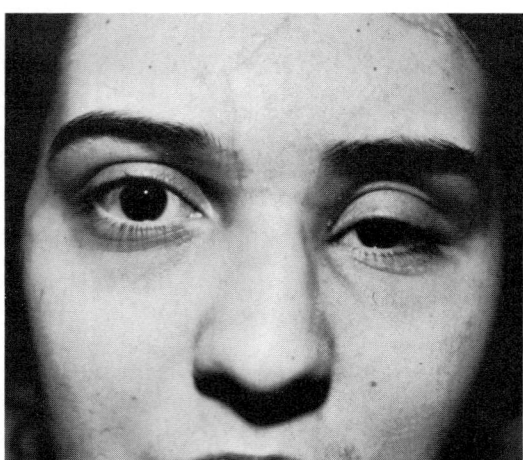

Figure 9-18 Blowout fracture of the orbit (patient looking straight ahead).

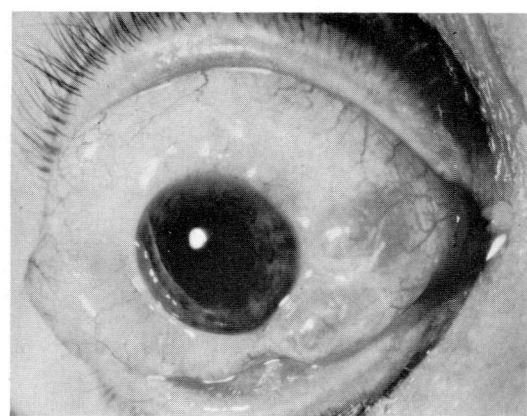

Figure 9-20 Emphysema involving the eye, resulting from fracture into the ethmoid sinus.

or cartilage graft. If a blowout fracture is associated with fractures of the facial bones and orbital rim, it is advisable for the ophthalmologist to work with the otolaryngologist or maxillofacial surgeon. Careful roentgen studies should be done. Because the bone is thin and fractures are difficult to demonstrate, both the Waters view and body section films should be used. Blowout fractures rarely occur into the ethmoid sinus. Fractures into either it or the maxillary sinus may allow air to infiltrate the tissues (emphysema), which, on palpation, exhibit a characteristic crackling or crepitation (Fig. 9-20).

BIBLIOGRAPHY

Burns

Cogan, D. G.: Lesions of the eye from radiant energy. J A.M.A. *142*:145, 1950.

Culver, J. F.: Visual aspects of radiation exposure. Mil. Med. *126*:667, 1961.

Grant, W. M., and Kern, H. L.: Action of alkalis on the corneal stroma. Arch. Ophth. *54*:931, 1955.

Hoffmann, D. H.: Eye burns caused by tear gas. Brit. J. Ophth. *51*:265, 1967.

Horwitz, I. D.: Management of alkali burns of the cornea and conjunctiva. Am. J. Ophth. *61*:340, 1966.

Hughes, W. F., Jr.: Chemical burns of the eyes. Arch. Ophth. *32*:432, 1944.

Penner, R., and McNair, J. N.: Eclipse blindness. Am. J. Ophth. *61*:1452, 1966.

Ryan, R. W.: Emergency treatment of chemical injuries of the eye. Arch. Indust. Hyg. *16*:250, 1957.

Symposium of the New Orleans Academy of Ophthalmology: Industrial and traumatic ophthalmology. St. Louis, The C. V. Mosby Co., 1964.

Lacerations of the Eyelid

Amdur, J.: Intermarginal suture for eyelid lacerations. Arch. Ophth. *69*:556, 1963.

Callahan, A.: Surgery of the Eye: Injuries. Springfield, Illinois, Charles C Thomas, 1950.

Smith, B.: Eyelid surgery. Surg. Clin. N. A. *39*:367, 1959.

Spaeth, E. B.: Closure of vertical lid lacerations. Am. J. Ophth. *61*:490, 1966.

Worst, J. G. F.: Method of reconstructing torn lacrimal canaliculus. Am. J. Ophth. *53*:520, 1962.

Foreign Bodies

Albert, D. M., Burns, W. P., and Scheie, H. G.: Severe orbitocranial foreign body injury. Am. J. Ophth. *60*:1109, 1965.

Bishop, J. W., and Morton, M. R.: Caterpillar hair keratoconjunctivitis. Am. J. Ophth. *64*:778, 1967.

Corley, J. A.: Reflections on the management of intraocular foreign bodies. Tr. Ophth. Soc. U. Kingdom *86*:803, 1966.

Fenton, R. H.: Power lawn mowers as a source of ocular injuries. Am. J. Ophth. *59*:312, 1965.

Hoefle, F. B.: Initial treatment of eye injuries. Arch. Ophth. *79*:33, 1968.

Laibson, P. R.: Inferior bullous keratopathy and unsuspected anterior chamber foreign body. Arch. Ophth. *74*:191, 1965.

Pfeiffer, R. L.: Localization of intraocular foreign bodies by means of the contact lens. Arch. Ophth. *32*:261, 1944.

Thorpe, H. E.: Foreign bodies in the anterior chamber angle. Am. J. Ophth. *61*:1339, 1966.

Abrasions and Superficial Lacerations of the Cornea

George, C. W., and Slack, W. J.: Corneal and scleral lacerations: a 5-year review. Am. J. Ophth. *54*: 119, 1962.

Perforating Injuries of the Eyeball

Bellow, J. G.: Observations on 300 consecutive cases of ocular war injuries. Am. J. Ophth. *30*:309, 1947.

Hull, F. E.: Management of eye casualties in the Far East Command during the Korean conflict. Tr. Am. Acad. Ophth. *56*:885, 1951.

Penner, R.: The liquid center golf ball. Arch. Ophth. *75*:68, 1966.

Wolter, J. R.: Removal of intraocular copper wire with a simple instrument. Am. J. Ophth. *78*:217, 1967.

Contusion of the Eyeball

Britten, M. J. A.: Follow-up of 54 cases of ocular contusion with hyphaema. Brit. J. Ophth. *49*:120, 1965.

Byrnes, V. A.: Elevated intravascular pressure as an etiologic mechanism in the production of eye injuries. Tr. Am. Ophth. Soc. *57*:473, 1959.

Gitter, K. A., Slusher, M., and Justice, J.: Traumatic hemorrhagic detachment of retinal pigment epithelium. Arch. Ophth. *79*:729, 1968.

Jarrett, W. H.: Dislocation of the lens. Am. J. Ophth. *78*:289, 1967.

Marr, W. G., and Marr, E. G.: Some observations on Purtscher's disease: traumatic retinal angiopathy. Am. J. Ophth. *54*:693, 1962.

Riffenburgh, R. S.: Contusion rupture of the sclera. Arch. Ophth. *69*:722, 1963.

Rodman, H. I.: Chronic open angle glaucoma associated with traumatic dislocation of the lens: a new pathogenetic concept. Arch. Ophth. *69*: 445, 1963.

Smith, M. E., and Zimmerman, L. E.: Contusive angle recession in phacolytic glaucoma. Arch. Ophth. *74*:799, 1965.

Weidentral, D. T., and Schepens, R. C.: Peripheral fundus changes associated with ocular contusion. Am. J. Ophth. *62*:465, 1966.

Wolff, S. M., and Zimmerman, L. E.: Chronic secondary glaucoma associated with retrodisplacement of iris root and deepening of the anterior chamber angle secondary to contusion. Am. J. Ophth. *54*:547, 1962.

Wolter, J.: Coup-contrecoup mechanism of ocular injuries. Am. J. Ophth. *56*:785, 1963.

Zimmerman, L. E.: Acute secondary open angle glaucoma ten years after contusion. Surv. Ophth. *8*: 26, 1963.

Orbital Injuries

Abrahams, I. W., and Dodd, R. W.: Orbital floor fractures: a combined procedure of early surgical management. Arch. Ophth. *68*:159, 1962.

Anderson, R. D., and Teague, D. A.: Blowout fractures of the orbital floor: the use of a stent in their repair. Am. J. Ophth. *56*:46, 1963.

Brown, O. L., *et al.*: Roentgen manifestations of blowout fractures of the orbit. Radiology *85*:908, 1965.

Converse, J. J., and Smith, B.: Symposium: midfacial fractures. Nasoorbital fractures. Tr. Am. Acad. Ophth. *67*:622, 1963.

Cunningham, J. D., and Marden, P. A.: Blowout fracture of the orbital floor. Arch. Ophth. *68*:498, 1962.

Jones, D. E. P.: Blowout fractures of the orbit. Tr. Ophth. Soc. U. Kingdom *86*:271, 1966.

Kazanjian, V. H., and Converse, J. M.: The Surgical Treatment of Facial Injuries. 2nd ed. Baltimore, Williams & Wilkins Co., 1959.

Kroll, M., and Wolper, J.: Orbital blowout fractures. Am. J. Ophth. *64*:1169, 1967.

Lloyd, G. A. S.: Orbital emphysema. Brit. J. Radiol. *39*:933, 1966.

Logan, W. C., and Gordon, D. S.: Traumatic lesions of the optic chiasma. Brit. J. Ophth. *51*:258, 1967.

Milauskas, A. D., and Fueger, G. F.: Serious ocular complications associated with blowout fractures of the orbit. Am. J. Ophth. *62*:670, 1966.

Nahum, A. M.: Facial trauma in automobile collisions. Tr. Am. Acad. Ophth. *69*:396, 1965.

Reeh, M. J., and Tsuyimura, J. K.: Early detection and treatment of blowout fractures of the orbit. Am. J. Ophth. *62*:79, 1966.

Smith, B., and Regan, W. F., Jr.: Blowout fracture of the orbit: mechanism and correction of internal orbital fractures. Am. J. Ophth. *44*:733, 1957.

Sugar, H. S., and Meyer, S. J.: Pulsating exophthalmos. Arch. Ophth. *23*:1288, 1940.

Chapter Ten

PRINCIPLES OF OCULAR SURGERY

This chapter is meant to orient physicians who are in branches of medicine other than ophthalmology in the principles of ocular surgery. The nature, the prognosis, and the significance of different operations are briefly discussed. No attempt is made to describe techniques in detail because eye operations rarely are performed by anyone but an ophthalmologist. The physician who wants more information, however, can obtain it from textbooks on ocular surgery.

CATARACT EXTRACTION

Cataract extraction is one of the most rewarding operations in the entire field of surgery. By restoring vision dramatically, it provides a new outlook on life for the elderly and a lifetime of vision for children.

General Principles

The history of cataract extraction dates to antiquity. For centuries, the accepted method was couching. It was done by inserting a needle into the eye to dislocate the opaque lens downward and backward into the vitreous cavity, thus providing a clear pupillary space.

Extracapsular Cataract Extraction. In 1745, Daviel revolutionized cataract extraction by introducing an extracapsular technique which is still widely used today, especially in young people. A large incision is made at the limbus through which the lens is removed after opening the anterior capsule. The posterior capsule is left in place. Because of its density and optical irregularities it may interfere with vision, necessitating a second operation, a capsulotomy (opening of the capsule), to produce a clear pupil (Fig. 10-1*A, B*). Even though the capsule may be clear and the vision good immediately after cataract extraction, it may opacify later because of debris, cell deposits, or even cell proliferation upon its surface.

Extracapsular extraction can be done only when a cataract is complete or mature (ripe). In such lenses the cortex is degenerative and fluid, and is readily irrigated from the eye after the hard nucleus is removed first, usually by external pressure upon the eyeball. If the cataract is incipient or immature, the lens cortex is viscid and tenacious; significant amounts of it remain adherent to the retained posterior lens capsule, and this may cause severe inflam-

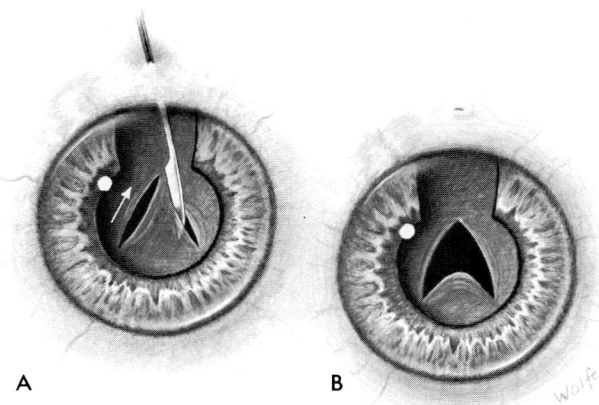

A   B

Figure 10-1 Incision of membranous posterior capsule (capsulotomy). *(A)* Creating an inverted V (arrow). *(B)* Resultant opening with clear pupil.

matory reactions even to the loss of an eye (phacoanaphylaxis).

Intracapsular Cataract Extraction. Developed near the turn of this century, intracapsular cataract extraction is now the most widely used operation for senile cataract. A large incision is made at the limbus, and the lens is grasped by a toothless forceps that pinches the capsule but does not tear it (Fig. 10-2*A, B*). Gentle traction upon the lens capsule and external pressure upon the eyeball rupture the zonule, or supporting ligament, of the lens and permit its removal intact within the capsule. Subsequent capsulotomy is thereby avoided. The lens may also be grasped and removed by the use of a suction cup (erisiphake) or by the increasingly popular cryoapplicator.

Originally the intracapsular procedure was accompanied by a high incidence of vitreous loss and wound complications because of the large incision, which extends over one half of the circumference of the limbus. These problems, however, have been largely eliminated by improved methods of anesthesia, by techniques for immobilizing the facial muscles (akinesia), and by refined methods of incision and wound closure made possible by the use of very delicate instruments, fine sutures, and specially developed needles.

The intracapsular method today is the operation of choice for the extraction of senile cataract, but it is rarely used for individuals under 30 years of age. In these younger individuals the zonular ligament supporting the lens is extremely tough, and the lens also is firmly attached near its

equator to the face of the vitreous (ligamentum hyaloideocapsulare). These lens attachments become significantly weaker throughout life, and after 30 years of age safe removal of the lens within its capsule can be accomplished. At an earlier age,

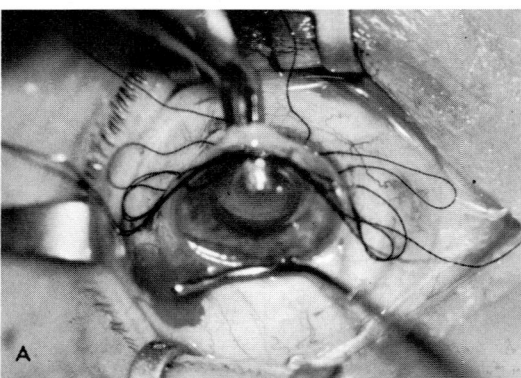

A

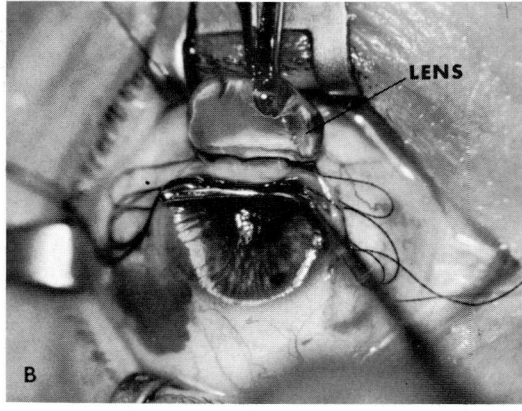

LENS

B

Figure 10-2 Intracapsular cataract extraction. *(A)* Capsule forceps applied to lens. *(B)* Delivery of lens through limbal incision.

vitreous is often lost because of the pressure required to rupture the zonule and through traction on the vitreous body due to the attachment of the lens to the face of the vitreous.

Vitreous loss is extremely serious and may result in degeneration of the globe, detachment of the retina, and wound complications, including corneal edema. Intracapsular lens removal has been greatly facilitated by the use of alpha-chymotrypsin, an enzyme that has a selective action upon the zonule, causing it to dissolve. Two or three minutes after injection of the enzyme behind the iris, the lens can be removed with little traction and minimal pressure. Although the zonule can be weakened at all ages, the ligamentum hyaloideocapsulare remains unaffected, and in the young it serves as a contraindication to the intracapsular method. The extracapsular type of extraction remains the operation of choice when the patient is under 30 years of age.

SENILE CATARACT. The great advantage of the intracapsular cataract removal is that it can be done any time a patient with a senile cataract is visually handicapped. The cataract need not be complete or "ripe," thus eliminating a prolonged period of progressive blindness during "ripening." Also, capsulotomy is avoided.

Indications for Surgery

Cataracts can be removed whenever the vision is sufficiently poor to interfere with everyday life. Visual acuity or a Snellen chart is not a reliable indication for surgery. For example, a lawyer or accountant might have excellent vision at 20 feet but still be unable to do the close work required by his profession. Surgery would be indicated, therefore, at an earlier time than for a laboring man who did little or no close work. Cataract extraction usually is not advised unless vision in both eyes is impaired, because an eye that has been operated on for cataract cannot be used with the unoperated fellow eye. When a cataract in one eye is removed, good visual acuity is obtained only by a strong spectacle lens of approximately 11 diopters to replace the optical power of the patient's own lens. The magnifying effect of this lens produces a retinal image that is of a different size than that of the fellow eye, and insurmountable diplopia

results. A contact lens may overcome the double vision but not every patient can tolerate one.

If good binocular vision is essential, unilateral cataract removal may be justified with the hope that it will be obtained by a contact lens for the operated eye. It is also often done if a cataract is complete to protect the eye against such possible complications of a hypermature cataract as dislocation with subsequent ocular irritation if posterior (and glaucoma if anterior); phacolytic glaucoma secondary to toxic substances from the cataract; and swelling of the lens, causing acute congestive (angle closure) glaucoma. Removing a mature cataract is also justified, even though vision in the other eye may be excellent, if the patient has a good life expectancy. Not only will his "side" vision be restored for driving a car and getting about, but also his eye will be protected and ready for correction and full usefulness in the future if the other eye should fail, which is likely.

Contraindications for Surgery

Associated Ocular Disease. A cataract should not be removed from an eye that is blind or nearly blind from other causes, because vision will not improve. For example, a patient may have had an unsuccessful operation for retinal detachment, or he may have an obstructed retinal artery or vein or an eye that has always been amblyopic. Senile macular degeneration is common in the elderly and should be excluded by careful preoperative examination. Such other signs of ocular pathology as marked iris atrophy, or signs of previous uveitis, suggest a guarded prognosis. Retinal function should be evaluated routinely before cataract extraction if the cataract is so advanced as to prevent viewing of the fundus. These tests, however, are somewhat crude and not entirely reliable. The patient's light field should be determined with a small, bright ophthalmoscope light. The field should be full and the patient should be able to tell the direction from which the light enters his visual field. He should be able to detect two lights that are 3 or 4 inches apart when they are held 2 feet from his eye. He should also be able to detect color when a red filter is held between his eye and the light. Gross defects in his visual field suggest retinal detachment or other severe retinal abnormality. Poor discrimination of two lights or of color suggests macular degeneration.

General Health. An elderly patient's general health, particularly his cardiovascular status, should always be evaluated preoperatively. If he has a life expectancy of a year or two, or even of several months, but his vision is poor, cataract extraction may be justified. The risks are small because the operation is done under local anesthesia, and the patient is ambulatory almost immediately. If he has diabetes, it should be well controlled, and diabetic retinopathy should be excluded, if possible, as a cause of vision loss. Unless terminal, a malignant tumor is not a contraindication, nor are previous episodes of coronary occlusions from which a patient has recovered. In the hospital a patient with cerebral atherosclerosis may become disoriented, but even on the first postoperative day he can be returned to his home environment where he usually recovers promptly.

The patient can see to get about with the operated eye in three to five days, provided he uses a cataract lens of approximate accuracy. Spectacles for reading are fitted in seven to nine weeks after surgery.

Technique for Cataract Extraction

Cataract extraction can be done under general or local anesthesia. Local anesthesia has many advantages, especially for the elderly, and is obtained by instilling an agent such as tetracaine hydrochloride, 1 per cent, into the conjunctiva, as well as by inserting a needle through the eyelid behind the eyeball and into the muscle cone to block the ciliary nerves and ganglion. This injection also paralyzes the extraocular muscles and prevents ocular movements. Anesthesia injected around the seventh nerve immobilizes the facial muscles and prevents forcible closing of the eyelids. Otherwise

the ocular contents might extrude and the eye might subsequently be lost. Improved methods of preoperative sedation are also safety factors.

Instruments used for cataract surgery have improved greatly. Incisions can be meticulously made and then tightly closed with fine sutures, thereby preventing postoperative wound complications. No longer must the patient be kept in bed for a week to ten days with his eyes covered and sandbags beside his head. Formerly this procedure subjected the elderly patient to the dangers of hypostatic pneumonia, circulatory disturbances, and other difficulties.

Complications. Complications during and following cataract extraction have been greatly reduced. Prolapse of the iris, formerly very common, rarely occurs because excellent wound closure is routine in present-day eye surgery. Postoperative infection may be prevented by the prophylactic use of antibiotics, both preoperatively and postoperatively, but if it does occur it can now be much more successfully treated. Postoperative iritis usually responds well to local and systemic steroids. Intraocular hemorrhage remains as a serious danger. Retinal detachment, although relatively rare, can be corrected by appropriate surgery. As a result, patients can be reassured that the prognosis in routine cataract extraction is extremely good. When the ophthalmologist recommends surgery, the general physician should not hesitate to support him.

Cataract Extraction in the Young Patient

In operations on individuals under 30 years of age, including children with congenital cataracts, the extracapsular method is the operation of choice. The extracapsular method is particularly adapted to the eye of the young patient because of his age; the nucleus of the lens is soft, permitting removal of the cataract through a small opening. A technique has been developed which permits aspiration of the lens through a No. 18 or No. 19 gauge needle. If the cataract is incomplete, a ripening operation can be done, consisting of incising the anterior lens capsule to permit the aqueous humor to enter the lens and liquefy the lens material. The lens is small and the fibers are loosely packed. This permits rapid action by the aqueous after the capsule has been opened. Removal of the lens material is readily accomplished after a few days. As with extracapsular extraction in the older patient, capsulotomy usually is needed.

Cataracts in young people often are referred to as soft cataracts because of the characteristics of the lens. Numerous causes for cataracts in this age group are mentioned in the literature (p. 123). Congenital and traumatic cataracts, however, are the commonest types in the young.

CONGENITAL CATARACTS

Congenital cataracts account for approximately 11 per cent of blindness in school children. The surgical treatment is more difficult and the results more unpredictable than in senile cataracts. Associated ocular anomalies such as microphthalmia, nystagmus, strabismus, myopia, aniridia, colobomas of the iris and lens, and systemic anomalies (such as rubella) require a guarded prognosis for good vision, even with a good surgical result. Associated mental retardation is not unusual. Attempt should always be made to determine the cause. Heredity is the most important single factor, but metabolic factors such as Lowe's syndrome, diabetes, hypocalcemia, and others should always be excluded.

Indications for Surgery. Ophthalmologists generally agree that surgery for bilateral complete cataract should be avoided until the child is at least 6 months of age and should not be done then if contraindicated by associated anomalies or severe systemic disease. If the cataracts are incomplete, but the child is developing normally and plays well, operation should be postponed until he is truly handicapped. This often becomes apparent when he is of school age and it is realized that he cannot do the work of his class. The decision to operate should be made jointly by the family, the teacher, the pediatrician, and the ophthalmologist.

SURGICAL TECHNIQUES FOR CATARACTS IN THE YOUNG

Optical Iridectomy. Iridectomy, which enlarges the pupil, may be effective if the lens opacity is dense and central. Light rays are then able to enter the eye through the clear portion of the lens peripheral to the opacity. Although the visual results are not as good as with other techniques, the procedure is safe and is of particular value in retarded children where excellent visual acuity is not as important as a safe operation.

Extracapsular Extraction. Several techniques of extracapsular extraction have been developed for operating on the young patient.

DISCISSION. This involves opening the anterior lens capsule with a sharp needle-like knife to permit access of the aqueous to the lens substance, which is then slowly digested. The operation has several disadvantages. Multiple operations usually are necessary. Residual lens material and postoperative reaction tend to promote adhesions between the iris and the absorbing lens material and capsule. A resulting dense membrane over the pupillary space is difficult to open for a good visual result. Secondary glaucoma of the pupillary block type also can occur.

LINEAR EXTRACTION. A 5 to 6 mm. limbal or corneal incision is made, the anterior capsule of the lens is opened, and the soft lens material is washed and massaged from the eye, leaving the posterior capsule intact. Because the incision is relatively large, wound complications and vitreous loss are not unusual.

ASPIRATION. The lens capsule is opened, and the soft lens material is aspirated through an opening in the corneoscleral wall that should be just large enough to admit a No. 19 gauge needle. If the cataract is incomplete, a preliminary opening is made in the lens capsule, allowing aqueous to render the lens material semifluid (Plate 33). Three days to two weeks later, when the lens is opaque, aspiration removes the lens material readily and quite completely. This technique avoids the repeated operations of discission and the wound complications of linear extraction.

ZIEGLER THROUGH-AND-THROUGH DISCISSION. This single procedure operation involves making an incision through the entire thickness of the lens, usually in the form of an upright V. It is advantageous if the lens is thin and membranous.

Complications. Secondary glaucoma is a common complication following congenital cataract surgery and usually results from adhesion of the iris to residual lens material. This obstructs the flow of aqueous from the posterior to the anterior chamber (pupillary block). The adhesions may be prevented by the postoperative use of atropine and phenylephrine to maintain wide pupillary dilatation. If the pupil dilates poorly preoperatively (a not unusual finding, especially in cataracts due to rubella), a sector iridectomy should be done before, or at the same time as, the cataract is removed. When glaucoma does occur, iridectomy should be done promptly. A dense pupillary membrane, usually with adherent iris, can be a serious complication. Incision may be difficult and dangerous.

Retinal detachment, another complication, occurs with significantly higher incidence than in senile cataract operations and may come on years later. It probably results from a generally poorly developed eye, one anomaly occurring with the other.

Prognosis. The prognosis is more guarded in congenital cataract than in senile because surgical complications are more common. Associated abnormalities, such as nystagmus and microphthalmia, nearly always are accompanied by poor retinal function and a comparable visual result. The postoperative course is more unpredictable for congenital cataract than for senile; in the latter a timetable usually can be outlined. Since the lens is removed extracapsularly, the time required for absorption of the remaining lens material and recovery from surgery is somewhat uncertain. Sooner or later most of the eyes need an incision of the posterior capsule. For a child with a significant visual handicap as a result of congenital cataracts, however, surgery should be done because the operation is relatively safe and successful. The parents, however, always should be informed of the somewhat guarded outlook.

GLAUCOMA SURGERY

The indications for surgery have been discussed in the chapter on glaucoma (p. 336). In brief, the treatment for narrow angle glaucoma is primarily surgical and is performed as early as possible at a time when peripheral iridectomy is curative. If first seen in the acute phase, the attack should be controlled by medical treatment and followed by peripheral iridectomy. If the disease has become chronic because of the formation of anterior peripheral synechiae with permanent angle closure, a filtering operation must be done. Chronic simple (open angle) glaucoma is operated on only after medical therapy fails to control the intraocular pressure and to prevent visual loss. A filtering operation is the procedure of choice to produce a permanent fistula through the corneoscleral wall. About 15 per cent of filtering operations fail and are accompanied by a significant number of complications in contrast with peripheral iridectomy, which has almost none.

Operations for Glaucoma

Peripheral Iridectomy. A small incision, approximately 3 mm. long, is made at the limbus beneath a flap of conjunctiva that has been reflected toward the cornea (Fig. 10-3). The iris root is made to herniate into the limbal incision where it is grasped by a forceps and excised. A hole is then formed in the iris to provide a new channel for aqueous to flow from the posterior to the anterior chamber. This eliminates the physiologic iris bombé of narrow angle glaucoma and allows the iris to flatten and drop away from the angle wall. Almost invariably the operation is curative and the eye is left in a normal state with an intact corneoscleral wall. Complications are extremely rare. The patient is able to be ambulatory immediately with only one eye patched, and the convalescent period is short.

Filtering Operations. These are done for chronic narrow angle glaucoma and chronic simple (wide angle) glaucoma. The most common of the many different techniques are:

TREPHINATION OF ELLIOTT. After a 6 or 8 mm. conjunctival flap is reflected to the limbus, a 1.5 mm. trephine is used to create a hole through the wall of the angle of the limbus (Plate 34). The underlying iris is excised (iridectomy) to prevent its coming

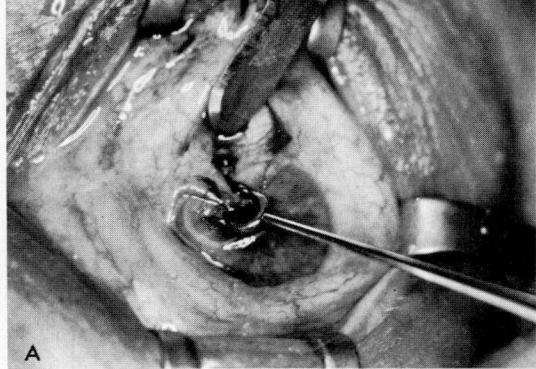

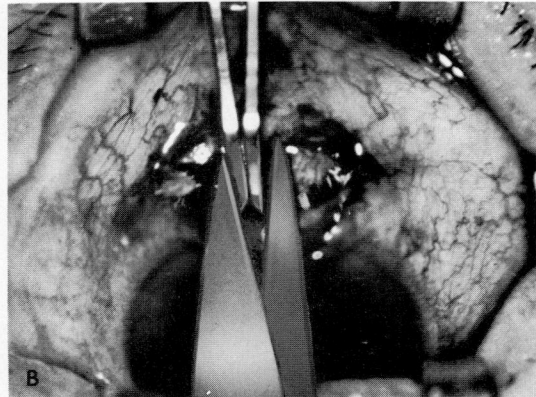

Figure 10-3 Peripheral iridectomy. *(A)* Iris herniated through small scleral incision. *(B)* Iris grasped by forceps and herniated portion excised.

forward to plug the trephine opening, and the conjunctival incision is sutured to provide an intact, subconjunctival space into which aqueous drains.

IRIDENCLEISIS. In this widely done filtering procedure, a conjunctival flap is reflected toward the limbus and a 6 mm. long incision is made into the anterior chamber. The iris is incarcerated within this incision so as to act as a wick to provide drainage of aqueous into the subconjunctival space.

SCLERECTOMY. A conjunctival flap is reflected toward the limbus and a small piece of sclera adjacent to it is removed with a punch. An iridectomy must also be done.

IRIDECTOMY WITH SCLERAL CAUTERY (THERMO-SCLERECTOMY, SCLEROTOMY WITH CAUTERY). An incision is made into the anterior chamber just behind the limbus after reflecting a conjunctival flap. The tip of a galvanocautery is applied along the lips of the scleral incision. Since heat

contracts collagen, the lips of the incision gape, and the opening remains as a fistula in a high percentage of eyes. An iridectomy always is done.

CYCLODIALYSIS. The incision is made through the sclera 4 or 5 mm. behind the limbus, and a spatula is inserted and carried forward between the ciliary body and sclera until the tip appears in the anterior chamber where it is swept first in one direction and then in the other to strip the ciliary body from its attachment at the scleral spur. Aqueous then drains into the suprachoroidal space where it is absorbed, presumably by the choroidal circulation. At times the operation probably lowers intraocular pressure by reopening the angle to restore normal drainage of aqueous. It is used for all types of glaucoma but is most effective for the type with angle closure following cataract extraction and delayed reformation of the anterior chamber.

CYCLODIATHERMY. Diathermy current is used to destroy a portion of the ciliary body and thus reduce the production of aqueous. Usually, this operation is used as a last resort.

CYCLOCRYOTHERAPY. This operation, still in developmental stages, embodies the same principle as cyclodiathermy except that cryo-techniques are used.

Prognosis

For narrow angle glaucoma the prognosis is excellent if simple peripheral iridectomy is done during the early phases, either during the interval after control of an acute attack (interval glaucoma) or before an acute attack has occurred (preglaucoma). Many ophthalmic surgeons feel it advisable to operate on both eyes, because a high percentage of patients develop acute glaucoma in the fellow eye within five years.

The prognosis is more guarded for narrow angle glaucoma treated by a filtering operation under adverse circumstances, such as during an uncontrollable acute attack when intraocular pressure is very high. The prognosis is also poor for chronic narrow angle glaucoma that necessitates a filtering operation. The tension may rise markedly, resulting in a devastating malignant postoperative glaucoma that is fatal to the eye in a high percentage of cases. Filtering operations may be accompanied by operative complications such as hemorrhage, vitreous loss, and trauma to the lens. Hemorrhage and infection can occur postoperatively. The anterior chamber may not reform for days or weeks, increasing the danger of adhesions and cataract formation. Late complications, such as cataract formation and intraocular infection from bacteria entering the eye through the filtering cicatrix during attacks of conjunctivitis, are not unusual.

Congenital Glaucoma

The treatment of infantile glaucoma is surgical. The prognosis for what used to be a blinding disease is now excellent. Goniotomy alone or combined with goniopuncture is effective in approximately 80 per cent of eyes. The operation is safe and preserves normal ocular function and appearance. Filtering operations for adult types of glaucoma are less effective in controlling pressure in infantile glaucoma and are accompanied by a higher incidence of serious complications, particularly vitreous loss. They are used, however, for reoperation after goniotomy has failed.

Goniotomy is done by inserting a specially made knife into the anterior chamber through the cornea within the temporal limbus (Plate 35). The tip is carried across the anterior chamber to the opposite angle where it is swept along the angle wall to incise the trabecula over one third or more of the circumference. The operation probably permits aqueous to escape through the canal of Schlemm and the aqueous veins. Goniopuncture, a somewhat similar operation, acts differently, creating a fistula (Plate 36). A puncture is made through the opposite corneoscleral wall rather than sweeping the angle. The two operations can be combined into one, termed goniotomy-goniopuncture, to utilize the mode of

action of each. Goniotomy is done first and, at the end of the sweep, a puncture is made through the angle wall to produce a fistula to obtain the combined effect of the two procedures. Either can control the pressure when done alone, but goniotomy is more effective than goniopuncture. If two or three goniotomy-goniopunctures fail, another filtering operation should be done. Iridectomy with scleral cautery is probably the safest and most effective.

Juvenile Glaucoma

This disease is treated like chronic simple glaucoma, but surgery usually is required because the disease tends to be severe and difficult to control by medical means. Goniopuncture is the procedure of choice because it is simple and does not deform the eye. It controls the intraocular pressure in about 50 per cent of eyes, and, although this percentage is low, it should be done once or twice before a more dangerous filtering operation, such as trephination, is performed. The prognosis for control of pressure in juvenile glaucoma is good unless associated anomalies, such as aniridia, are present.

RETINAL DETACHMENT

Retinal detachment, or more accurately, retinal separation, occurs when the sensory portion of the retina separates from the pigment layer. These layers are first recognizable when the optic vesicles invaginate to form the optic cup. The outer layer of the cup represents the future pigment layer of the retina, and the inner layer forms the sensory portion consisting of the rods and cones, ganglion cells, and nerve fibers. Throughout life, the two layers are loosely in contact, being firmly united only at the optic nerve and over the ciliary body. Any hole through the inner layer of the retina predisposes to retinal detachment by allowing fluid from the vitreous cavity to diffuse into the potential space between the two layers, causing them to separate. The holes, of varying sizes and shapes, usually are in the peripheral retina and must be sealed surgically for retinal detachment to be cured.

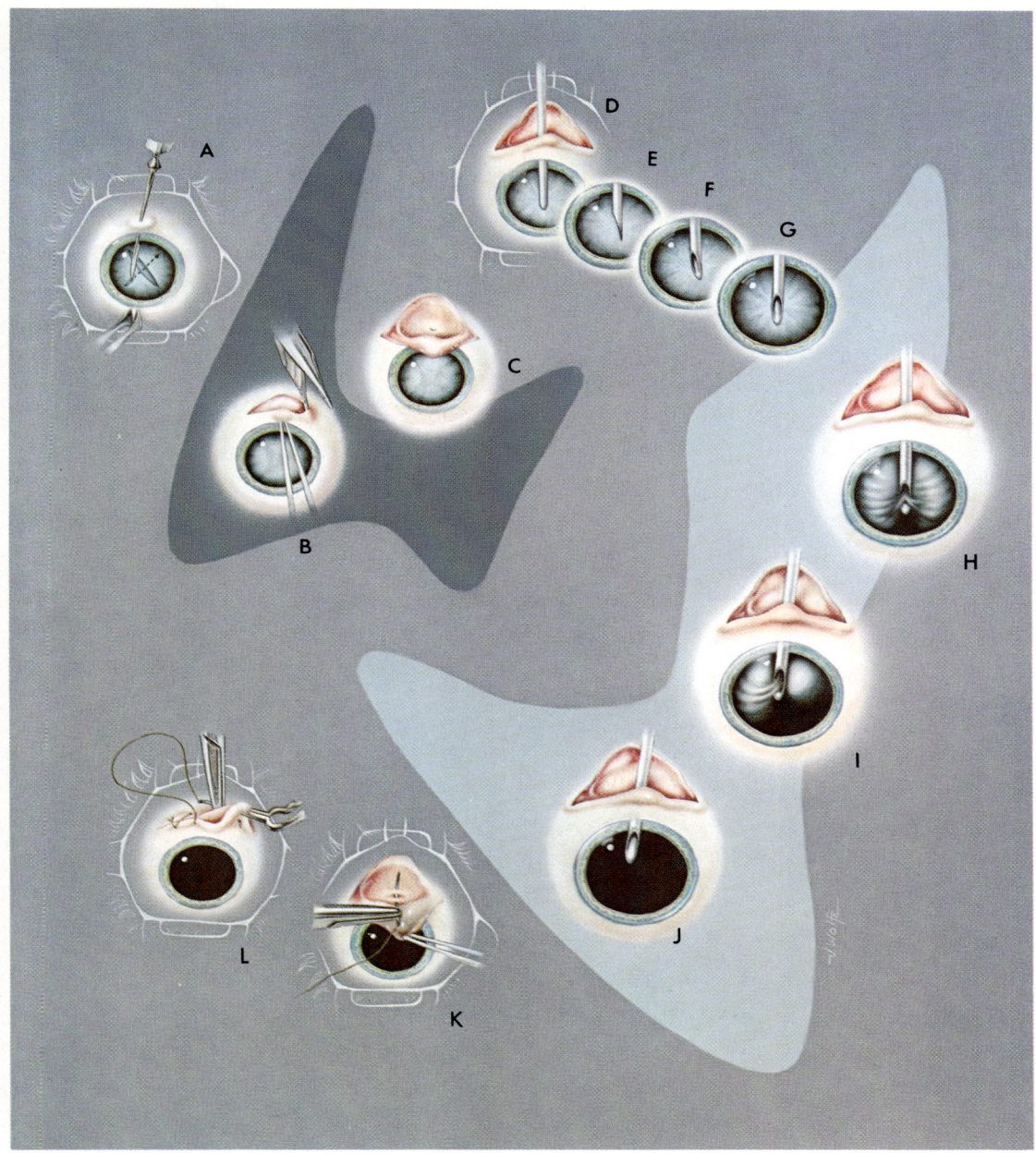

Plate 33 Discission and aspiration of soft cataracts (congenital, traumatic, diabetic, and others) in patients under 30 years of age. *(A)* When cataract is incomplete, a ripening operation is performed by making a large cruciate incision in anterior lens capsule with knife needle. If pupil dilates poorly, a preliminary complete iridectomy should be done beforehand. Three days to two or three weeks after ripening procedure, aspiration can be done. In eyes with complete cataract, ripening operation is unnecessary, and aspiration is done immediately after opening lens capsule. *(B)* Small conjunctival flap reflected to limbus. *(C)* Previously made puncture with Ziegler knife is visible after turning flap. *(D)* Thin-walled No. 19 needle inserted into anterior chamber, bevel down. *(E), (F), (G)* Needle rotated, turning aperture forward prior to aspiration of lens material to protect posterior lens capsule and vitreous face from damage by suction. *(H), (I), (J)* Physiologic saline gently pumped into and aspirated from anterior chamber to remove lens material. Tip of needle may be directed to any point in the anterior chamber to remove residual lens material. Care is taken to avoid traumatizing the iris by suction. Superior part of chamber aspirated last. *(K)* Gaping scleral puncture closed by 6-0 mild chromic catgut. *(L)* Conjunctival incision sutured with 6-0 mild chromic catgut. Wide pupillary dilatation must be maintained postoperatively by instillation of atropine, 1 per cent, and phenylephrine hydrochloride one or two times daily for several weeks. (Scheie, H. G.: The management of glaucoma and cataracts in children. *The Sight-Saving Review*, Summer, 1964.)

389

Since retinal holes may be multiple, a careful search must be made for them. Direct and indirect ophthalmoscopy and the Goldmann contact lens for viewing the retina should be used. The area of the hole is treated with diathermy current or a cryoapplicator, both of which irritate the overlying choroid and pigment layer of the retina, inducing scar tissue formation that seals the retinal hole.

Certain adjuncts are helpful in retinal detachment operations:

GRAVITY. This greatly affects a detached retina. A detachment of the upper half becomes more marked during the day while the patient is upright, but it settles at night. Proper positioning of the patient after the operation helps the retina to settle into place.

DRAINAGE OF SUBRETINAL FLUID. The fluid that lies between the two layers of the retina is drained at the time of surgery, which allows the two layers of the retina to come in contact where they heal.

IMPLANTS OF VARIOUS TYPES. These include plastic materials, preserved sclera, fascia lata, and other materials. They are used to indent the sclera, choroid, and outer layer of the retina inward toward the detached portion. The two layers of the retina must be in contact to permit sealing of the retinal hole.

VARIOUS SUBSTANCES INJECTED INTO THE VITREOUS. They increase vitreous volume and force the separated retina into position. Vitreous, spinal fluid, blood serum, saline, and air have all been used, but air probably is the most desirable.

Prognosis

The prognosis for a retinal detachment is guarded. Although present-day techniques produce reattachment of the retina in approximately 80 to 90 per cent of eyes, the visual outlook is uncertain. Visual acuity may be poor if the macular region of the retina has been detached for some time, or if, as a result of the cautery, secondary changes occur in the macula with loss of central vision. This may happen even years later.

CORNEAL TRANSPLANTATION

Transplanting a cornea from one person to another is a practical and widely accepted surgical procedure. The abnormal central portion of the cornea, usually containing scar tissue, is excised and replaced by clear, healthy donor cornea of the same size. Keratoplasty is indicated when poor vision has resulted from corneal scarring (Figs. 10-4, 10-5). Keratoconus and central scars do especially well, and such eyes should be operated on if the patient cannot tolerate contact lenses or obtain good vision with them.

Operative Procedure

The abnormal corneal tissue is excised and the donor tissue obtained by using a trephine, usually 6 to 8 mm. in diameter. The graft is sutured into place with multiple, fine, interrupted silk sutures.

Prognosis

Complications are few, except for graft reaction phenomena, which are prone to occur three to four weeks after surgery. The cellularity and vascularity of heavily scarred corneas make the reaction more severe. The use of ACTH and systemic and local corticosteroids has greatly improved the outlook. More than 90 per cent of eyes with central corneal scars and keratoconus heal well with clear grafts, whereas only a few eyes with severe chemical burns do well. In the future more clear grafts might be anticipated by the use of substances being developed to suppress graft rejection. Experimental work also is being done with the insertion of plastic buttons into eyes that appear hopeless. Although encouraging, this type of surgery is still experimental.

STRABISMUS

The management of strabismus is discussed in Pediatric Ophthalmology (p. 156).
(Text continued on p. 396)

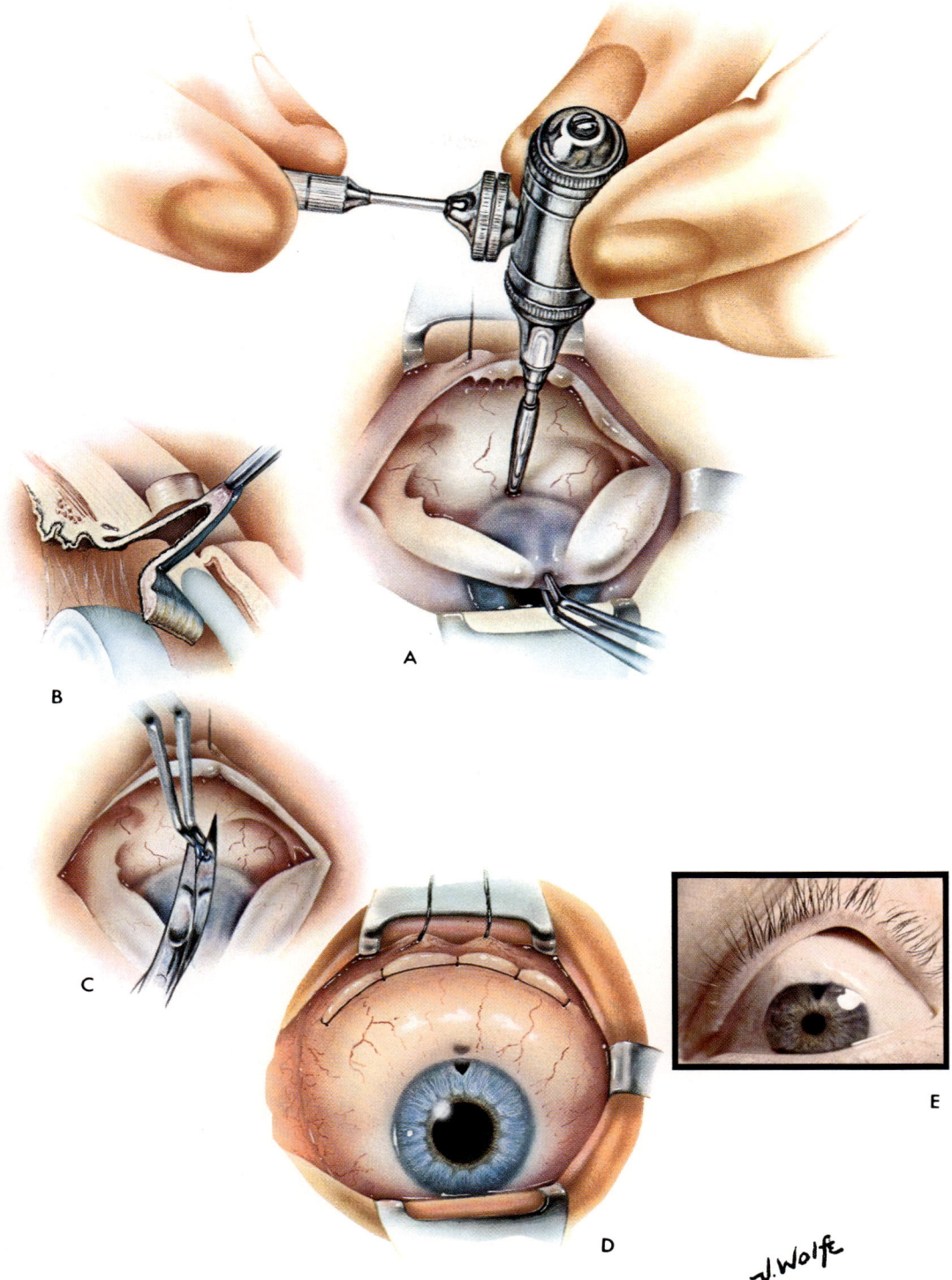

Plate 34 *(A)* Trephining through scleral wall with Gradle-Schiötz trephine. Trephine tilted forward to insure entering anterior chamber on corneal side. *(B)* Peripheral iridectomy performed. Trephine button remains hinged posteriorly. *(C)* Trephine button excised with sharply pointed scissors. *(D)* Appearance of eye following closure of conjunctiva. *(E)* Clinical postoperative photograph. (Scheie, H. G.: Filtering operations for glaucoma: a comparative study. *Am. J. Ophth.*, April, 1962.)

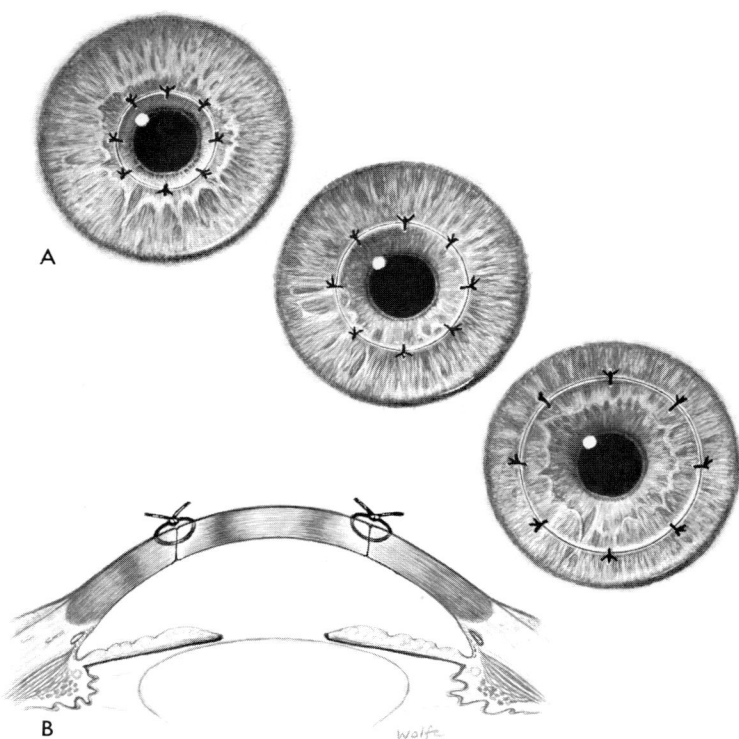

Figure 10-4 Corneal transplant. *(A)* Grafts of three different sizes. Interrupted sutures. *(B)* Sagittal section of cornea showing full-thickness graft.

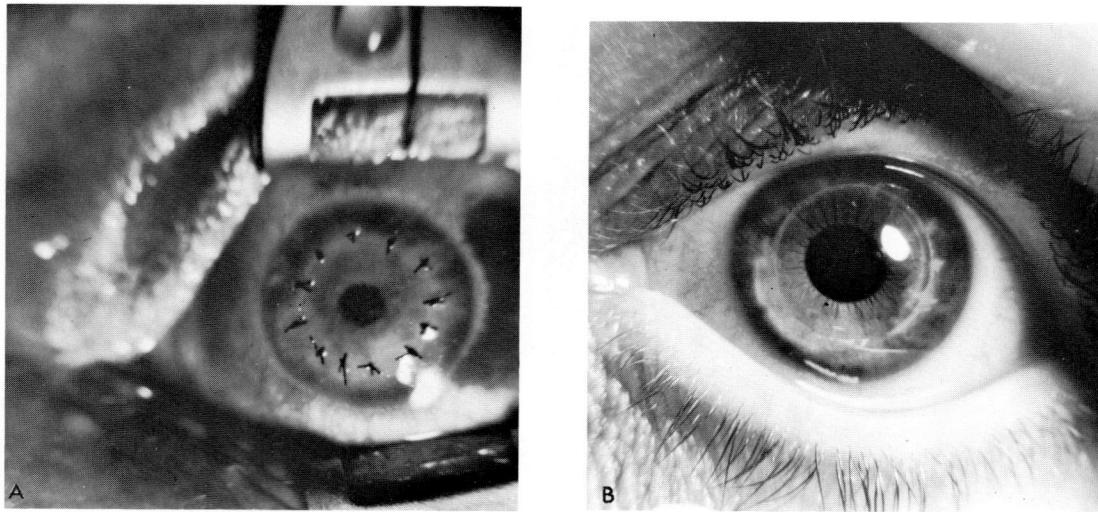

Figure 10-5 Corneal transplant. *(A)* Graft immediately postoperative. *(B)* Graft four weeks later.

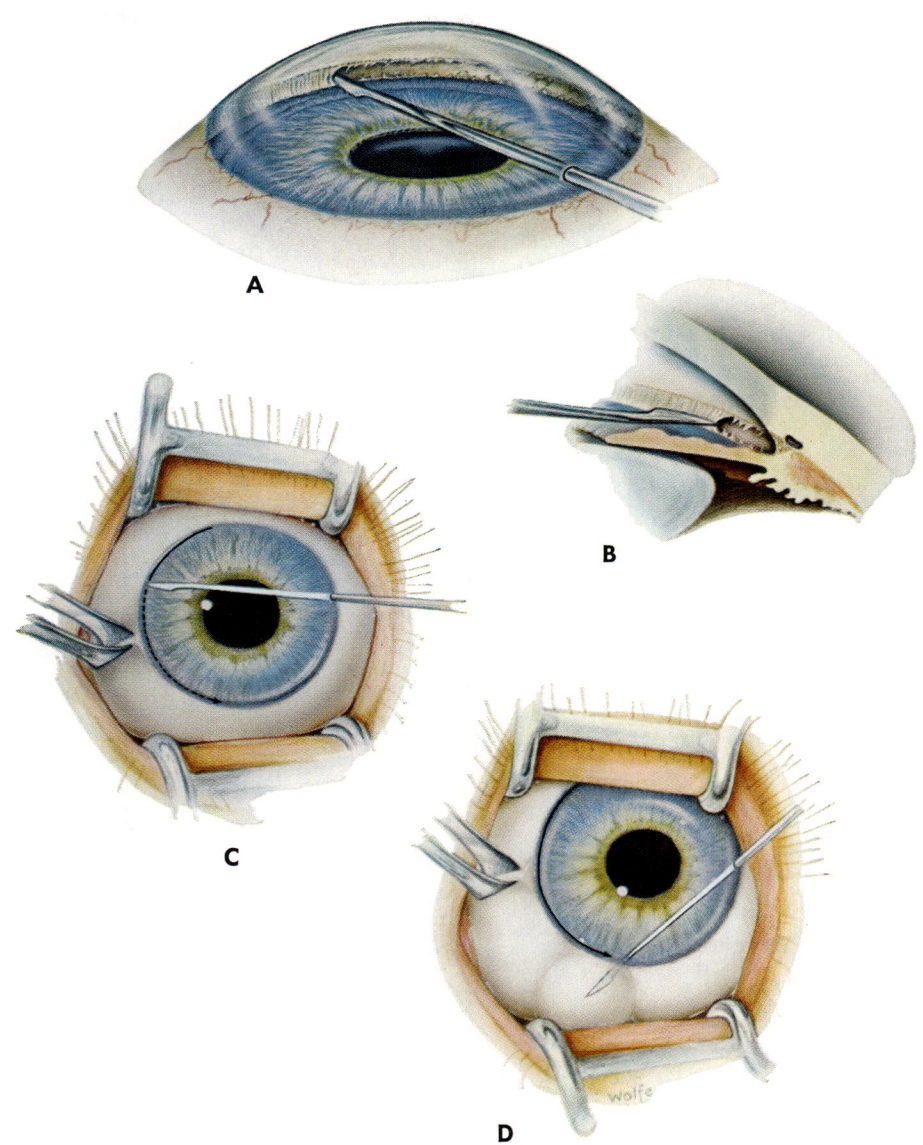

A

B

C

D

Plate 35 Goniotomy-goniopuncture for congenital glaucoma. *(A), (B), (C)* Goniotomy knife is inserted through cornea within temporal limbus and carried across anterior chamber. With tip of knife just behind opaque limbus, one third to one half of circumference of angle is swept. *(D)* Goniopuncture is performed upon completion of goniotomy. Because corneoscleral wall of infants is thin, knife blade is not rotated and no attempt is made to refill chamber. If bleeding occurs, all blood is removed before clotting occurs by immediately irrigating through site of entrance of goniotomy blade. (Scheie, H. G.: Indications for surgery in infantile and juvenile glaucoma. *Tr. Am. Acad. Ophth.,* July-August, 1963.)

Plate 36   Goniopuncture for juvenile glaucoma.   *(A), (B)* Oblique puncture with Ziegler knife needle for reformation of chamber after goniopuncture.   *(C)* Conjunctiva and Tenon's capsule ballooned with saline solution. *(D)* Tip of goniopuncture knife inserted through cornea within limbus temporally and carried across anterior chamber to corneoscleral wall at 6:00 o'clock. Puncture made in anterior trabecula with blade held parallel to iris.   *(E)* Knife is rotated, cutting edge forward, while still in subconjunctival space, and withdrawn into anterior chamber to create T-shaped opening. Knife again rotated in anterior chamber until blade is parallel with iris and then withdrawn from eye.   *(F), (G)* Anterior chamber filled with air or saline solution by No. 27 needle inserted into, but not through, previously made corneal tract. (Scheie, H. G.: Indications for surgery in infantile and juvenile glaucoma. *Tr. Am. Acad. Ophth.*, July-August, 1963.)

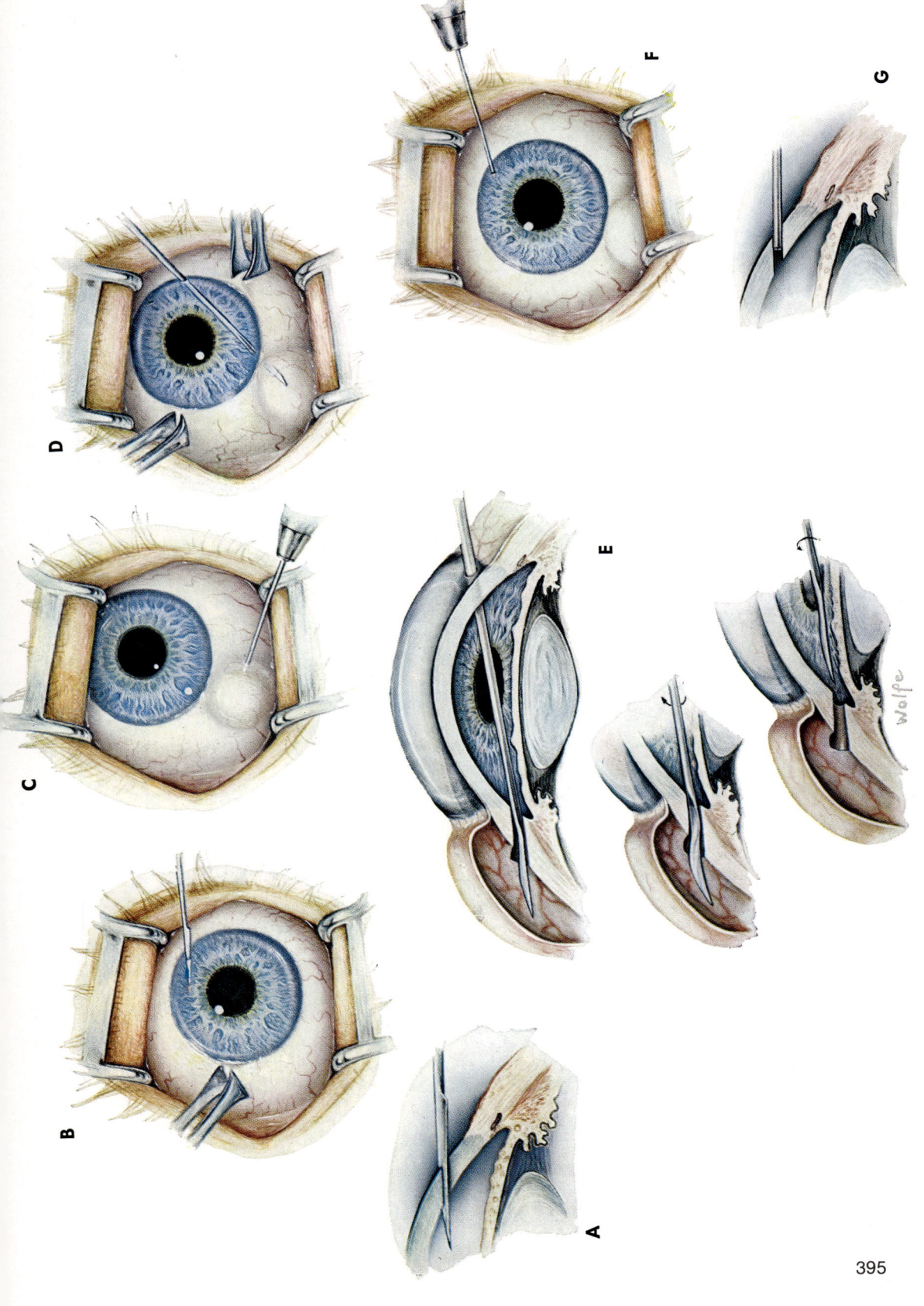

395

Surgery for strabismus is of the utmost importance because of its cosmetic and psychologic significance to the child. Binocular vision may or may not be obtained, but the effect of straightened eyes on psychologic well being cannot be overemphasized.

The operation should be done only if other approaches, such as spectacles or exercises, are ineffective. It can be done at almost any age, preferably before the child starts kindergarten. Children whose eyes are held straight by spectacles should have the operation deferred until later. The operation involves shortening or lengthening one or more of the horizontal rectus muscles. The parents should be told that more than one operation may be needed. The surgical approach should be conservative because it is simpler to carry out further surgery than to undo an overcorrection. Operations on muscles with vertical action, such as the superior and inferior recti or the oblique, are less common.

With present-day operative techniques, the eyes are not covered and the child usually is allowed to leave the hospital in a day or so.

PTERYGIUM

A pterygium is an overgrowth of epithelial tissue at the nasal or temporal limbus. Its stroma consists of thickened and degenerated connective tissue, elastic fibers, and blood vessels. Once it invades the cornea, it may progress toward, or even cross, the pupillary space. The treatment is surgical and several different techniques, such as simple excision with curettement of the cornea, have been devised. Sometimes the pterygium is transplanted under the conjunctiva into the inferior cul-de-sac with the hope that if it recurs, it will grow away from the cornea. Despite the varied approaches, a pterygium recurs frequently; however, this can be managed by excision, leaving a bare scleral base. Beta irradiation may be used, but this involves some danger of late cataract.

ENUCLEATION AND EVISCERATION

The only surgical treatment for a blind, painful eye is enucleation. Any other surgical procedure on the eye incurs the risk of sympathetic ophthalmia. Even though this condition is rare, the normal eye should not be endangered by operative attempts to save a nonseeing eye. Enucleation involves removing the globe while maintaining the integrity of the orbit as best as possible, so that a cosmetically satisfactory prosthesis may be inserted. Thus a dissection should be carefully done and a suitable implant inserted into the muscle cone to take up the dead space. Proper closure prevents shifting of the implant about the orbit and preserves the conjunctival cul-de-sac. As much mobility as possible is obtained following insertion of the prosthesis, which usually is fitted four to six weeks following surgery. The operation can be done under local or general anesthesia with little hazard.

Evisceration involves removing the contents of the globe while leaving the sclera in place. In the classic technique, the cornea and the contents of the globe are removed and an implant inserted in the scleral shell. The sclera is then sutured and the conjunctiva and Tenon's capsule closed over the sclera. This provides better motility of the prosthesis than does enucleation. It must be noted, however, that if there is any possibility of an intraocular tumor being present, the eye must be enucleated.

CHALAZIA

A chalazion may disappear without surgical interference, but if it continues to enlarge it can be removed simply and painlessly as an office procedure. Anesthesia is obtained by local drops and injection of procaine. A chalazion clamp, firmly closed on the lid with the chalazion centered in the open ring, everts the lid and prevents hemorrhage. The conjunctival surface of the tarsal plate is incised perpendicularly to the lid margin and parallel with the meibomian ducts. Usually gelatin-like or purulent material exudes through the incision. Pressure and sponging evacuates additional material, and the wall of the chalazion is curetted. After the clamp is removed, bleeding is controlled by pressure on the lids. Stitches are unnecessary, and usually the eye is patched for but a few hours.

Occasionally, if a chalazion erodes through the anterior surface of the tarsal plate, its contents lie beneath the skin of the lid. The skin as well as the tarsal plate must be incised to prevent recurrence. The incision through the skin should be made separately, parallel to the lid margin, and into the chalazion that is already open on its conjunctival aspect. Sutures usually are unnecessary.

CHANGES IN POSITION OF THE LID MARGINS

Relaxation of the lid septum results in spastic entropion, which almost always necessitates surgical correction. In some cases electrocautery (Ziegler) punctures through the skin surface into the lower lid may correct the condition. Some six to seven punctures are made about 5 mm. below the free lid margin to the depth of the tarsal plate; they should be 3 mm. apart. Subsequent scarring tightens the lid septum and prevents inversion of the lid margin. If this simple procedure fails, the lid septum should be tightened by plastic surgery. Ectropion (eversion of the lid) may require only shortening of the lid margin; if cicatricial, excision of scar tissue and possibly skin grafting may be necessary.

BIBLIOGRAPHY

Arruga, H.: Ocular Surgery. 3rd ed. New York, McGraw-Hill Book Co., 1962. Translated from 4th Spanish edition by Hogan, M. J., and Chaparro, L. E.

Atkinson, W. S.: Anesthesia in Ophthalmology. 2nd ed. Springfield, Illinois, Charles C Thomas, 1965.

Berens, C., and King, J. H.: An Atlas of Ophthalmic Surgery. Philadelphia, J. B. Lippincott Co., 1961.

Callahan, A.: Reconstructive Surgery of the Eyelids and Ocular Adnexa. Birmingham, Aesculapius Publishing Co., 1966.

Callahan, A.: Surgery of the Eye: Diseases. Springfield, Illinois, Charles C Thomas, 1956.

Castroviejo, R.: Cataract surgery: the handling of complications. Am. J. Ophth. 58:68, 1964.

Chandler, P. A.: Surgery of congenital cataract. Am. J Ophth. 65:663, 1968.

Chandler, P. A.: Surgery of the lens in infancy and childhood. Arch. Ophth. 45:125, 1951.

DeVoe, A. G., et al.: Symposium on Surgery of the Ocular Adnexa. St. Louis, The C. V. Mosby Co., 1966.

Fasanella, R. M. (ed.): Complications in Eye Surgery. 2nd ed. Philadelphia, W. B. Saunders Co., 1965.

Haik, G. M.: Symposium on Diseases and Surgery of the Lens. St. Louis, The C. V. Mosby Co., 1957.

Harms, H., and Mackensen, G.: Ocular Surgery Under the Microscope. Chicago, Year Book Medical Publishers, 1967. Translated and edited by Blodi, F. C.

Hawkins, W. R., and Schepens, C. L.: Choroidal detachment and retinal surgery. Am. J. Ophth. 62: 813, 1966.

Hill, H. F.: Cataract extraction with limited enzymatic zonulolysis. Arch. Ophth. 75:89, 1966.

Jones, L. T.: Conjunctivodacryocystorhinostomy. Am. J. Ophth. 59:773, 1965.

Kelman, C. D.: Atlas of Cryosurgical Techniques in Ophthalmology. St. Louis, The C. V. Mosby Co., 1966.

Kitano, S., and Goldmann, J. N.: Cytologic and histochemical changes in corneal wound repair. Arch. Ophth. 76:345, 1966.

McLean, J. M.: Atlas of Cataract Surgery. St. Louis, The C. V. Mosby Co., 1965.

McLean, J. M.: Atlas of Glaucoma Surgery. London, Kimpton, 1967.

Moore, J. G., and Youngman, P. M. E.: Secondary traumatic hyphaema. Brit. J. Ophth. 52:172, 1968.

Newell, F. W.: Advances in cataract surgery. Sight-Saving Review 30:69, 1960.

Paton, R. T., Smith, B., and Katzin, H. M.: Atlas of Eye Surgery. New York, McGraw-Hill Book Co., 1962.

Philips, S.: Ophthalmic Operations. 2nd ed. Baltimore, Williams & Wilkins, 1961.

Roper, K. L.: Anesthesia and akinesia in cataract surgery. Am. J. Ophth. 61:1278, 1966.

Scheie, H. G.: Aspiration of congenital or soft cataracts: a new technique. Am. J. Ophth. 50:1048, 1960.

Scheie, H. G., Rubenstein, R. A., and Kent, R. B.: Aspiration of congenital or soft cataracts: further experience. Am. J. Ophth. 63:3, 1967.

Spaeth, E. B.: Principles and Practice of Ophthalmic Surgery. 4th ed. Philadelphia, Lea & Febiger, 1948.

Stafford, W. R.: Sympathetic ophthalmia. Arch. Ophth. 74:521, 1965.

Stallard, H. B.: Eye Surgery. 4th ed. Baltimore, Williams & Wilkins, 1965.

Swan, K. C.: Iridectomy for narrow angle glaucoma. Am. J. Ophth. 61:601, 1966.

Tolentino, F. I., and Schepens, C. L.: Edema of posterior pole after cataract extraction. Arch. Ophth. 74:781, 1965.

Weiner, M., and Scheie, H. G.: Surgery of the Eye. 3rd ed. New York, Grune & Stratton, 1952.

Worthen, D. M., and Brubaker, R. F.: An evaluation of cataract cryoextraction. Arch. Ophth. 79:8, 1968.

Appendix I

Symptomatology of Eye Diseases

Knowledge of the history of any disease, as well as the physical findings, is essential in the diagnosis. In ophthalmology particularly, the chief complaint gives valuable clues, and before proceeding with an examination, the doctor should listen carefully to the patient's explanation of his disorder.

The physician will, of course, find it helpful to be aware of the characteristic symptoms of each disease entity. The general practitioner with little experience in ocular pathology should find this section especially helpful.

The patient's complaints may be both visual and nonvisual. The visual symptoms are those revealed by the patient as well as those the physician must elicit. The nonvisual symptoms may involve pain, fatigue, fullness of the eye, and others.

OCULAR SYMPTOMS, VISUAL

Loss of Vision. Patients describe impaired visual acuity in various terms. Emotional factors commonly lead to exaggeration, so a patient may state that he has lost the sight of one eye when the vision is only impaired. On the other hand, an occasional patient may overlook or minimize visual defects, describing as blurred or foggy vision what is truly a serious visual loss. Subjective complaints must always be checked against objective findings. The complaint of poor vision usually stems from loss of central visual acuity, for a patient is less apt to detect loss of peripheral field.

When the patient reports visual impairment, the examiner should determine when it occurred, whether the onset was sudden or gradual, and whether one or both eyes became affected. If both eyes are involved, the physician should determine which is now the worse, which failed first, and how much time elapsed between the two.

The actual onset of visual impairment does not always coincide with the time given by a patient. The visual acuity may have been deteriorating for months or years, becoming noticeable to the patient only when he happened to cover the good eye. In fact, he may not discover that he has a congenitally amblyopic eye until late in life. The discovery might be made only if something happens to the other eye, such as a cinder lodging in it or an injury to it. If the visual loss is discovered after some compensable accident, the patient may be even more convinced that it has just occurred. Since this involves medicolegal aspects, the physician must look for other signs of congenital amblyopia, such as a convergent strabismus. Peripheral portions of the visual field may deteriorate, and the patient may become aware of it only when the macular area of the retina becomes involved. Loss of central acuity may involve one or both eyes, a point of diagnostic importance. The loss may be sudden or gradual.

SUDDEN LOSS OR IMPAIRMENT OF VISION CONFINED TO ONE EYE. Sudden loss of vision in one eye usually occurs on a circulatory basis, but it may also result from inflammation. The former is more likely not only if the visual loss is sudden but also if it affects the entire visual field.

The following conditions should be considered:

1. Central vein obstruction (p. 246).
2. Closure of the central artery by thrombi, emboli, or spasm (p. 244); temporal arteritis (p. 315).
3. Massive vitreous or retinal hemorrhages from any cause, such as Eales' disease (p. 190), sickle cell anemia (p. 234), diabetes (p. 255), or various blood dyscrasias (p. 233).
4. Optic neuritis, papillitis, or retrobulbar neuritis (p. 304).
5. Detachment of the retina involving the macula (p. 286).
6. Uremic amaurosis.
7. Toxic amblyopia, e.g., methyl alcohol, quinine, lead (p. 309).
8. Embolic endophthalmitis (p. 244).
9. Thrombosis of internal carotid artery (p. 313).
10. Skull injuries, hemorrhage in optic canal (p. 362).

SUDDEN LOSS OR IMPAIRMENT OF VISION IN BOTH EYES. This is rare except from trauma. Most conditions that cause sudden unilateral loss of vision may affect both eyes successively, but rarely simultaneously except for injuries. Generally the sight of one eye is impaired more than that of the other.

The following conditions should be considered:

1. Optic neuritis, especially caused by the rare forms of the demyelinating diseases such as Devic's disease (neuromyelitis optica) (p. 305).
2. Uremic amaurosis.
3. Toxic amblyopia (p. 309).
4. Head injuries, concussion blindness (p. 374).
5. Hysteria and malingering (p. 435).
6. Migraine.

GRADUAL LOSS OR IMPAIRMENT OF VISION IN ONE EYE. Any disease affecting either the refractive media or the visual pathways

up to the optic chiasm can produce gradual impairment of vision in one eye. Refractive errors on a genetic basis or induced by diseases affecting the cornea, lens, uveal tract, retina, and optic nerve are to be considered. The use of a pinhole disc quickly and simply detects visual impairment caused by refractive errors (p. 409). The diagnosis of conditions other than refractive errors will develop from the objective findings.

The following conditions should be considered:

1. Refractive errors (p. 443).
   a. Myopia, hyperopia, and astigmatism. Visual impairment from hyperopia, unless marked, seldom occurs before the presbyopic age (p. 444).
   b. Myopia caused by lens sclerosis (p. 446).
   c. Refractive changes caused by changes in blood sugar in the diabetic (p. 255).
   d. Keratoconus (p. 118).
   e. Refractive changes resulting from dislocation or subluxation of the lens (p. 376).
   f. Refractive changes caused by lid pressure (p. 257), chalazia (p. 203), lid edema (p. 257), and ptosis.
   g. Refractive changes resulting from elevation of the retina (p. 263), orbital tumors (p. 272), central serous retinopathy (p. 30), and hemangioma of the choroid.
2. Cornea.
   a. Keratitis of any form (p. 187).
   b. Corneal dystrophies (p. 278).
   c. Allergic reactions of the cornea (p. 187).
   d. Changes of unknown character caused by drugs taken internally, e.g., chloroquine.
   e. Edema of the cornea (p. 188).
   f. Keratoconus (p. 118).
3. Lens.
   a. Opacification of the lens from any cause; nuclear sclerosis; cataract (p. 282).
   b. Change in position of the lens (p. 122).
4. Uveal tract.
   a. Inflammation, iritis, choroiditis, uveitis (p. 214).

b. Hemorrhagic diseases (p. 233); macular degeneration probably caused by subretinal hemorrhages (p. 284).

c. Tumors, primary and metastatic (p. 263).

5. Glaucoma. Generally the chronic simple, open angle type (p. 338); secondary glaucoma from any cause (p. 358).

6. Vitreous.

a. Any opacification of the vitreous; synchysis scintillans; snowball opacities (seldom cause visual impairment) (p. 281).

b. Hemorrhages into and from the retina (p. 26), choroid (p. 246) or skull (p. 364), or involving the subarachnoid space.

7. Retina.

a. Vascular lesions. Occlusion of a branch of the central retinal vein causes abrupt loss of vision, involving the affected retina, whereas occlusion of the whole vein causes more generalized sudden loss over the entire visual field. Similarly, a branch block of a retinal artery is not as sudden or as severe as the visual impairment caused by complete occlusion of the central retinal artery. Repeated small hemorrhages in the retina from hypertension, diabetes, and blood dyscrasias also cause vision to fail gradually, but central acuity is not affected until the macula is involved. Whether or not the patient has noticed gradual loss of vision may depend upon whether or not the macula is involved. Loss of peripheral vision might escape his notice until the macular region is affected by a hemorrhage (p. 287).

b. Macular degenerations. These can be considered quite properly as either retinal or choroidal diseases, since in many instances it is still uncertain whether they occur because of an abiotrophy of the visual elements or hemorrhages from the choroid on the basis of atherosclerosis. In the young the macular degenerations most commonly occur on a familial and, probably, a hereditary basis. In the elderly they are probably due to atherosclerosis of the choroidal vessels (p. 248).

c. Tapetoretinal degenerations. The most common are primary degeneration of the retina, secondary pigmentary degeneration, Laurence-Moon-Biedel syndrome, gyrate atrophy, choroideremia, and pigmentary degeneration sine pigmento (p. 131).

d. Toxic amblyopias. Among these are those due to tobacco, quinine, carbon bisulfide, and methyl alcohol. These affections may be included in the retinal diseases or the diseases of the optic nerve, depending upon the location of the action of the poison (p. 309).

e. Retinitis. This includes any inflammatory disease of the retina.

f. Retinopathies. These are included among the vascular lesions, but rather than being hemorrhages, their manifestations may be largely exudative or in the form of deposits of material in the retina resulting from abnormal metabolism. Hence the hypertensive (p. 236) and diabetic (p. 256) retinopathies may be placed in this group.

g. Tumors. Retinal tumors are both primary and metastatic (p. 265).

h. Detachment (p. 286).

8. Optic nerve (p. 298). Any disease involving the optic nerve up to the chiasm may give rise to gradual loss of vision in one eye. Beyond this point both eyes eventually are bound to be affected by disease of the visual pathways, although in the early stages one eye may escape.

a. Inflammation. Optic neuritis generally is sudden in onset (but not necessarily so) and produces a central scotoma. Repeated attacks with partial recovery are common in multiple sclerosis, leading eventually to serious permanent impairment of vision (p. 305).

b. Tumors. Pressure on any part of the optic nerve up to the chiasm produces impairment of conduction in the nerve fibers with resulting loss of parts of the visual field. The macular fibers are vulnerable to pressure and central scotomas may arise, especially if pressure occurs just behind the globe where the macular fibers run in the temporal periphery of the nerve (p. 292).

c. Papilledema. This rarely gives rise to visual loss per se, except for enlargement of the blind spot, but the edema and elevation of the retina may extend into the macula, giving rise to a cecocentral scotoma. Eventually, if the pressure is not relieved, vision is lost by constriction of the visual field resulting from optic atrophy (p. 300).

d. Optic atrophy. Optic atrophy from any cause obviously results in visual loss and is usually slowly progressive (p. 310).

GRADUAL LOSS OF VISION IN BOTH EYES. In nearly all the conditions listed under gradual loss of vision in one eye the second eye may later become involved. Some conditions, such as pigmentary degeneration of the retina, are always bilateral.

Spots Before the Eyes. Seeing spots, dust particles, specks, threads, and cobwebs in front of the eyes is common and generally of little pathologic significance. The vast majority of such complaints are caused by small opacities in the vitreous lying close enough to the retina to cast shadows on the photoreceptors, i.e., rods and cones. Under suitable illumination these become visible to the patient. Fine, dustlike opacities that may be sufficiently numerous to blur vision occur in inflammatory conditions of the choroid and retina. A thorough examination of the eye is necessary to differentiate harmless vitreous opacities from those associated with more serious disease (p. 416). The following conditions should be considered:

1. Vitreous opacities may be of no significance especially in myopic individuals and in the elderly.

2. Formed opacities, usually larger than those that are threadlike or dustlike, may be caused by ruptured retinal cysts or detachment of the vitreous from the retina. They may be harmless, but occasionally they may signify an operculum from a retinal tear or hole. Detachment of the retina may occur later.

3. Synchysis scintillans is a degenerative phenomenon (p. 281).

4. Snowball opacities are almost never visualized by the patient and seldom interfere with vision (p. 281).

5. Positive scotomas in the field of vision on occasion may be described as a spot in front of the vision of one eye (p. 426).

Flashes of Light (Sparks, Stars). The following causes are possible:

1. Scintillating scotoma of migraine.

2. Beginning detachment of the retina (p. 286).

3. Certain subjective phenomena known

as Moore's lightning flashes, or the phosphene of quick eye motion, are generally detected by the patient under conditions of complete dark adaptation, such as when rapidly moving the eyes from side to side upon awakening in the middle of the night in a dark room. The flashes are of no pathologic significance.

4. Any blunt force applied to the eye will cause light flashes because of mechanical stimulation of the retina (p. 376).

Loss of the Visual Field. The symptoms of visual field defects include curtained vision, shadows in front of sight, parts of an object not seen or disappearing, and words or letters seemingly missing in print.

The symptoms depend upon the extent, location in the field, and other characteristics of the defects. A hemianopia is often described as poor vision in the eye on the side of the field defect. Central field defects are noticed as such with blurred vision. Many diseases affecting the retina or optic nerve are detected by the patient as visual field defects, especially if the central vision is encroached on (p. 422).

The following conditions should be considered:

1. Detachment of the retina. The patient sees a cloud or curtain obstructing a portion of his visual field (p. 287).

2. Large vitreous or retinal hemorrhages (p. 246).

3. Large isolated choroiditis (p. 214).

4. Vascular lesions of the visual pathway.

Distorted Vision. In this condition letters or words look jumbled; lines, such as the edges of doorways, may be curved; parts of printed material look too small or too big. These complaints usually are caused by retinal disease that disrupts the even contour of the photoreceptors (rods and cones). Visual acuity may not be seriously impaired, but the distorted image is noted by the patient quite readily if he has good visual acuity. When the retinal image appears too big, the condition is called macropsia and when it appears too small, it is called micropsia.

The following conditions should be considered:

1. Central serous retinopathy (p. 30).

2. Flat detachment of the retina (p. 287).

3. Edema of the macula from any cause; small hemorrhages; trauma (p. 376).

Glare, Photophobia (Can't Tolerate Light). Photophobia may occur for no known reason. Albinos are especially photophobic if they have albinotic irides. Irritative disease of the conjunctiva or cornea, especially foreign bodies on the cornea, may induce photophobia. Acute inflammation of the iris likewise makes the eye sensitive to ordinary light.

The following conditions should be considered:

1. Acute conjunctivitis (p. 208).

2. Foreign bodies in the conjunctiva (p. 367) or cornea (p. 367).

3. All forms of keratitis (p. 187) or abrasions of the cornea (p. 370).

4. Acute iritis (p. 21).

5. Congenital glaucoma in infants (p. 355).

Inability to See in Dim Light (Night Blindness, Poor Dark Adaptation). All patients with pigmentary degeneration of the retina complain of impairment of dark adaptation. Some normal individuals, however, have congenitally poor dark adaptation. The majority of these have myopia without any observable disease. Vitamin A deficiency should also be considered. Special equipment may be needed to test for dark adaptation.

Colored Halos Around Lights. Some relatively harmless conditions can produce this symptom, but elevated intraocular pressure should always be suspected. Among the conditions are:

1. Attacks of elevated pressure in narrow angle glaucoma (p. 347), and occasionally in wide angle glaucoma (p. 338).

2. Conjunctival secretion in any of the bacterial (p. 196) or allergic (p. 186) forms of conjunctivitis.

3. Opacities in the cornea or bleb formation in the corneal epithelium.

4. Opacities in the lens, especially with nuclear cataracts (p. 381).

Colored Vision. Objects may have a different color with each eye, and normal people often observe this. It may be the effect of after-images or due to deposition of pigment in the lens in a developing nuclear cataract. After cataract extraction in one eye the patient may see blue much more intensely in that eye, because the lens that absorbed considerable quantities of the shortwaves of the spectrum has been removed. Digitalis may produce an intensification of the yellows, with the patient describing his vision as tinted yellow. This applies to both eyes.

Diplopia. Double vision; vision blurs with both eyes open but is clear in either eye when the other is closed. The patient usually recognizes double images when they are separate from each other, which happens in most ocular muscle paralyses. In muscle paresis, on the other hand, the images may not separate but partially overlap. The patient will describe blurring of vision with both eyes open but clear vision with either eye alone. On rare occasions double vision is monocular.

Conditions that must be considered include:

1. Ocular muscle paralysis, most commonly of the lateral rectus, which is innervated by the sixth cranial nerve (p. 333).

2. Monocular diplopia caused by changes in the lens, usually associated with cataract. This is rare.

3. Very rarely patients with comitant squint will experience monocular diplopia because of the retention of both normal and abnormal retinal correspondence.

4. Uncorrected high astigmatism may give rise to monocular diplopia (p. 449).

Objects Seem to Swim. The room appears to be moving; there is feeling of unsteadiness with the eyes open. This is part of vertigo. If mild, the sensation is one of unsteadiness; if severe, true vertigo with nausea is usually reported. The following conditions should be considered:

1. Any disturbance of the labyrinths (p. 326).

2. Disease of the central nervous system, producing nystagmus (p. 324).

3. Vertical ocular muscle imbalances may occasionally give rise to the same, but milder, symptoms (p. 461).

Color Blindness. Few color blind persons are aware of their defect until someone points it out to them. They may differentiate a green from a red traffic light and call cherries red and leaves green, but when given the usual tests for color vision they call different shades of red and green the same color but of slightly different intensity (p. 130).

Lack of Binocular Vision. Almost all persons whose visual axes have always been in alignment and whose visual acuity in both eyes is nearly the same and sufficient for the test targets used will show single binocular vision, i.e., use of both eyes together. If the visual axes are not aligned, the vision in one eye must be suppressed or the individual experiences diplopia. If a strabismus has been present, but corrected by glasses or surgery, alternation of the use of either eye may be continued. It may not be possible to train the individual to use both eyes together. If the vision of one eye is much poorer than that of the other, the two eyes cannot be used together even though the visual axes are aligned.

In spite of the absence of binocular single vision, an individual may still have fairly good depth perception, since many clues for perception of distances are monocular. Stereopsis, or depth perception by parallax, depends on single binocular vision; it results from the simultaneous stimulation of visual receptors in the two eyes, which are disparate, i.e., have slightly different visual directions. Although an individual may have good single binocular vision but not good stereopsis, he can be trained to improve his stereoscopic acuity. Stereopsis is as separate a sense as color vision. Some individuals whose stereoscopic acuity is tested under rigid conditions, where all clues other than disparateness of the images are excluded, never do acquire it, even though their eyes are otherwise normal. Obviously an individual should have excellent stereopsis in order to fly jets in formation. It is advisable, but not essential, to have single binocular vision for driving an automobile. Many one-eyed drivers, however, develop driving skill by using the monocular clues afforded them, but this requires training in the habitual use of one eye. Any patient, therefore, who has lost an eye or the vision in one eye should be especially careful when he starts to drive again.

Failure to Recognize Objects by Sight. Visual agnosia generally results from a lesion in Brodmann's area 18. The agnosia is for animate and inanimate objects only and does not interfere with the recognition of language symbols, since the memories of these are stored in another cortical area. For example, a patient cannot identify a watch by sight, but he can identify it and recognize it by some other sense, such as by hearing it tick or by feeling it when it is placed in his hands.

Mirror Writing. This is a common symptom that involves inverting words while reading and a slowing of reading speed. The pathologic physiology has not been determined.

OCULAR SYMPTOMS, NONVISUAL

Painful Symptoms

Foreign Body Sensation. Generally the patient is positive that he has something in his eye, usually beneath the upper lid; however, many conditions other than a foreign body may be causing the sensation. Although he usually states that the foreign body is under the upper lid, the sensation may be caused by movement of the lid over a foreign body embedded in the cornea, or by irritative lesions of the eyeball, such as corneal ulcer or conjunctivitis.

Suggested conditions that produce foreign body sensation are:

1. Foreign bodies in either lid or embedded in the cornea (p. 367).

2. Dried conjunctival secretion from conjunctivitis of any sort (p. 209).

3. Ingrown lashes rubbing the cornea; entropion (p. 113); trichiasis (p. 4); lash caught in punctum.

4. Superficial corneal inflammations (p. 212).

5. Corneal abrasions (p. 370).

6. Papillae in vernal catarrh (p. 186).

7. Bleb formation in cornea; corneal edema from raised intraocular pressure (p. 352); corneal dystrophies (p. 278).

Burning, Smarting. In all inflammatory and irritative diseases of the conjunctiva and the superficial layers of the cornea, the eyes burn and smart. This is a common complaint of persons such as students who get insufficient sleep and of persons who indulge too heavily in tobacco and alcohol. The complaint should always suggest the need for refraction. Elderly people whose conjunctival secretions are scanty and abnormal frequently complain of their eyes burning and smarting, as do persons who run low grade fever.

The most common conditions which produce burning and smarting are:

1. Uncorrected refractive errors (p. 444).
2. Conjunctivitis (p. 208).
3. Inflammatory disease of the cornea (p. 212).
4. Lack of sleep, overwork, excessive use of tobacco and alcohol.
5. Exposure to wind, dust, and occupational irritants; allergy to cosmetics.
6. Insufficient or abnormal conjunctival secretion in the elderly.
7. Sjögren's syndrome (p. 228).

Deep-Seated Aching, Boring, Throbbing Pain. Such pain commonly occurs in serious inflammations of the anterior uveal tract, i.e., the iris and ciliary body. It occurs during the course of corneal lesions and usually is evidence that the condition is getting worse and that the iris is involved. A patient with inflammatory disease of the choroid, the posterior part of the uveal tract, rarely complains of this type of pain. It may be produced, however, by inflammation of the orbital tissue or sinuses, and occasionally an iritis may produce it, not localized in the eye but referred to the teeth or the region of the antrum, giving rise to the suspicion of an infected tooth or an acute sinusitis.

Orbital periostitis and abscess can give extreme pain. Herpes zoster can give pain that occurs in the eye before any visible involvement of the eye and may persist long after the disease has run its course (p. 195). It is characteristically lancinating and spasmodic. Tic douloureux can be agonizing. Retrobulbar neuritis causes deep pain behind the eye, usually induced by ocular movement (p. 311). Aneurysms of the internal carotid or circle of Willis (p. 316) should always be considered in pains about or in the eye.

Tenderness, Soreness, Pain on Pressure. A complaint of soreness of the eyes usually means that the patient experiences pain on pressure, or tenderness. This usually indicates an inflammatory condition of the lids, such as a hordeolum on the eyelid. If the site of inflammation cannot be visualized, it can be determined by gentle pressure with a cotton-tipped applicator. Any inflammation of the anterior segment of the globe may cause tenderness, particularly in the nodular type of scleritis. Corneal foreign bodies will do the same thing. An acute sinusitis may cause tenderness of the ipsilateral eye. Both eyes may be tender in the presence of fever or during the course of a headache from any cause. Raised intraocular pressure rarely causes tenderness unless the pressure is very high with marked signs of congestion.

Some of the conditions which cause tenderness are:

1. Lid inflammations; styes (p. 203); chalazia (p. 203) in the beginning stage of infection.
2. Dacryoadenitis in mumps and measles (p. 207).
3. Dacryocystitis in the acute stage of infection (p. 206).
4. Orbital cellulitis, abscess, periostitis (p. 202).
5. Acute conjunctivitis, especially the purulent forms (p. 208).
6. Scleritis and episcleritis (p. 14).
7. Corneal foreign bodies (p. 367), abrasions (p. 370), ulcers (p. 214).
8. Iritis, and especially iridocyclitis. When the ciliary body is involved, tenderness becomes acute. This is a good way of gauging the progress of an inflammation of the anterior uveal tract (see also p. 214).
9. Sinusitis.
10. Fever.
11. Headaches from any cause.

Headache. Uncorrected errors of refraction, hyperopia, astigmatism, and presbyopia frequently cause headaches. The pain is referred to the eyes or to the brow and comes on after reading. Vertical muscle imbalances cause headaches along with a feeling of pulling in the eyes (to be described later). Early morning headaches are often present in open angle glaucoma because intraocular pressure increases during the night. Migraine headaches are typical, particularly if associated with scintillating scotoma or other field changes. Sinusitis is a common cause of headache. The severe headaches of raised intracranial pressure usually are associated with vomiting without nausea. Headaches may occur in any inflammatory condition of the eye and adnexa. The headache need not come from the eye itself but from an increased contractile state of the muscles of the head and may be occipital in location, owing to the occipitofrontalis muscle. Either high or low blood pressure may give rise to headaches around the eyes.

Painful Eyes (Pulling or Drawing Sensation). This expression is often used to describe discomfort or mild pain in the eyes, usually connected with reading or close work. It seldom indicates an inflammatory condition. The most frequent causes are uncorrected refractive errors and heterophoria, especially vertical muscle imbalances. The sensation can be readily experienced by anyone by placing a small prism, i.e., 2 to 4 P.D., in front of one eye with the base up or down.

Nonpainful Symptoms

Itching. Patients frequently rub their eyes when they are tired or strained from overuse. Marked itching, however, is nearly always a sign of allergy. It is becoming increasingly common in women from allergy to cosmetics, particularly sprayed applications. The various forms of "hair setting agents" are highly allergenic to some people. Accompanying signs of allergy in the conjunctiva should be looked for if the lids appear allergic. Healing wounds are often associated with itching, since the fibers involved in the mediation of pain also subserve the itch sensation, and itching may be induced by any stimulus whose threshold is just below that of the pain sense.

Tearing (Watering of the Eyes). Tearing, or watering of the eyes, may result from excessive formation of lacrimal fluid or from the inability of the normal tear passages to conduct the fluid out of the conjunctival cul-de-sac. All inflammatory conditions of the anterior segment of the eye lead to excessive formation of tears.

This is particularly true of inflammatory diseases or trauma to the cornea. The slightest irritation of the corneal nerves leads to a copious reflex secretion of tears so that the eye fills with fluid which overflows onto the cheeks. Emotional disturbances, pain, nausea, and exposing the eye to bright lights may cause excessive tear formation in the normal individual. Emotional tearing does not occur in the infant, even though they "cry" lustily. In the elderly, emotion, even though intense, often is not accompanied by weeping.

Tearing may be caused by malfunction of the nasolacrimal apparatus at any level. This can be relieved, in many instances, by surgical intervention. Ectropion permits the tears to pool in the lower cul-de-sac because they cannot drain through the displaced punctum. Eversion of the lower punctum without ectropion also may occur in the elderly because of relaxation of the tonus of the orbicularis muscle and redundancy of the skin of the lower lid. It is possible that excessive tear formation may exist with obstruction of the tear passages (see also p. 206).

The following common causes of tearing are listed:

1. Increased tearing from emotional states.

2. Increased tearing from general conditions, such as hyperthyroidism (p. 255), facial neuralgias, tic douloureux, and pain other than ocular.

3. Increased tearing from hypersecretion of the lacrimal gland caused by inflammation of the gland (p. 206) or by tumors (p. 263).

4. Increased tearing from irritation of the anterior segment of the globe caused by foreign bodies, misdirected lashes, corneal abrasions, and keratitis; tearing from allergic conditions of the conjunctiva and cornea.

5. Failure of the tears to reach the lacrimal passages caused by alterations in the lid margins, eversion of the punctum, blockage of the puncta, constrictions in the nasolacrimal ducts, and inflammation of the lacrimal sac. Impatency of the opening in the nose as a congenital defect or as the result of inflammatory processes.

Dryness. Elderly individuals frequently complain of dryness of the eyes, which is probably caused by a deficiency of tear formation as well as an alteration of the chemical and physical characteristics of the lacrimal secretion, which is analogous to the changes that take place in all mucous membranes with age. This symptom, when aggravated, is suggestive of Sjögren's syndrome, especially when the patient also complains of dryness of the mouth. Chronic conjunctivitis, leading to atrophy of the mucous glands in the conjunctiva, may eventually produce an alteration in the lacrimal secretion and lead to a feeling of dryness. Exposure of the conjunctival cul-de-sac as a result of changes in the position of the lids or their inability to close properly will produce the same sensation.

Therefore, the common causes of dryness are:

1. Chronic conjunctivitis, especially with conjunctival atrophy. This is caused by bacteria, exposure to chemical fumes, excessive smoking, and alcohol (p. 184).

2. Exposure of the conjunctiva caused by malposition of the lids (p. 366).

3. Failure of the lids to close properly, which could be a residual of Bell's palsy (p. 3), ectropion, (p. 113), and other conditions.

Sandiness, Grittiness. This symptom may occur alone or with dryness. The causes include those which are associated with dryness, but in general they suggest an alteration in the nature of the lacrimal secretion rather than a deficiency. Sandiness occurs frequently during an acute conjunctivitis because of an accumulation of mucus. Some people develop small yellow concretions in the conjunctiva, presumably a result of alteration in the metabolism of the conjunctival glands. These are hard, sandlike bodies embedded in the conjunctiva of the upper tarsus. When they erode through the epithelium, they rub against the cornea, producing this annoying sensation.

Bulging; Fullness of the Eyes. Patients may complain of a sensation of bulging of one eye during the development of a unilateral proptosis caused by an orbital tumor, but the majority who develop bilateral exophthalmos in Graves' disease usually have no such sensation, and only become aware of it through their friends or by looking in a mirror. Bulging of both lids, either of the whole lower lid or the upper lid near the inner canthi, occurs as an age change in some people. It is caused by relaxation of the septum orbitale, so that the orbital fat herniates into the lids. Fullness of the eyes is often complained of without any discoverable cause.

Twitching or Fluttering of the Lids. This is a common symptom caused by fibrillation of the orbicularis muscle. It is always unilateral and generally occurs in one and the same eye. Its cause is not known. The condition has been termed myokymia.

Heaviness of the Lids (Eyes Want to Close; Can't Open Eyes). This may be a symptom of fatigue in normal people, indicating that they are not getting sufficient sleep. The state of fatigue is felt first in the eyes; the lids feel heavy, want to close, and can be kept open only with a decided effort. The definition of drowsiness is "to be *heavy* with sleepiness." Drowsiness is also an expression of abnormal sleepiness, such as occurs in senility, encephalitis, and so forth.

Difficulty in getting the lids open occurs in ptosis from any cause. Unilateral ptosis occurring at any age should always create the suspicion of myasthenia gravis, particularly if the complaint increases as the day advances. Heaviness of the lids is complained of in any condition causing lid edema.

Dizziness. Dizziness or vertigo is seldom caused by disorders of the eyes, but most commonly arises from some disturbance of the inner ear. Meniere's disease must always be considered, as well as cerebellar disease. However, refractive errors and heterophoria on occasion can give rise to a sensation of dizziness more marked when the patient does close work. Nystagmus itself does not produce dizziness; for example, ocular nystagmus is never associated with dizziness, nor is nystagmus of central origin associated with dizziness unless mechanisms other than the ocular mechanisms producing the nystagmus are directly involved. Vestibular nystagmus, on the other hand, is always associated with vertigo, which is one of its hallmarks. When nystagmus is present without vertigo it is not of vestibular origin. The chief cause of vertigo related to the eyes themselves is paralysis of an ocular muscle. In the early stages this is a frequent complaint and is caused by diplopia.

Blinking. Parents frequently bring a child in for examination complaining that he has spells of blinking. The child himself rarely complains. In most cases this is a form of facial tic and disappears spontaneously. It is often mimicked by several children in a classroom after one child starts it. Calling the child's attention to the tic usually intensifies and prolongs it, and it may become a means adopted by the child of calling attention to himself. A frequent and often overlooked cause is the intertwining of long lashes of the upper and lower lids at the outer canthi. When these are cut the blinking stops. Unilateral blinking may be a sign of local irritation from any cause.

Squinting (Squeezing the Lids Together). The term "squint" to the ophthalmologist refers to a strabismus, whereas the laity use the term for narrowing the lid fissures. Normally the fissures are narrowed to cut down the intensity of light or to enable the patient to see better. The conditions causing the squinting are therefore those which cause glare, or refractive errors producing ametropia.

Lids Stuck Together. Abnormal or exces-sive ocular secretion due to any cause may dry during sleep, hardening on the lashes and gluing them together, making it difficult for the patient to separate his lids on awakening. An ointment instilled at bedtime is preventive.

Eyes Discharging (Full of Mucus or White Matter). This usually results from an inflammatory condition of the conjunctiva, but altered conjunctival secretion occurs in some noninflammatory conditions and the cause is not known. The altered secretion is in the form of white matter looking like a film of soapsuds. It is caused by overactivity of the meibomian glands which may produce an emulsion of the tears and meibomian oil. It does not indicate a state of vitamin A deficiency in the majority of patients who suffer from it, although a similar and perhaps identical type of altered secretion does occur in xerosis and xerophthalmia from severe vitamin A lack. In this case the secretion becomes adherent to the bulbar conjunctiva in spots (Bitot's spots) adjacent to the limbus.

Granulated Lids. The term is used by patients to indicate the dried secretion on the lashes found in the various forms of blepharitis (p. 203).

Eye Examinations

SHORT, PERTINENT HISTORY

Before proceeding with an examination of the eye, a pertinent history is always elicited. The patient's complaints and their duration are reviewed, as well as any other important ocular information such as previous diseases, injuries, or operations. Inquiry also is made about the patient's general health.

DISTANT AND CLOSE VISUAL ACUITY

The clinical testing of visual acuity indicates the function of the fovea, the most sensitive part of the retina. The size of the retinal image depends upon the size of the object and its distance from the eye. The farther an object, the smaller the retinal image. The angle that the image subtends at the nodal point of the eye is the visual angle. By combining the two factors of size and distance, it is possible to determine the minimum visual angle, that is, the smallest retinal image that can be seen. The so-called normal eye can identify an entire letter subtending an angle of 5 minutes of arc and any component of a letter subtending 1 minute of arc. Many persons, however, can resolve letters subtending a smaller visual angle.

408

Usually the patient reads a Snellen chart, or one of its modifications (Figs. II-1, II-2, II-3), at a distance of 6 meters. At this distance rays of light from an object are practically parallel, and no effort of accommodation is necessary to focus on the object. The Snellen chart is composed of letters of graduated sizes with the distance at which

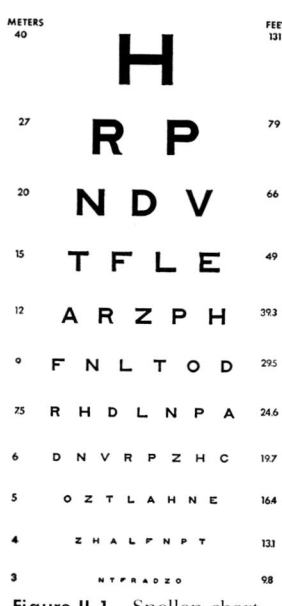

Figure II-1 Snellen chart.

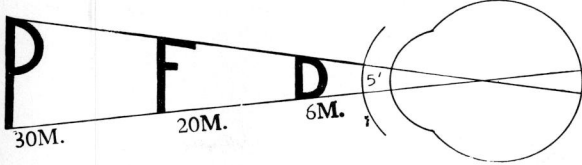

Figure II-2   The minimum visual angle is 5 minutes.

each size subtends an angle of 5 minutes indicated along the side. On some Snellen charts the angle of a whole letter subtends 4 minutes of arc instead of 5. If the patient reads the line of letters that subtends the angle of 5 minutes at 6 meters, his vision is expressed as 6/6*, which is the visual acuity recorded as the smallest line on which the majority of letters are read. The numerator of the fraction denotes the distance in meters (usually 6) at which the test is conducted and the denominator the distance at which the smallest letters subtend an angle of 5 minutes.

The vision of the normal eye is 6/6, although many persons have vision better than normal with an acuity of 6/5 or even 6/4. The vision of each eye should be tested separately with and without glasses. For example, if one or two letters are missed on the 6/6 line, this may be recorded as 6/6−1 or 6/6−2 respectively. If the largest letter on the chart, which generally is 6/150, cannot be seen, the patient may be brought closer to the chart and the distance at which the letter is seen is used as the numerator, for example, 3/150. Since usually there is only one large letter on each chart, the patient must be shown different charts on different visits.

If the largest letter cannot be seen at 1 meter, the patient is asked to count the examiner's fingers at a particular distance. The result is recorded as counting fingers at a particular distance. If the patient cannot count the fingers, he is asked whether or not he can see the examiner's

hand move. If he cannot, light is directed into his eye and he is asked to tell when he sees it. Then the light is thrown into his eye from different directions and he is asked to tell from what direction it comes. If the patient is able to determine when the light goes on and off, the notation "light perception present" is made. If the projection of the light is good, that is, the direction from which the light comes to the patient (right, left, above, or below) is discerned correctly, this also is noted. A patient is technically blind only when he has no light perception.

If the vision test is given in a room less than 6 meters long, a mirror image of an ordinary chart may be used. The chart is hung on the wall behind the patient who faces a mirror at the opposite end of the room in which the chart is reflected. The distance from the chart to the mirror and back to the patient is doubled, and thus a room of only 4 meters may be used.

The fraction that is used to denote visual acuity cannot be reduced. It is incorrect to reason that if 6/6 vision equals one, then 6/12 vision is only one half as good. Fractions denoting visual acuity do not represent fractions of visual functions. Near (reading) vision is tested by special charts (Fig. II-4).

With a pinhole disc, the examiner may roughly determine whether vision that is subnormal without glasses is caused by a refractive error or by other conditions. A cardboard disc with a small pinhole in the center is placed in front of the eye to be tested, while the other eye is occluded. The small aperture in the disc allows only a small pencil of rays to pass into the eye and through the axis of the dioptric system. The patient with the refractive error should read 6/6. If the pinhole fails to improve his

---

*Because the metric system conforms with other measurements in ophthalmology, such as the use of diopters to record lens strength, it is preferred to the foot-yard measure. To convert from feet to meters, divide roughly by three. For example, 6 meters correspond approximately to 20 feet, so 6/6 visual acuity is the same as 20/20.

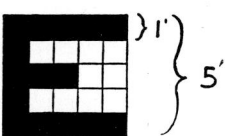

Figure II-3   Test letter of Snellen chart.

spectacles. These errors require further examination for refraction.

No. 1.

The eye is the organ of vision, and resembles a photographer's camera in its construction. The iris is the diaphragm, with a pupillary opening in the center, which adjusts itself to the amount of light by dilating or contracting. Like the camera, the vitreous chamber is darkened inside by the pigmented layer of the choroid. The retina, or nervous layer, is the sensitive plate of the camera, and receives the impression or image of the object. The crystalline lens is so adjusted by the aid of the ciliary muscle as to bring the light to a focus

0.37

No. 2.

on the retina. In order to accomplish its function successfully all the media of the eye must be transparent. These media are from before backwards the cornea, the aqueous humor, the crystalline lens, and the vitreous humor. Any haziness of one or more of these media will, of course, interfere with the visual function. The first essential, then, of perfect vision is an absolute transparency of all the media, and the second is an accurate focusing of the rays of light on

0.50

No. 3.

the retina through the adjustment of the crystalline lens. These impressions when received upon the retina are gathered up and concentrated, as it were, in the optic nerve. through which they are carried to the brain. In short-sighted persons the eye-ball is too long, and the light rays come to a focus in

0.62

No. 4.

front of the retina, while in far-sighted persons the eye-ball is too short, and the focal point, therefore, falls behind the retina. In either case a blurred image is received upon the retina. In order to

0.75

No. 6.

overcome this blurring, and thus correct the optical defect, the eye unconsciously makes an effort by which the ciliary muscle acts on the lens. This effort explains why eye-strain may

0.87

No. 8.

cause pain and discomfort. An optical correction for the refractive error is found in spectacle lenses. In near-sightedness a

1.00

No. 10.

concave spherical lens will cause the focal point to recede until it falls directly on the retina;

1.50

No. 12.

while in far-sightedness

2.00

Figure II-4 Reading chart.

visual acuity score, there is some other cause for the reduced vision, such as opacities in the ocular media or retina/optic nerve disease.

Myopia and similar conditions reduce vision, which can be improved with proper

EXTERNAL EXAMINATION

Examination of the eye and adnexa without special apparatus may yield valuable information for the diagnosis and subsequent treatment of patients with ocular difficulties secondary to systemic disease. The eye should be examined not only as an isolated organ but in relation to the total body and to possible systemic diseases. The eyes and adnexa may offer important clues to general health. Exophthalmos, for example, may suggest a diagnosis of Graves' disease; ptosis may suggest myasthenia gravis; nystagmus may suggest multiple sclerosis and encephalitis; and an Argyll Robertson pupil may suggest tabes dorsalis.

As in a general physical examination, a systematic routine should be followed. At first a comprehensive examination is time-consuming, but with increased experience the physician learns to perceive at a glance what once required prolonged scrutiny. The following routine examination is suggested.

Eyelids and Palpebral Fissures. In diffuse light, preferably daylight, the physician should note the general appearance, color, texture, swelling, position, and motility of the lids. Localized swelling should be inspected and palpated. Signs of inflammation and edema should be noted. The skin should be observed for any abnormalities such as edema, rash, thinning, or presence of abnormal vessels. Previous ocular injury might be suggested by the presence of scars on the lids, especially near the orbital rims.

The positions of the lids alter the size of the palpebral fissures, which should be equal. The lid margins should overlay the cornea above and below, with no exposure of sclera (Fig. II-5). Voluntary lid closure should be excellent. Involuntary blinking should be present and frequent. Both upper lids should elevate equally well on upward gaze and on downward gaze (Figs. II-6, II-7A, B, C). The lid margins should follow the globe synchronously with no delay (lid lag). The lid borders should be

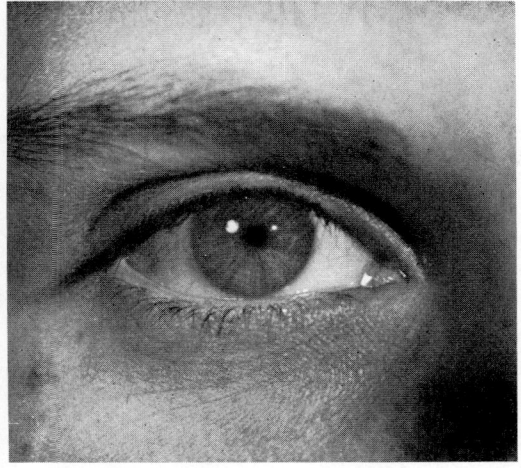

Figure II-5 Normal eyelids and adnexa. Note position of lower lid just below limbus. Also note highlights just off center of cornea.

in close apposition to the globe and neither inverted (entropion) or everted (ectropion). The skin between the two fissures covering the bridge of the nose may be normally excessive in amount and folded (characteristic in persons of certain races) or sometimes occur as a congenital anomaly in others (epicanthus).

Lashes and Eyebrows. Particular note should be made of the direction of the eyelashes (whether they are turned in, out, or misdirected), loss of lashes, or even of a localized patch of unpigmented eyelashes. The lash border should be scrutinized for any scales and hyperemia (blepharitis), or even for animal parasites.

Position of the Eyeballs. The prominence of the eyeballs varies widely in normal individuals. One eye displaced more than

1.5 mm. in front of its fellow eye is definitely abnormal. This can only be determined, however, by instrument measurements. Unless the difference in prominence is so great that there is no question about it, naked eye observations should not be relied on for the diagnosis of exophthalmos or enophthalmos. The examiner can be misled because the eye usually appears prominent in an orbit with a wide palpebral fissure and less prominent in one with a narrow fissure.

When the patient is looking straight ahead toward the horizon, his eyes should be on the same level and both axes apparently parallel. This can be simply observed by the corneal light reflexes from a pocket flashlight or ophthalmoscope that is held before the patient's eyes. If the reflection is in the same position in each eye, one can be reasonably sure that the eyeballs are aligned. The cornea is not a perfect sphere but an ellipsoid whose major axis frequently does not correspond to the visual line. Even though the eyes are in good alignment, therefore, the reflection may lie outside or inside the center of the pupil when the patient is looking straight ahead. This may give the false impression that the eyes are diverging, converging, or straight when, in reality, there may be a deviation of the visual axes.

A still more accurate method, the cover test, is to have the patient fix his eyes on a distant object and then to cover his right eye while observing any movement of his left eye. If no movement occurs, the eye is judged to be straight. The test is repeated with the other eye.

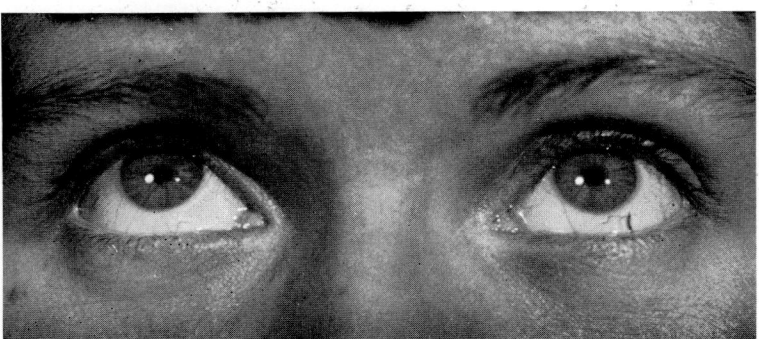

Figure II-6 Position of the lids on upward gaze. Note exposure of sclera below limbus and amount of iris covered by upper lid.

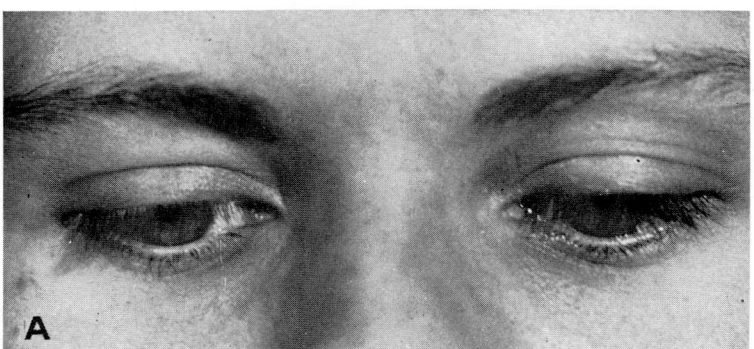

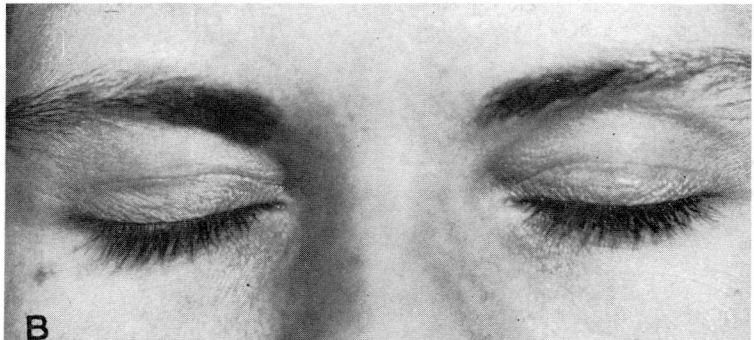

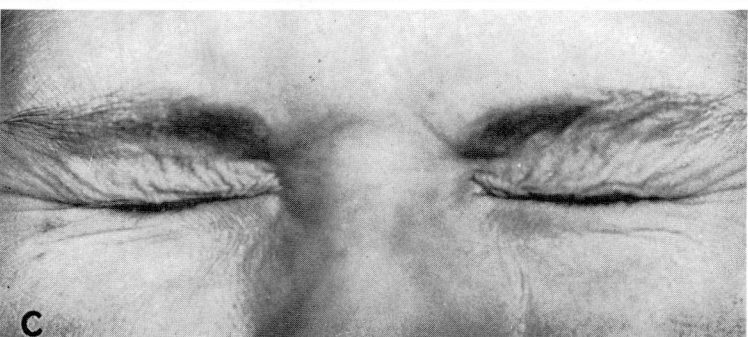

Figure II-7 *(A)* Position of lids on downward gaze. Note that upper lid closely follows the movement of the globe downward. *(B)* Position of lids on gentle closure. *(C)* Lids squeezed shut.

Motility of the Eyeballs. Ocular rotation and simultaneous eye movements should be determined. Normally they remain aligned over a wide range in all directions. Involuntary movements occur, at times normally, in extremes of gaze (end-position or physiologic nystagmus). Nystagmus, fine or coarse, slow or rapid, except at the end point, is observed. Occasionally a fine rotational nystagmus escapes observation until the fundus is examined by an ophthalmoscope, with which even small movements can be detected.

The convergence near point is the point closest to the patient on which both eyes can converge as an object is brought toward him. It normally is 50 to 70 mm. in front of the eyes. As soon as one eye begins to deviate outward, the limit of convergence has been reached.

Lacrimal Apparatus. The surface of the cornea and of the conjunctiva is moistened by tears and the secretion of the glands that line the lids. Excess or lack of tears should be noted. Tearing may be caused not only by excessive formation of fluid but also by obstruction of the passages that normally drain the eye. The position and patency of lacrimal puncta should be observed. Pressure should be exerted on the lacrimal sac to determine if it contains any secretion or pus. When either regurgitate from the puncta, the tear duct is blocked. Purulent material indicates that the sac is infected.

Bulbar Conjunctiva. The bulbar conjunctiva should be examined while the lids are held apart gently and before any manipulation might produce congestion of the conjunctival vessels. In the normal conjunctiva a few large and tortuous episcleral vessels usually are visible. Because the eyes look congested, women, especially, note their presence. To avoid the mistake of regarding such vessels as pathologic, the physician should be familiar with the common normal variations. Except for these vessels and occasional deposits of pigment, the sclera should be seen through the transparent bulbar conjunctiva as a porcelain-white color.

At either side of the limbus, but especially on the nasal side, a slightly raised, yellow area (pinguecula) may be seen in normal persons. It becomes more prominent with age, and, though often mistaken for a tumor, is composed of yellow elastic tissue. In some instances the pinguecula becomes cystic and causes a cosmetic blemish that is of no pathologic significance.

The conjunctiva may be pigmented with a discrete nevus, or more rarely a melanoma. A slightly gray appearance, especially in the lower cul-de-sac, suggests a history of using eyedrops containing silver salts (argyrosis). Edema of the conjunctiva (chemosis), emphysema with crepitus, and subconjunctival hemorrhage should be noted. Innocuous themselves, they may be manifestations of serious ocular and periocular pathology or injury.

Pathologic congestion of the bulbar conjunctiva should be recognized at once. There are two forms: superficial and deep congestion. Superficial congestion is characteristic of conjunctival irritation, whether by a foreign body, bacteria, or trauma. Only the superficial layer of bright, brick-red vessels is involved. These vessels are tortuous and are more evident at the periphery of the bulbar conjunctiva in the fornices than near the limbus (the junction of the cornea with the sclera). If the congestion is considerable, the small capillaries between the large vessels visible to the naked eye may be engorged, giving a diffuse redness to the whole conjunctiva. Petechial hemorrhages may be present. This superficial congestion gives rise to the lay term "pink-eye." It is generally caused by an acute infection of the conjunctiva.

Deep congestion always indicates an involvement of the cornea or of the deeper structures within the eye. It is seen in keratitis, iritis, and when a foreign body is embedded in the cornea. In the latter it signifies that the eye is sufficiently irritated to dilate the vessels supplying the iris and ciliary body. This form of congestion is found immediately around the limbus. The individual normal vessels in this area are too small to be seen by the naked eye, but when they are dilated they produce a diffuse red flush. With magnification they appear underneath the conjunctiva and do not move when the overlying conjunctiva is touched gently with an applicator. This form of congestion is called a ciliary flush.

If either superficial or deep congestion is

present, there is seldom any doubt as to its character. In severe inflammatory conditions of the eye, however, both forms often may be present together. Diagnosing an underlying disease by the type of congestion alone, therefore, is not always easy.

Palpebral Conjunctiva. At different ages the normal palpebral conjunctiva varies considerably in redness and in character. The normal palpebral conjunctiva likewise changes in appearance from the retrotarsal fold to the tarsal plates. In the retrotarsal fold it is loose and contains frequent follicles and large vessels. Over the tarsal plate the conjunctiva is firmly bound to the underlying tarsus, shows no follicles, and is characterized by yellow lines of the meibomian glands shining through the translucent overlying tissue.

The conjunctiva of the upper and lower lids should be inspected carefully. To expose the upper conjunctiva, the lid must be everted, a maneuver requiring a little practice, especially when an acute inflammatory condition is causing blepharospasm. The inspection may be done best if the physician faces the patient, whose head is supported by a headrest. The patient is asked to keep both eyes open while looking down.

With the thumb and forefinger of his right hand, the physician grasps the eyelashes of the upper lid, pulling the lid down and away from the globe (Fig. II-8A,B,C,D). He uses his left forefinger or an applicator to press against the upper edge of the tarsus through the skin while his right hand quickly pulls the eyelid up and over his left forefinger. He then removes his left forefinger and holds the lash border up and against the upper lid and orbital rim while he examines the tarsal conjunctiva. Once everted, the lid can be held in place by the left hand, leaving the right free for the necessary manipulation. To return the upper lid to its normal position, the physi-

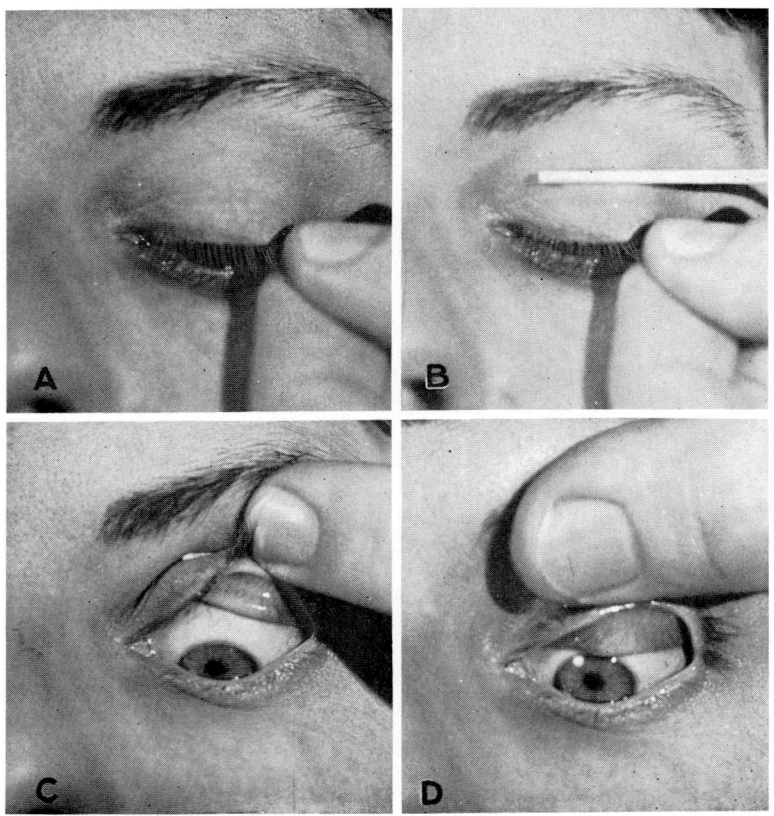

Figure II-8 (A) First procedure in everting upper lid. (B) Second procedure in everting upper lid. (C) Third procedure in everting upper lid. (D) Maintaining lid in everted position.

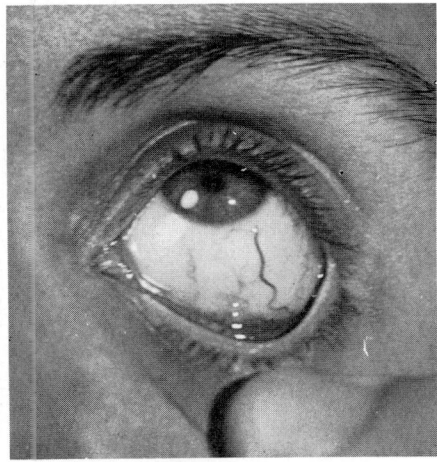

Figure II-9 Eversion of lower lid.

cian needs only to direct the patient to look up. The everted tarsal plate automatically goes back into place.

Occasionally the retrotarsal conjunctiva demands more careful scrutiny. To expose it thoroughly, the upper lid must be everted and a cotton-tipped applicator placed well in back of the everted tarsus and pressed down and forward to push the retrotarsal tissues into view. Although foreign bodies lodge here occasionally, the most common site in the upper lid is the groove formed by the sulcus above the lash border of the tarsal plate. The lower lid may be everted by pulling it down with the thumb and then pressing the thumb back gently toward the orbit (Fig. II-9).

Other External Examinations

The Cornea. The normal corneal surface is so perfect that it forms an excellent reflecting surface. Just as the finest ripple on a smooth lake becomes apparent by a break on the reflecting surface, so any defect in the cornea can be detected at once by a disturbance in its mirror-like reflection. The reflection of an examining light from the corneal surface should be carefully observed for any irregularities or any area of dullness. The physician should note the size of each cornea and compare one with the other while looking for any departure from the normal.

A pen-sized flashlight and a loupe for magnification can be used to observe

changes, such as scars, remains of empty vessels, deposits on the endothelial surface, and the like, that might be difficult to see with the unaided eye. Even foreign bodies on the cornea may be easily missed without good illumination and magnification.

Staining the cornea with fluorescein is an important means of detecting abrasions on the corneal surface. Convenient, sterile fluorescein strips or flourescein solution can be used. Whenever the corneal epithelium is broken, the underlying stroma stains a brilliant green, so that even pinpoint abrasions show up clearly, especially if a cobalt blue filter is used with illumination.

If it is difficult to examine the cornea because photophobia and blepharospasm secondary to an acute corneal lesion are present, a drop of local anesthetic may bring decided relief and allow a more thorough examination.

A detailed examination of the cornea, the anterior chamber, and the lens requires the use of a slit lamp and a corneal microscope. It is not expected that the student or general practitioner will have access to these instruments.

CORNEAL SENSITIVITY. It is important to determine whether or not the cornea is normally sensitive to touch, for if intracranial lesions involve the fifth nerve, corneal sensitivity frequently is impaired on the side of the lesion. Certain local conditions of the cornea, such as herpetic keratitis, are also characterized by loss of sensation. Thus, by determining corneal sensitivity, these conditions may be differentiated in part from other disease processes affecting the cornea.

To determine corneal sensitivity, the cornea is touched lightly with a wisp of cotton drawn out to a few threads while the lids are held apart. One eye and then the other should be tested for comparison. Care should be taken not to touch the lashes. The patient should be reassured that he will experience no pain and is requested to tell as soon as he feels the slightest touch. To make sure of this, the examiner should go through the motions several times without actually touching the cornea with the cotton.

Anterior Chamber. Although a detailed examination of the anterior chamber is difficult without the use of a slit lamp biomicroscope, a good light and the naked eye will give a general impression of chamber depth, clearness or cloudiness of the aqueous, presence of blood (hyphema), or accumulation of cellular exudate (hypopyon).

Iris. The color of the iris in each eye should be noted and particular attention paid to differences in color, texture, and pattern. New vessels on the iris, deposits on its surface, or tears that might have been caused by injury and adhesions of the iris to the lens, as well as other signs, should be detected.

The general appearance of the pupils, their size, shape, situation, and equality should be studied as the patient faces a diffuse light. Normal pupils are round, centrally placed, and, in a majority of persons, equal in size. Unequal pupils, however, are not of themselves a sign of disease, because 25 per cent of normal persons have them.

Pupillary reflexes should be tested. The most important test is for light reflex. With the patient facing a bright, even illumination, both his eyes are covered with two cards or with the palms of the observer. One card or palm is withdrawn and pupillary contraction noted. The pupil should contract briskly and promptly and the contraction should be maintained; this is a direct light reflex. The other pupil should contract simultaneously even though shielded from the light; this contraction is the consensual light reflex. The observer can note the contraction behind his palm or the card.

Next, the near-point reflex should be elicited by having the patient look into the distance and then at an object held about 6 inches from his nose and slightly below the horizon. During this procedure illumination should remain constant. Both pupils should contract. Usually near-point contraction is not as rapid or as marked as contraction to light. In some cases it may be advisable to test pupil reaction to various drugs such as cocaine, epinephrine, and Mecholyl.

Another reflex occasionally tested is pupil dilatation in response to painful stimuli. This is best elicited by pulling on a few hairs at the back of the patient's neck. Normally, both pupils should dilate.

Lens. The lens should be observed for deposits on its surface and opacities in its substance by obliquely placed illumination. The pupil must be dilated to see much of the lens, but some of the pupillary region may be seen without dilatation. It should be noted whether the lens appears in its normal position or if it has become subluxated and dislocated. Lens translucency diminishes greatly with age; if marked, it may indicate a cataract. Even though clear of discrete opacities, the lens in most elderly persons generally looks somewhat gray by oblique illumination.

OPHTHALMOSCOPY

The invention of the reflecting ophthalmoscope by Helmholtz in 1851 not only revolutionized ophthalmology but also offered the general physician the opportunity to obtain information of great diagnostic value by studying the fundus. Ophthalmoscopy should be part of the routine physical examination of every patient, and the physician should use the ophthalmoscope with the same ease as he uses the stethoscope. When the findings are uncertain or unusual, he may then call in an ophthalmologist, just as he would consult a cardiologist in a perplexing heart case. Ophthalmoscopic examination should be done with pupils dilated, especially if the periphery of the retina is to be studied.

Examination of the Ocular Media. To observe the patient's right eye with the direct ophthalmoscope, the observer holds the instrument in his right hand with the forefinger on the milled lens-selection disc and uses his right eye (Fig. II-10). The procedure is reversed for the patient's left eye (Fig. II-11). The patient should not wear his glasses except in refractive errors of high astigmatism or high myopia. The observer may wear his glasses. It is convenient to make the examination standing at the side of the patient. The patient should fix his eye upon a distant target. The resultant fundus view is magnified 15 × and

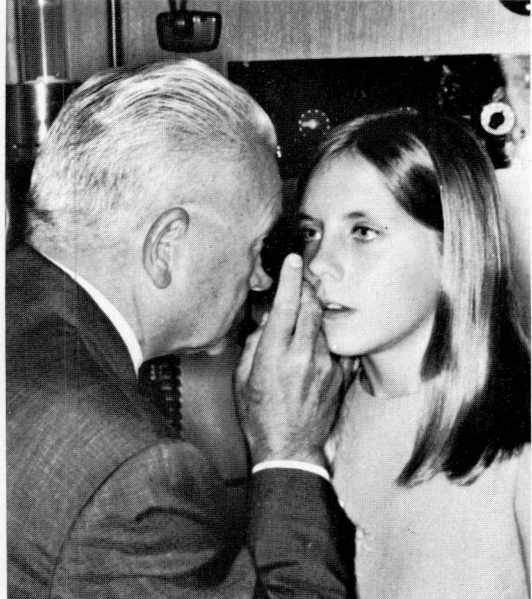

Figure II-10 Method of examining right fundus details with ophthalmoscope.

erect, i.e., all directions are seen as they actually exist.

With the lens setting at zero, light from the ophthalmoscope is directed into the patient's pupil about 6 inches from his eye. The normal fundus is seen as a red reflex.

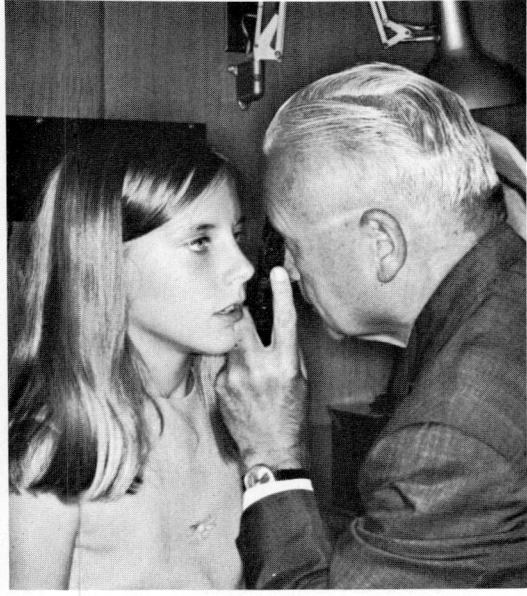

Figure II-11 Method of examining left fundus details with ophthalmoscope.

Opacities may be seen in the ocular media and should be localized and studied. Opacities are black since they obstruct the reflected light from reaching the observer's eye. With direct focal illumination the true color of the opacities is seen. To localize the opacities, the observer moves toward the patient until the opacity is in focus. When he is directly against the patient, the observer uses black or positive lenses. A +8 or +10 lens focuses corneal opacities, whereas lower power lenses focus progressively back. The retina focuses at zero, i.e., no lens effect, provided both patient and observer have no refractive error. Unintentional accommodative spasm by either patient or observer necessitates moving the lens setting toward the minus or red side for a clear focus.

Opacities also may be localized by their displacement when the eye is moved, usually up. Corneal opacities move up to a great degree, but anterior lens opacities move up to a much lesser extent. Posterior lens opacities move down to a small degree; vitreous opacities move down to a great degree.

Examination of the Fundus. In examining the fundus the pupil should be dilated as widely as possible and the patient brought to a darkened room. Excellent mydriatic agents are Cyclogyl, ½ per cent, or Mydriacyl, 1 per cent. These may be reinforced by Neosynephrine, 10 per cent. These should not, however, be instilled in eyes with very narrow angles (see Glaucoma, p. 347), and the only way to protect the patient with certainty is by gonioscopy. Some estimate of angles can be made, however, by illuminating the anterior chamber from the side with a penlight.

The optic disc should be examined first. It may be circular to oval but usually is vertically oval and pink, and the temporal area usually is a lighter pink. The center of the disc has a pale depression, the physiologic cup, the bottom of which may be mottled and gray, representing the fibers of the lamina cribrosa of the sclera. In chronic simple glaucoma, the cup may be large, with sharp, excavated borders. In optic atrophy the entire disc may be pale;

in papilledema or papillitis, it may be congested. Its size varies with the refractive error, being small in hyperopia and large in myopia.

The border of the disc may gradually merge into the surrounding retina without any clear-cut edge, or it may be demarcated sharply from the retina by a ring of white, the so-called white scleral ring or crescent. This is formed by exposure of sclera between the choroid and the opening for the optic nerve. Thickened retinal pigment epithelium may result in a black ring or crescent. In papilledema or papillitis and in hyperopic eyes, the disc border may be blurry.

The retinal arteries are red, the veins darker or bluer. The arteries are smaller than the veins in about a 4 to 5 proportion. The arteries have a thicker wall that gives a shiny, central, reflex stripe. Since both vessel walls are transparent, the observer is actually seeing a column of blood. Branching of the vessels is extremely variable. Various degrees of arteriosclerotic and hypertensive changes affect the vessels (p. 241). The observer should evaluate general and focal narrowing of the arterioles, the width and color of the arteriolar reflex stripe, and the nature of arteriovenous crossings.

The macular area is usually darker than the surrounding retina and is about 2 disc diameters from the disc on the temporal side. The small branches of the superior and inferior temporal vessels in the macular area converge toward it, but the macula itself is free from visible vessels. The very center is called the fovea centralis, which appears as a small area of darker red. A tiny light reflex can be seen at the center of the fovea, which is caused by reflection of the ophthalmoscopic light from the concave inner surface of the area. The reflex moves in the opposite direction as the ophthalmoscope is moved.

The periphery of the fundus is easily examined by having the patient move his eye in the direction to be observed: up for the superior quadrant, out for the temporal quadrant, and so forth. Combined with appropriate movements of the observer's head (Fig. II-12), the periphery can be seen directly with an ophthalmoscope up to 1.5 mm. from the ora serrata with a widely dilated pupil. Use of indirect ophthalmoscopy and indenting the overlying sclera by pressure permits visualization of the peripheral retina and adjacent ora serrata of the ciliary body. It is not uncommon in normal eyes to find the retinal pigment thin at the periphery, especially at the nasal side, but one should look for white areas or areas of unusual pigmentation, which are scars of previous inflammation. In this location signs of certain diseases, such as peripheral uveitis or pigmentary degeneration of the retina, are frequently found.

Fundus lesions should be measured and located. The size of a lesion is estimated by comparing it with the size of the disc, which averages 1.5 mm. Thus the size of a patch of choroiditis may be said to be 2 disc diameters. Similarly, lesions are located relative to the disc, e.g., 4 disc diameters from the disc at 11 o'clock. When a lesion is elevated, as in papilledema, the elevation may be measured by noting the most convex lens that clearly focuses on some nearby normal area of the fundus. The elevation is thus reported in diopters; 3 diopters is about 1 millimeter.

NORMAL VARIATIONS. Intelligent, curious observation and experience will ac-

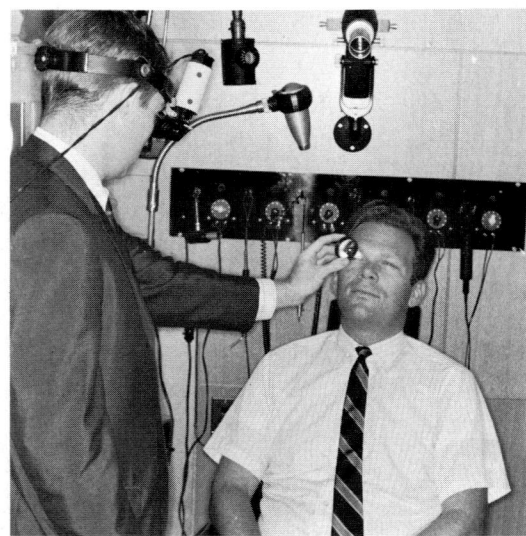

Figure II-12 Indirect ophthalmoscopy.

quaint the physician with the wide range of normal variations. Vessels are notoriously variable. They may have no apparent connection to the main tree, running from the temporal aspect of the disc to the macular area. Called cilioretinal vessels, they originate from the circle of Zinn, which is formed around the optic nerve in the scleral foramen by branches from the short posterior ciliary arteries. Cilioretinal vessels, therefore, are really anastomatic between the choroidal (ciliary) and retinal circulation.

A small tuft of connective tissue frequently is seen arising from the optic disc at its nasal side and projecting forward into the vitreous, which represents an embryonic remnant of the hyaloid artery or of the surrounding canal of Cloquet. If it is near the edge of the disc, the disc margins may appear blurred and even elevated. Unless associated with other defects, such persistent hyaloid remnants never interfere with vision.

Medullated nerve fibers may be seen on the fundus. Normally the myelination stops at the optic disc. At times some of the fibers carry their myelination past the disc into the retina and then appear as snowy-white patches in the retina, usually near the optic disc.

A normal variation in the disc, or more commonly in the peripheral fundus, are drüsen, which are small, round hyaline excrescences formed on Bruch's membrane.

The normal color of the fundus varies greatly, often in proportion to the general complexion of the patient's skin and hair. Fundal color components include the melanin of the retinal pigment epithelium and the choroidal stroma, and the blood mass in the retinal and choroidal vasculature. A fundus with prominent choroidal vasculature is known as a tessellated or tigroid fundus.

The macular region varies greatly among normal individuals. In some fundi the foveal reflex is distinct, whereas in many others the fovea is so shallow that no foveal reflex is seen. In blonde fundi especially, there may be nothing to mark the macular region except its location in relation to the optic disc and to the retinal vessels. In other fundi, especially brunets, the macular region is a dark area where the choroidal pigment shows through the retina. In some persons, especially young children and adult Negroes, a circular reflex surrounds the macular area and other reflexes may radiate from it. These are caused by light reflecting from the internal limiting membrane of the retina. They must not be confused with retinal edema or inflammatory changes.

Indirect Ophthalmoscopy. Indirect ophthalmoscopy differs from direct ophthalmoscopy chiefly in that it employs a high diopter condensing lens to form the retinal image, which is seen anterior to the eye (Fig. II-12). Light emerging from an emmetropic eye does so in parallel bundles that can be gathered by a lens to form an image at the principal focal plane of that lens. In an ametropic eye that converges (myopia) or diverges (hyperopia) light rays, there is no significant change in the picture obtained; this is because of the large power of the condensing lens usually employed (+20 to +30 diopters). The image is inverted, real, and capable of being seen on a semitransparent film held at the focal plane of the lens. The observer should use bifocal glass over each eye to reduce fatigue in viewing this image. Standard indirect ophthalmoscopes are used for this purpose.

The indirect ophthalmoscope offers a brilliantly illuminated, binocular, stereoscopic image that covers about ten times the area usually seen in the field of the direct ophthalmoscope. The image is smaller, about 3× as compared with 15× of direct ophthalmoscopy. The larger field of view gives a perspective to the whole fundus that is quite helpful in situations such as retinal detachment.

SPECIAL EXAMINATIONS OF THE EYE

Slit Lamp Biomicroscopy

The need for magnification in examining the anterior portion of the eyes, especially the cornea, led to the invention of the slit lamp biomicroscope and the corneal microscope, and their combination into one instrument (Fig. II-13). This diagnostic instrument is second in importance only to the ophthalmoscope. The slit lamp uses an intense narrow beam of focal light passing through a narrow slit and then through an adjustable condensing lens. The slit of illumination lights the tissue, which then can be observed with the biomicroscope. The tissue illuminated by the narrow beam is referred to as an optical section and is comparable to a slice cut by a microtome. The cornea and lens, transparent to ordinary diffused light, are seen to be composed of layers of different optical densities. These layers (the epithelium, Bowman's membrane, Descemet's membrane in the cornea, and zones in the crystalline lens) are, therefore, visualized as separate entities. Opacities and other pathologic details can be localized with great accuracy. Cells floating in the aqueous or vitreous, which are invisible by ordinary illumination and magnification, may be seen, and their presence may give evidence of intraocular inflammation at a stage when it may be discovered by no other means. Even the increased protein content of the aqueous that is caused by the early dilatation of blood vessels in inflammatory conditions can be detected (the Tyndall phenomenon) as the light traverses the anterior chamber. In a nor-

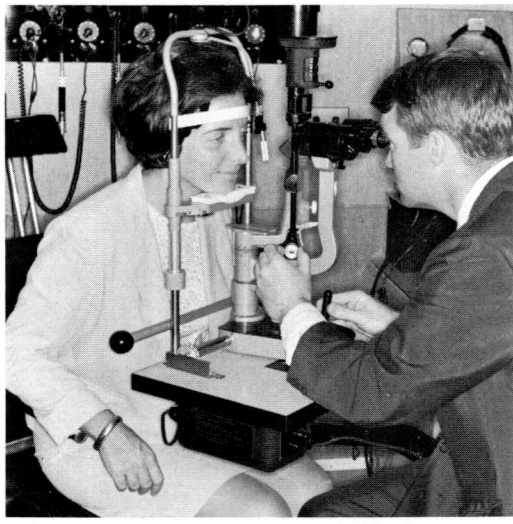

Figure II-13   Slit lamp biomicroscopic examination.

mal person the aqueous humor is clear or optically empty, but with increased protein content the beam of light becomes visible. This is spoken of as an aqueous flare.

Usually the slit lamp biomicroscope is suitable only for examining the tissues of the front of the eye, including the anterior third of the vitreous chamber. However, special contact lenses have been devised which permit the angle and even the retina to be seen. For more complete works on the subject, the reader is referred to a volume such as *Biomicroscopy of the Eye*, by M. L. Berliner.

Measurement of Intraocular Pressure

Finger Tension.   Intraocular pressure may be roughly estimated by palpation of the eyeball through closed lids. The patient is directed to look down toward the floor and to keep both eyes steady. The examiner places two forefingers on the upper lid over the globe and exerts pressure alternately with each forefinger while the other rests on the globe. Just enough pressure should be exerted to indent the globe slightly, a procedure which may be done without pain unless inflammation is present. After a number of normal eyeballs have been palpated by this method, the normal resistance of the globe to indentation will be learned. A comparison then can be made with eyeballs that are either too hard or too soft. Determining intraocular pressure this way is of value only where the tension is markedly increased or diminished. In many cases of chronic, simple glaucoma, the pressure is too slightly elevated to be detected by this means, but the method is still of value in comparing the patient's eyes.

Tonometry.   The only accurate method of determining intraocular pressure is by use of a reliable tonometer (p. 340). The Schiötz instrument consists of a footplate, curved to fit the average normal cornea, with a metal plunger in the center for holding various weights (Fig. II-14). Topping the plunger is the short, curved arm of a lever whose long arm is a pointer for reading positions on a scale that tops the tonometer. When the ocular end of the plunger fits flush with the curved footplate resting on the cornea, the pointer is at zero on the scale. Before the plunger in-

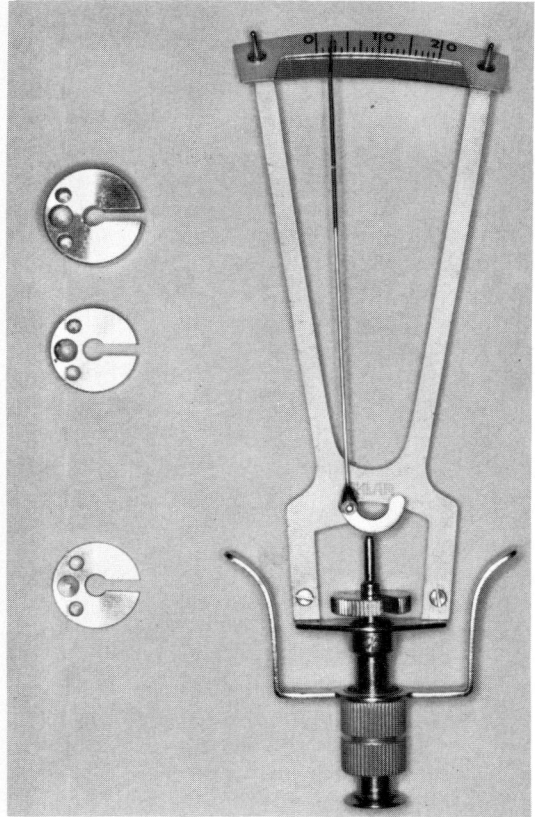

Figure II-14 Schiötz tonometer with extra weights.

position and asked to look directly upward, preferably at some fixed object. With the tonometer in his right hand, the physician stands beside the patient and separates the lids to keep them from contact with the eyeball. The instrument is placed gently in a vertical position, directly over the cornea, and the plunger allowed to exert its full weight. If the instrument is held steady, the pointer will stay fixed at one of the scale markings. Occasionally it will oscillate about one half of a millimeter either way because of alterations of internal pressure caused by the arterial pulse in the eye.

If the reading with the 5.5 gm. weight is between 3 and 6 on the scale, this reading may be used. If the reading is below 3, the 7.5 gm. weight should be added and the reading taken again. If the reading still falls below 3, the 10 gm. weight should be used. The readings are converted to an equivalent in millimeters of mercury from the graph furnished with the instrument.

Many patients find it difficult to relax during the procedure but the readings are only valid when he is relaxed. Care must be observed that he does not squeeze his lids while the tonometer is being used, because squeezing raises the internal pressure. Care must also be observed when the footplate is applied to the cornea so as to avoid any abrasion of the epithelium.

APPLANATION TONOMETRY.   Another simple and reliable method for measuring intraocular pressure is applanation tonometry. It may be performed with a minimum of corneal trauma immediately following a routine slit lamp biomicroscope examination. Applanation tonometry measures the force necessary to flatten a corneal surface of constant size. With the use of the Goldmann applanation tonometer (Fig. II-15), the exact measurement of the small flattened surface is made with the microscope of the slit lamp. The force necessary to flatten this standard area of cornea is measured directly as the pressure.

Procedure.   The Goldmann tonometer is mounted on the slit lamp biomicroscope. After the cornea is anesthetized by one or two drops of local anesthetic agent such as Ophthaine, 0.5 per cent, the tear fluid is

dents the eye, the pointer remains flush with the footplate and at zero, no matter what weight is added to the plunger. When placed on a normal eye, the plunger indents it to a certain distance, depending upon the weight and resistance. The pointer moves accordingly on the scale. Each instrument is accompanied by a graph that expresses the scale readings in millimeters of mercury of internal pressure within the eye. Since many factors determine the relation between the indentability of the eye and the actual pressure inside the eye, these readings do not represent the actual intraocular pressure. One such factor is ocular coat elasticity, which varies in individuals and at different ages. Determining internal pressure by instrument is far more accurate than by fingers. Accurate, standardized instruments are now on the market.

TONOMETRY TECHNIQUE.   With his eyes anesthetized from one or two drops of Pontocaine, 1 per cent, or Ophthaine, 0.5 per cent, the patient is placed in a supine

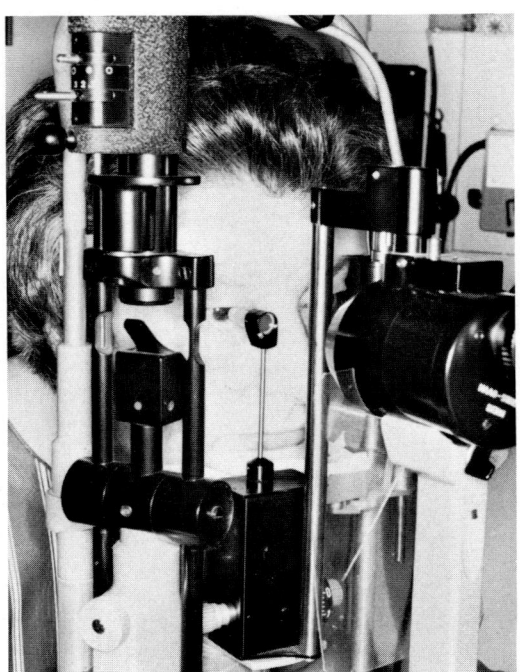

Figure II-15 Applanation tonometry (close-up photo).

stained with a moistened fluorescein paper strip inserted into the lower cul-de-sac. The patient and examiner sit in their usual positions at the slit lamp biomicroscope. After the tonometer is placed on the slit lamp, the prism is cleansed with distilled water, and the drum is set at 1.0 gm. A cobalt blue filter is placed in front of the fully opened diaphragm of the slit lamp in order to illuminate the prism with a diffuse beam of blue light. The angle between the illumination device and the microscope should be about 60 degrees so that the image appears bright and free of reflection.

The patient is instructed to look straight ahead as the slit lamp is moved forward until the prism just makes contact with the cornea. On contact the limbus of the cornea glows with a blue light. The lids should not touch the prism since this may produce errors in subsequent readings. If necessary the lids should be retracted manually, avoiding pressure on the globe.

After contact with the cornea, the two fluorescein semicircles are seen through the microscope. Their steady pulsation indicates that the instrument is in the correct position. The height and control lever of the microscope should be adjusted so that two semicircles of equal size are in the middle of the field of view. Pressure on the eye is increased by turning the calibrated dial on the tonometer until the inner borders of the two semicircles just touch each other and overlap with each pulsation of the eye. The amount of pressure applied is read on the measuring drum. This reading, multiplied by ten, is an estimate of the intraocular pressure in millimeters of mercury.

If the instrument is too far away from the cornea, the two semicircles cannot be made to overlap. If the instrument is too far forward, the semicircles cannot be separated. These adjustments should then be made with the control lever. Even when corneal astigmatism is present, intraocular pressure can be measured precisely by rotation of the prism.

Great accuracy is achieved with the applanation tonometer since the average error does not exceed ±0.5 mm.Hg. Scleral rigidity is not taken into account since the small volumetric displacement of 9.56 mm. increases the intraocular pressure only by about 2.5 per cent. Although massage decreases intraocular pressure, no massage effect is produced by repeated measurements, so a decrease in intraocular pressure is not caused by such measurements.

Visual Fields

With the peripheral retina the eye can perceive objects not in the direct visual axis. This visual field may be examined by perimetry. Its purpose is to detect vision that is defective within the visual field, as well as to define the outer limits of the visual field. The interpretation of the visual fields is important for diagnosis of a disease, in localizing its visual pathway, and in noting its progress or remission. Consequently, careful, repeated tests of the visual fields may be most valuable.

When the visual axis of one eye is directed to a point in space, other objects within a given area of fixation are perceived by the eye. The outer limits of this space depend upon the distance from the fixation point, the intensity of illumination, and the size and color of the test object (visual angle subtended). Colored objects offer less stimulus to the retina than white objects of the same size. The sensitivity of the retina is greatest at the fovea and falls off rapidly away from this point. Thus objects may be so small that they fail to stimulate the retinal receptors in the periphery of the retina, but become effective stimuli when they are brought sufficiently close to the macular region or the fovea. It is of the utmost importance when examining a patient that these factors are kept constant.

The visual field has been defined by Traquair as an island of vision in a sea of blindness (Fig. II-16). Perimetry determines the coastline of this island and the contour elevations (levels of retinal sensitivity) throughout the island. Near the center of the island is a mountain peak representing the fovea. Acuity is highest at the top (Fig. II-17). If different sized test objects are selected, it is as possible to map out contours of retinal sensitivity (isopters) as to measure contours of height or elevation above the seacoast in a geodetic survey

(Fig. II-18). In recording the visual field, the isopter is expressed as a fraction, which is the size of the object over the distance. For example, if a 3 mm. white object is selected and the perimeter has a radius of 330 mm., the isopter is recorded as the field for 3/330 white. A separate field is taken for each eye.

Confrontation Method. The seated patient faces the examiner 1 meter away. With his left eye covered, the patient is instructed to look with his right eye at the left eye of the examiner, whose own right eye is closed. The examiner brings his hand midway between the patient and himself and explores the peripheral boundaries of the visual field throughout its circumference. If he and the patient look steadily at each other's eye, and if the patient tells the examiner as soon as he sees the hand come into the field of vision, a rough estimate of

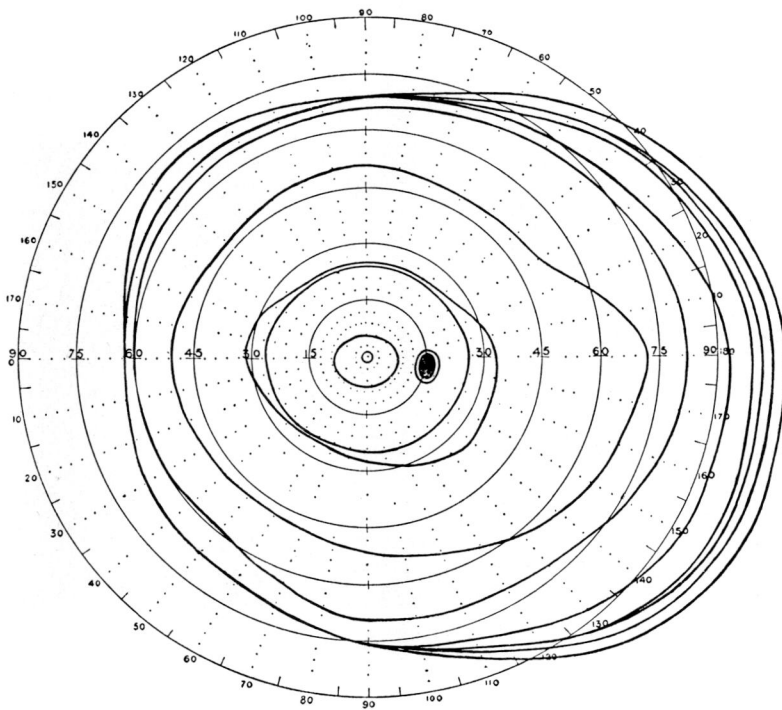

Figure II-16 Chart of visual field of right eye, showing isopters from periphery inward to center for 160/1000, 80/1000, 40/1000, 20/1000, 10/1000, 5/1000, 5/2000, 3/2000, 1/2000, 1/4000, and 0.63/4000. (Traquair: *Clinical Perimetry*, 5th ed. Courtesy of Henry Kimpton, London.)

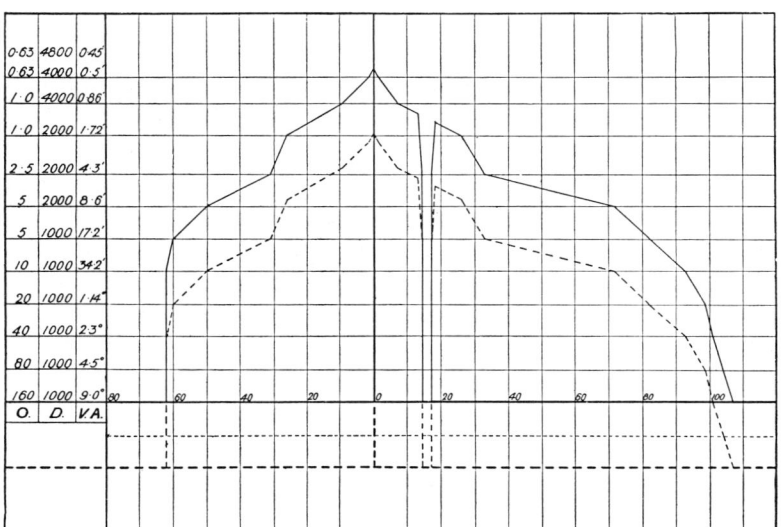

Figure II-17   Field of vision charted along horizontal meridian from data in previous figure. (Traquair: *Clinical Perimetry*, 5th ed. Courtesy of Henry Kimpton, London.)

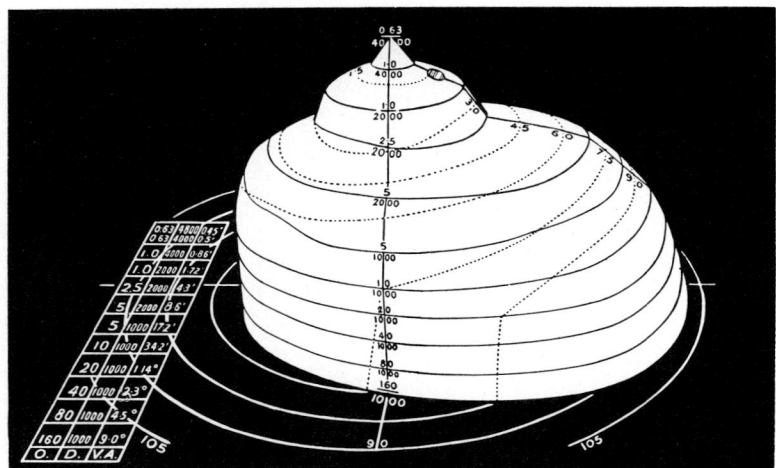

Figure II-18   Model of field of vision in three dimensions. Note steep nasal and more sloping temporal periphery. (Traquair: *Clinical Perimetry*. 5th ed. Courtesy of Henry Kimpton, London.)

the patient's visual field may be obtained. If the examiner's visual field is normal, the patient's field should correspond to it.

Tangent Screen Method. This method (p. 292) is most useful in detecting retinal changes within 30 degrees of fixation, the arc where most of the retinal changes occur. The tangent screen is usually constructed of 2 square meters of cork, linoleum, or black felt. The center of the screen is marked with a small, bright object from which radiate circles marked at 5-degree intervals up to 30 or 40. The area of the blind spot should be indicated on each side of fixation. Test objects vary in size from 1 mm. to 50 mm., but generally the smaller sizes are used. The central portions of the visual field are best tested as follows. With the patient seated 1 to 2 meters from, and in a direct line with, the fixation object on the tangent screen, a test object is brought in from the periphery. The patient acknowledges when he sees it, the point is marked on the board, and the test proceeds in all meridians. The blind spot should be outlined carefully. The findings are charted, including the size and color of the test object and the distance from the screen. Each eye is tested separately with the other eye occluded.

Perimetry. A perimeter may be used to assess the peripheral visual field. The usual perimeter consists of a metal arc of a circle, marked off in degrees and pivoted on a stand that can be revolved 360 degrees. The light source is attached to the perimeter and rotates with the arc, so that

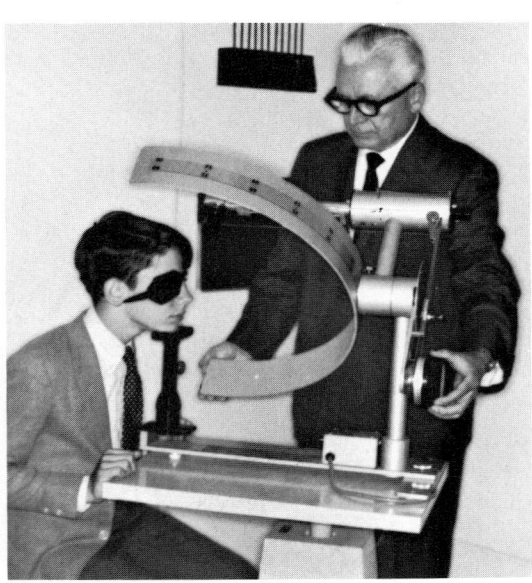

Figure II-19 Perimetry.

illumination remains uniform in all meridians. A chin and head rest support the patient's head (Fig. II-19). He closes one eye and fixes the other on a central mark. The examiner brings in a test object from the periphery toward the center of the arc and instructs the patient to indicate when he is aware of it. The examiner must make sure that the patient keeps his gaze

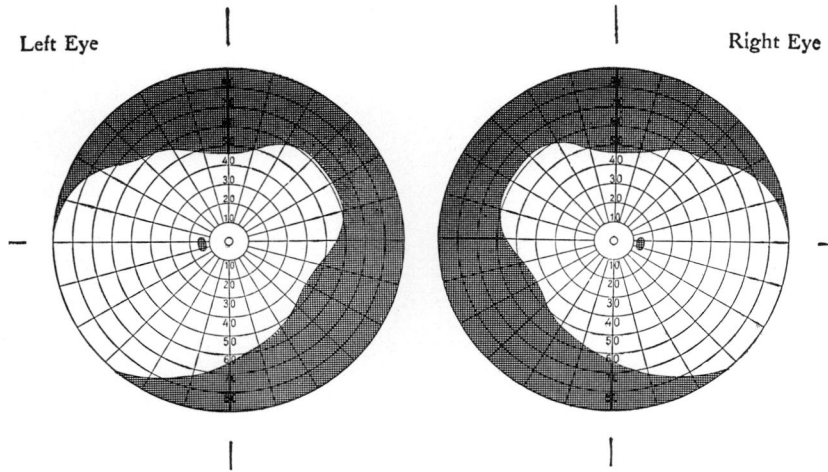

Figure II-20 Chart for recording peripheral field. Unshaded area is extent of normal field.

riveted upon the fixation mark, for many people find this difficult and tend to glance directly at the test object. Each eye is tested separately, and the findings are recorded on charts (Fig. II-20).

Scotometry. This is the examination of the central visual field for scotomas, areas of diminished retinal sensitivity. It is employed chiefly to map out the blind spots and to determine scotomas within the 15 to 50 degree area around fixation. Color fields (blue, red, and green), as well as the fields for black and white, are sometimes useful.

DISTRIBUTION OF NERVE FIBERS

A general knowledge of the arrangement of nerve fibers is needed to interpret field defects.

Retina. If a vertical line were drawn through the center of the optic papilla, dividing the retina in two, the arrangement of the nerve fibers coming from the nasal side would differ from that of the nerve fibers coming from the temporal side.

Fibers on the nasal side are in straight lines, but fibers on the temporal side follow an arcuate course from the periphery of the disc, curving over and under the papillomacular bundle which they surround (Fig. II-21).

Light stimulus is sent up the optic nerve fibers to their final cell stations in the visual cortex around the calcarine fissure. Having no sensory receptors (rods and cones), the papilla, which is the exit of the optic nerve fibers from the eye, is insensitive to light. Stimuli confined to this area, therefore, give no response. In the field of vision, this is represented by a scotoma, the so-called *blind spot of Mariotte.*

The macular region, the region of most distinct vision, contains mostly cones and sends fibers into the optic nerve. They lie together in the distinctive papillomacular bundle. If cut with a knife, these fibers would produce a lesion at the margin of the optic disc, resulting in nerve fiber bundle defect. Cells in the upper temporal periphery send all of their fibers into the upper half of the optic nerve; cells in the lower half of the temporal periphery send their fibers into the lower half of the optic nerve. In this way, a horizontal raphe is established.

Nerve fiber bundle defects in the temporal fibers are always limited by a horizontal line in the field of vision on the nasal side (see illustrations of typical nerve fiber bundle defects in the left visual fields Fig. II-22A, B).

Optic Nerve. When fibers enter the optic nerve, their arrangement is strictly maintained up to the final cell stations in the calcarine cortex; that is, fibers from the upper half of the retina lie in the upper half of the optic nerve; those from the lower

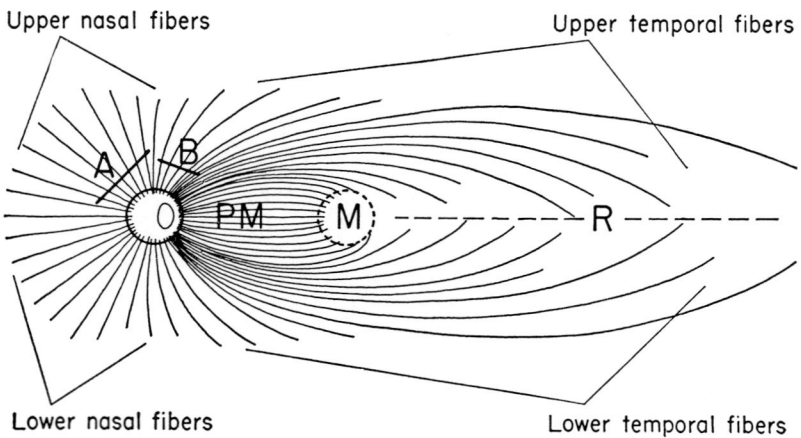

Upper nasal fibers   Upper temporal fibers

Lower nasal fibers   Lower temporal fibers

Figure II-21 Schematized distribution of left retinal nerve fibers. PM, papillomacular bundle; M, macula; R, raphe formed by meeting of fibers from upper and lower temporal quadrants; *A*, lesion of upper nasal fibers; *B*, lesion of upper temporal fibers. (Adler, F. H.: *Physiology of the Eye.* The C. V. Mosby Co., St. Louis, Mo.)

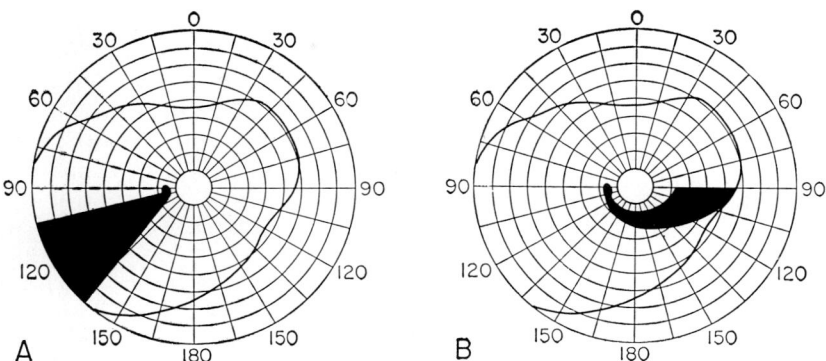

Figure II-22 *(A)* Fan-shaped scotoma resulting from a lesion of the upper nasal fibers.   *(B)* Scimitar-shaped scotoma resulting from a lesion of the upper temporal fibers as shown in Figure II-21.

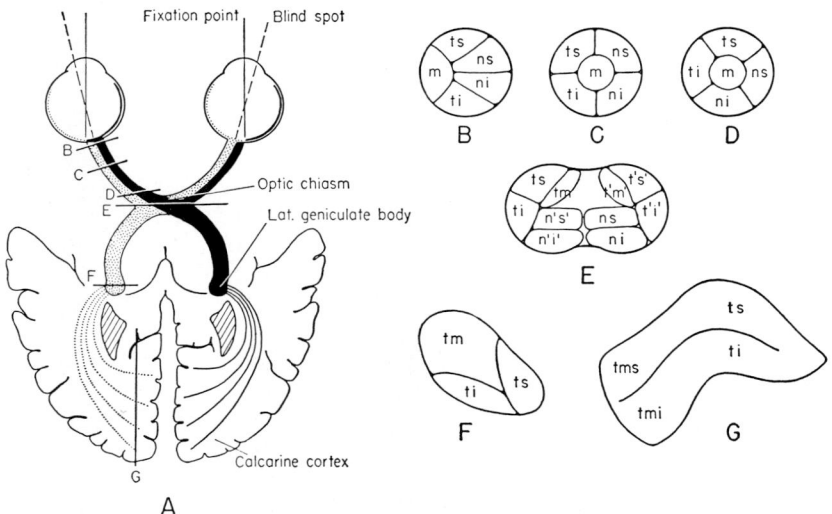

Figure II-23 Diagram of visual nerve paths and representative cross sections showing distribution of nerve fiber bundles at different levels of the pathway. A, visual pathways; B, optic nerve behind eye; C, optic nerve behind entrance of central vessels into the nerve; D, optic nerve in front of its entrance into chiasm; E, optic chiasm; F, lateral geniculate body; G, calcarine cortex; ts, fibers from temporal superior quadrant of extramacular retina; t's', fibers from temporal superior quadrant of extramacular retina of other eye; ti, fibers from temporal inferior quadrant of extramacular retina; t'i', fibers from temporal inferior quadrant of extramacular retina of other eye; ns, fibers from nasal superior quadrant of extramacular retina; n's', fibers from nasal superior quadrant of extramacular retina of other eye; ni, fibers from nasal inferior quadrant of extramacular retina; n'i', fibers from nasal inferior quadrant of extramacular retina of other eye; m, fibers from macula; tm, fibers from temporal half of macula; tms, fibers from temporal superior quadrant of macula; tmi, fibers from temporal inferior quadrant of macula. (Adler, F. H.: *Physiology of the Eye*. The C. V. Mosby Co., St. Louis, Mo.)

half of the retina lie in the lower half of the optic nerve, and so on through the chiasm, optic tracts, and optic radiations. The papillomacular bundle, as it runs in the optic nerve behind the globe, lies very close to the temporal periphery of the nerve and only as it passes back in the nerve does it gradually come to lie centrally (Fig. II-23).

Chiasm. In man about 75 per cent of the fibers from each optic nerve cross to the opposite side in the chiasm. If a vertical line were drawn through the fovea, the fibers from the temporal half of the retina would not cross at the chiasm, whereas the fibers on the nasal half of the line would all cross to the opposite side and enter that optic tract. Plate 37 shows the arrangement of fibers in the chiasm. The crossed fibers from the lower inner retinal quadrant of the right optic nerve cross in the anterior part of the chiasm and form a knee where the left optic nerve terminates. From there they pass to the lower inner quadrant of the left optic tract. Fibers from the lower inner retinal quadrant of the left optic nerve cross similarly. Also, somewhat similarly arranged is the knee of the fibers from the upper inner, or nasal, retinal quadrants of both right and left optic nerves in the back of the chiasm, but this is not of such clinical importance.

Suprachiasmal Pathway. Beginning with the chiasm, the fibers from the left and right halves of the retinas of the two eyes form the left and right optic tracts. Each optic tract, therefore, receives impulses from the temporal half of the ipsilateral retina and from the nasal half of the contralateral retina. After the fibers have emerged from the lateral geniculate body, where a new neuron begins, they enter the temporal lobe where they spread out into what is known as *Meyer's loop* (Fig. II-24). Because the fibers spread around the ventricle, those that come from the upper quadrant of each retina separate from those that come from the lower quadrant of each retina. A lesion in this region produces an isolated quadrantanopia, or a defect in the corresponding quadrants in each visual field. After traversing Meyer's loop, the fibers come together again and form the optic radiation (Fig. II-25), which proceeds back to the calcarine fissure (Fig. II-26). The upper lip of the calcarine fissure represents the superior quadrant of each half retina, whereas the lower lip of the calcarine fissure receives impulses from the lower quadrant of each half retina. The macular fibers end in the calcarine region at the extreme occipital or posterior pole and are probably not represented bilaterally.

TYPES OF PATHOLOGIC FIELD DEFECTS

Six types of pathologic field defects are:
1. Concentric contraction.
2. Local contraction.

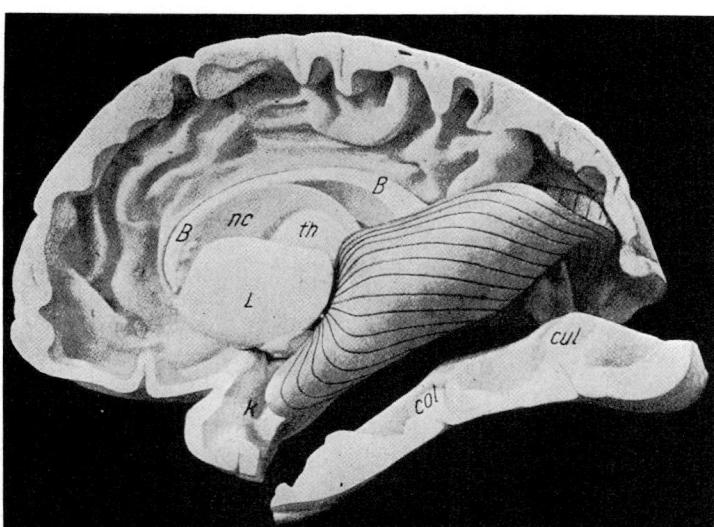

Figure II-24 Meyer's loop. This is represented by striated fibers just above K. K, temporal bend of optic fibers; B, corpus callosum; L, lenticular nucleus; nc, nucleus caudatus; th, thalamus; col, gray matter of collateral fissure, cul, highest level of gray matter of collateral fissure. (Pfeifer: *Kurzes Handbuch der Ophthalmologie.* Vol. 6. Julius Springer, West Berlin.)

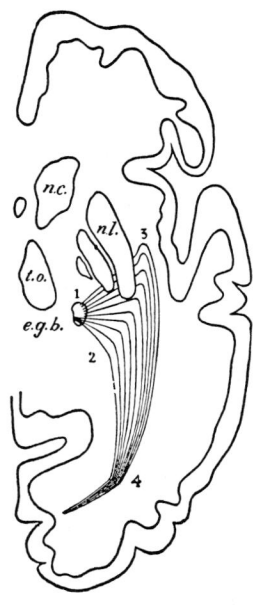

Figure II-25 Schematized course of a part of the optic radiation corresponding to a vertical cross section through the retina.

e.g.b. = external geniculate body.

t.o.　= thalamus opticus.

n.c.　= nucleus caudatus.

n.l.　= nucleus lentiformis.

1 = optic radiation after leaving external geniculate body, situated immediately behind internal capsule.

2 = superior part of optic radiation, running directly backward.

3 = inferior part of optic radiation, forming Meyer's loop.

4 = close relationship between optic radiation and convex surface of brain.

(Kestenbaum: *Clinical Methods of Neuro-ophthalmologic Examination*. Grune & Stratton, New York, 1961.)

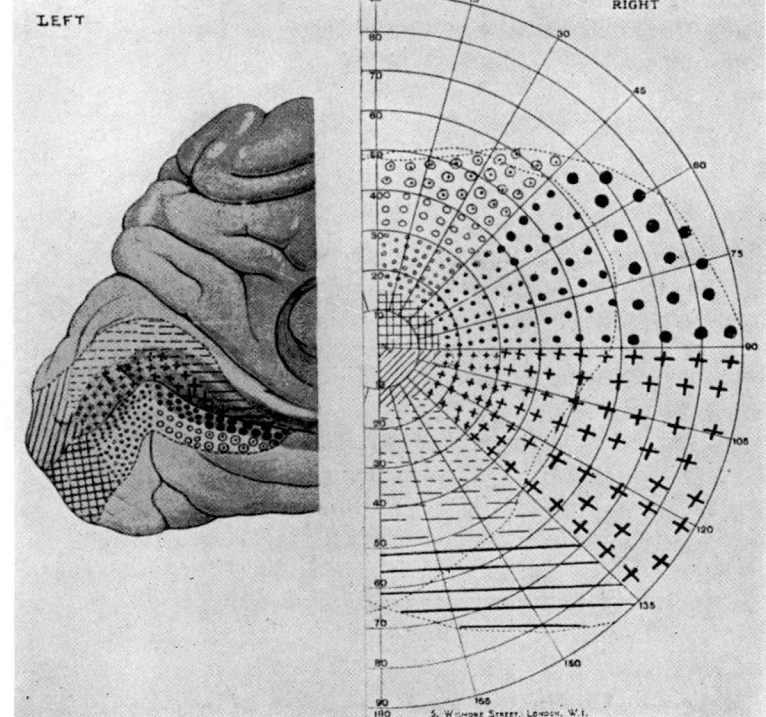

Figure II-26 Cortical retina (Gordon Holmes). Calcarine fissure is represented as widely opened. Macular area is relatively large, and peripheral area relatively small. (Traquair: *Clinical Perimetry*, 5th ed. Courtesy of Henry Kimpton, London.)

3. Sector defect: a local contraction bounded by two radii forming a sector.

4. Quadrant defect: a sector defect bounded by a vertical and a horizontal radius.

5. Hemianopia: this term designates a defect occupying half of each visual field, usually a vertical half. It is preferable to reserve the term for bilateral field defects produced by a single lesion, which must be chiasmal or suprachiasmal. True hemianopia, therefore, is always a defect of the binocular field. When a quadrant of each field is affected, quadrant hemianopia, or quadrantanopia, is present. This may be homonymous or crossed, bitemporal or binasal, upper or lower. Hemianopic defects are either congruous or incongruous, i.e., alike in the two fields or more marked in one than in the other. The line of the vertical meridian of the field, separating the blind from the seeing portion, may divide the fixation area (fovea) or may pass around it to include it in the seeing field. In this case the fixation area is said to be spared; an example would be the sparing of the macula in occipital lobe lesions.

6. Scotoma: an area of depressed vision within the field margin, surrounded by an area of depressed or normal vision.

The general physician is chiefly interested in the field defects seen in chronic simple glaucoma because his diagnosis largely depends on them and on those arising from lesions of the optic nerve, the chiasm, or the optic tract and radiation above the chiasm. Defects characteristic of glaucoma and of optic nerve disorders are discussed elsewhere (pp. 336 and 298). Defects from lesions of the visual pathways from the chiasm upward affect both the subgeniculate pathway, the part from the chiasm to the lateral geniculate body, i.e., the optic tract; and the suprageniculate pathway, the part from the lateral geniculate body to the calcarine cortex, i.e., the optic radiation.

Lesions of the Chiasm. Lesions of the chiasm are always hemianopic and 70 per cent show bitemporal hemianopia. Usually they result from a pituitary tumor. Pressure on the underside of the chiasm from such a spacetaking lesion begins to depress the visual field in the upper temporal quadrant where the isopters may show contraction toward the center (Figs. II-27, II-28). The more peripheral isopters may show no change whatever; the earliest change is always a restriction of the smaller isopters within the 30 degree circle in the upper, temporal quadrant. Such changes usually can be detected only from tangent screen examination (p. 292). All the earliest field changes are in the central area of the field and not at the periphery. The lower temporal quadrant then fails below peripherally. The lower, and then the upper, nasal quadrant finally becomes depressed, and the field extinguished.

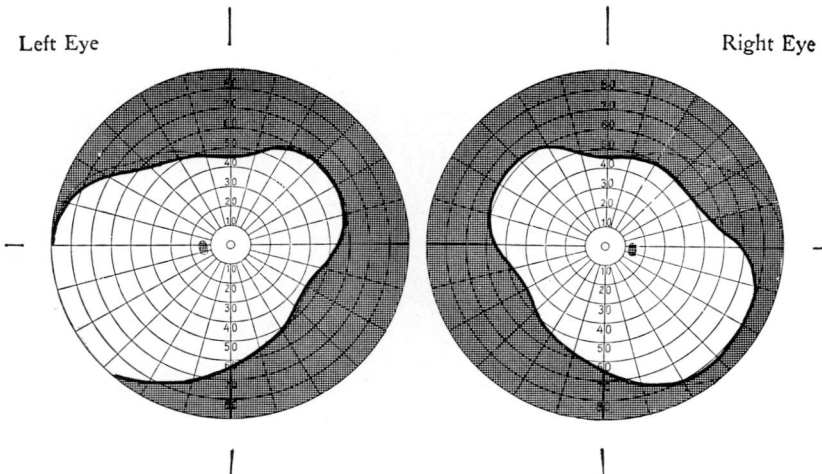

Left Eye

Right Eye

Figure II-27 Bitemporal hemianopia, early stage of depression of right upper temporal field. Peripheral fields.

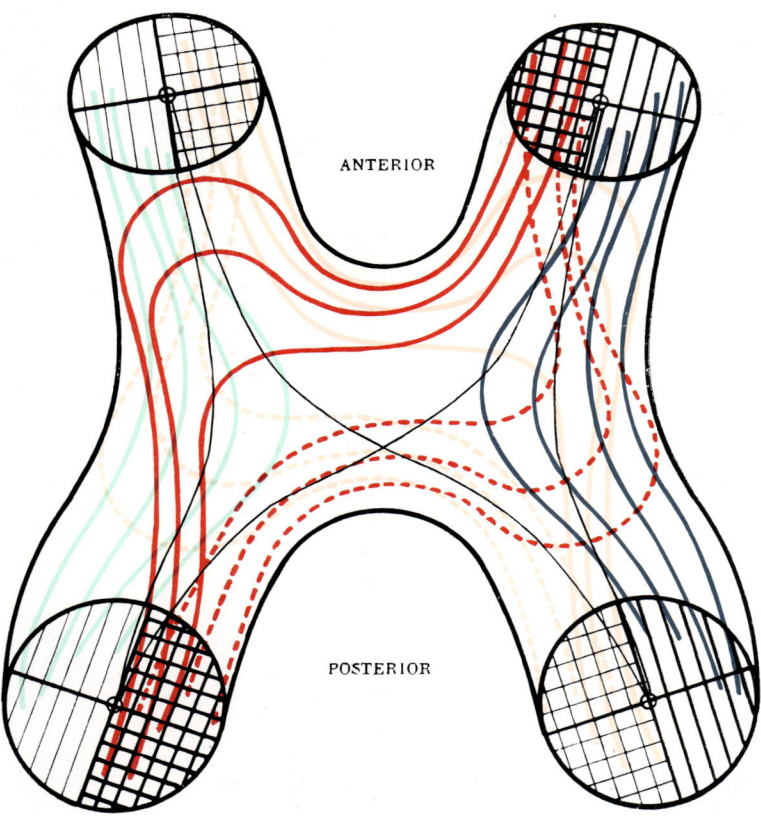

ANTERIOR

POSTERIOR

Plate 37 Diagram to show probable arrangement of chiasmal crossing. To avoid confusion, fibers from right optic nerve are colored brightly; those from left nerve, faintly. Crossed fibers from lower inner retinal quadrant of right optic nerve (continuous red line) cross anterior part of chiasm and form the knee in termination of left optic nerve. They then pass to lower inner quadrant of left optic tract. Crossed fibers from upper inner quadrant of right optic nerve (broken red line) pass backward along same side of chiasm to its posterior angle and then across its posterior part to upper inner quadrant of opposite tract. Uncrossed fibers (blue) are expanded so that dorsal fibers lie innermost. At each side of chiasm crossed fibers from both sides mingle with uncrossed fibers of the same side. Thin black lines indicate position of macular fibers. These fibers occupy a relatively large area in posteroventral part of chiasm, and thus are easily affected by interference from below and behind. (Traquair: *Clinical Perimetry*. 5th ed. Courtesy of Henry Kimpton, London.)

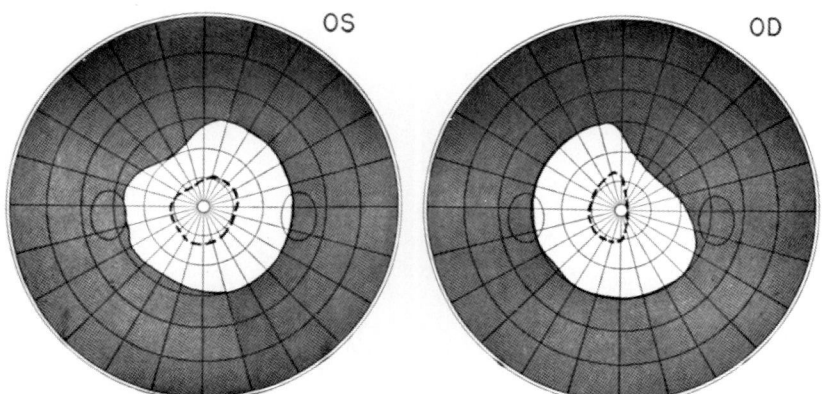

Figure II-28   Bitemporal hemianopia, early stage. Central fields.

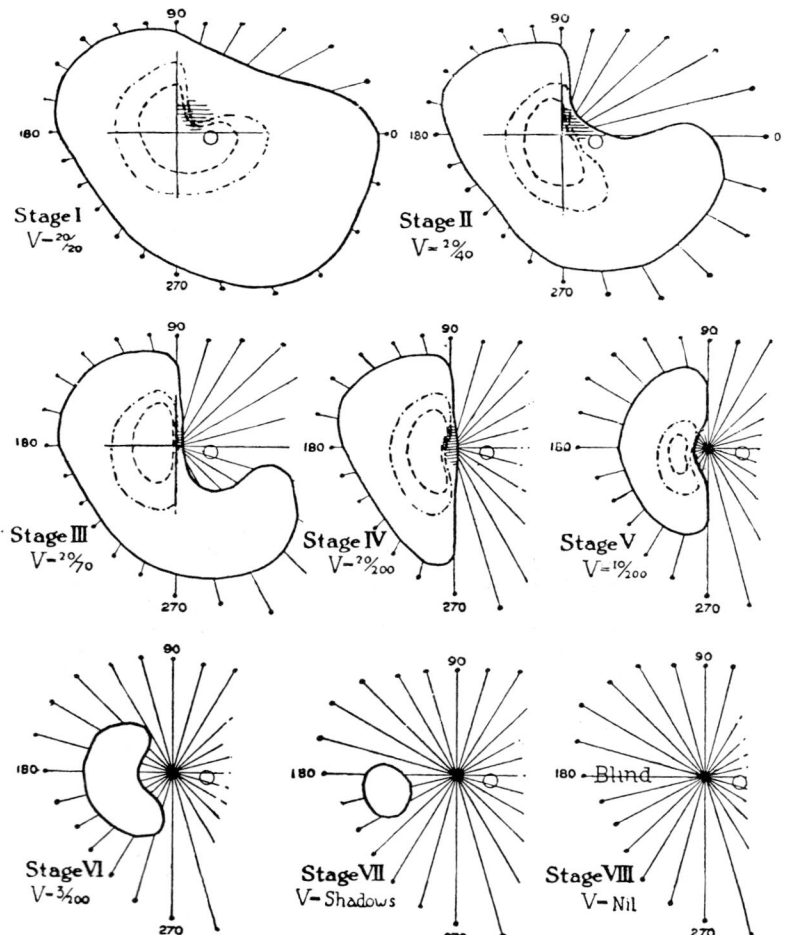

Figure II-29   Stages of progressing field defect in right field in pituitary disease. (Cushing and Walker.)

In this manner the changes in field progress regularly through the quadrants, clockwise in the right eye and counterclockwise in the left (Fig. II-29). These changes always affect both fields but usually to different degrees, so that one field presents a more advanced stage than the other. The disparity may be small, or it may be so extreme that one field is entirely wiped out and the patient blind in that eye, whereas the changes may be so slight in the other eye as to escape any detection but by a meticulous search. At times the progress of the defect seems to halt. Its chief pause occurs when the temporal field has practically disappeared (Fig. II-30). A second pause may occur when the temporal field and lower nasal quadrant have disappeared, leaving a fairly clean-cut upper nasal quadrant with steep edges.

Such changes may be regarded as typical of those arising from interference with the chiasmal pathways. The character of the field changes can be interpreted from the anatomic arrangement of the fibers in the chiasm. The usual lesion that affects the chiasm is a pituitary tumor or cyst. Since this comes from beneath the chiasm, the first fibers caught will be those near the midline at the bottom of the chiasm. These are the crossing fibers which come from the lower nasal quadrant. When they are pressed, the initial defect is loss of the upper temporal part of each field, causing a temporal slant. This is diagnostic of pituitary lesions in general.

Suprachiasmal Pathway. The characteristic field change caused by the lesions above the chiasm affecting the optic tract or optic radiation is homonymous hemianopia (Fig. II-31). Lesions between the chiasm and the lateral geniculate body (optic tract) produce field changes that differ somewhat from those produced by lesions of that part of the pathway extending from the lateral geniculate body up to, and including, the occipital cortex (optic radiation).

Incongruity. Usually the field of one eye is affected more than that of the other eye (Fig. II-31), and only when the interference extends and becomes more severe late in the disease do the field changes in the two eyes become congruous.

Macula Not Spared. Tract hemianopia usually is caused by a tumor that tends to involve the posterior angle of the chiasm where the macular fibers cross. The macular fibers are thus affected, and the line of demarcation between the seeing and the blind halves of the field runs directly through the macula. The maculas are not spared. In lesions of the occipital cortex and posterior part of the optic radiation, however, the macular areas are frequently spared (p. 297).

Onset Gradual. The onset of tract lesions usually is gradual and the course progress-

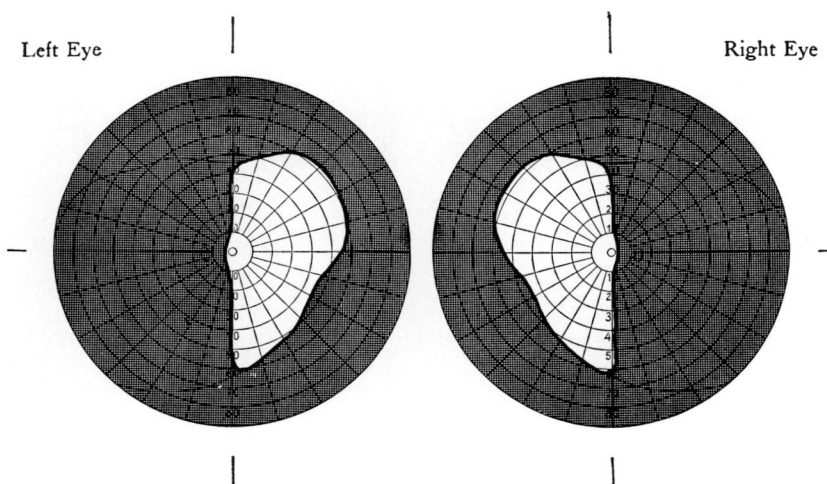

Left Eye

Right Eye

Figure II-30 Later stage of Figure II-29, showing complete bitemporal hemianopia. Peripheral fields.

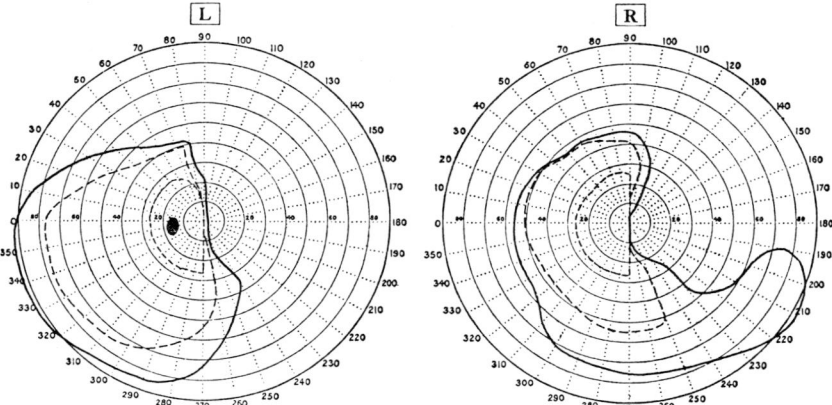

Figure II-31 Homonymous hemianopia, incongruous, referable to tract interference. Neurologic diagnosis: tumor of midbrain. Objects 10/330, 1/330, 1/2000. R.V. 6/6 part; L.V. 6/12. Fixation area divided for small object. (Pa., 1923.) (Traquair: *Clinical Perimetry*, 5th ed. Courtesy of Henry Kimpton, London.)

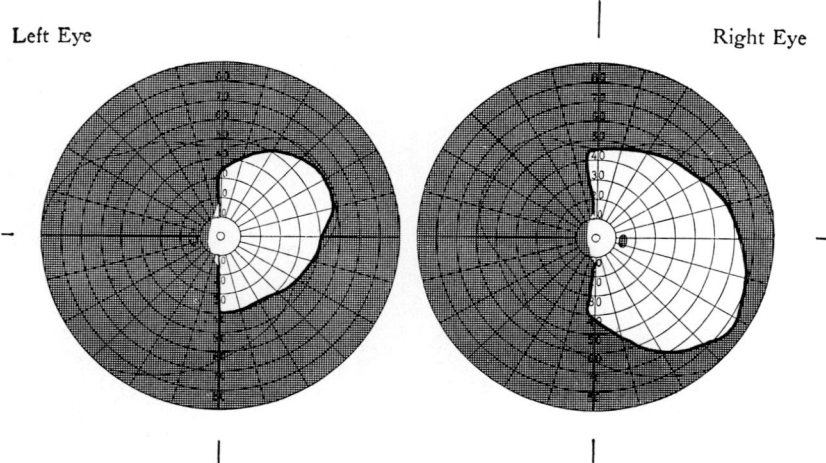

Figure II-32 Homonymous hemianopia, congruous. Compare with Figure II-31.

ive. In contrast, lesions that affect the suprageniculate part of the pathways are frequently congruous (Fig. II-32). They may be quadrantic or hemianopic defects, but for the most part they are identical in the two fields. The more congruous they are, the more likely is the lesion found in the occipital cortex or near the cortex. Sparing of the macula is common with lesions that affect the cortex. This is particularly true of vascular lesions, which constitute the majority of lesions of the occipital lobe. Nearly all of the field changes from vascular lesions come on suddenly and are more extensive than those from tumors.

Emotional Disturbances

Functional disturbances of psychosomatic origin are probably more common in the eye than in any other organ of the body, and they are sometimes very difficult to differentiate from organic diseases. The eyes, particularly, seem to serve as a locus on which the emotionally upset individual focuses his attention. Psychosomatic ocular complaints run the gamut of symptoms from vague aches and pains to complete blindness.

It is important to detect psychosomatic ailments of the eyes because the very examination that detects organic disease tends to concentrate the patient's attention further on his eyes, giving him new symptoms at each examination.

In his zealous attempt to find a cause for the patient's complaints, such as error of refraction or muscle imbalance, the ophthalmologist may completely miss the true cause of the patient's symptomatology. As a result, the patient, unrelieved of his symptoms by the prescription of the ophthalmologist, travels from office to office. The patient may be encouraged in useless eye exercises, aniseikonic lenses, or some form of quackery. Generally the more absurd the treatment, the more rapid is the response of this type of patient, but it is usually short-lived and the patient again returns with his symptoms.

The same rules of common sense apply in ophthalmology as in general medicine. Symptoms that are excessive, i.e., beyond the degree usually produced by the abnormality found and particularly if one is present, should arouse suspicion. A

multiplicity of complaints likewise indicates an emotional background. Whenever a patient has been thoroughly examined by a competent ophthalmologist and nothing abnormal is found, the patient should be suspected of having a psychosomatic difficulty.

Many persons with psychosomatic difficulties consult their family physicians first. If the doctor recognizes the signals of emotional difficulties and treats his patient accordingly, or refers him to a psychiatrist, the person can save time and expense and be returned to health.

Malingering. The malingerer usually has the same complaints as the psychosomatic patient; in addition, the history gives an immediate clue to the emotional drive that produced his complaints. It will be an obvious, purposeful one, i.e., to avoid something unpleasant, such as military duty, or to capitalize on an injury.

It is often far simpler to suspect the malingerer than the psychosomatic, but malingering may be more difficult to detect and prove. A good reason in the patient's history should raise the index of suspicion of the examiner. The following tests may assist in detecting and proving the condition.

TOTAL BLINDNESS. Some time during the examination, the examiner may lead the patient across the room and deliberately into an obstacle. If the patient carefully avoids the obstacle, he has some vision. Similarly the opticokinetic nystagmus response, if present, indicates some vision. This response is elicited by placing a rotating drum with alternate vertical black and white lines in front of the patient. The seeing patient who looks at the drum inhibits his eye movements and a jerk nystagmus results. (The slow component arises from fixation on the moving object.) A piece of cloth 20 by 2 inches with alternating red and white squares each 2 inches wide may be substituted for the drum. A bright light flashed into the eyes usually makes a patient wink if he has light perception. A light reflex of the pupils can occur in a blind person, but it is rare. It may occur in bilateral lesions above the region of the geniculate bodies.

PARTIAL LOSS OF VISION OF BOTH EYES. Vision should be recorded from each eye and then repeated on different charts and at different distances. Rarely can the malingerer make the results fit the acuity initially recorded.

PARTIAL OR COMPLETE LOSS OF VISION OF ONE EYE. To test the vision of the allegedly injured eye, the patient may be led to believe that the healthy one is being examined. If the patient wears glasses for distance, that correction should be placed in the trial frame. A plano lens is inserted in the frame in front of the injured eye and a +3.00 D in front of the normal eye. The patient is then asked to keep both eyes open and read the test letters. If he continues to read the chart with the good eye blurred, he must be using the injured eye. If there is any question concerning the results of these tests, an ophthalmologist should be consulted.

Tests for Color Sense

Color vision is evaluated in routine examination of applicants for some jobs. A number of states include color testing in the examination of driver applicants. Red-green color blindness is the commonest form and exists in about 4 per cent of all males and in about 0.4 per cent of all females. Color vision may be disturbed in diseases of the fovea and optic nerve and in some nutritional deficiencies, particularly avitaminosis A. Ishihara test plates are commonly used to detect color blindness (Plate 38).

Gonioscopy

Gonioscopy is a method of examining a hitherto inaccessible portion of the eye, the angle of the anterior chamber, by using a specially made contact lens, focal illumination, and a microscope. Except for the contact lens, the principles are the same as for slit lamp biomicroscopy (p. 419).

The angle of the anterior chamber ordinarily cannot be seen because light rays emanating from the drainage angle undergo total internal reflection from corneal curvature. A contact lens eliminates the corneal curve and allows light to be reflected from the angle so that its structures can be seen in detail. Gonioscopy may be performed with the patient seated or recumbent.

Various lenses may be used. The Allen-Thorpe, Goldmann, and Zeiss lenses have mirrors by which the angle is examined with reflected light. They are indirect gonioscopic lenses. The patient is examined while seated at the slit lamp, using its light source and magnification.

For examination with the Koeppe contact lens, the patient's head must be in a nearly horizontal position. The angle is viewed through a hand-held microscope with a lamp that gives bright focal illumination, such as a Barkan illuminator, held in the other hand. The Koeppe lens gives better magnification of the details of the angle and can be used more quickly than contact lenses. Whichever is used, however, the space between it and the eye must be filled with a clear fluid, either physiologic saline or methylcellulose solution, 1 or 2 per cent.

Gonioscopy is most useful in glaucoma. By permitting evaluation of angle width (distance of root of iris from trabecula) and study of the tissues of the angle of the glaucomatous eye at various stages, gonioscopy has contributed a great deal to our knowledge and treatment of the disease. It is of value too in many conditions besides glaucoma that may involve tissues of the angle of the anterior chamber. For example, intraocular foreign bodies hidden in the recess of the angle can be seen only through gonioscopy. It is helpful also in the study of tumors of the iris. With the pupil widely dilated, the area behind the iris (posterior chamber), including the ciliary processes, zonule, and equator of the lens, can be seen in most people.

Procedure. Ability to do a gonioscopic examination depends upon recognizing the gonioscopic appearance of the anatomic landmarks. With the patient in a supine position, a local anesthetic is instilled in the eye to be examined, the goniolens (Koeppe) is placed over the cornea and the patient's head is rotated to the same side as the eye being examined. The goniolens is lifted slightly from the nasal aspect of the eye to permit sterile saline solution to flow between the cornea and lens, filling the space. The patient is then directed to

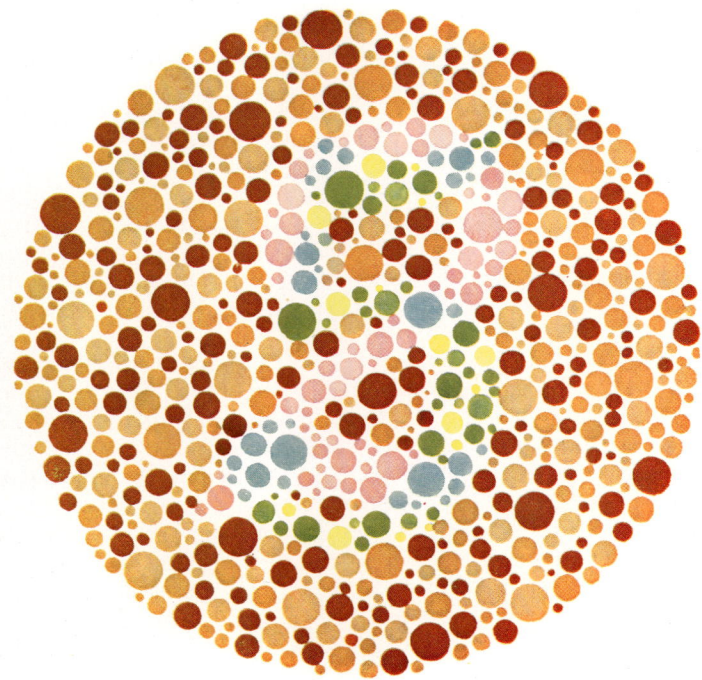

Plate 38 Hidden figure chart for detection of color blindness. The normal eye sees a figure 5, the color blind eye sees a figure 2. (Copied by permission from Ishihara: Series of Plates Designed as Tests for Color Blindness. Tokyo, 1920.)

fix his gaze upon a specific target on the ceiling while gentle pressure is applied to the goniolens to keep it in place, and the examiner is able to view the anterior chamber contents and the angle with a hand microscope and the Barkan focal illuminator. The entire circumference should be evaluated thoroughly.

Transillumination of the Eye

Transillumination of the eye is often helpful in the diagnosing of intraocular tumors. Intense light placed on the sclera behind the ciliary body will be transmitted to the interior of the eye where it produces a red reflex in the pupil. Solid masses of tissue, such as an intraocular tumor, especially a melanoma containing pigment, will intercept the light when it is placed over the tumor, and thus diminish or prevent the red reflex. This is of particular value in retinal detachment. The fluid beneath the detachment does not interfere with the red reflex, but if a tumor is present, a common cause of detachment, the light might be impaired. Hence, transillumination affords a means of differentiating serous retinal detachments from those caused by pigmented intraocular tumors. Transillumination also may reveal atrophy of the pigment layer of the iris or ciliary body. Normally the pigment lining the back surface of the iris prevents light from coming through the body of the iris. When the pigment is atrophic, transillumination will show the area as a light red spot in the body of the iris where the pigment has been lost.

The principle of transillumination is to provide, at the sclera, a sharply demarcated beam of light shielded from the eyes of the observer. The light then enters the sclera to illuminate the interior of the eye. The end of the transilluminator is curved to fit the scleral surface and is usually pressed back into the conjunctival cul-de-sac after appropriate local anesthesia. The instrument must be placed at least 8 mm. back of the limbus, because the area in front of this is occupied by the ciliary body that normally cuts off entering light. The examining room must be completely dark, and the eyes of the examiner must be partly dark-adapted for accurate observations.

Ultrasonography

Ultrasonic waves have a frequency above the hearing range of the human ear, i.e., all vibrational waves above approximately 20,000 cycles per second. When an ultrasonic beam strikes an interface between tissues of different acoustic impedance, a portion is reflected and forms an echo (Fig. II-33). The remainder passes through the structure being examined until it meets another similar interface. The acoustic impedance of a structure depends on its density and on the velocity of the sound passing through it. In the human eye the cornea, the anterior and posterior surfaces of the lens, and the posterior bulbar wall produce clearly identifiable echoes. The normal aqueous and vitreous are acoustically homogeneous and produce no echoes. The retrobulbar tissue, which is mostly fat, produces numerous echoes of irregular amplitude.

Ultrasonography is a useful diagnostic aid in evaluating serous retinal detachments, solid retinal detachments, and other intraocular pathologic conditions, especially if the media is not clear as in vitreous hemorrhage or leukokoria. Intraocular and extraocular foreign bodies may be diagnosed with ultrasound. Ultrasound is useful also for evaluating unilateral proptosis from the standpoint of orbital tumors and for measuring axial lengths of both intraocular and retrobulbar areas.

Fluorescein Funduscopy

Since 1960 the specialized technique of observing the retinal vasculature morphologically and physiologically has been used increasingly.

The fundus is examined following the intravenous injection of fluorescein. Rapid serial photography records the arterial, arteriovenous, venous, and late venous phase of retinal circulation.

This additional test helps to differentiate fundus lesions and to explain the under-

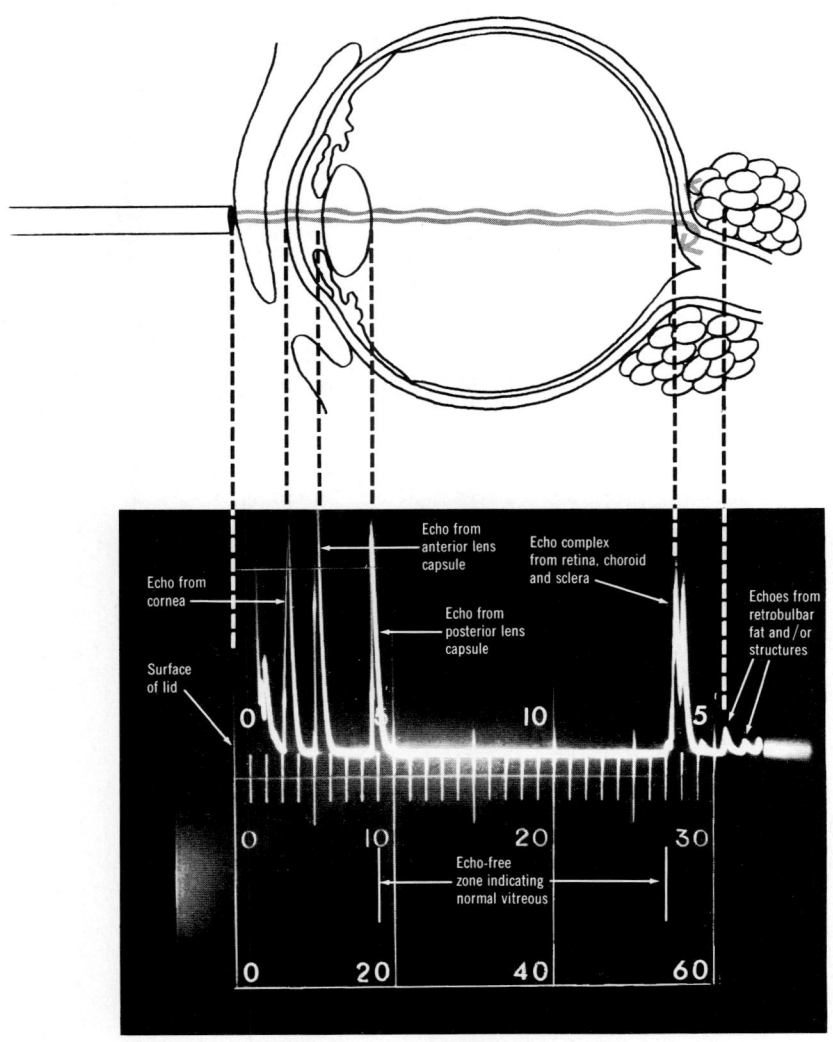

Figure II-33 Typical anterior-posterior ultrasonic record from normal eye. Note that axial length, read from corneal echo to the posterior wall echo, is 24 millimeters. (From *Physician's Manual.* 'EKOLINE 12' Ophthalmic Ultrasonoscope. Smith Kline Instrument Co., 1967. Used by permission.)

lying disturbed physiologic condition in certain diseases affecting the retinal vasculature. It can be helpful in diagnosing certain choroidal diseases because some cause permeability of vessels with escape of dye into the tissues and others do not.

BIBLIOGRAPHY

Adler, F. H.: Physiology of the Eye. 4th ed. St. Louis, The C. V. Mosby Co., 1963.

Apt, L.: Diagnostic Procedures in Pediatric Ophthalmology. Boston, Little, Brown & Co., 1963.

Barkan, O., Boyle, S. F., and Maisler, S.: On the genesis of the glaucoma: an improved method based on slit lamp microscopy of the angle of the anterior chamber. Am. J. Ophth. *19*:209, 1936.

Berliner, M. L.: Biomicroscopy of the Eye. Vols. I, II. New York, Paul B. Hoeber, 1949.

Carr, R. E., and Gouras, P.: Clinical electroretinography. J.A.M.A. *198*:173, 1966.

Duke-Elder, S.: System of Ophthalmology. Vol. 7, The Foundations of Ophthalmology. St. Louis, The C. V. Mosby Co., 1962.

Gloster, J.: Tonometry and Tonography. International Ophthalmology Clinics. Boston, Little, Brown & Co., 1965.

Goldmann, H.: Slit lamp examination of vitreous and fundus. Brit. J. Ophth. *33*:242, 1949.

Harrington, D. O.: The Visual Fields. 2nd ed. St. Louis, The C. V. Mosby Co., 1964.

Heyman, A., Karp, H. R., and Bloor, B. M.: Determination of retinal artery pressures in diagnosis of carotid artery occlusion. Neurology *7*:97, 1957.

Linksz, A.: Physiology of the Eye. Vols. I, II. New York, Grune & Stratton, 1952.

Norton, E. W. D., *et al.*: Fluorescein fundus photography. Tr. Am. Acad. Ophth. *68*:755, 1964.

Rosenthal, M., and Fradin, S.: The technique of binocular indirect ophthalmoscopy. Highlights of Ophth. Vol. IX, No. 3, 1966.

Scheie, H. G.: Width and pigmentation of the angle of the anterior chamber. Arch. Ophth. *58*:510, 1957.

Scott, G. I. (ed.): Traquair's Clinical Perimetry. St. Louis, The C. V. Mosby Co., 1957.

Shaffer, R. N.: Stereoscopic Manual of Gonioscopy. St. Louis, The C. V. Mosby Co., 1962.

Thiel, R.: Atlas of Diseases of the Eye. Vols. I, II. Amsterdam. Elsevier Publishing Co., 1963. (First English edition translated and edited from sixth German edition by D. Guerry, W. J. Geeraet, and H. Wiesinger.)

Zuckerman, J.: Diagnostic Examination of the Eye. 2nd ed. Philadelphia, J. B. Lippincott Co., 1964.

Appendix III

Optical Defects of the Eye

PHYSIOLOGIC OPTICS

Refraction. To understand the common optical difficulties of the eye and how spectacles correct them, it is necessary to review a few elementary facts of physiologic optics. Optical difficulties are spoken of as errors of refraction. The examination of the eye for such abnormalities is called refraction of the eye.

In optical terminology refraction refers to deflection of light from a straight path as it passes from one medium into another of different optical density. A ray of light is bent at the surface between the two media. The amount of deflection depends upon the difference in density of the two media and upon the angle of incidence of the ray at the point where it passes from one medium into the other.

In Figure III-1, I and II represent two transparent media of different optical densities separated by the surface at AB. The line XY is perpendicular to this surface. If a ray of light enters in the direction of XY, it suffers no deflection at the surface AB, although the denser medium slows up the velocity of the ray. If any other ray, such as CO, strikes the surface AB at other than a right angle, it bends. This bending is called refraction. If Y is the denser medium, the ray CO bends toward the perpendicular XOY and continues in the direc-

tion of OD instead of the direction OD′, from which it originated. The angle COX is the angle of incidence and the angle DOY is the angle of refraction.

Regardless of the angle at which the ray CO enters the second medium, the angle of refraction always bears a constant relationship to the angle of incidence: $\frac{\text{sine } i}{\text{sine } r} = K$. If E and F are equidistant from the surface AB separating the two media, the distance XE is equivalent to the sine of the angle COX and the distance FY is

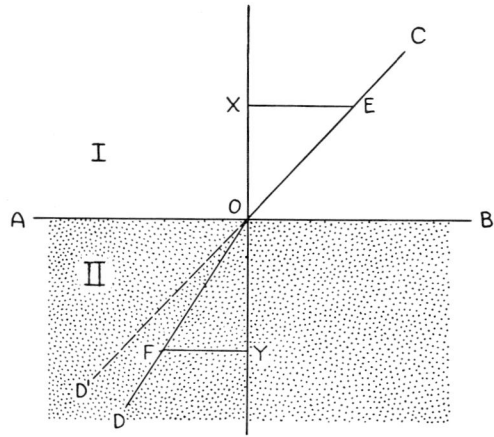

Figure III-1 Passage of ray of light from one medium into another of greater optical density.

equivalent to the sine of the angle YOD, provided these angles are small. $\frac{XE}{FY} = K$. If the first medium is air, whose density is taken as unity, and the second medium is denser than air (e.g., water or glass), the constant K equals the index of refraction of the second medium. The index of refraction of water is 1.33 and of crown glass, from which most optical lenses are made, 1.5. The refractive index of the cornea is 1.33 and of the crystalline lens about 1.42. The aqueous and vitreous, being approximately the same density as water, have an index of refraction of about 1.33. How a ray of light bends as it passes from air into a medium of greater optical density depends upon the density of the second medium and upon the angle at which the ray strikes the surface between the two media.

Glass Prisms. In Figure III-2 the line CO represents an entering ray striking the surface of the optical prism of glass. XY is perpendicular to the surface of the prism on the side at which the ray enters; X'Y' is perpendicular to the surface of the prism on the side from which the ray emerges. The ray CO is refracted toward the perpendicular XY at point O and therefore is bent down toward the base of the prism. On emerging from the prism at the point F, it undergoes further refraction, in this instance away from the perpendicular X'Y', because the ray is now leaving a medium of greater density and going into a medium of lesser density. The ray therefore emerges in the direction of FG. The amount of the

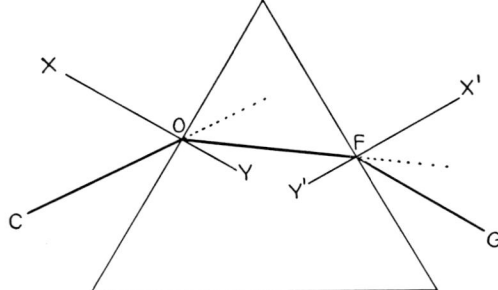

Figure III-2 Refraction through a glass prism.

refraction depends upon the angle at which the ray CO enters the prism.

Lenses. When one or both surfaces of the refracting medium are curved, a lens is formed. A convex lens can be thought of as being made up of an infinite number of truncated prisms with their bases toward each other above and below an optic axis. When a ray of light enters the lens through the optic axis, it suffers no refraction in a line perpendicular to the surfaces of the lens. Any other ray undergoes refraction at the surface in the same way that rays are refracted in a glass prism. The rays, therefore, bend toward the base of the prism and on emerging from the lens cross the optic axis at some point.

In Figure III-3, ray AC, on passing through the lens, emerges in the direction of A' and intersects the optic axis at the point PHI. If rays AC and BD are parallel to the optic axis and, therefore, parallel to each other when they enter the lens, the point PHI is called the posterior principal focus of the lens. This point is determined by the optical density of the lens and by its surfaces of curvature. Assuming that all lenses have the same density or

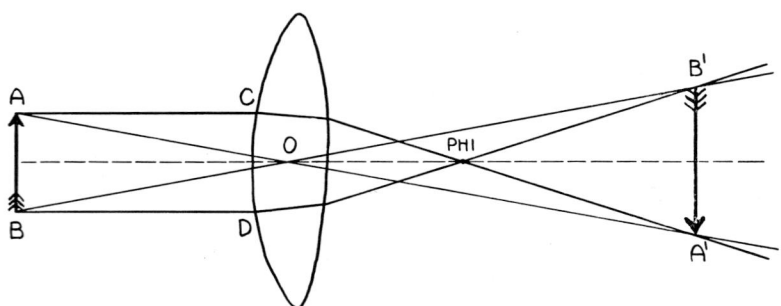

Figure III-3 Image formation by a convex lens.

TABLE III-1 FOCAL LENGTH OF VARIOUS DIOPTER STRENGTHS

Diopter Strength	Focal Length
1	1 meter
2	0.5 meter
5	0.2 meter (20 cm.)
0.5	2 meters
0.2	5 meters

index of refraction, a more deeply curved lens focuses the rays of light closer to it than one with a lesser degree of curvature. The power of the lens is determined by the distance of the posterior principal focus from the back surface of the lens. This distance is called the posterior principal focal distance or, more commonly, focal length. The stronger the lens, the shorter this distance. The unit of lens strength is known as the diopter (Table III-1).

A *concave* lens may be thought of as a series of truncated prisms whose bases are directed away from one another. *Convex* lenses, "plus lenses," converge rays of light passing through them to a focus behind the lens. Concave lenses, "minus lenses," diverge rays of light passing through them so that no real focus is formed behind the lens, but instead a virtual focus is formed in front of the lens on the same side as the source of the light.

Under appropriate conditions, convex lenses form a real inverted image of objects in space. In Figure III-3 from the point A rays emerge in all directions. The ray AC, being parallel to the optic axis, crosses the optic axis behind the lens at the point PHI and proceeds further in that direction toward the point A'. Ray AO, which passes in through the center of curvature of the lens, does not bend and continues to the point A'. At A' the rays AA' and CA' come to a focus and form an image of the point A. Two rays of light from the point B give a similar focus of this point at B'. If AB is an arrow, therefore, its image is formed at A'B' and is inverted and magnified.

The size of the image produced through a convex lens depends upon the distance of the object from the lens and upon the strength of the lens. Concave lenses do not form real images back of the lens, but by geometric construction a virtual image is

formed in front of the lens. This virtual image is erect and smaller than the object.

REFRACTION BY THE EYE

The eye can be considered an optical instrument having a number of surfaces of different curvature and refractive indexes. Most of the refraction is accomplished at the surface of the cornea, for here the rays enter from air, whose index of refraction is 1.0, into the cornea (1.33). The cornea acts as a convex lens (Fig. III-4). After passing through the cornea, the rays emerge into the aqueous, which has practically the same index of refraction. They then strike a second medium of greater optical density, namely, the lens (1.42). As the rays emerge from the lens into the vitreous (1.33), they enter a medium of lesser density and are therefore slightly diverged. After being bent by these surfaces, the rays come to a focus on the retina if the eye is normal and if the entering rays are parallel to the optic axis.

Theoretically, rays of light are parallel only when they come from infinity, but for practical purposes they may be considered parallel when they come from a distance of

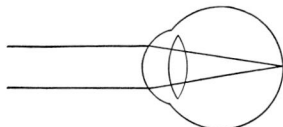

Figure III-4 Refraction by normal emmetropic eye.

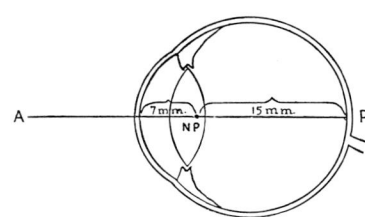

Figure III-5 Refraction by human eye, showing posterior principal focus at the retina when eye is emmetropic, or normal. AP, optic axis; P, posterior principal focus; NP, nodal point.

6 meters or more. If the eye is optically normal, therefore, rays of light 6 meters or more from the eye should come to a focus on the retina, which is then the posterior principal focus of the eye (Fig. III-5). Such a state in the eye is called *emmetropia*.

Accommodation

All objects closer than 6 meters from the emmetropic eye send rays of light to the eye which are not parallel but divergent, and the closer the object is to the eye, the more divergent is the bundle of rays that reaches the eye. Such rays, therefore, focus behind the retina and cause a blurred retinal image unless some mechanism increases the length of the eyeball, i.e., pushes the retina back to the focus of the rays or increases the refractive power of the eye. The latter occurs in accommodation. The dioptric or refractive power of the eye can be increased by changing the curvature of the crystalline lens in the eye.

The exact mechanism of accommodation is not fully understood. It is known that contraction of the ciliary muscle, which is supplied by the parasympathetic third nerve, results in increased curvature, particularly of the anterior surface of the lens. This gives the eye greater dioptric power than it has in the resting state, so that divergent rays of light coming from less than 6 meters now are focused on the retina. The reflex mechanism is so well adjusted that normal individuals are not aware of the process as they focus on objects of varying distances from the eye. How ciliary muscle contraction effects an increase in the curvature of the lens is still disputed.

Young and von Helmholtz assumed that the lens is elastic and that contraction of the ciliary muscle, particularly the circular fibers of the ciliary muscle, draws the ciliary processes together so that the zonule of Zinn is relaxed. The zonule is a sheet of tissue made up of numerous fibers that support the lens in its capsule. When the lens is taken out of the eye in its capsule, it is more circular than when it is confined in the eye during the nonaccommodated state. When the zonule relaxes, the lens capsule, which is elastic, tends to force the lens to assume a more spherical form, causing its anterior surface to become more convex, and thus increases its optical power.

Contraction of the ciliary muscle causes a change in refractive power of the crystalline lens from the earliest age at which accommodation can be measured up to about 45 or 50 years of age.

Presbyopia. The power of accommodation gradually weakens with age and is known as presbyopia. Although a very slight loss can be measured at 15 years of age, this does not become important until around 45 years of age. When accommodation becomes less than the 3 diopters needed in the emmetropic individual for ordinary reading at 33 cm., and the near point recedes until reading is possible only at 40 or 50 cm., the individual begins to have trouble reading fine print and usually complains, also, of headache and visual fatigue. The size of the retinal image is too small for very small letters to be distinguished. The recession of the near point is responsible for the characteristic difficulty of older persons who must hold reading matter farther and farther away from the eyes. When the newspaper has to be held at arm's length, the individual usually seeks relief. Spectacles of the weakest convex glass which permits the patient to read at the customary distance should be prescribed. Stronger spectacles tend to further weaken accommodation.

Loss of accommodation may occur other than by presbyopia. Certain diseases, especially diphtheria, produce toxins which may permanently paralyze the ciliary muscle.

AMETROPIA

Most people have ametropic eyes, i.e., optical defects which do not permit parallel rays of light to fall exactly on the retina. Such eyes are said to have refractive errors. The defects can be caused by changes in the curvature of the refracting surfaces; by changes in the index of refraction of the transparent tissues through which the light has to pass; by alterations in the distance of the various refracting surfaces from one another, for example, the distance of the lens from the cornea; and by changes in the axial length of the eye.

From infancy, the eye seems to follow a plan of development that aims toward a state of approximate emmetropia. Eyes whose refracting surfaces have a high refractive power develop a short axis, and those with low refractive power develop a long axis. Emmetropia results from an adequate correlation between axis length and refractive power. The average length of the emmetropic eye varies from 22 to 25 mm. Heredity plays an important role in the final outcome as to whether the adult eye will be emmetropic or ametropic. The chances are much in favor of children inheriting the refractive pattern of their parents. This is particularly true of myopia (near-sightedness), but applies as well to hyperopia (ineptly termed far-sightedness by the laity), and to astigmatism. The amount of ametropia is determined by the strength of convex or concave lens necessary to bring the focus of parallel rays onto the retina. Thus a hyperopia of 2 diopters means that a convex lens of 2D. was necessary to bring parallel rays onto the retina; a myopia of 2 diopters would require a concave lens of 2D.

Hyperopia

If the eyeball is too short from front to back, the retina lies in front of the posterior principal focus of the eye. Parallel rays of light therefore come to a focus behind the retina and produce blurred diffusion circles on it. Such an eye is called hyperopic or hypermetropic (Fig. III-6A, B). Some degree of hyperopia is present in most infants at birth, but as the eye grows this disappears or tends to lessen. The eye of a normal infant should therefore be slightly hyperopic, i.e., between 0.5 and 1 diopter. The hyperopic individual, if he is less than 45 years of age, may correct his optical defect by accommodation, provided that the hyperopia is not so excessive as to make this impossible.

Causes. The shape of the eye and the curvature of its refractive media, as well as the tendency of these factors to develop in certain ways during growth, are undoubt-

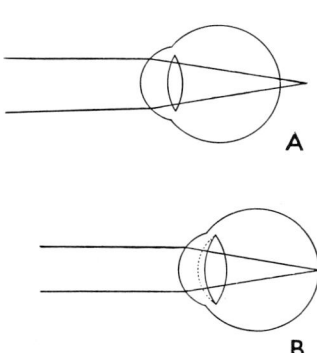

Figure III-6 The hyperopic eye. *(A)* With accommodation relaxed. *(B)* Effect of accommodation on parallel rays.

edly inherited. A special type of hyperopia is that seen in aphakia (absence of the crystalline lens, e.g., as the result of operation for cataract). When the lens is removed from an eye that was emmetropic before the crystalline lens became opaque, a convex spectacle lens of approximately 10 diopters must be placed in front of the eye to compensate for the loss.

Symptoms. Young hyperopes do not lose acuity in distant vision. If the hyperopia is not marked, i.e., over 1.50D., the acuity may not be impaired throughout adult life. Both young and older individuals may suffer from eyestrain, since the additional amount of accommodative effort required for close work causes pain after long use, blurring of the print, sleepiness while reading, and headaches. When these symptoms are severe, reading may become impossible and, in some individuals, troublesome nervous symptoms may develop.

In hyperopia of high degree, the distance acuity also may be poor without spectacles, and in the majority of cases of extreme hyperopia, i.e., 10D. and over, the eye is otherwise defective to such a degree that normal vision cannot be obtained even with spectacles.

In children hyperopia frequently causes convergent strabismus, called accommodative esotropia or "cross-eyes."

Treatment. To determine the amount of hyperopia present in a person under 46 years of age, a cycloplegic drug should be instilled in the eye to paralyze accommodation. In children under six, atropine should be used. Determinations made without the use of a cycloplegic drug are merely approximations of the refractive error. In low degrees of hyperopia the patient may not experience any symptoms. If the error is compensated by accommodation and producing no symptoms, spectacles need not be prescribed. If the error is sufficient to cause symptoms when the patient reads, it may be corrected partly by prescribing convex spectacles for reading only. These frequently are spoken of as rest spectacles.

As the person gets older and his accommodation begins to fail, more and more of the total hyperopia has to be corrected. The patient is instructed to use his spectacles not only for reading but also for distance. By the time he reaches 45 to 50 years of age, cycloplegic drugs no longer are necessary to paralyze the ciliary muscle. Such a person has to receive both a full correction of his hyperopia for distance and a further correction for his presbyopia. This may be accomplished either by his being prescribed two sets of spectacles, one for distance and one for near vision, or by the presbyopic correction being ground into the lower half of the lens used for distance. The latter lenses are called bifocal. Most people prefer to have these, rather than constantly having to change their spectacles. Trifocals, or spectacles with three different focal distances, i.e., distance, reading, and intermediate, are sometimes prescribed. The intermediate is for use in occupations requiring detailed vision at 2 to 3 feet.

Myopia

If the axial length of the eyeball is so long that the posterior principal focus of the eye lies in front of the retina, myopia, or nearsightedness, results (Fig. III-7*A, B, C*). Parallel rays of light are focused in front of the retina and, after crossing, form blurred diffusion images on the retina. The young

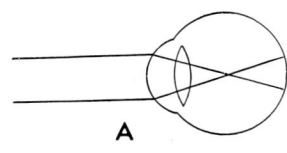

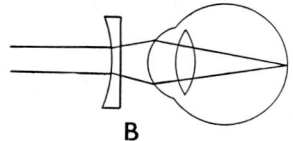

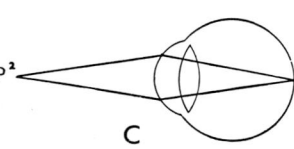

Figure III-7 Myopia. *(A)* Parallel rays cross in front of retina. *(B)* Effect of concave lens on parallel rays. *(C)* Divergent rays from punctum remotum, P², focus on retina without use of accommodation.

individual cannot overcome this defect by accommodation. No mechanism exists in the myopic eye to diminish the refractive power and send focused rays back to the retina. The myope, therefore, invariably has poor distant visual acuity. He may improve his distance acuity to a certain degree by squeezing his lids together in a stenopeic slit. In very bright light, contraction of the pupil may cut down the size of the diffusion circles on his retina. He experiences no difficulty in reading unless the degree of myopia differs in each eye, or unless the myopia is complicated by astigmatism (p. 449). Rays of light from a finite distance diverge when they strike the eye, and hence some point can be found from which these rays fall on the retina of the myope without accommodation, depending upon the degree of myopia. If myopia measures exactly 3 diopters, rays of light from the position of the usual reading distance (33 cm.) fall exactly on the retina and the patient is able to read without accommodating at all.

Causes. In the higher grades of myopia the axial length generally varies from 27 to 36 mm. For this reason this type of myopia has been called axial myopia. The most important cause of axial myopia is heredity. The normal eye assumes about 75 per cent of its full growth at 4 years of age. In myopia the eyes continue to grow at an abnormal rate, especially during adolescence. Some authorities have attributed myopia to the close use of the eyes during school age, but there is no good evidence that the use of the eyes in any way changes the degree of myopia or in any way is detrimental to eyes having an ordinary degree of myopia. Myopia up to 5 diopters generally does not seem to cause any abnormal changes in the eye, but if the myopia increases above this amount ("progressive myopia"), the eyes may show certain serious degenerative signs.

Symptoms. In most myopia the only symptom is defective distant vision. A refractive error of low degree is noticed only when maximal acuity is required. Many myopes are not aware of their visual defect until their visual acuity is tested. If the myopia is of considerable degree, the patient becomes aware that he does not see as a normal person does. Myopes seldom complain about reading since there is no strain upon the accommodation.

Because of this fact and because the retinal images in uncorrected myopia (i.e., without spectacles) are larger than in emmetropia, the myope often can do fine work with greater ease than can a person with emmetropia.

Objective Changes. The myopic eye usually has a deep anterior chamber. Its abnormal length may cause the eye to appear more prominent than normal. If one eye only is highly myopic, the physician frequently may mistake these eyes as having unilateral Graves' disease. There is a tendency to divergent strabismus in myopia. As the myopia increases, ophthalmoscopic examination of the fundus shows the following changes:

1. There is loss of pigment in the pigment epithelium, so that the choroidal vessels generally become visible.

2. The disc appears large and often has a white, crescent-shaped area on the temporal side where the sclera is exposed, which is the so-called myopic conus (Plate 26G). This appears because, as the eye increases in size, the optic nerve enters it from the nasal side at a more acute angle than normal. The white crescent may not be limited to the temporal side of the nerve but sometimes may surround it completely.

If the myopia is still more advanced, degenerative changes occur in the retina. The pigment epithelium in the macular region atrophies further and appears as a lighter area. It may become the seat of hemorrhages (Plate 26H). The blood vessels are pushed to the nasal side of the optic disc and bend over at the margin, somewhat resembling a glaucoma cup. The retina in the neighborhood of the disc, especially on the temporal side, atrophies and exposes the white sclera which stretches and bulges backward (called a posterior staphyloma). All these changes result from inner coats of the eye thinning and stretching as it enlarges (Fig. III-8). Further retinal degeneration results in thinned-out areas throughout the fundus and occasionally in holes in the retina formed either spontaneously or as the result of trauma. Such holes, especially in the periphery, cause the type of retinal detachment to which myopic eyes are especially liable. Other degenerative changes occur in the vitreous, which becomes liquefied, showing dustlike or threadlike opacities by ophthalmoscopic examination. When the myopia has reached 10 diopters or more the degenerative changes usually prohibit the vision being corrected to normal with spectacles. Such eyes are subject to further changes which materially deteriorate the vision. The prognosis then is usually serious.

Treatment. The treatment of myopia includes, first of all, correction of the error by concave lenses. Full correction is prescribed for low and moderate errors and is usually less than the full correction for higher degrees of myopia. The exact refractive error should be determined in all patients less than 46 years of age while they are under a cycloplegic. Beyond this age cycloplegia no longer is necessary because of the normal loss of accommodation. Some ophthalmologists believe that the correction by spectacles prevents further progress of myopia. This probably is not true, however, even if spectacles are worn constantly. The myope should wear his spectacles whenever he wishes to get distinct distant vision. He may have to wear them all the time if the myopia is unequal in the two eyes or is associated with astigmatism. Many ophthalmologists now consider optical correction only a means of relieving poor vision. Hence they prescribe the particular correction that may be worn most comfortably when maximal vision is desired, and they allow the patient to go without spectacles for the rest of the day.

If the myopia increases rapidly and in considerable amount, especially in a child, some restriction in using the eyes generally is advised. Some ophthalmologists have urged that children with myopia above a certain degree be placed in special classes for children with defective vision. They insist also that these children be taken out of school entirely during the periods in which the refractive error is progressing. There is no good evidence, however, that doing this in any way mitigates the difficulties or prevents the children from becoming more myopic. It seems unfortunate, therefore, to separate them from normal children unless some other pathologic condition is present which makes the corrected vision so defective that the myopes cannot keep up with their classes.

A healthy regimen should always be prescribed for high myopes, including proper diet and outdoor exercise. They should be instructed to read under proper conditions, i.e., good light and good posture. Children with rapidly developing myopia who are overweight should have a basal metabolic test and other tests for glandular imbalance. They frequently lose their excessive weight at adolescence and their myopia seems to advance at a lesser rate. Parents often ask about the value of certain eye exercises because of the claims of well advertised schools of nonmedical practitioners. They should be told that while such exercises are not harmful, they have absolutely no effect on the condition. This fact has been demonstrated by carefully controlled studies. If the constant use of spectacles in myopia were insisted upon less, such claims would lose much of their popular appeal.

A chief danger to which a myopic eye is exposed is retinal detachment. Myopia in itself actually may not cause detachment, but retinal degeneration, with which it is associated, makes the retina liable to tears. High myopes should be cautioned against violent sports such as boxing, football, and high diving, which frequently involve trauma to the eyes. When the eye has suffered from myopic chorioretinal degeneration, treatment is of no value.

Children who are myopic should be examined once a year, preferably before the beginning of the school term.

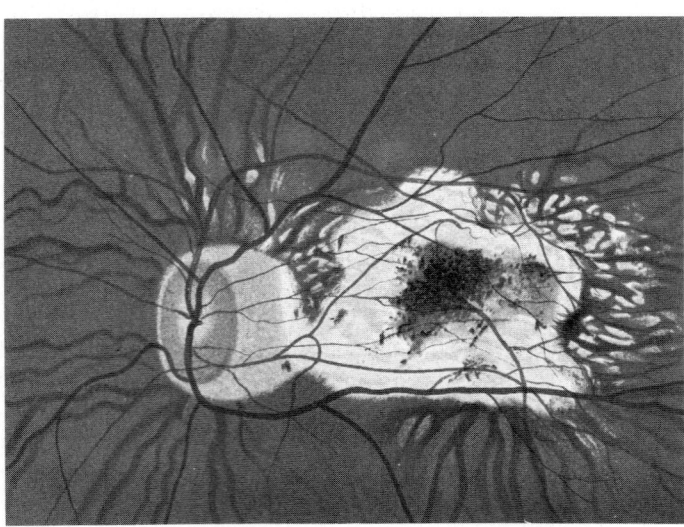

Figure III-8 Posterior staphyloma and advanced myopic degeneration of posterior pole of eye. (Frost: *Fundus Oculi.* The Macmillan Co., New York.)

In astigmatism, refraction is not the same in different meridians of the eye. Since the condition nearly always results from curvature of the cornea, it can best be explained to the patient in the following terms. In the normal eye the cornea has the curvature of the inside of a kitchen bowl, i.e., spherical. If the eye is astigmatic, the curvature of the cornea is elliptical or like that of a kitchen spoon, in which one meridian has a certain curvature that is different from the meridian at right angles to it. The corneal curvature can be measured using a keratometer (Fig. III-9). In regular astigmatism the refraction in each meridian is regular, but it differs in the two principal meridians, which are placed at right angles to each other. Astigmatism is corrected by means of a cylindrical lens that is ground so as to refract rays of light entering the eye in one meridian only. Very few people have only a simple astigmatism. It usually is associated with some degree of hyperopia or myopia. The final correction, therefore, is composed of the glass that corrects the hyperopia or the myopia, plus the cylindrical lens that corrects the astigmatism.

Causes. Nearly all astigmatism is a congenital condition in which heredity is the only known factor. Changes in amount and in the axis of astigmatism occur during growth, just as do changes in the axial length of the eye, but they usually are slight. They also may occur throughout life, necessitating new spectacles from time to time.

Symptoms. The lower grades of astigmatism produce symptoms of eyestrain. These vary greatly and usually have no relation to the degree of error. In fact patients with less than 1 diopter of astigmatism not only complain of headaches and pain after using the eyes, but often suffer just as much after any activity that requires prolonged attention at a distance, such as the theater or driving. This is due to clear vision being unobtainable at any distance unless the correct spectacles are worn. In high astigmatism the images are so blurred that the person makes no effort to clear them by accommodation. In the lower astigmatic errors, the images, while somewhat distorted, are still seen well enough to stimulate an almost constant effort of accommodation. Clear vision never actually results, however, and the patient suffers from asthenopic symptoms from the use of his accommodation.

Treatment. The astigmatic patient must wear his spectacles at all times if he is to obtain relief from his symptoms. Eyes of patients less than 46 years of age always should be examined with a cycloplegic to determine accurately the amount and the axis of the astigmatism. This should be done every year or so to determine if any changes are needed.

METHODS OF REFRACTION

Subjective Method. The subjective method involves having the patient distinguish between the effects of various lenses on the visibility of letters on the Snellen chart. It is applicable only to patients old enough and possessing sufficient intelligence to cooperate. Hence it is of little value in children less than 7 to 8 years of age or in adults of low intellect. In persons less than 46 years of age who have the power of accommodation, the ciliary muscle should be paralyzed with a cycloplegic before testing.

Objective Methods. The objective methods of refraction include examination with the ophthalmoscope (p. 416) and with the retinoscope.

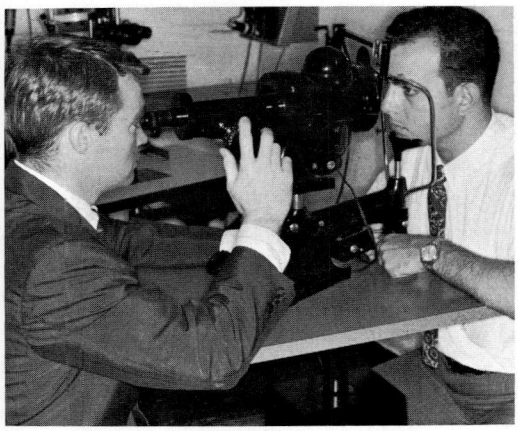

Figure III-9 Measurement of corneal curvature, using keratometer.

Prescription of Spectacles

The type of test or combination of tests depends upon the age and the intelligence of the individual patient as well as upon other factors.

In children under 6 it is seldom possible to obtain cooperation for a subjective refraction. If the vision can be obtained, this is recorded and examination under atropine is carried out; the drug should be instilled three times on the day previous to the examination and once on the morning of the examination. The findings of retinoscopy and ophthalmoscopy are recorded. The vision then is obtained with this correction and, if possible, a subjective test is carried out. A later appointment is made for some time after the atropine has worn off, which usually takes a week to ten days, and the findings are then checked by subjective examination if possible.

It is a good rule that spectacles shall be prescribed only if the patient has symptoms of eyestrain or a definite defect in vision which should be improved by correction. A moderate and sometimes considerable amount of hyperopia may exist without producing any symptoms and without decreasing visual acuity, until the presbyopic age approaches. The same occasionally is true of moderate degrees of hyperopic astigmatism, but these patients usually complain of asthenopia. A person in whom a refractive error is discovered in routine physical examination, but who is absolutely free from symptoms of eyestrain, should not be subjected to the expense and inconvenience of spectacles.

Patients with symptoms of eyestrain, however, in whom a refractive error of any considerable degree is found, should have most accurate correction with spectacles. The habit of holding a book close to the eyes so commonly seen in children cannot be considered an indication for spectacles. It must be emphasized that persons with errors of refraction so small that good vision may be obtained by an effort of accommodation are the ones most often subject to the eyestrain complex. If simple hyperopia of very low degree, not over 0.75 diopter, is discovered, it is questionable whether or not it should be corrected. If the history of symptoms after close work is definite, however, it may be advisable to try giving the full correction for close work only. Most myopes require correction for clear distant vision. In low degrees of myopia, i.e., 0.25 to 0.50 diopter, difficulty in distant vision may not be noticed. The patient then should decide if he wants the correction.

In general it is sufficient if spectacles are prescribed for use only for the symptom responsible for poor vision or eyestrain. For example, a hyperope who has symptoms only after reading needs to wear spectacles only for this purpose. In accommodative asthenopia with little or no refractive error, it may be necessary to prescribe glasses to relieve even the normal strain on accommodation. Patients with refractive errors should be examined about every two years. With children during the growing period, and especially with myopes as previously stated, it may be wise to bring the child back once a year for a checkup. Emphasis should be placed on correct light and posture during reading.

Contact Lens. Contact lenses have been replacing ordinary spectacles increasingly as the fitting has improved and especially since the development of the small corneal lens, which covers only a small portion of the cornea and is inserted without fluid. Although learning to tolerate a contact lens requires considerable motivation, since in reality it is a foreign body in the eye, many individuals wear these lenses with comfort throughout the major portion of the day. The average wearing time without undue irritation is around eight hours. The lenses are worn mainly for cosmetic reasons but also are useful in sports.

The medical indications for their use include keratoconus (in which they are highly successful), high degrees of ametropia, after cataract extraction, and aniridia. They are contraindicated in any disease of the anterior segment, such as conjunctivitis, keratitis, iritis, and angle closure glaucoma.

As the number of people wearing contact lenses increases, however, ophthalmologists are encountering an increasing number of complications from their use. Most of these are the result of trauma in insertion or removal, but some are from ill-fitting lenses and from attempts to wear them too long at one time. Corneal abrasions frequently are seen, and, rarely, a serious keratitis or infected ulcer.

The difficulties and dangers inherent in their use prevent their replacing ordinary lenses for the majority of persons. The patient who wants contact lenses should be under the care of an ophthalmologist and be advised not to be fitted by a non-medical practitioner without supervision.

BIBLIOGRAPHY

Black, R. K., Jay, B., and MacFaul, P.: The concept of degenerative myopia. Proc. Roy. Soc. Med. *58*: 109, 1965.

Donders, F. C.: On the Anomalies of Accommodation and Refraction of the Eye. London, New Sydenham Society, 1864. Translated by W. D. Moore, published by Haarlem, Bohn, 1962.

Duke-Elder, S. W.: The Practice of Refraction. St. Louis, The C. V. Mosby Co., 1965.

Fonda, G.: Management of the Patient with Subnormal Vision. St. Louis, The C. V. Mosby Co., 1965.

Gettes, G. C.: Practical Refraction. New York, Grune & Stratton, 1957.

Girard, L. J.: Corneal Contact Lens. St. Louis, The C. V. Mosby Co., 1964.

Heaton, J. M.: Pain in eyestrain. Am. J. Ophth. *61*:104, 1966.

Hiatt, R. G., Costenbader, F. D., and Albert, D. G.: Clinical evaluation of congenital myopia. Arch. Ophth. *74*:31, 1965.

Lancaster, W. B.: Refraction and Motility. Springfield, Illinois, Charles C Thomas, 1952.

Riffenburgh, R. S.: Onset of myopia in the adult. Am. J. Ophth. *59*:925, 1965.

Ruben, M.: The use of corneal lenses in developmental anisometropia. Proc. Roy. Soc. Med. *58*:112, 1965.

Rubin, M. L.: Optics and visual physiology. Arch. Ophth. *73*:863, 1965; *75*:836, 1966; *78*:77, 1967.

Sloane, A. E.: Manual of refraction. Boston, Little, Brown & Co., 1961.

Appendix IV

Physiology

THE CORNEA

Chemistry. Fractional chemical analysis of the cornea is highly significant, for when the epithelial and endothelial layers and stroma are analyzed separately they yield greatly different values from the whole cornea. For example, over 90 per cent of the cornea is acellular stroma with low lipid content, but the epithelium and endothelium are cellular with high lipid content. This explains their permeability to fat-soluble substances. The epithelial cells also contain more ascorbic acid than does the stroma, but less glutathione, the significance of which is not clear. In addition, the epithelium is high in acetylcholine, the concentration decreasing after postganglionic section of the fifth nerve.

About 60 per cent of the dry cornea is protein, largely collagen but also albumin and globulin. Particles above a molecular weight of 500,000, such as macroglobulins or β-lipoproteins, are absent possibly because of diffusion barriers from the limbal vessels. Older patients and those with abnormal lipid metabolism commonly have arcus senilis, a gray ring within the limbus. Histochemically, arcus senilis consists of a deposit of cholesterol, phospholipids, and neutral fat. Its presence does not appear to correlate well with serum cholesterol levels. The polysaccharides—keratin sulfate, chondroitin-4 sulfate, and chondroi-

tin—act as an interlamellar cement. The constituents of beef cornea are summarized in Table IV-1.

Metabolism. The energy requirements of the cornea are supplied primarily by glucose, which is metabolized in several ways. Sixty-five per cent of the glucose follows the Embden-Meyerhof glycolytic pathway leading to the formation of lactic or pyruvic acid. Glycolysis can proceed in the presence or absence of oxygen, but in the cornea it is much more rapid when oxygen is absent (anaerobically). A small amount of the pyruvate is oxidized to carbon dioxide and

TABLE IV-1   PER CENT OF CONSTITUENTS OF BEEF CORNEA AND SCLERA*

Constituent	Sclera	Cornea	Corneal Epithelium
Water	72.2	81.1	80.5
Solids	27.8	18.9	19.5
Inorganic matter	0.7	0.17	—
Organic matter	27.1	18.7	—
Mucoid	2.3	—	—
Collagen (gelatin)	22.1	18.4	—
Elastin (albuminoid)	1.5	—	—
Albumin and globulin	0.6	0.15	trace
Water-soluble extractives	0.5	0.13	—
Lipids (ether-soluble)	0.1	0.04	4.3†
Nucleic acid	low	low	8.5†

*Adapted from Krause, A. C.: The Biochemistry of the Eye. The Johns Hopkins Press, 1934.

†Dry tissue.

452

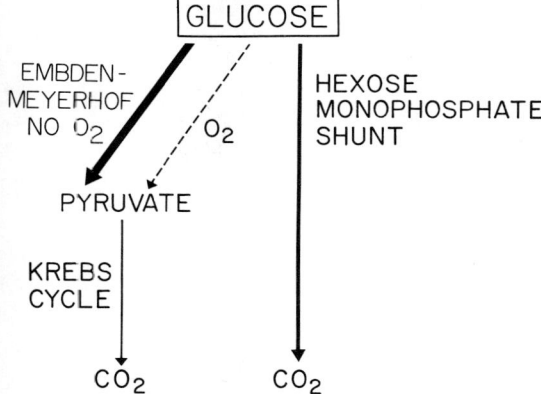

Figure IV-1 Pathways of glucose metabolism in the cornea.

water by the tricarboxylic acid (citric acid or Krebs) cycle. One third of the glucose is oxidized to carbon dioxide by the hexose monophosphate shunt. The fate of glucose is summarized in Figure IV-1.

The epithelium accounts for most of the high uptake of oxygen in the cornea. Since the normal cornea is avascular, four sources of oxygen are available: precorneal film, aqueous humor, limbal capillaries, and palpebral conjunctival capillaries when the lids are closed (Fig. IV-2). Although endothelium may derive most of its oxygen from aqueous, not enough oxygen can diffuse through the stroma to meet the needs of the epithelium. The cornea may derive some of its oxygen requirements from the limbal and conjunctival capillaries, particularly when the lids are closed during sleep. Most evidence, however, implicates the oxygen from the air via the precorneal film as the largest supplier of oxygen to the cornea.

Permeability. Permeability of the cornea is important because the avascular cornea, particularly centrally, receives its nutrition from diffused substances; also, drugs penetrate the cornea by this means and permeability contributes to the maintenance of intraocular pressure. The most important factor in the permeability of the cornea to a substance is relative lipid and non-lipid solubility. The corneal epithelium, with its high lipoid content, is permeable to fat-soluble substances (non-polar or symmetrical compounds). Water-soluble (polar or asymmetrical) molecules, on the other hand, penetrate the epithelium poorly, but traverse the stroma well. The permeability of the endothelium resembles that of the epithelium. Other less important factors are pH, tonicity, size of the molecule, and the electrical charge of the particle. These play roles in permeability, but probably exert their effects by altering the lipid/non-lipid solubility of a substance. Water, though a polar compound, penetrates all layers of the cornea equally well in both directions.

Kinsey has proposed an explanation for the penetration of many of the topical alkaloid drugs that are used in ophthalmology. Basically he suggests that many of

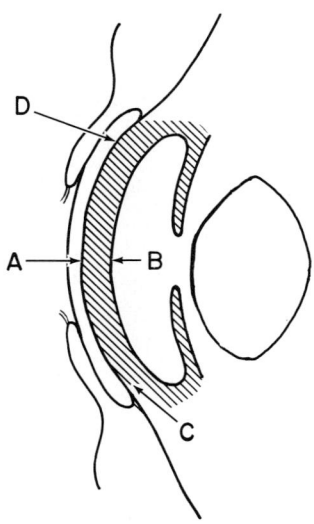

Figure IV-2 Sources of oxygen available to cornea: *A*, precorneal film; *B*, aqueous humor; *C*, limbal capillaries; *D*, palpebral conjunctival capillaries.

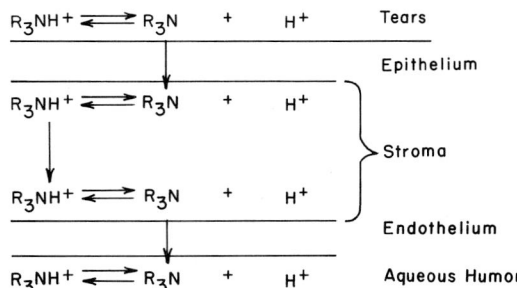

Figure IV-3 Proposed mechanism of penetration of cornea by alkaloid drugs.

the drugs are capable of changing their charges and, therefore, their lipid or water solubility at the critical areas in the cornea. An example for the alkaloid, homatropine, is presented in Figure IV-3.

Turgescence. The cornea normally keeps its water content at a relatively deturgescent state (about 75 per cent of its weight). This is probably maintained by a metabolic pump (i.e., an active transport mechanism) involving oxygen, which keeps the cornea relatively dehydrated. Neither the site of the pump (in the epithelium, endothelium, or both) nor the substance actively transported is known. That the integrity of the endothelial layer is essential for deturgescence is evident from the clinical condition, Fuchs' dystrophy. In this situation primary disease of the endothelium allows edema of the overlying corneal stroma and epithelium. A paradoxical active mechanism that pumps sodium *into* the cornea has been described, but is felt not to be related to corneal dehydration. An alternate explanation of corneal deturgescence offered by Langham suggests that cohesive forces within the components of the corneal stroma balance the imbibition pressure and are maintained by aerobic glycolysis. Corneal swelling would result if the forces of cohesion decreased. Much investigation is necessary to explain thoroughly all of the mechanisms of corneal deturgescence.

Transparency. Corneal transparency is essential for a clear retinal image and good vision. Transparency is maintained by the anatomical structure of the cornea and by its relative deturgescence. The anatomical factors are a precorneal tear film, which provides a smooth, regular, refractive surface; the absence of a keratinized layer of cells in the epithelium; the uniform and regular arrangement of epithelial and endothelial cells; the lack of blood vessels and pigment; the same index of refraction of the epithelial and endothelial cells and Descemet's membrane; and the lattice arrangement of collagen fibrils that provides transparency in the direction of the incident light, but that eliminates by destructive interference the light striking the lattice obliquely.

Wound Healing. Repair of corneal epithelium following abrasion begins almost immediately by two processes: migration of cells to cover the denuded area and mitosis to restore the normal number of epithelial cells. Cell migration occurs first, and if the epithelial defect is small, the reparative process may be limited to migration. Areas of 2 to 3 sq. mm. may be completely covered within 24 hours.

When the wound is deeper and involves Bowman's membrane and the stroma, formation of keratocytes and migration of fibrocytes from the limbus are stimulated, with resultant. scar formation. Numerous drugs, such as local anesthetics and sympathomimetics, can retard mitosis and delay healing.

Vascularization. Since the normal cornea has no blood vessels, their presence suggests present or past corneal disease. The mechanism of corneal vascularization is not entirely clear. It is generally agreed that edema, although not a cause, is an essential condition for vascular invasion. Corneal edema, however it originates, results either in a breakdown of the ground substance lying between the lamellar or individual collagen fibrils of the stroma, or in a general weakening of the structure of the tissue. Vascularization is then induced by unidentified chemical substance(s) called "vessel stimulating factor" (VSF). Apparently forming in damaged tissues, VSF may be capable of stimulating the growth of capillaries or neutralizing a normally present, growth-inhibiting substance.

THE LENS

The anatomy and growth characteristics of the lens, discussed elsewhere (p. 69), are unique in the body. The lens is completely surrounded by a capsule. This stains like other basement membranes and has glycolytic activity independent of other parts of the lens. A lens epithelium normally is present only beneath the anterior capsule. New lens fibers are constantly formed throughout life from the epithelium at the equator. The fibers lose their nuclei, migrate toward the nucleus of the lens, and compress older fibers in an onionskin-like arrangement.

Composition. The lens contains a higher

percentage (35 per cent) of protein than any other structure in the body. The remaining constituent of the lens is primarily water, both bound and unbound. Lens protein has been classified into four groups based on solubility differences: albuminoid, alpha crystallin, beta crystallin, and albumin or gamma crystallin. According to recent investigations, classic groups of proteins have similar charges, but can be differentiated into possibly 20 subunits with gel-filtration, disc electrophoresis, and ultracentrifugation. Very little is known about the mechanism of protein synthesis except that protein production decreases with the age of the animal.

Lens protein has similar antigenic properties in different species. At least five to ten different antigens are shared by vertebrate lenses, and there is an antigenic cross reaction with other vertebrate lenses. Evidently lens material is isolated from a vascular supply in an early embryologic stage, possibly before immune tolerance develops.

Metabolism. The lens metabolizes slowly. Glucose, the primary if not sole substrate, is metabolized to a large extent (85 per cent) by the Embden-Meyerhof pathway of glycolysis to form lactic acid. Only a small part of the lactic acid is metabolized to carbon dioxide and water by the tricarboxylic cycle. Much of the remaining glucose is catabolized through the hexosemonophosphate pathway, but this avenue is limited by the small amount of oxygen available from the aqueous. In the rat lens glucose is converted to sorbitol and then to fructose. However, the significance of this series of reactions is unknown.

High concentrations of glutathione and ascorbic acid, both potential hydrogen carriers, have been found in the lens. The exact nature of their function is unknown, but it is evident that they play a role, perhaps a related one, in lens metabolism.

Principal cation concentrations in the interior of the lens resemble those in the interior of a cell. Potassium concentration is almost 25 times that in the aqueous, whereas sodium concentration is only one seventh of that in the aqueous. The maintenance of these ionic relationships is related to the presence of Na_1K-ATPase. When this enzyme is inhibited by cardiac glycosides, low temperature, glucose deficiency, or inhibitors of glycolysis, there is loss of potassium and gain of sodium, uptake of water, and loss of transparency.

Optical Properties. The single most important characteristic of the lens is its excellent transmission of light. No significant absorption of light occurs between 420 and 760 mμ. The small particles of the lens scatter little light because they are in a high degree of order, a paracrystalline state. Diffraction and reflection by large particles are greatly reduced by the regularity of the fiber structures.

The total refractive power of the lens is greater than if the index of refraction were uniform throughout. The lens can be thought of as having a central, biconvex core of high refractive index surrounded on either side by a concavoconvex lens of considerable less density (Fig. IV-4). The convergent effect of the nucleus, therefore, will more than offset the diverging power surrounding it.

Cataracts. Since the lens is isolated from a blood supply early in the embryonic development, its reactions to physical and chemical insults are extremely limited. Unlike other tissues, its reactions are not typically inflammatory. Instead, water and electrolyte content change and fibers opacify. Numerous, diverse insults, therefore, lead to the same end result: loss of transparency

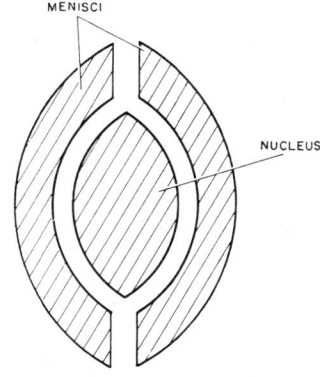

Figure IV-4 Artificial division of the lens into two portions having different refractive indices. (From Adler, F. H.: Physiology of the Eye. 4th ed. St. Louis, The C. V. Mosby Co., 1965.)

of the lens and cataract formation. The sites of initial lens opacification may vary with the nature of the insult, the onset and duration of its action on the lens, and on known and unknown heritable factors.

Clinically, cataracts are found after direct mechanical trauma, such as perforating injuries; after ionizing radiation; after use of chemicals such as MER-29, a hypocholesterolemic agent; and after prolonged use of corticosteroids. Cataracts may be congenital, with a history of a maternal infection such as rubella in the first trimester of pregnancy, or more often without such a history. The commonest known cause for congenital cataracts is heredity. Lens opacities can be found in association with other diseases such as diabetes mellitus and retinitis pigmentosa. By far the commonest cataracts, seen in middle or old age (presenile or senile cataracts, respectively), usually have no known cause.

Lens changes (cataracts) can be produced experimentally in animals by a variety of techniques. Diets high in certain sugars, such as galactose or xylose, invariably lead to lens opacities. High levels of galactose in the aqueous of infants with galactosemia, a human inborn error of metabolism, are associated with cataracts. Such diabetogenic agents as alloxan, dehydroascorbic acid, and diphenylthiocarbazone experimentally lead to cataracts that are well correlated with blood sugar levels. Diets deficient in proteins, particularly the amino acids tryptophan, phenylalanine, valine, and histidine, are also associated with cataracts.

A number of chemical changes occur in both natural and experimental cataracts. In most instances the significance of these changes, especially as to cause or effect, is not clear. In early senile cataracts the water content of the lens increases; this is followed by a decrease in water, total weight, and total protein. The high ratio of potassium to sodium is markedly reduced. Free amino acids may be decreased early and increased later. Calcium is increased. Glutathione and probably ascorbic acid are lost. Decreased oxygen consumption is involved. The pathogenesis of cataracts, particularly the senile variety, must still be considered unknown.

THE VITREOUS

The vitreous body is a gel-like structure that fills the eye behind the lens. The early development and structure of the vitreous are discussed elsewhere (p. 68).

Vitreous is mostly water. Collagen fibrils give it gel properties and a nonuniform, fibrillar structure in which three types of fibers of different sizes have been identified. The collagen fibrils are subject to destruction by several enzymes, one of which, alphachymotrypsin, is utilized clinically to weaken the collagenous zonular fibers prior to extraction of a cataractous lens. When the fibrils of the vitreous are destroyed, the vitreous is liquified permanently, for fibrils do not regenerate.

Hyaluronic acid, a mucopolysaccharide, contributes greatly to vitreous viscosity and is thought to be derived from the hyalocytes on the surface of the vitreous body.

Besides the many proteins found in aqueous humor, the vitreous contains two of its own, mucoid and vitrein. The latter is a residual protein that is similar to collagen except for the carbohydrate to which it is bound. Vitreous has considerably less glucose and phosphate than the aqueous, possibly owing to the utilization of glucose and phosphate by the retina.

EXTRAOCULAR MUSCLES

The physiology of extraocular muscles differs widely from that of other muscles in the body. Extraocular muscles have the smallest ratio of any muscle in the body in the number of muscle fibers innervated by each nerve fiber. Since only five to ten muscle fibers are supplied by each nerve fiber, precise gradations in eye mobility are possible.

Extraocular muscles are characterized also by an extremely rich vascular supply; a short refractory period (less than 1 msec., as compared with 2 msec. for other facial muscles); a short twitch period of 7.5 to 10 msec., comparable with other muscles performing fine work; an increase in fusion frequency (the extraocular muscles will respond without a maximal mechanical output to stimuli at high frequencies of 75 cycles/sec., as compared with other muscles that will respond maximally at 30 to 50 cycles/sec.); and extraocular muscles have tone and electrical activity in the primary position, whereas other muscles have neither tone nor electrical activity when at rest. These and other differences between extraocular muscles and skeletal muscles are summarized in Table IV-2.

Recently researchers have attempted to correlate saccadic (fast, phasic twitch) and tonic (slow) eye motions with two anatomical types of muscle fibers. The two types of eye movements are summarized in Table IV-3.

At least two (perhaps three to five) kinds of extraocular muscle fibers have been described by use of light and electron microscopy. One anatomical type, *Feldenstruktur*, appears to be involved with slow-graded contractions, whereas another, *Fibrillenstruktur*, appears to be involved with the twitch response. This is summarized in Table IV-4.

The gross anatomy of the six extraocular muscles of the eye has already been discussed (p. 49). These muscles rotate the eyeball around its center of rotation within the globe.

Because the eye is firmly supported by orbital fascia, ligaments, and orbital fat, early investigators felt that the center of rotation in man represented a fixed point. Accordingly, they believed that the muscles rotated the globe around three axes, each of which passed through the center of rotation. The axes of Fick, as they are still termed, are the X, or horizontal axis, rotation around which elevates or depresses the globe; the Y, or anteroposterior axis, rotation around which produces torsion, a clockwise or counterclockwise turning of the globe; and a Z, or vertical axis, rotation

around which produces purely horizontal movement (Fig. IV-5).

The plane containing the X and Z axes was thought to pass through both the center of rotation and the equator of the eye in the primary position. This was termed Listing's Plane, or the equatorial plane. The Y axis supposedly ran through the center of rotation at right angles to Listing's plane.

It was later demonstrated, however, that translatory movements, sometimes of considerable magnitude, do occur, and that there is no fixed, stationary center of rotation. In horizontal movements the point around which the globe rotates moves in a semicircle in the plane of rotation. The locus of these points is called the space centrode.

The following list summarizes movements of a single eye:

1. Rotation about the Z, or vertical, axis.

a. Abduction — rotation of the eye temporally.

b. Adduction — rotation of eye nasally.

2. Rotation around the X, or horizontal, axis.

a. Sursumduction (supraduction, elevation) — rotation of eye upward.

b. Deosursumduction (infraduction, depression) — rotation of eye downward.

3. Rotation around Y, or anteroposterior axis.

a. Incycloduction (intorsion) — tilting of superior pole of cornea nasally.

b. Excycloduction (extorsion) — tilting of superior pole of cornea temporally.

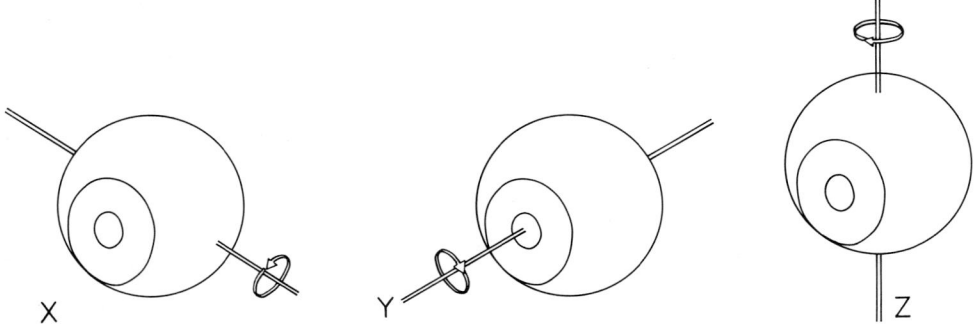

Figure IV-5 Diagram showing Fick's axes.

TABLE IV-2 ELECTRICAL ACTIVITY OF OCULAR MUSCLE COMPARED WITH THAT OF SKELETAL MUSCLE*

Characteristic	Ocular Muscle	Skeletal Muscle
Amplitude at rest	20 to 150 μV	0
Duration at rest	1 to 2 msec.	0
Frequency at rest	Up to 150/sec.	0
Amplitude during activity	400 to 600 μV	100 to 3000
Duration during activity	1 to 2 msec.	5 to 10 msec.
Frequency during activity	Several hundred/sec.	5 to 30/sec.
Minimal rate of stimulation to produce maximal tetanus	250/sec.	50/sec.
Minimal number of shocks to produce maximal tetanus	20 to 30/sec.	10/sec.

*From Adler, F. H.: Physiology of the Eye. 4th ed. The C. V. Mosby Co., 1965.

TABLE IV-3 THE BASIC TYPES OF EYE MOVEMENTS IN MAN*

Description	Saccadic	Tonic
Function	Bring image on the fovea by one or more rapid movements; may occur in trains with intervals of 100 to 150 msec.	Maintains image on fovea when the head moves; stabilization, vergence. Response to the movements of the image across the retina.
Synonyms	Phasic, jerky, version, ballistic, exploratory.	Smooth tracking, pursuit, following.
Reaction time and velocity	Conjugate movements: reaction time 150 to 250 msec.; velocity 200 to 500 degrees per second. Disjunctive movements: none.	Conjugate movements: velocity up to 40 degrees per second, linearly related to target velocity. Disjunctive movements: reaction time about 160 msec.; velocity about 25 degrees per second; velocity is first a function of stimulus amplitude and then assumes an asymptotic decline until a final level is reached in a total time of 800 msec.
Characteristics	Ballistic — preset, follows inevitable course.	Guided — under continuous control; precise match between target and eye velocity. Conjugate tonic movements depend on saccade to bring about fixation.
Neuromuscular fiber system	Fibrillenstruktur (twitch).	Feldenstruktur (tonic).

*From Jampel, R. S.: Multiple motor systems in the extraocular muscles of man. Invest. Ophth. 6:290, 1967.

Factor	Slow, Multinucleated, Striate Fibers (Feldenstruktur)	Fast-Twitch Striate Fibers (Fibrillenstruktur)
Physiology		
1. Response to stimulation.	Slow, maintained, graded contraction; (?) no action potentials displayed; graded, multiple junctional potentials.	Rapid transient contraction, action potential, all-or-none impulse activity, end-plate potentials.
2. Nerve velocity.	2 to 8 meters per sec. (frog).	8 to 40 meters per sec. (frog).
3. Fusion frequency.	30 stimuli per second.	350 stimuli per second.
Anatomy		
1. Myofibrils.	Large, irregularly separated, poorly defined; incomplete sarcoplasmic reticulum; no transverse tubules and triads; located in outer core of muscle.	Small, regularly separated (by sarcoplasmic reticulum), punctate, well defined; abundant sarcoplasmic reticulum, transverse tubules, and triads present; located in inner core of muscle.
2. Nerve endings.	Multiple, small, irregularly distributed motor terminals ("en grappe"); no invaginating sarcolemmal folds under nerve terminals; decreased sole plate sarcoplasm.	Large individual end-plate ("en plaque"); invaginating sarcolemmal folds, extensive sole plate sarcoplasm.
3. Nerve diameters.	3 to 8 μ (cat's superior oblique).	Over 8 μ (cat's superior oblique).
Pharmacology		
1. Acetylcholine.	Contracture.	No effect.
2. Succinylcholine.	Increases resting tension.	Decreases twitch response.
3. Epinephrine.	(?) Increases tension.	(?) No effect.
4. Curare.	Decreases muscle tension.†	Decreases twitch response.
5. Edrophonium and neostigmine.	Increases muscle tension.	Increases twitch response.

*From Jampel, R. S.: Multiple motor systems in the extraocular muscles of man. Inv. Ophth. 6:289, 1967.
†Under unique conditions increases muscle tension.

Rotations about the Z and X axes can be performed voluntarily, but the rotations about the Y axis, or torsions, are involuntary.

Actions of the Individual Muscles (Table IV-5)

Because muscle action varies with the starting position of the globe, these actions are usually discussed as they apply to the eye in the primary position (straight ahead) as well as for other stated positions. (Main actions are italicized.)

When the eye moves from one position to another, certain muscles act together in rotating the globe and are termed *agonists*, whereas other muscles act in an opposite direction and are termed *antagonists*. The superior rectus and the inferior oblique are agonists in elevation of the globe. In the primary position the superior rectus is the more effective elevator and its effectiveness increases in abduction, whereas the inferior oblique becomes the more effective eleva-

tor in adduction. Similarly the inferior rectus and superior oblique are agonists for depression, the superior oblique and the superior rectus for intorsion, the inferior oblique and the inferior rectus for extorsion, the lateral rectus and the superior and inferior obliques for abduction, and the medial rectus and the superior and inferior recti for adduction.

The antagonistic groups of muscles are the medial and the lateral recti, the superior and inferior recti, and the superior and inferior obliques. If the direct antagonists were to contract simultaneously and with equal force (cocontraction), there would be little rotary movement; the primary movement would be of the globe back into the orbit. Occasionally this occurs clinically, but by far the more common situation is a reciprocal inhibition of the direct antagonist of the contracting muscle. Thus, *Sherrington's law* states that the increase in contraction (or the converse) in a muscle does not proceed simultaneously in its antagonist. Two antagonistic muscles may contract at the same time, but in one it may be with increasing intensity, whereas in the other with decreasing intensity. This phenomenon allows a finely graded response and steady movements.

TABLE IV-5   ACTIONS OF THE INDIVIDUAL MUSCLES

Muscle	Action in Primary Position	Other Positions	Action
Medial rectus	*Adduction*	Elevation Depression	*Increase in elevation* *Increase in depression*
Lateral rectus	*Abduction*	Elevation Depression	*Increase in elevation* *Increase in depression*
Superior rectus	*Elevation* Intorsion Adduction	Abduction Adduction	*Elevation* Adduction Intorsion
Inferior rectus	*Depression* Extorsion Adduction	Abduction Adduction	*Depression* Adduction Extorsion
Superior oblique	Depression Intorsion Abduction	Adduction Abduction	*Depression* Intorsion
Inferior oblique	Extorsion Elevation Abduction	Abduction Adduction	*Extorsion* Abduction *Elevation*

When the two eyes move together, the term *version* is used if the movement of the two eyes is in the same direction, and the term *vergence* if the movement of the two eyes is in opposite directions. Versions are conjunctive movements, whereas vergences are disjunctive movements.

Versions. To describe the direction of gaze, the proper prefix is attached to the basic word version. For example, looking to the right is dextroversion, to the left is levoversion, looking up is sursumversion, down is deosursumversion. Not only are there muscles within the same eye that act as agonists or antagonists, but in opposite eyes there are muscles that act together, termed yoke muscles (Table IV-6).

Thus in dextroversion the lateral rectus of the right eye and its yoke muscle in the left eye, the medial rectus, are the prime muscles responsible for the movement. *Hering's law* states that in all voluntary movements of the eye, equal and simultaneous innervation flows from the central nervous system to the muscles of both eyes gazing in a particular direction. It must be remembered, however, that Table IV-6 presents only the prime muscles for each version, but that numerous muscles are involved in each gaze. For example, in dextroversion in the right eye there is contraction not only of the lateral rectus, but also of the other muscles involved with abduction—the superior and inferior obliques—and relaxation of their antagonists. Accordingly, in the left eye all the adductors contract—the medial, superior, and inferior recti—with relaxation of their antagonists.

Vergences. Vergences refer to the movement of the two eyes in opposite directions. Convergence is a movement of the eyes toward each other, while divergence is a movement away from each other. Vertical and torsional vergences are rarely seen.

CONVERGENCE. Convergence appears late phylogenetically in the species and also late developmentally in the human. Infants show little convergence until the third month of life. The voluntary aspect of convergence is developed to varying degrees in people; many people are unable to converge without a near point on which to fixate. Accommodation and miosis are associated with convergence in the near point reaction (p. 444).

The pathways for convergence are not known with certainty. In the primate, simultaneous stimulation of both frontal or both occipital eye fields has produced convergence. In man stimulation of the frontal cortex has produced convergence. The near response was obtained in lightly anesthetized macaques by unilateral stimulation of areas 19 and 22 of the cerebral cortex. Conducting fibers could be traced from areas 18 and 19 to the tectum of the midbrain where they terminated, whereas other fibers could be traced as far as the level of the inferior colliculi. The latter fibers were thought to carry inhibitory fibers to the abducens center, which would inhibit the lateral rectus during the act of convergence. Although the fiber tracts have never been localized, clinical evidence suggests that they reach the nucleus of the third nerve by way of the anterior brachia and superior colliculi rather than by the pons. Thus lesions of the superior colliculi associated with paralysis of vertical gaze rather than horizontal gaze are more likely to be seen with loss of convergence, as in Parinaud's syndrome. No subcortical centers subserving convergence have been identified.

TABLE IV-6 YOKE MUSCLES

Right Eye	Left Eye	Version
Medial rectus	Lateral rectus	Left
Lateral rectus	Medial rectus	Right
Superior rectus	Inferior oblique	Up and right
Inferior rectus	Superior oblique	Down and right
Superior oblique	Inferior rectus	Down and left
Inferior oblique	Superior rectus	Up and left

Four types of convergence have been recognized. Tonic convergence refers to the tone in the medial recti in the primary position from birth on. It is generally excessive in childhood and diminishes with age. Proximal convergence is induced by a sense of nearness of an object. Accommodative convergence is that portion of convergence that is initiated by the stimulus to accommodation. Just how closely accommodation and convergence are related is not clear. Various authors have described them as completely independent or inseparable. Clinically the relationship of the accommodative convergence to accommodation is expressed as a ratio (AC/A). An easy way to measure this ratio is to determine the phoria at a given distance, add a known plus or minus lens, and again measure the phoria. The amount of change in the phoria per diopter change in accommodation is the AC/A ratio. In most people the AC/A ratio is constant over all viewing distances, the average figure being 3.5 Δ/D. Fusional convergence attempts to keep an object of regard on the foveae of both eyes.

DIVERGENCE. The question of whether divergence is an independent, active process or merely a manifestation of inhibition of convergence tone has not been settled. No anatomic pathways for active divergence have been found in the human and, until recently, most of the observed phenomena of divergence have been explained as inhibition of convergence tonus and elasticity of the lateral recti and fascia. On the other hand, evidence is accumulating that divergence results from an active innervation of both lateral recti. The measurement of electrical activity from a lateral rectus muscle clearly shows impulses during divergence. Also, the clinical entity of divergence paralysis is best explained by an active divergence mechanism. Divergence paralysis can be elicited by the bifoveal fixation of a midline objective as it is withdrawn from the eyes. At the point diplopia develops, the separation of the objects is measured. If now the object is moved laterally either to the right or to the left, but still the same distance from the eyes, the separation of the objects remains the same as when the object was in the midline. This situation is pathognomonic for divergence paralysis and is best explained by active divergence.

Proprioception

Muscle spindles have been found in humans, apes, and goats, but not in monkeys, dogs, rabbits, or cats. There is abundant evidence that conditions in humans that put muscles on stretch will increase the sensory nerve output from the muscle and will increase the motor firing of extraocular muscles. However, this proprioceptive mechanism does not provide man with a sense of position of the globe. When he is placed in a completely dark room and his eye movements are stimulated through a reflex mechanism, such as turning his chair or moving his globe passively by a forceps on an anesthetized conjunctiva, he is completely unaware of either his eye movements or their position in space.

Muscle Pain

Pain from an extraocular muscle ordinarily is not elicited by cutting it or passing a needle through it. Severe pain can be elicited, however, by pulling on an extraocular muscle (e.g., by passing a suture under the superior rectus), by depriving it of blood supply, or by bruising. Muscle pain is thought to be due partially to deprivation of oxygen and accumulation of lactic acid.

MEASURING ELECTRICAL PHENOMENA

Electrical phenomena in and around the eye have been measured with increasing frequency in recent years, especially by use of the microelectrode technique of intracellular recording of potentials. Only the more clinically applied techniques will be discussed here.

Electromyography (EMG). The recording of action potentials from the surface of muscle need only be briefly mentioned, since the significant findings in extraocular muscles and the differences between extraocular muscles and other skeletal muscles have already been discussed.

Electro-oculograph (EOG). This is based on the observation that the electrical potential of the cornea is positive when compared to that of the fundus. The source of this difference in potential is unknown, but thought to be related to the metabolic activity of the pigment epithelium and/or the outer segments of the rods. Clinically one may make use of the corneal-fundal potential by attaching electrodes at the outer and inner canthi of the eye. The eye then will behave like a dipole oriented in the anteroposterior axis, and movements of the eye around a vertical axis will cause changes in the measured potential. Therefore, electro-oculography is a sensitive sensor of small horizontal movements of the eye of even less than 1°. In addition, chloroquine toxicity, vitamin A deficiency, shallow pigment epithelium detachments, and other conditions may often be detected early by measuring the difference in electrical activity between the light-stimulated and nonstimulated eye.

Electroretinography (ERG). This is a measurement of evoked potentials occurring between the cornea and the retina. In man, ERG is usually recorded as the difference in potential between an electrode in a corneal contact lens and a second electrode applied to the forehead. The general form of an ERG consists in four primary waves (Fig. IV-6): an "a" wave, which is the initial negative deflection occurring

after a short latency period following the onset of illumination; a "b" wave, which is a positive deflection of short duration that follows the "a" wave; a "c" wave, which consists of an initial increase, then a decrease, in potential occurring over a long period; and a "d" wave, or "off" effect, which occurs after the stimulus is withdrawn and is followed by a gradual return to the resting potential.

Recently, with the use of computers, more subtle wavelets within the "a" and "b" waves have been defined. The sources of the various waves are not known with certainty, except that the retinal layers extending from the inner plexiform layer out to the pigment epithelium seem to be involved in the production of the ERG. The ganglion cell layer and nerve fiber layer, therefore, do not appear to play a role in the ERG, and local destruction of either of these two layers (e.g., glaucoma) does not produce any abnormalities in the ERG.

Not only are the sources of the waves of the ERG obscure, but so also is their significance. The "a" wave becomes increasingly prominent with increasing intensities of light, whereas the "b" wave is more prominent in the dark-adapted state. One of the early "b" wavelets, known as

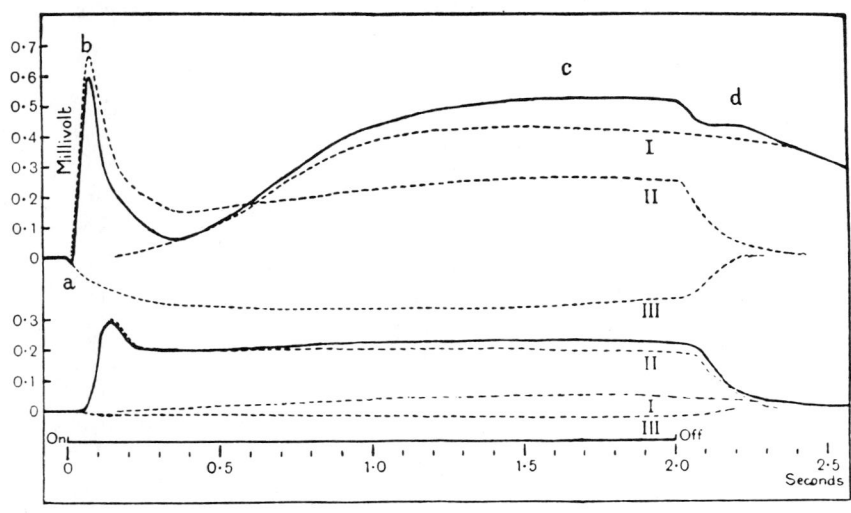

Figure IV-6   General form of an ERG. (Granit, 1933.)

B photopic, however, appears more responsive in photopic conditions.

Aside from research value, the ERG has not proved to be an extremely important clinical tool. Its use has generally been limited to detecting diseases involving widespread retinal pathology, such as occlusions of the central retinal artery or vein, retinal detachments and abiotrophies, hypovitaminosis A, siderosis, chalcosis, diabetic retinopathy, anemia, and chloroquine toxicity. A computerized method that averages transients has been used to distinguish between various cone pigment dysfunctions.

LACRIMAL SYSTEM

The anterior aspect of the normal globe is covered by a precorneal tear film. Wolff was the first to suggest that the film is a three-layered structure, each layer arising from a different set of glands (Fig. IV-7).

The most superficial layer is oily. Its principal function appears to be to retard evaporation markedly from the underlying layers and, therefore, to maintain corneal thickness. It also may attract foreign particles, which may then be wiped away by the eyelids. The sources of this layer are the meibomian or tarsal glands, which empty at the lid margins, and perhaps the glands of Zeis and Moll.

The intermediate watery layer moistens the eye and washes away foreign particles. It contains lysozyme, an antibacterial enzyme, and other proteins. Its sources are multiple. The main palpebral gland (orbital lobe) and the accessory palpebral gland (palpebral lobe) are principal contributors. Others are accessory lacrimal glands of Krause and Wolfring and scattered glands in the plica, caruncle, and within the orbit.

The inner, mucoid layer seems to be involved with corneal nutrition. It arises primarily from the conjunctival goblet cells but probably also from the crypts of Henle in the upper lid and the glands of Manz that surround the limbus.

Tearing may be divided into four types.

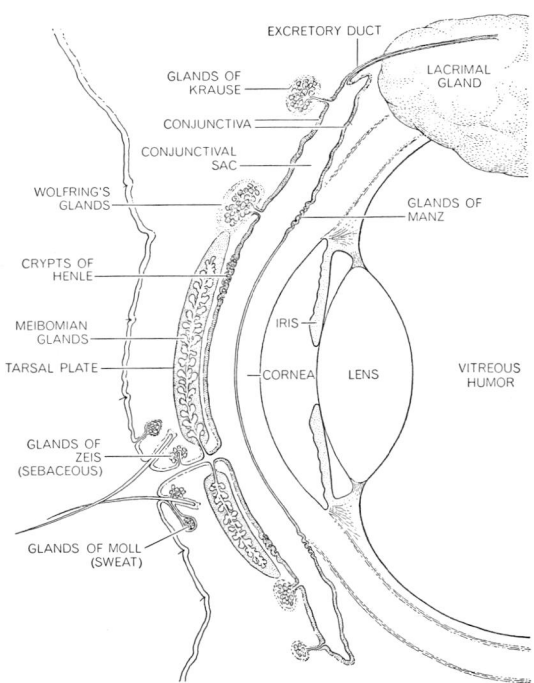

Figure IV-7 Glands that produce tears sheathe eye when lids close. Lacrimal gland (top) helps form watery substance in tears, along with glands of Krause and Wolfring. Crypts of Henle and glands of Manz produce a mucoid layer. Tarsal and meibomian glands, and glands of Moll and of Zeis, help to make oily layer. (From Tears and the Lacrimal Gland, by S. Y. Botelho. Copyright © 1964 by Scientific American, Inc. All rights reserved.)

First, there is *basic secretion*, which occurs continuously and independently of either the afferent or efferent nerve supply of the lacrimal system. *Reflex tearing* may follow stimulation of the olfactory (strong odors), optic (bright light), or trigeminal (irritation of the eye) nerves (Fig. IV-8). The efferent pathway of this reflex arc is via the parasympathetic nerve that arises in the pons above the superior salivatory nucleus and travels with the facial nerve, synapses in the sphenopalatine ganglion, and reaches the lacrimal gland in the zygomatic nerve. The relationship of the sympathetics to lacrimation is far from clear. The sympathetics arise in the hypothalamus, descend to the thoracic areas, synapse in the superior cervical ganglion, and reach the lacrimal gland by several pathways. Various authors feel that stimulating this system will increase, decrease, or not affect lacrimal secretion. Some of the discrepancies may be due to species differences. *Psychogenic tearing* appears unique to humans. It is rarely present at birth, and most infants do not display it until a month has elapsed. *Tearing in response to secretagogues*, such as mecholyl and pilocarpine, is the fourth type of secretion.

Clinical measurement of lacrimal secretion or composition is generally not very accurate or specific; the methods modify the amount of secretion, and the tears from all sources are measured together. The Schirmer No. 1 test, originally described in 1903, is the one most commonly used. It consists of folding a strip of Whatman No. 41 filter paper, 5 × 35 mm. long, 5 mm. from one end, and inserting it into the unanesthetized inferior cul-de-sac. The amount of wetting is measured after a specified time (usually five minutes).

Tears are usually isotonic or slightly hypertonic to plasma (0.90 to 1.01 NaCl equivalent). The pH of tears is similar to

TABLE IV-7 COMPOSITION OF TEARS*

Substance	Percentage
Total solids	1.8
Total protein	0.669
Albumin	0.394
Globulin	0.275
Nonprotein nitrogen	0.051
Total nitrogen	0.158
Urea	0.04
Sugar†	(0.065)
Na_2O	0.6
K_2O	0.14
Chlorine	0.394
NaCl	0.65

*From Ridley, F., and Sorsby, A. (eds.): Modern Trends in Ophthalmology. New York, Paul B. Hoeber, Inc., 1940.

†Glucose found to be 4.1 mg./100 ml. by Gasset *et al.*: American Journal of Ophthalmology, March, 1968.

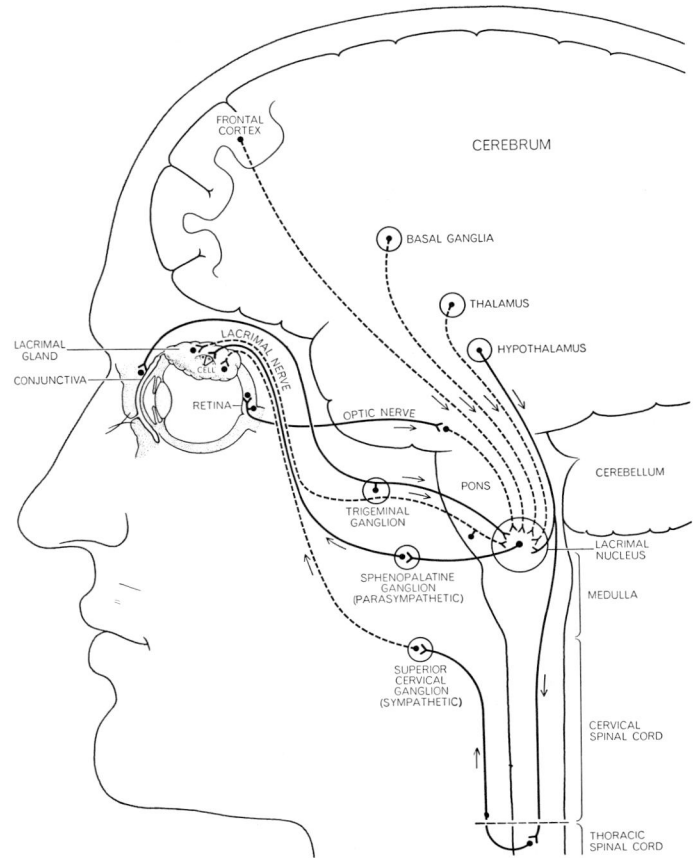

Figure IV-8 Nerve connections of lacrimal gland and accessory regions of eye and brain that apparently contribute to formation of tears are represented schematically. Fibers from lacrimal nucleus in brainstem carry motor impulse to neurons in sphenopalatine ganglion, a knot of nerves shown by a circle. The fibers that carry impulses from this ganglion to lacrimal gland are part of parasympathetic system. Sensory fibers connect lacrimal nucleus with lacrimal gland by way of trigeminal ganglion. Such fibers in optic nerve may carry impulses to lacrimal nucleus from retina. The unknown role of some fibers, such as those between lacrimal gland and superior cervical ganglion (sympathetic system), is indicated by broken lines. (From Tears and the Lacrimal Gland, by S. Y. Botelho. Copyright © 1964 by Scientific American, Inc. All rights reserved.)

that of blood, varying from 7.0 to 7.4, although samples may vary from 5.2 to 8.4. A relatively high concentration of proteins (0.67 per cent) lowers the surface tension of tears for better wetting. One of these proteins, the enzyme lysozyme, rapidly destroys many bacteria. Chloride and potassium ions are elevated in tears and may reflect an active transport mechanism. Table IV-7 summarizes Ridley's data.

RETINAL METABOLISM

Measurable energy changes in the retina result from various metabolic processes such as the basal metabolism of retinal cells, the destruction and resynthesis of visual pigments, the transmission of nerve impulses through and from the retina, and the active transport of substances through the retina.

The retina has the highest rate of respiration of any tissue in the body. Carbohydrate metabolism is the chief source of energy. Only recently has a large supply of glycogen, glycolytic, and glycogenic enzymes been demonstrated in human retinas, particularly in Müller's cells and fibers. Enzymes active in the citric acid cycle are present in the retina, and this cycle is thought to be the principal pathway for the oxidation of pyruvate and lactic acids. The oxidative systems are not active enough, however, to prevent an accumulation of lactic acid.

Many studies of the effects of light on retinal metabolism are equivocal. Recent work, however, shows an increase in the rate of metabolism and in the activity of the enzyme succinodehydrogenase in the inner segments of the rods and cones. The metabolism of the retina along with that of the brain is unique because of the formation of ammonia. It has been shown that the rate of ammonia formation is higher during aerobic glycolysis than anaerobic glycolysis, and higher in the light-adapted retina than the dark-adapted one. The source and significance of ammonia formation is unknown, but it is thought to be related to the breakdown of visual pigments. The pH of the retina shifts from 7.3 in the dark-adapted state to 7.0 in the light-adapted, a change that has stirred considerable controversy.

NATURE OF LIGHT

Light is a sensation produced by a particular group of wavelengths of the electromagnetic energy spectrum. These wavelengths are capable of being transmitted through the ocular media to the receptor cells of the retina where they are absorbed and thereby initiate a neuroelectrical response that is propagated to the occipital cortex. The radiation involved in the phenomenon of light has wavelengths from about 400 mμ to 700 mμ—an extremely small band of the electromagnetic spectrum that extends from cosmic radiation (wavelength 10^{-12} cm.) to long radio waves (wavelength 10^8 cm.).

$$1 \text{ Ångström unit} = 1\text{Å} = 10^{-1} \text{ m}\mu = 10^{-8} \text{ cm.} = 10^{-10}\text{m.}$$

Electromagnetic radiation travels at 186,000 miles/sec. (3.0×10^{-10} cm./sec.) in a vacuum. When radiation enters an atmosphere, its velocity is reduced by $1/n$, where n equals the index of refraction of that atmosphere.

The nature of light has been a source of interest and controversy for many years. Newton conceived of light as a series of perfectly elastic and fast-moving bodies or corpuscles. On the other hand, Huygens felt that phenomena such as reflection could best be explained by a wave theory of light. More recently, Planck and Einstein postulated that the energy in a light beam, instead of being distributed in the electric and magnetic fields of an electromagnetic wave, was concentrated in small packets or photons. Some of the wave picture was retained in this theory, however, so a photon was still considered to have a frequency (v), and the energy of a photon (e) was proportional to its frequency.

(1) $e \propto v$

(2) $e = hv$

where H = Planck's constant

since

(3) $\lambda = \dfrac{c}{v}$

where λ = wavelength

c = velocity

then

(4) $e = \dfrac{hc}{\lambda}$

Currently most physicists feel that light appears dualistic. The phenomena of light propagation (e.g., reflection, refraction, and so forth) may be best understood by the electromagnetic wave theory. The interaction of light with matter (e.g., emission, absorption, and so forth) may be best explained in corpuscular terms.

To be perceived as light, electromagnetic radiation must be transmitted through the cornea, aqueous humor, lens, vitreous humor, and inner layers of the retina with minimal reflection or absorption. However, the retinal cells responsible for the conversion of light energy into nerve impulses should absorb light to a high degree with little transmission or reflection. How much light reaches the retina depends upon a number of factors, including the intensity, wavelength, and direction of the incident light, the size of the pupil, and the transmission through the ocular media.

The cornea is opaque to radiation of less than 293 mμ, but longer ultraviolet rays, particularly 315 mμ and greater, penetrate. Radiation in this spectrum can cause ultraviolet keratitis and conjunctivitis. Radiation from 400 to 1250 mμ will be transmitted almost perfectly through the cornea. The clinical significance of this differential transmission through the cornea is that most of the harmful ultraviolet radiation is filtered from the inner eye by the cornea, but infrared radiation can penetrate the cornea and cause deleterious effects at the lens (e.g., glassblowers' cataracts) or at the retina (e.g., eclipse burn).

Light Measurements. An arbitrary unit, which is defined as a *candle* of certain thickness that burns a given amount of wax in a given time, emits one candle power of light energy. If one thinks of a candle at the center of a sphere and cuts out a circle on the surface of that sphere so that the apex is the candle and the base on the surface of the sphere is equal in area to the square of the radius of the sphere, then the unit solid angle resulting will contain 1 *lumen* of light. Since the surface of the whole sphere is $4\pi r^2$, one candle power contains 12.56 lumens (Fig. IV-9).

If 1 lumen of light falls on a surface of 1 square foot, the *lumination* of that surface is 1 foot candle. Luminance depends on light reflected from a surface. One *lambert* is the luminance of 1 square centi-

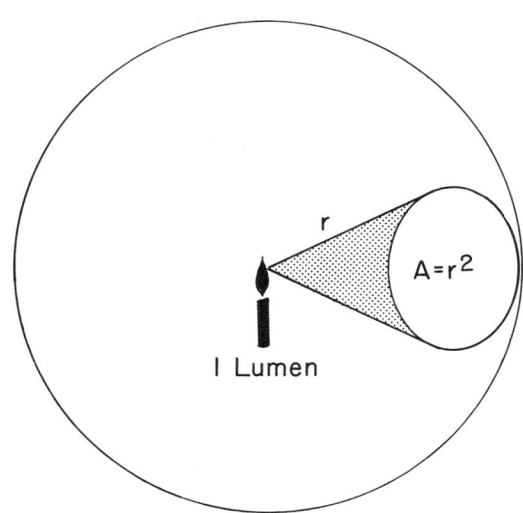

Figure IV-9 A lumen of light. Amount of light emitted within a unit solid angle whose apex is a light of one candle power and whose base area is equal to the square of its radius.

meter of surface that reflects 1 lumen of light. It is more common to deal with *millilamberts* or *microlamberts*.

PHOTOCHEMISTRY OF VISION

As mentioned earlier, wavelengths between 400 and 800 mμ excite the eye and initiate the complex process of sight. After light is transmitted through the ocular media, it is absorbed by pigments in the rod and cone cells of the retina. How a light signal is converted to an electrical signal that is sent down the neural pathways to the central nervous system is little understood at present.

The first pigment to be extracted from the retina of vertebrates was rhodopsin, which Boll called "visual purple" in 1876. Found in human rod cells, rhodopsin is a magenta or red-purple pigment in the dark. Under the influence of light, it bleaches rapidly through orange-colored intermediary compounds to a mixture of the yellow all-*trans* retinene and the colorless protein scotopsin (Fig. IV-10*A*). At this point *trans*

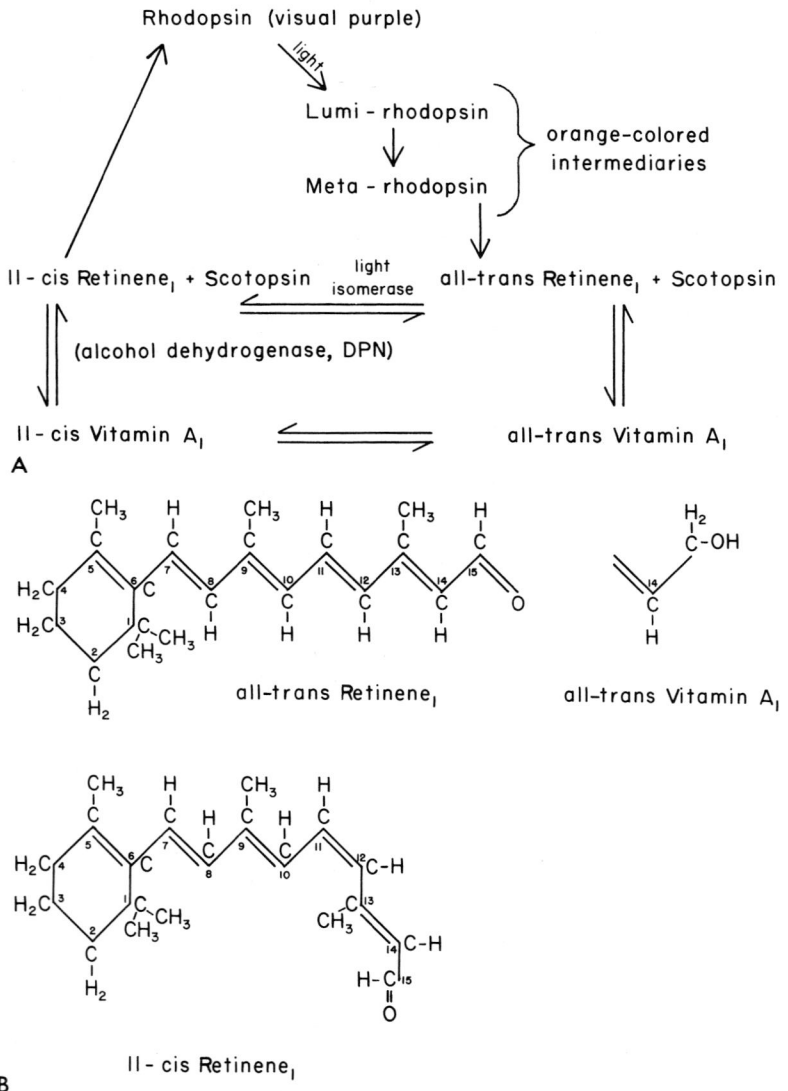

Figure IV-10 (*A*) Effect of light on rhodopsin and its reformation. (*B*) Chemical structures of all-*trans* and 11-*cis* retinene₁, and all-*trans* vitamin A₁. Only 11-*cis* retinene is incorporated into rhodopsin.

retinene may follow one of two pathways. It may be chemically reduced from retinene, the aldehyde, to *trans* vitamin A, the alcohol. The all-*trans* vitamin A is then converted to an 11-*cis* form and, under the influence of alcohol dehydrogenase and DPN, is oxidized to 11-*cis* retinene. The 11-*cis* retinene can also be converted directly from all-*trans* retinene under light or in the presence of enzyme retinene isomerase. Rhodopsin is then resynthesized from the union of 11-*cis* retinene and scotopsin. Of all possible isomer forms of retinene, the 11-*cis* configuration is the only one suitable for the formation of rhodopsin (Fig. IV-10*B*).

Rods and their pigment, rhodopsin, are the basis of the mechanism for dark-adapted, or scotopic, vision. Accordingly, when the light absorption curve of rhodopsin and the visibility curve of the dark-adapted eye are compared, they are found to be similar, but not identical (Fig. IV-11). The maximum sensitivity of the dark-adapted eye is to light of 510 mμ, whereas the maximum absorption of light by rhodopsin is to light of 497 mμ. When corrections are made for light that is selectively absorbed by the various components of the ocular media and for differences in the energy levels of light, an excellent fit of the curves occurs.

In the cones are three photosensitive pigments—blue, green, and red—formerly referred to collectively as iodopsin. Recent

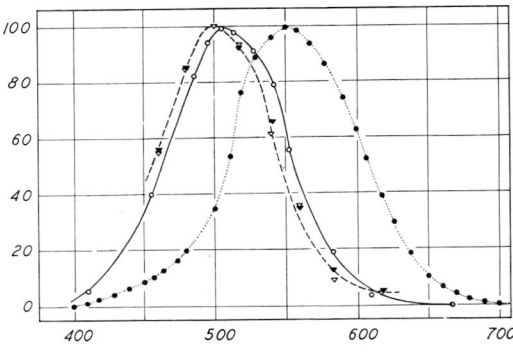

Figure IV-11 Visibility curves and absorption spectrum of rhodopsin. Open circles and continuous line are a recording of the relative effectiveness of the spectrum at the lowest intensities arranged so that the maximum effectiveness is 100. Filled circles and broken line are a recording of the effectiveness of the spectrum at high intensities of illumination. (From Adler, F. H.: Physiology of the Eye. 4th ed. St. Louis, The C. V. Mosby Co., 1965.)

work on human and monkey retinas has demonstrated that each cone has one of the three pigments with maximum absorptions of 455 mμ (blue-sensitive), 535 mμ (green-sensitive), and 570 mμ (red-sensitive). Thus far, only in the latter two pigments has retinene been demonstrated.

Light Adaptation (Photopic Vision). When a dark-adapted eye is suddenly exposed to moderate light, its sensitivity immediately falls. This adaptation is thought to occur through two processes: a fast or alpha adaptation that is almost complete in 0.05 sec., and a slow or beta adaptation that is complete in about 50 sec. The alpha process is thought to be related to a nervous mechanism, because any part of one retina may be stimulated. The beta process is probably related to a photochemical process because it is restricted to the area stimulated. The photopic eye is most sensitive to light of 550 mμ.

Dark Adaptation. Dark adaptation is the transition of the retina from the light-adapted or photopic state to a dark-adapted or scotopic state. In the dark-adapted state the eye increases its sensitivity to light about 100,000 times. Although the visual acuity or ability of the eye to resolve patterns is maximal under photopic conditions, its ability to detect small intensities of light is maximal under scotopic conditions.

Dark adaptation in humans is measured by determining the threshold of the minimum amount of light that can barely be detected. First, the eye is exposed to a standard bright light to insure adequate light adaptation. Then the light is turned off, and a selected area of the retina is stimulated with a light of increasing intensity until it can be faintly detected by the subject. The course of dark adaptation is plotted, with time in minutes, on the abscissa, and the log of the light intensity, in microlamberts, on the ordinate. Light intensity usually is expressed logarithmically because of the wide variation in intensity.

Maximum sensitivity to light is approached at about 30 minutes (Fig. IV-12), but it is reached completely only after an hour in the dark.

In comparing dark adaptation curves between one individual and another, or on the same individual at different times, certain variables must be controlled. The region of the retina stimulated is crucial. Figure IV-12 shows the dark adaptation curve for an area 20 degrees from the fovea. In this curve two distinct parts can be recognized: the initial increase in sensitivity, or fall in intensity of light, that flattens out at about five or seven minutes and is due to adaptation of the cones; and a second, more gradual fall in intensity due to adaptation of the rods. As one stimulates areas closer to the fovea, which has cones only, the second phase of the curve becomes increasingly less prominent until there is only the early depression of intensity.

The intensity and duration of the preadapting light will modify the ensuing dark adaptation. As they increase, the slope of the dark adaptation curve becomes less steep (Fig. IV-12). The wavelength of the preadapting light is also important. One can more readily adapt to darkness after exposure to longwave light, such as red, than after exposure to shortwave light, such as blue. This is why radiologists who want to remain dark-adapted wear red goggles in bright light. How red goggles affect dark adaptation is not clear, but it may be that they prevent the shorter wavelengths from reaching the rods, which are stimulated by blue light under dim light conditions.

The wavelength of the stimulating light is another important variable. The light-adapted eye is most sensitive to light of 550 mμ, but the fully dark-adapted eye will appreciate yellow-green light most sensitively at 510 mμ (blue-green). This change in maximum sensitivities of the light-adapted and dark-adapted eye is known as the Purkinje shift.

In addition to affecting retinal adaptation, light will change the size of the pupil. Retinal adaptation and pupillary response counteract one another, thus maintaining homeostasis. Under reduced illumination, therefore, the retina becomes increasingly sensitive to light, whereas the pupil decreases the sensitivity by dilating and allowing more light to enter the eye.

COLOR VISION

The basic mechanism of color vision is not completely understood, but two theories predominate: Young-Helmholtz's and Hering's.

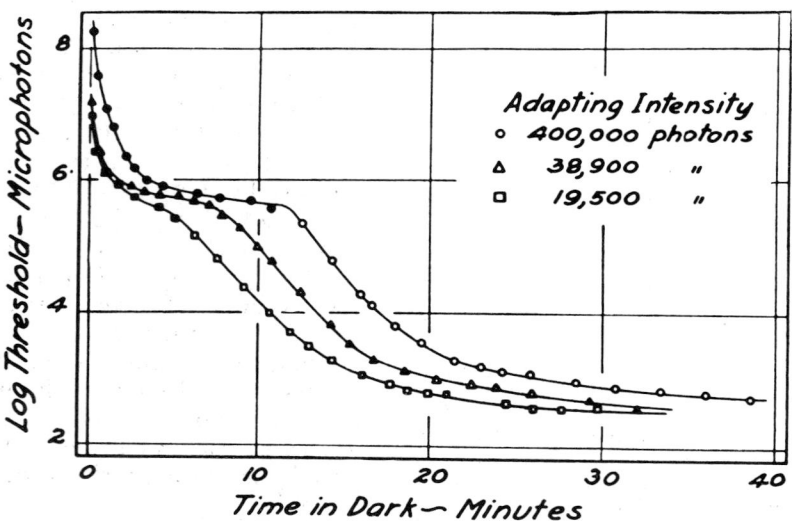

Figure IV-12 The course of dark adaptation. Since the abscissas are in log units, it is evident that the increase in sensitivity caused by dark adaptation is several thousandfold. Complete adaptation of the cones takes place in the first few minutes, and is followed by the more gradual adaptation of the rods, indicated by the break in the curve around ten minutes. (Hecht.)

Briefly, the Young-Helmholtz, or tri-chromatic, theory states that there are three different visual receptors in the retina, each receptor being sensitive primarily at a different wavelength. The appreciation of white results from the stimulation of all three receptors; black indicates lack of stimulation. There is considerable evidence that three different color sensitive pigments exist in the cones of the retina. Recently the cone cells of the carp have been impaled with microelectrodes, resulting in three distinct groups of cells being identified with maximal electrical responses at three different wavelengths — red-sensitive at 611 mμ, green-sensitive at 529 mμ, and blue-sensitive at 462 mμ. In a limited number of experiments with monkey and human cones, the light absorption characteristics of individual cells have been determined and appear to fall into three groups in accordance with the Young-Helmholtz theory.

The other major theory is the Hering, or opponent-process, theory. Three reversible processes are assumed to occur in the retina. The first has to do with the sensation of red and green. If the reaction proceeds in one direction, there is the sensation of red; if it proceeds in the opposite direction, there is green. Similarly there is a process involving the opposition of yellow and blue, and another involving black and white.

Strong evidence exists for both theories. Current feeling is that the trichromatic theory may account for the receptor stage of color vision, whereas the opponent-process theory may be involved with neural interaction at higher levels in the visual system.

People with defective color vision are described in terms of the trichromatic theory. Trichromats have all three color pigments and normal color vision. Anomalous trichromats apparently have all the color pigments but a deficiency or lack of sensitivity to one of them. A protanomalous person has a decreased sensitivity to the first substance, or red-sensitive pigment. Deuteranomalous and tritanomalous persons show decreased sensitivities to the second, or green-sensitive, pigment and third, or blue-sensitive pigment, respectively. Patients who have been called color blind completely lack the activity of one of the pigments and, therefore, are dichromats. Protanopes lack the first substance; deuteranopes lack the second substance; and tritanopes lack the third substance. Monochromats have only one cone pigment; hence, they are color blind.

INTRAOCULAR PRESSURE

The pressure within the globe is the highest in the body except for the arterial system. The average intraocular pressure for the human is about 15 mm. Hg above atmospheric pressure; the normal range is 10 to 22 mm. Hg; and a range of 22 to 25 mm. Hg is considered suspiciously high. All eyes with pressures of 25 mm. Hg or greater, however, are not necessarily abnormal or glaucomatous. Nor are all eyes with pressures under 25 mm. Hg normal. The individual variation of ocular tissues to elevated intraocular tension is considerable. A patient may have continual increases in intraocular pressure but with none of the other signs of glaucoma, such as cupping of the optic disc or changes in the visual fields. On the other hand, "normal pressures" may continually be recorded in a patient with progressive field changes. This "low tension glaucoma" may reflect an unusual intolerance of the ocular structures to intraocular pressures usually well tolerated, abnormalities in ocular rigidity, or measurements of pressure during low points of wide diurnal variations.

Intraocular pressure can be measured in three ways: palpation, tonometry, and manometry. Digital palpation is the least reliable method and is useful only for estimating large deviations from normal. Its use should be restricted to eyes with external ocular infections and to uncooperative patients, such as infants, where there is a contraindication to general anesthesia. Tonometric techniques are used almost exclusively in the clinic for estimating intraocular pressure. The most accurate means, however, is manometry. This consists of inserting a needle into the anterior, posterior, or vitreous chambers and connecting the needle by tubing to a sensitive pressure transducer. The method has limited clinical use, but it is an extremely accurate procedure in the laboratory. Manometric techniques can demonstrate changes in intraocular pressure of as much as 5 mm. Hg varying with respiration, and 1 to 2 mm. Hg varying with pulse beats.

Intraocular pressure also varies diurnally. Characteristically the pressure is highest in the morning when a person awakes, and it gradually falls during the day to reach a minimum at about 5 to 7 p.m. Although this variation seldom exceeds 3 or 4 mm. Hg in the normal eye, patients with chronic, simple glaucoma may exhibit wide pressure swings. The physiologic basis for the diurnal pressure variation is not entirely clear.

The intraocular pressure is intimately involved with aqueous humor dynamics (Fig. IV-13). About 80 per cent of the aqueous is present in the anterior chamber and the remainder in the posterior chamber. Attempts to explain the mechanisms of formation of aqueous have been clouded by several factors: the differences in techniques in measuring the constituents of the aqueous and particularly the unreliability of some of the earlier techniques; the marked differences in concentrations of substances in various species; and the difference in concentrations of substances in the anterior and posterior chambers.

Out of the mass of contradictory data is growing a concept of the formation of

aqueous. Apparently three processes are occurring between particles in the blood and in the aqueous: diffusion, ultrafiltration, and active transport. *Diffusion* refers to the tendency of molecules to distribute themselves uniformly throughout a solution. When unequal concentrations of a solution are separated by a membrane that is soluble to the solute, particles will move in both directions across the membrane, but the net movement of particles will be from the side of the higher concentration to the lower at a rate proportional to the differences in concentration. The situation is a bit more complex if the membrane between two solutions is permeable to some of the solutes, but not to others (i.e., a semipermeable membrane). For example, if an aqueous solution containing salt and protein is separated from pure water by a membrane permeable to water and salt, but not to the larger protein molecules, the process of *dialysis* will occur. In this situation the salt will travel down the concentration gradient into the pure water. Water molecules, on the other hand, will move in the opposite direction since they are in 100 per cent concentration on the side of the pure water and something less than that on the other side. The protein particles will not migrate because of the selective impermeability of the membrane.

When a hydrostatic pressure is applied to the side containing protein to accelerate the transfer of salt particles, the process is called *ultrafiltration*. Finally the terms *active transport* or *secretion* refer to the transfer of particles at the expense of cellular energy. Characteristically this process requires a substrate (e.g., glucose), an oxidizer (e.g., oxygen), and a series of enzymes which may be inhibited by cold, anoxia, or metabolic poisons.

To summarize our present state of knowledge about aqueous formation we may state that aqueous is constantly being formed and its contents altered by diffusion and ultrafiltration occurring between the capillaries of the iris and ciliary body and the aqueous. In addition, good evidence exists for the presence of active transport in the ciliary body.

The concentrations of most substances in the aqueous are approximately equal to their plasma levels (Table IV-8). Some substances, such as glucose and urea, are present in lower concentration in the aqueous

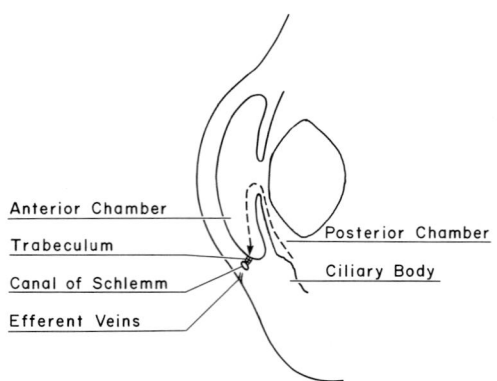

Anterior Chamber

Trabeculum

Canal of Schlemm

Efferent Veins

Posterior Chamber

Ciliary Body

Figure IV-13 Path of aqueous.

TABLE IV-8 COMPARISON OF THE CHEMICAL COMPOSITION OF AQUEOUS HUMOR AND BLOOD PLASMA OF THE RABBIT (MILLIMOLES/KG. H_2O)*

Substance	Aqueous Humor	Plasma
Na	143.5	151.5
K	5.25	5.5
Ca	1.7	2.6
Mg	0.78	1.0
Cl	109.5	108.0
HCO_3	33.6	27.4
Lactate	7.4	4.3
Pyruvate	0.66	0.22
Ascorbate	0.96	0.02
Urea	7.0	9.1
Reducing value (as glucose)	6.9	8.3

*From Davson, H. M. (ed.): The Eye. New York, The Academic Press, 1962.

than in the plasma. Utilization of these substances by the tissues of the eye or loss of the substances into the posterior portion of the globe may account for the differences in concentration. Other substances, such as ascorbic acid and hyaluronic acid, are present at much higher levels in the aqueous and are thought to be elaborated by active secretion. Chloride and bicarbonate concentrations vary among different species. These differences in ionic concentrations have prevented the acceptance of a universal theory for the production of aqueous.

BIBLIOGRAPHY

General

Adler, F. H.: Physiology of the Eye. Clinical Application. 4th ed. St. Louis, The C. V. Mosby Co., 1965.

Bonting, S. L.: Physiological chemistry of the eye. A review of papers published during 1966. Arch. Ophth. 78:803, 1967.

Bonting, S. L.: Physiological chemistry of the eye. A review of papers published during 1965. Arch. Ophth. 76:607, 1966.

Bonting, S. L.: Physiological chemistry of the eye. A review of papers published during 1964. Arch. Ophth. 74:561, 1965.

Davson, H. M. (ed.): The Eye. Vol. 1. Vegetative Physiology and Biochemistry. Vol. 2. The Visual Process. Vol. 3. Muscular Mechanisms. Vol. 4. Visual Optics and the Optical Space Sense. New York, The Academic Press, 1962.

Krause, A. C.: The Biochemistry of the Eye. Baltimore, The Johns Hopkins Press, 1934.

Linksz, A.: Physiology of the Eye. Vol. 1. Optics. Vol. 2. Vision. Vol. 3. Physiology. New York, Grune and Stratton, 1952.

Pirie, A., and Van Heyningen, R.: Biochemistry of the Eye. Springfield, Illinois, Charles C Thomas, 1956.

Ridley, F., and Sorsby, A. (eds.): Modern Trends in Ophthalmology. New York, Paul B. Hoeber, Inc., 1940.

Smelser, G. K. (ed.): The Structure of the Eye. Proceedings of symposium at 7th International Congress of anatomists, 1960. New York, Academic Press, 1961.

Cornea

Brown, S. I., and Mishima, S.: The effect of intralamellar water-impermeable membranes on corneal hydration. Arch. Ophth. 76:702, 1966.

Cogan, D. G.: Corneal vascularization. Invest. Ophth. 1:253, 1962.

Duke-Elder, S.: System of Ophthalmology. Vol. VIII, Part II. Cornea and Sclera. St. Louis, The C. V. Mosby Co., 1965.

Farris, R. L., Takahashi, G. H., and Donn, A.: Oxygen flux across the in vivo rabbit cornea. Arch. Ophth. 74:679, 1965.

Harris, J. E.: Current thoughts on the maintenance of corneal hydration in vivo. Arch. Ophth. 78:126, 1967.

Lambert, B., and Donn, A.: Effect of ouabain on active transport of sodium in the cornea. Arch. Ophth. 72:525, 1964.

Maurice, D. M.: Clinical physiology of the cornea. In Trevor-Roper, P. D. (ed.): Diseases of the Cornea. Internat. Ophth. Clinics, Vol. 2, No. 3, Boston, Little, Brown & Co., 1962.

Maurice, D. M.: The structure and transparency of the cornea. J. Physiol. 136:263, 1957.

Maurice, D. M., Zauberman, H., and Michaelson, I. C.: The stimulus to neovascularization in the cornea. Exper. Eye Res. 5:168, 1966.

Symposium on the cornea. Invest. Ophth. 1:1, 1961.

Tschetter, R. T.: Lipid analysis of the human cornea with and without arcus senilis. Arch. Ophth. 76:403, 1966.

Zucker, B. B.: Hydration and transparency of corneal stroma. Arch. Ophth. 75:228, 1965.

Lens

Bellows, J. G.: Cataract and Anomalies of the Lens. St. Louis, The C. V. Mosby Co., 1944.

Devi, A., and Raina, P. L.: Change of proteins and amino acids in the lens of the eye with progressive age and cataract formation. Current Sc. 35:13, 1966.

Harris, J. E. (ed.): Symposium on the Lens. St. Louis, The C. V. Mosby Co., 1965.

Kinoshita, J. H.: Cataracts in galactosemia. Invest. Ophth. 4:786, 1965.

Kinoshita, J. H.: Carbohydrate metabolism of lens. Arch. Ophth. 54:360, 1955.

Lerman, S.: Metabolic pathways in experimental sugar and radiation cataract. Physiol. Rev. 45:98, 1965.

Lerman, S.: Cataracts: Chemistry, Mechanisms and Therapy. Springfield, Illinois, Charles C Thomas, 1964.

Lerman, S., et al.: Further studies on the metabolism of xylose by the rat lens. Acta. Ophth. 43:764, 1965.

Lerman, S., Zigman, S., and Sa'at, Y. A.: Further

studies on nucleic acid metabolism in the lens. Am. J. Ophth. *59*:243, 1965.

Maisel, H., and Goodman, M.: The ontogeny and specificity of human lens proteins. Invest. Ophth. *4*:129, 1964.

Spector, A.: Methods of isolation of alpha, beta and gamma crystallins and their subgroups. Invest. Ophth. *3*:182, 1964.

Symposium on the Lens. Exper. Eye Res. *1*:291, 1962.

Symposium on the Lens. Invest. Ophth. *4*:377, 1965.

Vitreous

Berman, E. R., and Michaelson, K.: The chemical composition of the human vitreous body as related to age and myopia. Exper. Eye Res. *3*:9, 1964.

Extraocular Muscles and Electrical Phenomena

Bach-y-Rita, P.: Neurophysiology of extraocular muscles. Invest. Ophth. *6*:229, 1967.

Burian, H. M., and Jacobson, J. H. (eds.): Clinical Electroretinography. Proceedings of the third international symposium held October, 1964. Oxford, Pergamon Press, Ltd., 1966.

Hess, A.: The structure of vertebrate slow and twitch muscle fibers. Invest. Ophth. *6*:217, 1967.

Jacobson, J. H.: Clinical Electroretinography. Springfield, Illinois, Charles C Thomas, 1961.

Jampel, R. S.: Multiple motor systems in the extra-ocular muscles of man. Invest. Ophth. *6*:288, 1967.

Lacrimal System

Botelho, S. Y.: Tears and the lacrimal gland. Scient. Am. *211*:78, 1964.

Gasset, A. R., *et al.*: Tear glucose detection of hyperglycemia. Am. J. Ophth. *65*:414, 1968.

Jones, L. T.: The lacrimal secretory system and its treatment. Am. J. Ophth. *62*:47, 1966.

Last, R. J.: Wolff's Anatomy of the Eye and Orbit. 5th ed. Philadelphia, W. B. Saunders Co., 1961.

Mishima, S.: Some physiological aspects of the pre-corneal tear film. Arch. Ophth. *73*:233, 1965.

Mishima, S., *et al.*: Determination of tear volume and tear flow. Invest. Ophth. *5*:264, 1966.

Norn, M. S.: Lacrimal apparatus tests. Acta Ophth. *43*:557, 1965.

Retina and Sensory Mechanisms

Bonting, S. L., and Bangham, A. D.: On the biochemical mechanism of the visual process. Exper. Eye Res. *6*:400, 1967.

Brown, P. K., and Wald, G.: Visual pigments in single rods and cones of the human retina. Science *144*:45, 1964.

deReuck, A. V. A., and Knight, J. (eds.): Colour Vision-Physiology and Experimental Psychology. Boston, Little, Brown & Co., 1965.

Dowling, J. E., and Wald, G.: The biological function of vitamin A acid. Proc. Nat. Acad. Sc. USA *46*:587, 1960.

Granit, R.: Sensory Mechanisms of the Retina. London, Oxford Univ. Press, 1947.

Granit, R.: Components of the retinal action potential in mammals and their relation to the discharge in the optic nerve. J. Physiol. *77*:207, 1933.

Graymore, C. N. (ed.): Biochemistry of the Retina. New York, The Academic Press, 1965.

Hecht, S., Shlaer, S., and Pirenne, M. H.: Energy, quanta and vision. J. Gen. Physiol. *25*:819, 1942.

MacNichol, E. F., Jr.: Three-pigment color vision. Scient. Am. *211*:48, 1964.

Marks, W. B., Dobelle, W. H., and MacNichol, E. F., Jr.: Visual pigments of single primate cones. Science *143*:1181, 1964.

Pitt, G. A. J.: Modes of action of vitamin A—the present-day outlook. Biochem. J. *90*:35, 1964.

Riggs, L. A.: Electrical evidence on the trichromatic theory. Invest. Ophth. *6*:6, 1967.

Rushton, W. A. H.: Densitometry of pigments and cones of normal and color defective subjects. Invest. Ophth. *5*:233, 1966.

Stiles, W. S.: The directional sensitivity of the retina. Ann. Roy. Coll. Surgeons England *30*:73, 1962.

Wolken, J. J.: Vision: Biophysics and Biochemistry of the Retinal Photoreceptors. Springfield, Illinois, Charles C Thomas, 1966.

Intraocular Pressure and Aqueous

Becker, B.: Ouabain and aqueous humor dynamics in the rabbit eye. Invest. Ophth. *2*:325, 1963.

Becker, B.: Carbonic anhydrase and the formation of aqueous humor. Am. J. Ophth. *47*:342, 1959.

Bonting, S. L., Simon, K. A., and Hawkins, N. M.: Studies on sodium-potassium-activated adenosine triphosphatase. I. Quantitative distribution in several tissues of the cat. Arch. Biochem. *95*:416, 1961.

deBerardinis, E., *et al.*: The chemical composition of the human aqueous humor in normal and pathological conditions. Exper. Eye Res. *4*:179, 1965.

Draeger, J.: Tonometry—physical fundamentals, development of methods and clinical application. New York, Hafner Publishing Co., 1966.

Friedenwald, J.: Contribution to the theory and practice of tonometry. Am. J. Ophth. *20*:985, 1937.

Kinsey, V. E., and Reddy, D. V. N.: Chemistry and dynamics of aqueous humor. *In* Prince, J. H. (ed.): The Rabbit in Eye Research. Springfield, Illinois, Charles C Thomas, 1964.

Macri, F. J.: The pressure dependence of aqueous humor formation. Arch. Ophth. *78*:629, 1967.

Pohjola, S.: Glucose content of the aqueous humor in man. Acta Ophth. Suppl. *88*:80, 1960.

Simon, K. A., Bonting, S. L., and Hawkins, N. M.: Studies on sodium-potassium-activated adenosine triphosphatase. II. Formation of aqueous humor. Exper. Eye Res. *1*:253, 1962.

Thomas, R. P., and Riley, M. W.: Acetazolamide and ocular tension: mechanism of action. Am. J. Ophth. *60*:241, 1965.

Appendix V

Pharmacology

A great variety of drugs are either useful in treating ocular disease or have toxic effects that involve the eye. Accessibility and ease of observation have made the eye an ideal organ for the study of many drug effects, particularly those on the autonomic nervous system. Effects of adrenergic and cholinergic stimulating or blocking agents and of parasympathetic or sympathetic denervation are easily studied by observing changes in the iris, ciliary body, and intraocular pressure. Other drugs of ophthalmologic interest, including carbonic anhydrase inhibitors, osmotic diuretics, and cardiac glycosides, also alter the intraocular pressure.

The eye and its adnexa are subject to both specific and nonspecific inflammatory diseases. Most antibiotics, antiviral and antifungal agents, and corticosteroids have been used to treat these with varying results and not without complications. Prolonged use of topically applied corticosteroids, for example, may elevate the intraocular pressure. Other groups of drugs, including antihistaminics and anticoagulants, are of clinical or experimental interest in ophthalmology. It is not unusual to find that drugs used to treat ocular as well as systemic diseases have toxic effects on the eye.

DRUGS INFLUENCING THE AUTONOMIC NERVOUS SYSTEM

The autonomic nervous system consists of two major anatomical divisions: the parasympathetic (craniosacral) and the sympathetic (thoracolumbar). Functionally the division is not absolute. Autonomic nerves innervate the muscles of the iris and ciliary body as well as the blood vessels of the eye, excluding the branches of the central retinal artery, which apparently are not innervated. The iris musculature, unlike most smooth muscle, is derived embryologically from ectoderm. Only the sphincter or circular muscle of the iris becomes well defined anatomically. The dilator or radial muscle consists of smooth muscle fibers continuous with the outermost portions of the anterior layer of iris epithelial cells, from which they originate. Like smooth muscle throughout the body, the sphincter and dilator muscles receive a parasympathetic and sympathetic innervation; clinically, however, the parasympathetic innervation of the sphincter and the sympathetic innervation of the dilator are most important. Pupillary tone is maintained primarily by the sphincter, since the dilator is structurally weaker. The smooth muscle of the ciliary body is innervated by both types of nerve fibers, but the tone is maintained by the parasympathetics, with the sympathetics causing slight relaxation. The blood vessels of the conjunctiva, iris, ciliary body, and choroid, as well as those of the skin, are constricted by sympathomimetic agents and dilated by parasympathomimetic agents. These have little effect on the noninnervated retinal vessels.

Alteration of Cholinergic Effects. Since the eye is an excellent organ for studying the effects of autonomic drugs, the mechanisms by which they alter neurohumoral transmission of nerve impulses and influence the neuroeffector cells will be reviewed. Acetylcholine is the neurohumoral substance involved in transmission of the nerve impulse at four major sites in the nervous system. These are (1) the synapse of the preganglionic nerves on both sympathetic and parasympathetic ganglion cells; (2) the synapse of the axon of motoneurons at the motor end-plate of skeletal muscle; (3) the synapse of the postganglionic fiber of parasympathetic ganglion cells on smooth muscle and glands, as well as postganglionic sympathetic fibers to sweat glands and arrectores pilorum muscles; and (4) certain synapses in the central nervous system. The first two sites frequently are referred to as nicotinic, since nicotine in low doses stimulates them. The third site usually is referred to as muscarinic, for the alkaloid muscarine, like acetylcholine, stimulates these effector cells. The effect of acetylcholine at muscarinic sites is blocked by belladonna alkaloids, such as atropine or synthetic substitutes. The nicotinic sites at the motor end-plate are blocked by succinylcholine, decamethonium, or tubocurarine. At the ganglionic sites acetylcholine is blocked by tetraethylammonium or hexamethonium. In contrast to the drugs which block or mimic the effects of acetylcholine by acting at the receptor site, the anticholinesterase agents potentiate its effects by blocking the enzyme acetylcholinesterase, which normally destroys acetylcholine rapidly.

Alteration of Adrenergic Effects. The sympathetic nervous system has two types of receptor sites, alpha and beta. The alpha receptors are excitatory (e.g., vasoconstriction), whereas the beta receptors usually are inhibitory (e.g., vasodilation, ciliary body relaxation), except in the heart, where stimulation of beta receptors causes an increase in contractility and rate.

Stimulation of the postganglionic sympathetic nerves produces alpha or beta effects, depending on the relative number of alpha and beta receptors in the organ innervated. The major neurohumoral transmitter in postganglionic sympathetic nerves is the catecholamine norepinephrine. When given exogenously, its primary effect is on the alpha receptor. Epinephrine, a catecholamine derived from norepinephrine, is found predominantly in chromaffin tissue (i.e., the adrenal medulla). When it is given exogenously, it may act on both alpha and beta receptors, with the response depending on the ratio of alpha to beta receptors in the tissue and on the dose administered. Isoproterenol, apparently not a naturally occurring catecholamine, is the most potent stimulator of beta receptors known.

The precursor of norepinephrine, dopamine, is of interest to ophthalmology, for it is found in significant amounts only in the basal ganglion and the retina. In both tissues evidence suggests that it may function as a neurohumoral transmitter. The absence of dopamine from the basal ganglion in parkinsonism suggests a causative relationship. The clinical manifestations of this disease have been experimentally reduced by giving dopa, the precursor of dopamine. Unlike dopamine, dopa can penetrate the blood-brain barrier, and that which reaches the dopamine-deficient neurons found in parkinsonism is able to be converted to dopamine, the missing neurotransmitter. The defect in these neurons associated with the basal ganglion appears to be in the conversion of tyrosine to dopa. Functional abnormalities of the retina associated with changes in dopamine content currently are unknown.

Adrenergic effects may be simulated or blocked by a large number of drugs. Agents such as phenylephrine (Neosynephrine) primarily interact directly with the receptor to produce adrenergic effects, whereas ephedrine and hydroxyamphetamine release norepinephrine from nerve terminals and produce most of their adrenergic effects secondarily. Cocaine potentiates or produces adrenergic effects by blocking the transport of catecholamines back into the sympathetic postganglionic fibers. The active transport of catecholamines into the postganglionic fiber is responsible for terminating their action during synaptic transmission.

Dibenamine and phentolamine specifically block alpha receptors; dichloroisoproterenol and the newer drug, propanolol, block beta receptors by preventing the interaction of catecholamines with the receptor. Adrenergic effects also may be blocked by depleting catecholamines from the nerve terminals. Reserpine does this by blocking the uptake of catecholamines back into the nerve terminals and the granules where they are stored. Guanethidine also depletes catecholamines but does so by actively causing their release from the storage granules.

Bretylium blocks adrenergic effects not by depleting but by preventing the release of catecholamines from the nerve terminal. Agents that block the uptake of tyrosine, the precursor of norepinephrine, or that interfere with its conversion to norepinephrine, also will prevent synaptic transmission involving adrenergic receptor sites. The only well-known example of this type of agent is an experimental compound, alpha-methyl-para-tyrosine, which inhibits tyrosine hydroxylase, the rate-limiting

enzyme in the conversion of tyrosine to norepinephrine.

Alpha-methyldopa, used widely as an antihypertensive, also blocks adrenergic effects, but does this by being taken up into the nerve where it is converted into alpha-methyl-dopamine by the same enzyme system used to synthesize norepinephrine. This compound is stored in the granules like norepinephrine and is released by nerve impulses into the synaptic cleft. It is unable, however, to combine with the receptors in a way to cause depolarization. The derivative of alpha-methyldopa, alpha-methyl-dopamine, and similarly acting compounds are referred to as false neurotransmitters.

Monoamine oxidase and catechol-o-methyl transferase are the major enzymes in metabolizing catecholamines, but they have little physiologic importance in terminating the action of catecholamines during synaptic transmission. Monoamine oxidase acts primarily intracellularly, whereas catechol-o-methyl transferase is found extracellularly. Inhibitors of both these enzymes have been described. Pyrogallol

TABLE V-1 SITE OF ACTION OF REPRESENTATIVE DRUGS INFLUENCING GANGLIA AND NEUROEFFECTOR SITES

Drug Action	Neuroeffector Sites			Autonomic Ganglia
	Adrenergic	*Cholinergic Autonomic*	*Neuromuscular*	
Release neurohumoral transmitter.	Ephedrine, Hydroxyamphetamine Reserpine.* Guanethidine.*			
Interfere with destruction of neurohumoral transmitter.	MAO and COMT inhibitors.	Anticholinesterase agents.	Anticholinesterase agents.	Anticholinesterase agents.
Stimulate postsynaptic sites.	Norepinephrine, Epinephrine, Isoproterenol, Phenylephrine.	Acetylcholine, Muscarine, Pilocarpine	Acetylcholine, Nicotine (initial effect).	Acetylcholine, Nicotine (initial effect).
Block postsynaptic sites.	Dibenamine and phentolamine block alpha receptors; dichloroisoproterenol blocks beta receptors.	Atropine; synthetic atropine-like drugs.	Succinylcholine, Decamethonium, Tubocurarine.	Tetraethyl-ammonium, Hexamethonium.

*Adrenergic blockade is major effect.

inhibits catechol-o-methyl transferase but has no clinical applicability. Iproniazid, nialamide, and other drugs that inhibit monoamine oxidase are used to treat depressions. Although the overall mechanism of their clinical action is unknown, they do increase the intracellular content of catecholamines.

Table V-1 summarizes the effects of some of the drugs just discussed.

Parasympathomimetic Agents. Used topically on the eye for their muscarinic effects, these agents cause miosis, contraction of the ciliary body resulting in increased accommodation, dilatation of the conjunctival and uveal blood vessels with a decrease in the blood-aqueous barrier, and increased facility of outflow of aqueous. The latter of these is the most obscure. The increased facility of outflow has been attributed variously to the pull of the iris and ciliary body upon the scleral spur to stretch the trabecular meshwork, dilatation of the collector channels and veins peripheral to the canal of Schlemm, and a direct effect on muscarinic sites in the trabecular meshwork.

Parasympathomimetic agents may be divided into two groups: congeners of acetylcholine and cholinomimetic alkaloids. Four drugs that are congeners of acetylcholine are methacholine, carbamylcholine, bethanechol, and furthrethonium. Currently some of them are used clinically. All have a quaternary nitrogen, and, therefore, they poorly penetrate lipid membranes such as the corneal epithelium. In addition, the high concentration of acetylcholinesterase in the nerve plexus of the cornea, iris, and ciliary body rapidly limits the effect of exogenously applied acetylcholine. By direct application onto the surface of the iris, however, this drug has been used to cause pupillary constriction after cataract extraction.

Methacholine is hydrolyzed by acetylcholinesterase at one third of the rate of acetylcholine; therefore its action in decreasing intraocular pressure in open angle glaucoma is too brief to be of much use clinically. A 2.5 per cent solution of methacholine commonly is used to test for denervation supersensitivity of the iris, which is discussed later in this section. Carbamylcholine is not hydrolyzed by any cholinesterases and may be used as a 0.75 to 3 per cent solution in place of pilocarpine when patients have developed allergy or tolerance to that drug. Systemic administration may be hazardous because carbamylcholine not only acts at muscarinic sites but also has the most marked nicotinic effect of any of the parasympathomimetic agents. This probably is associated with the ability of carbamylcholine to release acetylcholine from nerve terminals.

Bethanechol, 1 per cent, has been used in the therapy of open angle glaucoma, but it has no advantages over pilocarpine or carbamylcholine. Furthrethonium, which also is not hydrolyzed by acetylcholinesterase, was used for glaucoma some years ago. Its use was abandoned, however, because in many instances it caused conjunctival irritation with obstruction of the canaliculi and lacrimal duct.

Of the three agents in the group of cholinomimetic alkaloids (muscarine, arecoline, and pilocarpine), only pilocarpine is used clinically in the United States. Muscarine is the prototype for the parasympathomimetic agents. Until it was synthesized a few years ago only crude preparations were available. Like the congeners of acetylcholine, muscarine has a quarternary nitrogen that is associated with poor lipid membrane permeability. This, in addition to its impure form, has limited its use in ophthalmology. Arecoline has stimulatory effects at nicotinic and central nervous system sites as well as muscarinic sites. It has been used topically for the therapy of glaucoma in certain European countries, but it is very irritating. Pilocarpine is by far the most widely used parasympathomimetic agent for the treatment of glaucoma. It was extracted originally from the leaves of a tropical shrub, *Pilocarpus jaborandi*, and its action on the pupil and ciliary muscle was reported as early as 1875. It is stable, almost exclusively muscarinic, and penetrates the cornea well when used topically. A solution of 0.5 to 4 per cent usually is prescribed.

Anticholinesterase Agents. These agents block the action of the cholinesterase enzymes, thereby preventing destruction of acetylcholine, which then builds up at both nicotinic and muscarinic sites. The results of systemic administration of anticholinesterase agents depend upon the dose, the relative excess and types of cholinesterases at the synaptic area, and the predominate tone of the organ. Two types of cholinesterases are known:

1. True, or acetylcholinesterase, which hydrolyzes acetylcholine more rapidly than other choline esters and is associated with neural elements and red blood cells. Acetylcholine appears to be its physiologic substrate.

2. A heterogeneous group of enzymes called nonspecific or butyrocholinesterases. These hydrolyze butyrylcholine or other long-chained choline esters more rapidly than acetylcholine. Their function or physiologic substrates are unknown, but they are made by the liver and are found in the plasma and in glial cells.

In ophthalmology anticholinesterase agents are used topically to produce the same muscarinic effects seen with parasympathomimetic agents. They generally are used when parasympathomimetic preparations have proved to be inadequate or where tolerance has developed. Since they allow acetylcholine, the naturally occurring neurohumor, to act at the receptor site, their effect usually is greater than that seen with the nonphysiologic cholinomimetics. Topical application may involve systemic absorption. In many pa-

tients treated topically with anticholinesterases, the serum and red blood cell cholinesterases are decreased. With frequent application these agents may produce gastrointestinal toxicity, usually diarrhea. Bradycardia and bronchospasm occur less frequently. Ocular side effects include iris cysts at the pupillary border (which rarely interfere with vision), brow ache secondary to spasm of the ciliary body and sphincter pupillae, and engorgement of the blood vessels of the conjunctiva, iris, and ciliary body. The engorgement of the iris vessels may be sufficient to compromise an already narrow angle and thereby precipitate angle closure glaucoma.

Acetylcholinesterase has two closely apposed reaction sites, the anionic and the esteratic (Fig. V-1). The anionic site has a negative charge and forms a weak ionic bond with the quarternary nitrogen of acetylcholine.

Agents such as edrophonium that act exclusively at the anionic site are rapidly reversible. Thus, although edrophonium is used for diagnostic purposes, as in myasthenia gravis, its action is too brief to be useful therapeutically.

The esteratic site forms a covalent bond

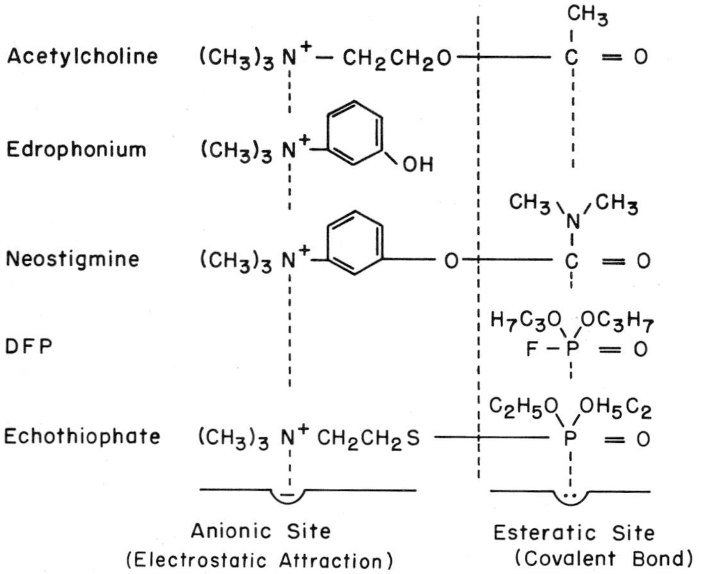

Figure V-1 Structure and site of action of cholinesterase inhibitors.

with the esteratic carbon of acetylcholine, thus allowing the choline portion to split off. With the acetate from acetylcholine, the covalent bond is relatively weak and easily hydrolyzed by water. The bond to the carbamyl ion of such drugs as physostigmine is more stable, however, and carbamyl ester compounds form the group of slowly reversible anticholinesterase agents. Several such substances are well known.

Physostigmine (eserine) was the first miotic used in the treatment of glaucoma and still is occasionally prescribed. It may be used to supplement the action of pilocarpine in chronic simple glaucoma and to cause miosis during an acute attack of narrow angle glaucoma. Over long periods of time it tends to produce an irritative follicular conjunctivitis. Neostigmine (prostigmine), a synthetic analogue of eserine, also may be used to treat glaucoma, and it is the standard drug for the therapy of myasthenia gravis against which newer agents are compared.

Demarcarium bromide consists of two neostigmine molecules attached together. Demarcarium is so structured that it may attach at two anionic and esteratic sites, a property making it a longer-acting and more potent agent than the other carbamyl ester compounds. It is widely used.

Another group of anticholinesterase agents are the organophosphorous compounds. Their action is irreversible because of the strong covalent bond formed between the esteratic site and the phosphorous portion of the organophosphorous molecule. Many compounds of this class have been synthesized and are used as insecticides. Two compounds, diisopropyl phosphorofluoridate (DFP) and echothiophate, are used in the United States in the treatment of glaucoma. DFP was developed during World War II, when it was first used in clinical trials. It forms an extremely stable bond at the esteratic site only. It is no longer commonly used, however, since it is unstable in aqueous solution and must be given in peanut oil, which tends to blur the patient's vision. Furthermore, a very small amount of moisture entering the oily solution, such as tears on the eye-dropper, causes hydrolysis of the DFP. Echothiophate, an organophosphorous nucleus attached to thiocholine, is stable in aqueous solution. It forms bonds at both the anionic and esteratic sites. The thiocholine portion is split off rapidly, but the bond at the esteratic site is very stable for long periods. Echothiophate usually is administered every 12 hours as a 0.06 to 0.25 per cent solution.

Because use of the long-acting organophosphorous agents may result in toxic effects due to systemic absorption or accidental poisoning, pharmacologists have devised compounds able to reverse their action. Hydroxyl amine ($HONH_2$) was observed to react with the organophosphorous moiety attached to the esteratic site. The phosphoro-esteratic site bond is weakened and ultimately breaks. Based on this observation, a number of other compounds have been synthesized that fit the cholinesterase-organophosphorous complex sterically. The most commonly used of these agents is pralidoxime (2-PAM), which has been given subconjunctivally and intracamerally to reverse the effects of DFP and echothiophate. Theoretically, after the organophosphorous compound has been present for a few hours, pralidoxime is unable to cause reversal, for a molecular rearrangement occurs making the complex nonreactive with it. The apparent reversal reported clinically may well be due to the inherent sympathomimetic action of pralidoxime.

Antimuscarinics. These drugs block the muscarinic action of acetylcholine or other parasympathomimetic agents. They paralyze the sphincter of the iris, causing pupillary dilatation (mydriasis), and block accommodation by paralyzing the ciliary muscle (cycloplegia).

Atropine, a belladonna alkaloid, is the prototype drug. It is used where maximum paralysis of the ciliary body is indicated. This includes the treatment of anterior uveitis as well as the refraction of young children, especially those with accommodative esotropia. Atropine is extremely long-acting, with mydriasis and cycloplegia lasting from 7 to 12 days. Synthetic substances acting for shorter periods may be used for refraction and fundus examination. These include homatropine, cyclopentolate, and tropicamide.

Homatropine, an atropine-like compound used in 1 to 5 per cent solution to produce mydriasis and cycloplegia, requires one to two days for complete recovery. Cyclopentolate (Cyclogel), available in 0.5 to 2 per cent solution, produces cycloplegia and mydriasis in 20 to 30 minutes with recovery in from 2 to 24 hours. A well-known, but rare, side effect is the precipitation of a transient, acute psychosis in children. Tropicamide (Mydriacyl) has the most rapid onset of action, approximately 15 minutes, and its effect usually lasts only from one-half to four hours. It is useful in refraction, for fundus examination, and in photography.

The synthetic drugs are remarkably free from side effects. Atropine, however, frequently causes toxic reactions, particularly when it is used to obtain cycloplegia in young children. They include a rash, particularly over the face, neck, and upper part of the trunk; a hot, dry, and flushed skin; thirst; and tachycardia. They reverse rapidly on cessation of the drug. Significant overdoses can result in delirium and a high temperature. In adults who use atropine for conditions such as anterior uveitis, contact dermatitis is not uncommon. In those patients sensitive to atropine, scopolamine may be substituted. This drug is similar to atropine in its effect on the eye, with the duration of cycloplegia lasting up to seven days, but the incidence of idiosyncratic reactions, however, is higher than with atropine.

Sympathomimetic Agents. These drugs are used to dilate the pupil for funduscopic examinations when cycloplegic drugs are not desired; to supplement cycloplegic drugs for maximal dilatation, especially to prevent posterior synechiae in chronic anterior uveitis; and to treat open angle glaucoma by decreasing aqueous secretion and increasing the facility of outflow. Additionally, many proprietary eye preparations contain sympathomimetic agents to cause constriction of the conjunctival vessels and thereby whiten the eye.

Both epinephrine and phenylephrine (Neosynephrine) are used because they act directly on the alpha receptors in the eye. Epinephrine in a 1 or 2 per cent solution penetrates the eye with incredible speed. It is used in the therapy of open angle glaucoma either alone or combined with the parasympathomimetic or anticholinesterase agents. It apparently decreases aqueous formation by decreasing the blood flow through the ciliary processes and also increases the outflow facility. Progressive increase in the facility of outflow seems to occur with continued therapy. A firm understanding of how epinephrine increases outflow is lacking. Currently, however, it appears related to stimulation of adrenergic receptors in the angle structures, but irrefutable evidence for this has not been obtained, and other mechanisms may be involved. Many patients develop a local hypersensitivity to the degradation products of epinephrine, and plaques of conjunctival pigmentation are not unusual.

Phenylephrine, also a direct-acting sympathomimetic amine, is used for its alpha effect on the dilator muscle of the iris to produce pupillary dilatation. Occasionally it is combined with the anticholinesterase agents to help prevent the formation of iris cysts that are associated with such drugs; possibly it acts by reducing the traction of the sphincter muscle of the iris on the epithelial layer of the iris. In cases of sympathetic denervation of Müller's muscle, as seen in Horner's syndrome, applying phenylephrine to the conjunctiva elevates the lid.

Indirect-acting sympathomimetics include ephedrine and hydroxyamphetamine (Paredrine). Both act by releasing norepinephrine from the nerve terminals. They have been used for pupillary dilatation, but only hydroxyamphetamine is available currently.

Adrenergic Blockade. Adrenergic effects may be blocked by several methods. These include directly interfering with the reaction between catecholamines and the receptor substance, either alpha or beta; preventing the release of catecholamines by nerve stimulation, either by depleting the nerve terminal of its stores or by stabilizing the membrane of the nerve terminal so that the catecholamines cannot be released; preventing the uptake or conversion of tyrosine to a catecholamine; and synthesizing a false neurotransmitter. A number of drugs of this group have been tried in the treatment of glaucoma. In general they lower intraocular pressure, but the results have not been sufficiently encouraging to justify continuing their use.

Dibenamine is a specific and long-acting alpha blocker that is believed to decrease aqueous formation. It was used before carbonic anhydrase inhibitors and osmotic diuretics to decrease the intraocular pressure in acute glaucoma. For satisfactory results intravenous administration was required, and this was commonly followed by thrombophlebitis or tissue necrosis. Orthostatic hypotension occurred in most patients, requiring them to remain in bed for at least 24 hours. Confusion and even hallucinations in older patients were not uncommon. Tolazoline, also an alpha blocker, is used primarily for its *direct* vasodilating effect. It may be given by retrobulbar injection to dilate the central retinal artery in arterial occlusions. Although the ergot alkaloids also block alpha receptors, they usually are used for their *direct* stimulatory (vasoconstrictive) effect on smooth muscle. This may be observed as a miosis. Most commonly, they are used to relieve migraine. The ergot alkaloids, ergotamine particularly, is believed to relieve the headache by directly causing vasoconstriction of the cranial arteries. The symptoms of migraine have been attributed to an increased pulsation of those vessels.

Reserpine and guanethidine both deplete the intracellular stores of catecholamines. Both are able to decrease the intraocular pressure, although the mechanism is not known. When guanethidine is applied topically as a 10 per cent solution, miosis and a decrease in intraocular pressure occur. A transient mydriasis and an increase in pressure may occur first, secondary to the initial sympathomimetic effects of guanethidine. The decrease in intraocular pressure is seen in both normal and glaucomatous eyes, and an increase in facility of outflow has been demonstrated. Guanethidine also has been employed for lid retraction due to an apparent increased sympathetic tone as seen in Müller's muscle in hyperthyroidism. When applied topically

the stimulation of Müller's muscle is decreased, since there is a lessened release of norepinephrine from the adrenergic nerves that innervate it, and the upper lid lowers.

The agents that form false neurotransmitters include alpha-methyldopa. After this drug is given, the systemic arterial pressure is reduced, accompanied by a slight reduction of intraocular pressure. This drug is of no therapeutic value in ophthalmology.

Ganglionic Blockade. This group of drugs is largely of theoretical interest in ophthalmology. They decrease systemic blood pressure and through this action might favorably influence hypertensive retinopathy. Mydriasis and conjunctival injection occur with systemic administration. Tearing and accommodation are decreased. The intraocular pressure also is decreased, probably due to diminished aqueous secretion that is most likely secondary to the fall in blood pressure. An important side effect has been blindness from very precipitous decreases in blood pressure.

Neuromuscular Blockade. The extraocular muscle and tensor tympani contain both fast and slow muscle fibers. This is unique for mammalian musculature, for all other muscles have only fast fibers. These two types of fibers differ innervationally, histologically, biochemically, and pharmacologically. In lower vertebrates, such as the frog, these two types of muscle fibers are anatomically separate (i.e., rectus abdominus is slow, gastrocnemius is fast). Therefore, they have been studied most widely in that animal. Neuromuscular blocking agents may be (1) competitive blockers, typified by d-tubocurarine, which compete with acetylcholine for receptor sites at the subneural apparatus of the motor end-plate, and (2) depolarizing blockers, which cause an initial depolarization at the receptor site as does acetylcholine, but this persists and spreads to adjacent regions of the muscle fiber so that it becomes unexcitable. It remains so even after the depolarization is terminated. Decamethonium and succinylcholine are the two commonly used agents of the second type.

Both types of agents produce flaccid paralysis of fast muscle fibers. Decamethonium and succinylcholine produce a prolonged contracture of slow muscle, whereas d-tubocurarine produces flaccid paralysis of slow muscle. With mixed muscles, such as the extraocular, the use of d-tubocurarine results in a flaccid paralysis with little effect upon intraocular pressure. The depolarizing type of agents, such as succinylcholine, however, paralyzes the twitch response characteristic of fast muscle, and at the same time markedly increases the overall tone of the muscle due to contracture of the slow muscle fibers. Depolarizing agents, therefore, may cause a marked rise in intraocular pressure by increasing extraocular muscle tone. This can be very dangerous to the eye during intraocular surgery.

The anesthesiologist should know which patients are receiving anticholinesterase agents topically. Succinylcholine depends upon butyrocholinesterases to hydrolyze it to succinate and acetate ions, and thereby to terminate its activity. In many patients receiving anticholinesterases topically, the serum butyrocholinesterase is depressed, and if succinylcholine is given to these patients, prolonged apnea may result. Likewise, several familial forms of atypical butyrocholinesterases will not hydrolyze succinylcholine. Before he uses this agent, the physician should be aware of any family history that the patient may have of prolonged apnea associated with the use of succinylcholine.

Evaluation of Autonomic Denervations. Cannon, in his law of denervation, stated, "When in a series of efferent neurons a unit is destroyed, an increased contractility to chemical agents develops in the isolated structure or structures, the effect being maximal in the part denervated." This commonly is known as supersensitization. These effects are easily observed in pupillary responses following sympathetic or

parasympathetic denervation of the eye. Adie's (tonic) pupil (p. 18), because of its response to methacholine (Mecholyl), is thought to result from a partial parasympathetic denervation. The pupil constricts to a 2.5 per cent methacholine solution, a concentration less than a quarter of that normally causing constriction. This phenomenon of supersensitivity is explained, at least for some cholinergic sites, by the spread of receptor sites over the effector cell after the nerves have degenerated. This results in a greater area sensitive to parasympathomimetic agents. Although Adie's syndrome usually is considered the prime example of such supersensitivity, the phenomenon also has been noted after trauma to the orbit or eye and has been associated with chronic iritis.

The classic example of sympathetic denervation is Horner's syndrome. This may be due to preganglionic denervation of the superior cervical ganglion or to destruction of the ganglion or its postganglionic fibers. Many times the type of denervation can be identified pharmacologically by studying the responses to a variety of drugs. The preganglionic type (decentralization) has a nonspecific supersensitivity to both direct- and indirect-acting sympathomimetics and, as a result, a concentration of 1:1000 epinephrine, which normally does not cause mydriasis, may cause dilatation of the decentralized pupil. Since the nerve fibers from the ganglion to the iris are intact and contain catecholamine in the decentralized type, tyramine, hydroxyamphetamine, and other indirect-acting sympathomimetics

TABLE V-2   RESPONSE OF THE IRIS TO SYMPATHOMIMETICS

	Normal	Decentralized	Denervated
Direct acting sympathomimetic, e.g., epinephrine 1:1000.	0	+ or −	+
Indirect acting sympathomimetic, e.g., hydroxyamphetamine 1%.	+	+	0
Cocaine.	+	+	0

+ = dilatation; 0 = no response

will cause mydriasis. Cocaine, 2 per cent solution, normally causes mydriasis and also gives mydriasis in a sympathetically decentralized iris. Sympathetic denervation of the iris is also associated with supersensitivity. This apparently consists of the decentralization response to epinephrine plus the effect normally seen with cocaine. (Since there are no longer postganglionic fibers to take up the catecholamine, the same effect is achieved as when cocaine is given.)

Supersensitivity in the denervation type of Horner's syndrome is only to direct-acting sympathomimetics. It usually is more marked than that seen with decentralization. Although the application of these principles is of pharmacologic interest, roentgenograms of the chest clinically differentiate the more serious causes of Horner's syndrome (in general, initially preganglionic) from the benign (ganglionic) (Table V-2).

OCULAR HYPOTENSIVE AGENTS OTHER THAN AUTONOMIC DRUGS

A variety of substances other than autonomic drugs are used to lower the intraocular pressure. Some are used for long-term therapy; others only for acute phases of glaucoma.

Carbonic Anhydrase Inhibitors. Carbonic anhydrase is found in many organs of the body, including the kidney, eye, and gastric mucosa. It catalyzes the reaction between carbon dioxide and water to form carbonic acid. The dissociation of carbonic acid to hydrogen and bicarbonate ions is instantaneous and independent of enzymatic acceleration. Where found, carbonic anhydrase seemingly is involved in secretory processes.

After sulfa drugs were introduced for clinical use, one side effect noted was a metabolic acidosis. Studies revealed that sulfonamides inhibited carbonic anhydrase, preventing the secretion of hydrogen ions into the urine in exchange for sodium. This led to the development of a group of drugs having greater specificity and effectiveness than sulfonamides in inhibiting carbonic anhydrase. These agents are used in the treatment of glaucoma. A dose sufficient to inhibit almost all the carbonic anhydrase enzyme of the ciliary body causes aqueous secretion to be reduced approximately in half. Since the outflow of aqueous is unchanged, the intraocular pressure falls. This mechanism is not yet precisely understood. The most obvious one, however, is reduction in secretion of bicarbonate ion into the posterior chamber. This would reduce the amount of osmotically active substances in the aqueous and, therefore, less water would be drawn into the posterior chamber. In the rabbit, bicarbonate is in excess and is the most osmotically important anion when compared with plasma. In man, however, chloride seems to be the anion in excess. Other suggested mechanisms include a vasoconstriction of the ciliary arteries, stimulation of beta receptors in the eye, and a general poisoning of active transport.

Acetazolamide (Diamox), available in 250 mg. tablets given two to four times per day, is the most widely used carbonic anhydrase inhibitor. Other preparations include methazolamide (Neptazane), effective in one fourth to one third the dose of acetazolamide, ethoxzolamide (Cardrase), effective in one fourth to one half the dose, and dichlorphenamide (Daranide), effective in two fifths to four fifths the dose. When orally administered, the ocular effects of these drugs are noted in one to two hours and persist four to six hours. A "sequel" form of Diamox is available so that one dose of 500 mg. is released over an 8 to 12 hour period. The kidney excretes the drugs unchanged. Side effects include paresthesias, anorexia, gastrointestinal disturbances, skin eruptions, bone marrow depression, confusion, hypokalemia, and ureteral stones with renal colic.

Carbonic anhydrase inhibitors are most useful for short-term therapy, such as in secondary glaucomas and for acute attacks of narrow angle glaucoma. They are used for long-term therapy of chronic simple glaucoma, but there is a high failure because of intolerable side effects and their inability to control the intraocular pressure in many instances. They may be used to lower intraocular pressure preoperatively and thereby possibly help to reduce vitreous volume so as to prevent vitreous loss. Postoperatively they may be used to treat flat anterior chambers by reducing aqueous secretion and allowing wound leaks to seal.

Osmotic Diuretics. When the osmolarity of the blood is increased, water is drawn from the tissues to maintain osmotic equilibrium. In the eye, fluid is drawn from the aqueous and probably from the vitreous as well, which rather markedly reduces intraocular pressure. An ideal agent should not penetrate tissues well, should be metabolized or excreted slowly, and should be of a low molecular weight to permit as small a dose as possible. The most commonly used substances are urea, mannitol, and glycerol. About equally effective in reducing the intraocular pressure, they are especially useful in acute stages of narrow angle glaucoma. The reduced pressure allows the iris musculature to respond to miotic agents, with opening of the angle. Osmotic agents also are useful in intraocular surgery in reducing the intraocular volume, thereby helping to prevent vitreous loss and other complications. Their brief action makes them of little or no use in chronic simple (open angle) glaucoma, but they can be of great value in some secondary glaucomas, especially with traumatic hyphemas.

Urea is administered intravenously (oral therapy is effective but unpalatable) as a 30 per cent solution in 10 per cent invert sugar for a total of 1 to 1.5 gm./kg. of body weight. The invert sugar prevents hemolysis of red blood cells. It must be given slowly into a large vein to prevent thrombophlebitis and given with extreme care to prevent extravasations that can cause tissue necrosis and sloughing. The intraocular pressure usually falls within one half hour, and the hypotensive effects persist for five hours. The anterior chamber may deepen by up to 0.2 mm. after the infusion. Urea penetrates into the eye slowly. Two hours after infusion the aqueous concentration is only about one third that of the plasma. With the usual dose of urea and normal renal function, the blood urea nitrogen requires 24 hours to return to normal levels.

Unfortunately intravenous urea therapy is accompanied by certain problems. Marked reduction in the cerebrospinal fluid pressure often causes a severe headache, which is more marked if the infusion is given rapidly. If nausea and vomiting, which frequently occur, are not controlled by antiemetics, surgery may have to be postponed. Long operative procedures may require catheterization because of the associated diuresis. Acute pulmonary edema may occur in elderly patients with borderline cardiac compensation.

Mannitol has a molecular weight approximately three times that of urea, but unlike urea remains exclusively in the extracellular fluid. Therefore, its osmotic effect per gram as compared with urea is greater than that postulated on a molar basis. As with urea, its maximum hypotensive effect occurs in one half hour and lasts six hours. The usual dose is 2 gm./kg. as a 20 per cent solution that must be given intravenously, for mannitol is not absorbed from the gastrointestinal tract. It also is not metabolized and is excreted by glomerular filtration. Diuresis and headache may be as severe as with urea, but mannitol does not cause tissue necrosis when infiltrated.

Glycerol is the easiest to use and the best tolerated of these agents. The usual dose is 1 to 1.5 gm./kg. of body weight given orally as a 50 per cent solution with lemon juice. It is rapidly absorbed from the gastrointestinal tract and distributes through body water at about one sixth the rate of urea. It is a naturally occurring component of lipids and is metabolized by the body as a carbohydrate. After oral administration, the intraocular pressure begins to drop in 10 minutes and is lowest by 30 minutes. Hypotension persists for approximately five hours. The most annoying side effects are nausea and headache. Recently a new oral hyperosmolar agent, isosorbide, has been tried clinically. It is similar chemically to mannitol, but like urea it distributes throughout the body water. Since it is not metabolized, it may be used in patients who are on limited caloric intake, where glycerol may be contraindicated. Headaches and other side effects occur, but the incidence of nausea is much lower than with glycerol. The drug should be used with care, however, because its long-term intracellular effects have not been investigated.

Cardiac Glycosides. Although not accepted clinically because of possible toxic effects, digitalis preparations decrease intraocular pressure. This drug presumably blocks the Na—K activated ATPase of the ciliary body that is required for aqueous secretion. To obtain any effect requires full digitalization, and with it aqueous production can be decreased by as much as 45 per cent. A slight additive effect occurs when digitalis preparations are used with acetazolamide. Topical ointments also are effective, but their use is associated with a painful keratopathy.

Oral Contraceptives. The agent, norethynodrel with mestranol (Enovid), produced a statistically significant decrease in intraocular pressure in double-blind studies on patients with open angle glaucoma. The decrease occurred irrespective of whether or not the individuals were on standard glaucoma medications simultaneously. The effects persisted for as long as six weeks after oral contraceptives were terminated. Insufficient knowledge of side effects in older age groups does not warrant its routine use as an adjunct to standard glaucoma therapy at the present time.

Alcohol. The consumption of 50 ml. of alcohol (ethanol) in the form of whiskey has little effect on intraocular pressure in normal individuals. In patients with open angle glaucoma, however, this amount of alcohol causes a decrease of up to 30 mm./Hg. within one hour, which has been reported to persist for up to two to three hours. Besides not being therapeutically useful, consumption of alcohol by the patient before examinations may obscure the diagnosis of glaucoma.

CHEMOTHERAPEUTIC AGENTS

Ocular tissues are subject to the same bacteria, viruses, fungi, and parasites that produce infections elsewhere in the body. Additionally, organisms that produce systemic infections may have unique effects on ocular tissue (i.e., herpes simplex infection of the cornea), whereas other organisms such as the trachoma virus and adenovirus type 8 that produces epidemic keratoconjunctivitis primarily involve ocular tissues. However, the same chemotherapeutic agents are useful in ocular infections as are used in infections elsewhere in the body. Because of the accessibility of the eye and the high incidence of superficial extraocular infections, topical chemotherapy usually is the method of choice. The anterior chamber may be reached by topical drugs, but intraocular infections in general are treated by combining systemic and topical drugs. Epithelial abrasions facilitate the penetration of topical chemotherapeutic agents into the anterior chamber, and the breakdown of the blood aqueous barrier that accompanies intraocular inflammation facilitates system chemotherapy.

Antibacterial Agents. The general principles of antibacterial therapy discussed in most textbooks of medicine are applicable to ophthalmology, and the reader is referred to those sources. Antibacterial agents are administered topically whenever feasible, utilizing agents too toxic for systemic use. This avoids the chance of the patient becoming sensitized to commonly used systemic agents. The notable exceptions to this general rule are chloramphenicol and sulfonamides, for there is evidence to suggest that these penetrate the eye more effectively than other antibacterials. In bacterial infections of deeper ocular tissues and in dangerous superficial infections, such as Pseudomonas corneal ulcers, systemic antibiotics are combined with topical agents.

Table V-3 lists the frequently used antibacterials, their dose, spectrum, and side effects.

Antifungal Agents. As in other fields of medicine, ophthalmology is encountering an increase in the incidence of fungal diseases associated with the widespread use of antibiotics and steroids. Fungal infections may involve the cornea, the uveal tract, or give a picture of an endophthalmitis. No particular fungi have a predilection for the eye. The diagnosis usually is made late, after there is no response to antibacterial therapy. Fungi are slow-growing organisms, and their response to antifungal agents that block their metabolism is likewise slow. Much of the damage to ocular tissue is not due to direct invasion of the fungi, but to the production of toxins that continue to destroy tissue even after the fungi have been destroyed.

Superficial fungal infections, such as

keratitis, usually are treated by a combination of systemic and topical therapy; for deep infections topical therapy is useless. Amphotericin B, which has a rather broad spectrum, is the most effective agent available for clinical use. It appears to attach to the fungal cell membrane and to block the transport of materials into the cell while allowing potassium and smaller molecules to leave. The final result is a blockade of cellular respiration and utilization of glucose. Amphotericin B may be used topically as a 1 to 3 per cent solution or as a 3 per cent ointment, but for deep or severe infections it must also be given systemically, since its penetration is extremely poor. The systemic dose is given intravenously over a six hour period starting at 0.25 to 0.40 mg./kg. per day diluted in dextrose and distilled water. The dose is increased gradually until toxic signs appear. Then it is decreased slightly and maintained at that level, hopefully at least 1 mg./kg. per day, but not over 1.5 mg./kg. per day. Toxicity is manifested by headache, nausea, vomiting, and increasing blood urea nitrogen. Occasionally the drug may be injected intracamerally, but such injections are associated with a moderately severe inflammatory reaction and generally are to be avoided.

Nystatin is a second wide-spectrum, antifungal agent that is especially useful against Candida. It is used topically. Systemic administration generally is not helpful because adequate intraocular levels are not attained. Intraocular administration causes a severe inflammatory response and therefore is hazardous. Thimerosal and iodide may be used topically in fungal keratitis. Sulfacetamide, in a solution of 15 per cent or greater, is effective against Nocardia and Actinomyces.

Antiviral Agents. In 1962 the antimetabolite 5-iodo-2'-deoxyuridine (IDU) was used clinically without ill effect to inhibit virus multiplication, and thus it became the first useful antiviral agent available. In some types of cancer cells it blocks the final phosphorylation of thymidine and its polymerization into DNA. On the basis of this evidence, investigators felt that it might be active against various nucleotide kinases and polymerases that are required for specific viral DNA formation and are stimulated in cells by viral infections. Apparently IDU inhibits the viral-induced

enzymes with some selectivity but does not affect the normal synthetic processes that form DNA in the cell. Tissue repair, therefore, proceeds normally in the presence of IDU.

IDU has been used to treat herpes simplex (dendritic) keratitis. It can be prescribed as a 0.1 per cent solution or ointment (its maximum solubility), although higher concentrations would be desirable. This concentration, although nontoxic to the corneal epithelium, is only slightly higher than that needed to inhibit the most sensitive herpes simplex viruses. More resistant virus strains do not respond. Since continued presence of antimetabolite is necessary to prevent virus multiplication, IDU must be given frequently day and night to be effective. Failure to respond to it possibly can be explained by virus strains that have acquired resistance to it, just as bacteria have to antibiotics. Furthermore, the poor penetration of IDU into ocular and other tissues might allow herpes simplex keratitis to reactivate as a result of the excretion of active virus from the tissues not affected by the drug.

IDU also has been suggested to prevent reactivation of virus multiplication in the epithelium when steroid therapy is deemed necessary. Experimental evidence has shown that the disciform keratitis and herpes simplex iritis may result from toxic or allergic response to the virus products. These conditions can be suppressed with steroids, but viral reactivation always is a threat. Some investigators claim that combined therapy is effective in preventing reactivation.

Other antiviral agents include cytosine arabinoside and the thiosemicarbazones. The former appears to block the metabolism and incorporation of cytosine similarly to the way that IDU blocks thymidine. It has advantages and disadvantages over IDU. Viruses resistant to IDU remain sensitive to cytosine arabinoside and highly potent concentrations of it can be prepared. Unfortunately it is less selective than IDU, can damage normal corneal cells, and, in high concentrations, causes marked corneal toxicity.

(*Text continues on page 492*)

TABLE V-3 FREQUENTLY USED ANTIBACTERIALS

Drug	Dose	Spectrum	Side Effects
Penicillin G.	200,000 to 400,000 U. q. 4 to 6 hrs. (o.)†; 300,000 U. q. 4 to 6 hrs. (i.m.); may go as high as 20,000,000 U./d.	Gm+ cocci and bacilli; Gm− cocci; spirochetes.	Hypersensitivity – usually rash and/or fever, occasionally serum sickness; less commonly anaphylactoid reactions; generally safest of all antibiotics.
Penicillin V (V-Cillin, Pen-Vee); semisynthetic penicillin.	250 mg. q.i.d.	Gm+ cocci and bacilli; Gm− cocci; less effective than penicillin G but more stable in acid of the stomach.	Hypersensitivity as with penicillin G.
Phenethicillin (Syncillin, Chemipen, Maxipen); semisynthetic penicillin.	125 to 250 mg. t.i.d.	Gm+ cocci and bacilli; Gm− cocci; less effective than penicillin G, but more stable in acid of the stomach.	Hypersensitivity as with penicillin G.
Ampicillin (Polycillin, Penbritin); semisynthetic penicillin.	500 to 1000 mg. q. 6 hrs. (o.); 500 mg. q. 6 hrs. (i.m.).	Gm+ organisms sensitive to penicillin G as well as a variety of Gm− rods; e.g., *H. influenza, E. coli, S. typhosa,* etc. Used for therapy of intraocular spirochetes.	Hypersensitivity as with penicillin G; elevation of SGOT.
Cloxacillin (Tegopen, Orbenin); semisynthetic penicillin.	500 to 1000 mg. q. 4 to 6 hrs. (o.); 1000 mg. q. 4 to 6 hrs. (i.m.)	Penicillin G resistant staphylococci.	Hypersensitivity as with penicillin G.
Methicillin (Staphcillin, Dimocillin); semisynthetic penicillin.	1 to 2 gm. q. 4 to 6 hrs. (i.m.).	Penicillin G resistant staphylococci.	Hypersensitivity, as with penicillin G; leukopenia, neutropenia, nephritis, superinfections with Gm− bacteria.

Drug	Dosage	Spectrum / Uses	Toxicity
Nafcillin (Unipen); semisynthetic penicillin.	500 to 1000 mg. q. 4 to 6 hrs. (o.); 500 to 1000 mg. q. 4 to 6 hrs. (i.m.).	Penicillin G resistant staphylococci.	Hypersensitivity as with penicillin G.
Oxacillin (Resistopen, Prostaphlin); semisynthetic penicillin.	500 to 1000 mg. q. 4 to 6 hrs. (o.) or (i.m.).	Penicillin G resistant staphylococci.	Hypersensitivity as with penicillin G; gastrointestinal complaints, anorexia, nausea, etc.; elevation of SGOT.
Tetracyclines: chlortetracycline* (Aureomycin), oxytetracycline* (Terramycin), tetracycline* (Achromycin); Demethylchlortetracycline (Declomycin).	250 to 500 mg. q.i.d. (o.) 150 to 225 mg. q.i.d. (o.)	Gm+ cocci, Gm- bacilli and cocci; rickettsia; psittacosis and lymphogranuloma group viruses.	Gastrointestinal disturbances, hepatic toxicity (during pregnancy), renal toxicity from outdated drug (Fanconi-like syndrome), mucous membrane toxicity, discoloration of teeth in children, superinfections.
Streptomycin.	250 to 500 mg. q.i.d. (i.m.).	Gm- organisms and tubercle bacilli, occasionally Gm+; resistance development is rapid; usually used in combination with another antibiotic.	Vestibular damage, dose-related deafness is seen rarely, hypersensitivity usually is manifest as a rash, occasionally urticaria, angioneurotic edema, or exfoliative dermatitis; eosinophilia with long-term therapy.
Chloramphenicol* (Chloromycetin).	250 to 500 mg. q. 6 hrs. (o.); also available (i.m.) and (i.v.).	Gm- bacilli (Proteus and Pseudomonas may be resistant), rickettsia, moderately effective against Gm+ cocci and bacilli, and Gm- cocci.	Gastrointestinal upsets, hematopoietic depression, "Gray syndrome" in the newborn, superinfections, especially Monilia.
Neomycin.*	8 to 16 gm. for 1 to 2 d. (o.) to prepare for bowel surgery; 10 to 15 mg./kg. per day (i.m.) rarely used.	Similar to streptomycin; not effective against Pseudomonas.	Parenterally; ototoxicity and nephrotoxicity; low incidence of allergic skin reactions with topical use.

(Table continued on following page.)

TABLE V-3   FREQUENTLY USED ANTIBACTERIALS (*Continued*)

Drug	Dose	Spectrum	Side Effects
Polymyxin B* (Aerosporin).	For Pseudomonas especially; (i.m.) or (i.v.) up to 2.5 mg. kg. daily.	Most Gm− organisms, especially Pseudomonas.	Nephrotoxicity, mild neurotoxicity.
Kanamycin (Kantrex).	7.5 to 15 mg./kg. daily (i.m.) or (i.v.); 1 gm. q. 4 hrs. (o.) to prepare for bowel surgery.	Similar to neomycin.	Similar to neomycin.
Bacitracin.*	Not absorbed (o.); rarely used (i.m.).	Gm+ cocci and bacilli.	Nephrotoxicity with parenteral use.
Colistin* (Colymycin).	2.5 to 5 mg/kg. (i.m.) daily.	Gm− organisms, especially Pseudomonas (not Proteus).	Nephrotoxicity; mild neurotoxicity.
Erythromycin* (Erythrocin, Ilotycin, Ilosone).	250 to 500 mg. q. 6 hrs. (o.).	Gm+ cocci and bacilli; Neisseria and Spirochetes.	Adverse effects are rare; cholestatic hepatitis with estolate salt (Ilosone).
Novobiocin (Albamycin, Cathomycin).	250 to 500 mg. q. 6 hrs. (o.); rarely used.	Staphylococci, Pneumococci, Clostridia, Neisseria, *H. influenza*, and some Proteus.	Skin eruptions, fever, jaundice, and gastrointestinal disturbances.
Ristocetin (Spontin).	25 mg./kg. per day (i.v.); rarely used.	Gm+ cocci and bacilli (includes penicillin resistant staphylococci), tubercle bacilli.	Phlebitis, fever, skin eruptions, thrombocytopenia, bone marrow depression.
Vancomycin (Vancocin).	2 to 4 gm. daily (i.v.); rarely used.	Gm+ cocci and bacilli (includes penicillin resistant staphylococci).	Phlebitis, fever, skin eruptions, nephrotoxicity, ototoxicity.

Drug	Dosage	Spectrum	Side Effects
Oleandomycin (Matromycin); triacetyloleandomycin (Cyclamycin. TAO).	250 to 500 mg. q. 6 hrs. (o.).	Gm+ cocci and bacilli; Neisseria and H. influenza.	Cholestatic hepatitis (triacetyloleandomycin); gastrointestinal disturbances.
Cephalothin (Keflin).	500 to 1000 mg. q. 6 hrs. (i.m.) or (i.v.).	Gm+ cocci (includes penicillin resistant staphylococci), Gm− cocci and bacilli, except Proteus and Pseudomonas.	Pain, phlebitis, drug rash, reversible neutropenia.
Lincomycin (Lincocin).	500 to 1000 mg. q. 6 hrs. (o.); 500 mg. q. 12 hrs. (i.m.) or (i.v.).	Gm+ cocci (including penicillin resistant staphylococci) except S. faecalis.	Diarrhea, pruritus vulvae and ani, abnormalities of liver function, superinfections.
Gentamycin* (Garamycin).	0.4 mg./kg. q. 6 hrs. (i.m.).	Gm+ cocci, Gm− bacilli, including Pseudomonas.	Vestibular toxicity, nephrotoxicity, phototoxicity
Sulfonamides: sulfisoxazole* (Gantrisin); sulfamethoxypyridazine (Kynex); sulfisomidine (Elkosin); sulfadimethoxine (Madribon); sulfacetamide* (Sulamyd): triple sulfa: sulfadiazine, sulfamerazine, sulfamethazine.	Usually 1 to 2 gm. to start, then 1 gm. q. 6 hrs.	Gm+ cocci and bacilli; Gm− cocci and some bacilli; psittacosis and lymphogranuloma group viruses, especially trachoma.	Crystalluria, hypersensitivity reactions including Stevens-Johnson syndrome, blood dyscrasias.

*Commonly used topically.
†(o.)=orally.

Drugs such as IDU have been considered for the systemic therapy of smallpox, but the experimental results have not been encouraging. The thiosemicarbazones, however, of which methisazone is the most extensively studied, when given systemically can prevent smallpox in contacts of active cases. It blocks viral multiplication late in the growth cycle, even after the viral DNA has been formed, but its precise mechanism of inhibition is not understood. Its clinical usefulness against smallpox has been demonstrated, and it is being evaluated in vaccinia and chickenpox.

Antiparasitic Agents. Toxoplasmosis is the commonest ocular inflammation in the United States that is caused by a parasite (pp. 142 and 200). Infections are seen most frequently in the neonatal period. In adults the diagnosis usually is much more difficult since positive titers to the organism occur in a large percentage of the population. The treatment in both neonate and adult is the same, consisting of a combination of pyrimethamine and sulfadiazine. Pyrimethamine is a potent folic acid antagonist that also is used to treat malaria. Since the infection is primarily a retinitis, pyrimethamine should be highly effective because it concentrates in the retina. The strains of Toxoplasma, however, vary in their sensitivity to this drug. The slowest-growing and the resistant strains are not affected by a clinically tolerable dose. As a result, response to therapy differs greatly between patients.

A strong synergism exists between sulfadiazine and pyrimethamine. Sulfadiazine blocks the conversion of para-aminobenzoic acid to intracellular folic acid by Toxoplasma. The organism, therefore, cannot produce the intracellular folic acid and its derivatives that are necessary for existence. Folic acid may be substituted by the organism, but less effectively. Pyrimethamine, on the other hand, blocks the conversion of the initial folic acid derivatives to the required derivatives. In man, folinic acid can be substituted at this stage without changing the effect of pyrimethamine on the Toxoplasma organism, but the effects of folic acid antagonism will be reversed. Combined therapy,

therefore, affects the metabolism of the organism at two different stages by interfering with the production of the required enzymatic cofactors. The usual dose of these drugs is 50 mg. of pyrimethamine with 4 gms. of sulfadiazine daily for one to three weeks. Blood counts should be done, and if depression occurs, folinic acid should be added to the therapy.

Steroids also are used with the above drugs to decrease the size of the inflammatory response and the resultant scar. The antibiotic, spiramycin, also has been used to treat Toxoplasma infections. Whereas it is not as effective as pyrimethamine, neither is it as toxic. It has been used in combination with pyrimethamine, but the effect of the combination may not be greater than that achieved by either drug alone.

CORTICOSTEROIDS

The corticosteroids and ACTH have dramatic anti-inflammatory effects on the eye. ACTH stimulates the adrenal cortex to produce corticosteroids and, therefore, only indirectly affects inflammation. ACTH has certain disadvantages: it causes severe metabolic changes since it stimulates aldosterone production, and it must be given either intramuscularly or intravenously, because it is a polypeptide. The synthetic, orally administered corticosteroids are all glucocorticoids with anti-inflammatory effects and generally have replaced ACTH. The glucocorticoid effect is closely related to the anti-inflammatory effect. Mineralocorticoids (i.e., aldosterone) may have anti-inflammatory effects, but are not suitable for such use because of associated salt-retaining properties.

Cortisone was the first commercial corticosteroid that could be used either topically or orally. Hydrocortisone (Cortisol), the major glucocorticoid secreted by the adrenal, was soon discovered to be more potent, and after that synthetic compounds such as prednisone, prednisolone, and others became available. Each had greater anti-inflammatory and less salt-retaining properties than the naturally occurring substances. Prednisolone has four times the glucocorticoid activity of cortisol with 80 per cent of the mineralocorticoid activity. Prednisone has less activity. Three newly synthesized compounds are now the most widely used and have no mineralocorticoid activity. These are methylprednisolone, which has five times the glucocorticoid activity of cortisol; dexamethasone, with 30 times the activity; and triamcinolone, with five times the activity.

The anti-inflammatory steroids are used in the eye to decrease the following:

1. Cellular and protein leakage into the aqueous during inflammation.

2. Tissue infiltrations and edema, which, for the retina, may result in improved vision.

3. Collagen formation and to diminish postinflammatory neovascularization.

Corticosteroids are used topically to treat allergic ocular diseases, such as vernal conjunctivitis and drug sensitivity blepharitis or conjunctivitis; to treat nonpyogenic inflammations, such as episcleritis or interstitial keratitis; and to reduce scar formation associated with corneal burns, especially due to alkali. They can be used systemically to treat various nonpyogenic inflammations of the posterior segment of the eye, including sympathetic ophthalmia and sarcoidosis; to treat inflammatory reactions involving the anterior segment not controlled by topical medications, including herpes zoster ophthalmicus and sarcoidosis; and to treat inflammations involving the optic nerve, such as papillitis or retrobulbar neuritis. Steroid therapy may induce all the changes of hypercortisonism. Even topically applied corticosteroids suppress the adrenal gland. Corticosteroid therapy also involves such hazards as potentiation of herpes simplex and other viral diseases, increased susceptibility to fungal infections, and possible increased spread of bacterial infection. When used systemically, corticosteroids can reactivate old choroidal tuberculosis.

A specific ocular complication of local therapy may be the increase in intraocular pressure that occurs in genetically predisposed individuals (p. 359). Posterior subcapsular cataracts may occur with long-term systemic administrations. Recently, a new anti-inflammatory steroid, hydroxymethylprogesterone, has been described. This drug is active when used topically for superficial inflammatory conditions and does not raise intraocular pressure. Its lack of effect on intraocular pressure may result from its failure to penetrate ocular tissue significantly, since to date no beneficial effect on anterior uveitis has been reported.

TOXIC EFFECTS OF DRUGS

The major toxic effects of the topical drugs have been mentioned earlier. This section discusses a few commonly used drugs given systemically that are associated with frequent or disastrous toxic effects on the eye.

Alcohol. The effects of ethyl alcohol usually are mild and of little consequence. With prolonged ingestion and decreased food intake, an amblyopia may occur (p. 309). The consequence of methyl alcohol ingestion, however, is much different. In those patients who survive the severe acidosis accompanying methyl alcohol ingestion, a primary optic atrophy with blindness frequently occurs.

Antimalarials. Although used in low doses to suppress malaria, drugs such as chloroquine now are used in much higher doses to treat rheumatoid arthritis and lupus erythematosus. Two complications occur. Chloroquine may be deposited in the corneal epithelium, giving the appearance of fine white dots in a whirl pattern. Patients with this manifestation frequently complain of halos around lights. The corneal deposits clear when the drug is discontinued, or may occasionally disappear spontaneously while the patient is still taking the drug. A more severe problem, pigmentary degeneration of the retina, begins centrally with a fine pigmentation of the macula and a central scotoma with a less dense central area (bull's-eye). This may progress to a complete pigmentary degeneration. The retinal changes are not reversible once a scotoma has occurred, but ERG depression is reported to occur before clinically recognizable signs, and at that time the changes are still reversible.

Quinine may produce a sudden loss of the visual field up to 5 degrees around fixation in the susceptible individual. This is not dose-related, and visual loss, or much of it, may be transient. If permanent, a marked optic atrophy occurs.

Cardiac Glycosides. (See Neuro-ophthalmology, p. 309).

Psychotherapeutic Agents. Although many drugs of this group are associated with mild visual disturbances, especially with blurred vision, the phenothiazines particularly are toxic. Chlorpromazine produces granular axial opacities in the subcapsular area of the lens, with similar granular changes in the posterior portion of the corneal stroma. These changes are dose-related and usually occur in patients who receive a minimum of 1000 gms. of the drug. Thioridazine has been shown to produce night blindness and a pigmentary retinopathy when used in high doses (1000 mg. daily). This drug, along with other phenothiazines, is stored in high concentrations in the choroid of pigmented animals. Apparently, when present in such high concentrations, these drugs can be toxic to retinal receptor elements. The changes produced by thioridazine are related to the amount and duration of drug dosage.

BIBLIOGRAPHY

Busch, H., and Lane, M.: Chemotherapy. Chicago, Year Book Medical Publishers, Inc., 1967.
Ellis, P. P.: Ocular pharmacology and toxicology. Arch. Ophth. 78:534, 1967.
Ellis, P. P.: Ocular pharmacology and toxicology. Arch. Ophth. 76:117, 1966.
Ellis, P. P., and Smith, D. L.: Handbook of Ocular Therapeutics and Pharmacology. St. Louis, The C. V. Mosby Co., 1966.
Goodman, L. S., and Gilman, A. (eds.): The Pharmacological Basis of Therapeutics. 3rd ed. New York, The Macmillan Co., 1965.
Gordon, D. M. (ed.): Medical Management of Ocular Disease. New York, Hoeber Medical Division, Harper & Row, 1964.
Grant, W. M.: Toxicology of the Eye. Springfield, Charles C Thomas, 1962.
Havener, W. H.: Ocular Pharmacology. St. Louis, The C. V. Mosby Co., 1966.
Leopold, I. H. (ed.): Ocular Therapy. Vol. I and Vol. II. St. Louis, The C. V. Mosby Co., 1966 and 1967.
Leopold, I. H. (ed.): Symposium on Ocular Therapy. Vol. III. St. Louis, The C. V. Mosby Co., 1968.
Leopold, I. H., and Keates, E.: Drugs used in the treatment of glaucoma. Clin. Pharm. and Therap. Part I. 6:130, 1965.
Leopold, I. H., and Keates, E.: Drugs used in the treatment of glaucoma. Clin. Pharm. and Therap. Part II. 6:262, 1965.
Leopold, I. H., and Krishna, N.: Local use of anticholinesterase agents in ocular therapy. In Koelle, G. B. (ed.): Cholinesterases and anticholinesterase agents. Heffter-Heubner Hanbuch der Exp. Pharmak. Suppl. 15. Heidelberg, Springer-Verlag, 1963.
Macri, F. J.: Pharmacology and toxicology of ophthalmic drugs. Arch. Ophth. 80:506, 1968.
Maren, T. H.: Carbonic anhydrase. Physiol. Rev. 47:709, 1967.
Paterson, G., Miller, S. J. H., and Paterson, G. D. (eds.): Drug Mechanisms in Glaucoma. Boston, Little, Brown & Co., 1966.
Potts, A. M.: The effects of drugs upon the eye. In Root, W. S., and Hofmann, F. G. (eds.): Physiological Pharmacology. Vol. II. Part B. p. 329 ff. New York, Academic Press, 1965.
Schwartz, B. (ed.): Corticosteroids and the Eye. International Ophthalmology Clinics, Vol. 6, No. 4. Boston, Little, Brown & Co., 1966.
Trendelenburg, U.: Supersensitivity and subsensitivity to sympathomimetic amines. Pharmacol. Rev. 15:225, 1963.

INDEX

Page numbers in *italics* indicate illustrations.

495

5